Operational and Medical Management of Explosive and Blast Incidents

David W. Callaway • Jonathan L. Burstein
Editors

Operational and Medical Management of Explosive and Blast Incidents

Springer

Editors
David W. Callaway
Carolinas Medical Center
Charlotte, NC
USA

Jonathan L. Burstein
Harvard Medical School
Beth Israel Deaconess Medical Center
Boston, MA
USA

ISBN 978-3-030-40654-7 ISBN 978-3-030-40655-4 (eBook)
https://doi.org/10.1007/978-3-030-40655-4

This Springer imprint is published by the registered company Springer Nature Switzerland AG
The registered company address is: Gewerbestrasse 11, 6330 Cham, Switzerland

To my boys, those rough men who stand ready in the night to step into harm's way, so that we may sleep soundly at night. May this book guide you as you care for our warriors.
To my girls, Jenny, Elizabeth, and Lilianna, for whom I would give it all.
And to my mother, who taught me that the strong protect the weak.

David W. Callaway

I wish to dedicate this book to Dr. Joseph "Joe" Waeckerle, a towering figure in disaster medicine and emergency medicine. His shoulders are those of the giants.
I wish to thank my clinical and governmental colleagues for their support of me in this endeavor and for what they do every day to preserve life, limb, and safety.
Finally, but hardly least, I wish to thank my family. Without them, where would I be?

Jonathan L. Burstein

Preface

Welcome to the most comprehensive textbook in print on the management of explosion-related injuries. This ambitious project brought together world experts from across military and civilian systems and across different medical subspecialties to provide the definitive resource for those engaged in the care of victims of explosions. We, the editors, hand-selected each author based upon their contribution to the science of blast injury, their experience caring for victims of explosions, or their expertise in system design. Each author team is comprised of legends, pioneers, and experienced frontline providers.

This work is the culmination of 2 years of labor from scientists, clinicians, and operators around the globe. As the editors, we would like to start with a note of thanks to the men and women who have taken time from their clinical practice, their intra-deployment downtime, and their families to join together and craft the most comprehensive book to date on the management of explosion-related injuries. Warriors, healers, scientists, and teachers all united by Hippocrates' "purity of purpose" to share their knowledge. You have all sworn that the bloody and personal lessons you have learned in places like Baghdad, Helmand, Tel Aviv, Boston, and Madrid will inform our future trauma and emergency responders.

Much has been written about the complex pathophysiology and physics of blast injuries. However, there are few resources that offer a bridge between cutting-edge blast science, clinical care for severely injured patients, and the operational knowledge required to actually implement systems-level strategies that reduce morbidity and mortality. Responders must understand individual effects, community impact, and system impact. And systems must support responders.

The health system response to explosive incidents is complex. We cannot predict every variable – blast type, health system bed capacity, disruptions in EMS response, or weather. As a result, at the system level, there is no best practice. There is only good practice, emergent response, and resilience. In order to succeed, responders must be part of dynamic, multidisciplinary teams that are experts within their field but also understand the importance of their individual role in a broader system. This textbook, unlike any other in print, offers a blueprint for creating these high-functioning teams.

We took on this project with the very ambitious goals of being able to craft a text that could be used at a variety of levels. First, the comprehensive nature of the book serves as a one-stop source for health system leaders and emergency managers – military and civilian – searching for guidance on how to best prepare for the increasing likelihood of explosive mass casualty incidents. Second, the specialty-specific sections are designed to be accessible across specialties in order to allow professionals to build integrated response plans. Finally, each section is designed to provide the most cutting-edge science and practice recommendations within a given specialty. The authors did an amazing job balancing these competing priorities.

The introductory section of the book is a must read for anyone involved in trauma care or the management of emergency and trauma systems. This section provides a comprehensive overview of the critical role that civilian and military trauma systems play in response to mass casualty incidents related to explosions. The introduction also provides an overview of the most cutting-edge science in blast biophysics and pathophysiology from authors who have helped to create the current blast injury taxonomy and are global leaders in research and development efforts on blast injury.

This book is subsequently divided into sections that address point of injury care through emergency department, operating theater, and intensive care unit. Each section specifically addresses the unique operational components of responding to an explosive incident as well as the most cutting-edge clinical care recommendations. Understanding that the operational context often shapes the clinical response, the chapters are designed to offer lessons learned from both international military experience and civilian response to terrorist attacks. The clinical chapters, all written by authors with hands-on experience caring for victims of explosions, lay out the best practices and evidence-based guidelines (where available) for the clinical care of explosion victims with complex poly-trauma. Case studies from civilian and military events augment these chapters and add ground truth to the recommendations.

This book includes perspectives and experiences from around the globe. As such, language occasionally varies. For example, the interchange of Mass Casualty Event (MCE) and Mass Casualty Incident (MCI). To the extent possible and where intent was consistent, we left native definitions in place to remain true to the authors local experience and to demonstrate the complexity of the challenges faced during global responses. Ultimately, we believe that this book offers new insights that will help prepare our health systems, our clinicians, and our operational teams to respond more effectively to individual and populations who are victims of an explosion. These scenarios are increasingly common and increasingly complex. Willful, or hopeful, ignorance is not an option. We must always be studying. We must always be practicing. We must always be improving. Otherwise, people will suffer.

From DC

Like many of the authors, the entirety of my medical career has been spent striving to understand how to better provide care for the victims of crisis; be it war, terrorism, violent crime, or disaster. The hours that I spent talking with these authors and reviewing their work were both inspirational and educational. I hope the reader garners as much from it as the editors.

From JB

In the 30 years I have practiced emergency medicine and disaster medicine, it is seldom that I have encountered such a dedicated, knowledgeable, and selfless group of people as I have in the creation of this book. Bravo Zulu to all.

Charlotte, NC, USA — David W. Callaway
Boston, MA, USA — Jonathan L. Burstein

Contents

Part V ICU Management

Part VI Special Considerations

Contributors

Craig R. Ainsworth, MD, MAJ Burn Center, Clinical Division, US Army Institute of Surgical Research, JBSA Fort Sam Houston, San Antonio, TX, USA

Isaac Ashkenazi, MD, MPA, MNS, Colonel (Res.) Israel Defense Forces, Yehud, Israel

International Expert for Disaster Management & Crisis Leadership, Faculty of Health Sciences, Ben Gurion University of the Negev, Yehud, Israel

Emory University, Rollins School of Public Health, Atlanta, GA, USA

David C. Asseff, CDR, USN (Ret), MD, MTMH Department of Anesthesiology, University of California, Davis, Sacramento, CA, USA

Avi Benov, MD, MHA Israel Defense Forces Medical Corps, Ramat Gan, Israel

Department of Surgery, The Azrieli Faculty of Medicine, Bar-Ilan University, Safed, Israel

Paul Biddinger Center for Disaster Medicine, Department of Emergency Medicine, Massachusetts General Hospital, Boston, MA, USA

Moran Bodas, MPH, PhD Sheba Medical Center, Gertner Institute for Epidemiology and Health Policy – The Israel National Center For Trauma and Emergency Medicine Research, Chaim Sheba Medical Center, Ramat-Gan, Israel

The Department of Emergency Management & Disaster Medicine, School of Public Health, Sackler Faculty of Medicine, Tel-Aviv University, Tel-Aviv, Israel

Matthew J. Bradley, MD, CD R, MC, USN Department of Surgery, Walter Reed National Military Medical Center, Bethesda, MD, USA

Jeremy W. Cannon, MD, SM Division of Traumatology, Surgical Critical Care & Emergency Surgery, Perelman School of Medicine at the University of Pennsylvania, Philadelphia, PA, USA

Department of Surgery, Uniformed Services University, Bethesda, MD, USA

Edward J. Caterson, MD, PhD Division of Plastic and Reconstructive Surgery, Brigham and Women's Hospital, Boston, MA, USA

Howard R. Champion, MD, FRCS, FACS Professor of Surgery, Uniformed Services University of Health Sciences, Bethesda, MD, USA

SimQuest. And, Annapolis, MD, USA

Rittik Chaudhuri, MD, PhD Center for Law Enforcement Medicine, Johns Hopkins Medical Institutions, Baltimore, MD, USA

Sarita Chung, MD Division of Emergency Medicine, Department of Medicine, Boston Childrens Hospital, Boston, MA, USA

Scott D. Deitchman, MD, MPH, Rear Admiral (Ret.) RADM (Ret), US Public Health Service, Duluth, GA, USA

Uniformed Services University of the Health Sciences, National Center for Disaster Medicine and Public Health, Duluth, GA, USA

Robert W. DesPain, MD Department of General Surgery, Walter Reed National Military Medical Center, Bethesda, MD, USA

Robert (Bob) Dobson Emergency Services London, London, UK

Nicholas D. Drakos, MD, FACEP, MA J, US Army Department of Emergency Medicine, Womack Army Medical Center, Fort Bragg, NC, USA

Brian J. Eastridge, MD Department of Surgery, Trauma and Emergency General Surgery, University of Texas Health Science Center at San Antonio, San Antonio, TX, USA

William Eisenhart, EMT-P Yale University Physician Assistant Program, New Haven, CT, USA

Henry Falk, MD, MPH Environmental Health, Emory University, Rollins School of Public Health, Atlanta, GA, USA

Meg S. Femino Emergency Management, Department of Health Care Quality, Beth Israel Deaconess Medical Center, Boston, MA, USA

Andrew David Fisher, MPAS Texas Medical Command, Texas Army National Guard, Austin, TX, USA

Jacob J. Glaser, MD, FACS Department of Trauma and Emergency Surgery, San Antonio Military Medical Center, San Antonio, TX, USA

Elon Glassberg, MD, MHA Israel Defense Forces, Ramat Gan, Israel

Department of Surgery, The Azrieli Faculty of Medicine, Bar-Ilan University, Safed, Israel

Uniformed Services University of the Health Sciences, Bethesda, MD, USA

Bradley Michael Golden, DO Department of Emergency Medicine, Medical College of Georgia at Augusta University, Augusta, GA, USA

Jennifer M. Gurney, MD Department of Surgery, Joint Trauma System, US Army Institute of Surgical Research/San Antonio Military Medical Center, San Antonio, TX, USA

Alexander Hart, MD Department of Emergency Medicine, Beth Israel Deaconess Medical Center, Boston, MA, USA

Guyon J. Hill, MD Department of Emergency Medicine, C. R. Darnall Army Medical Center, Fort Hood, TX, USA

Department of Pediatrics, Dell Children's Medical Center, Austin, TX, USA

John B. Holcomb, MD Department of Surgery, UT-Health/Memorial Hermann Hospital, Houston, TX, USA

Brandon R. Horne, MD Department of Orthopaedics, Wright-State University Boonshoft School of Medicine, Dayton, OH, USA

Steven J. Hudak, MD Department of Urology, UT Southwestern Medical Center, Dallas, TX, USA

Ameen M. Jamali, MD Center for Law Enforcement Medicine, Johns Hopkins Medical Institutions, Baltimore, MD, USA

Donald H. Jenkins, MD Department of Surgery, Division of Trauma and Emergency Surgery, UT Health San Antonio, San Antonio, TX, USA

Alex P. Keller IV, MD, DiMM, FAWM Military and Emergency Medicine, Uniformed Services University, United States Air Force, Athens, GA, USA

David R. King, MD, FACS, LTC, US Army Harvard Medical School, Division of Trauma, Emergency Surgery, and Surgical Critical Care, Boston, MA, USA

Knight Surgical Research Laboratory, Boston, MA, USA

Massachusetts General Hospital and Harvard Medical School, Boston, MA, USA

Ricky C. Kue, MD, MPH, FAEMS, FAWM Medical Corps, Vermont Army National Guard, Colchester, VT, USA

Boston University School of Medicine, Boston, MA, USA

Ofer Lichtman, EMT-P Rancho Cucamunga Fire Department, Rancho Cucamonga, CA, USA

Geoffrey Ling, MD, PhD Division of Neuro Critical Care, The Johns Hopkins Hospital, Baltimore, MD, USA

Yevgeniy Maksimenko, MD, MA, NREMT-P, FP-C United States Air Force, Medical Corps, Brookline, MA, USA

Department of Emergency Medicine, Boston Medical Center, Boston, MA, USA

Alexander D. Malloy, DO Division of Trauma, Department of Surgery, Brooke Army Medical Center, San Antonio, TX, USA

Drew Maurano, PA-C Department of Emergency Medicine, The George Washington University Hospital, Washington, DC, USA

Justin C. McCarty, DO Center for Surgery and Public Health, Brigham and Women's Hospital, Boston, MA, USA

John G. McManus, MD, MCR, MBA, FACEP, FAAEM, FSEM Augusta University, Evans, GA, USA

Richard McNutt, MD Combined Army/Civilian Emergency Medicine Residency, Department of Emergency Medicine, Augusta University Medical Center, Augusta, GA, USA

Ethan A. Miles, MD Maneuver Center of Excellence, Fort Benning, GA, USA

Charles E. Needham, BS, MS Needham Consulting, LLC, Albuquerque, NM, USA

William J. Parker, MD Department of General Surgery, Walter Reed National Military Medical Center, Bethesda, MD, USA

Ann Payne, MRCPsych, MA (CBT), FFSEM Department of Psychiatry/ University College Cork (UCC), St. Stephen's Hospital, Glanmire, Cork, Ireland

Kobi Peleg, MPH, PhD Sheba Medical Center, Gertner Institute for Epidemiology and Health Policy – The Israel National Center For Trauma and Emergency Medicine Research, Chaim Sheba Medical Center, Ramat-Gan, Israel

The Department of Emergency Management & Disaster Medicine, School of Public Health, Sackler Faculty of Medicine, Tel-Aviv University, Tel-Aviv, Israel

Jacob R. Peschman, MD Department of Surgery, The Medical College of Wisconsin, Milwaukee, WI, USA

James P. Phillips, MD, FACEP Department of Emergency Medicine, The George Washington University Hospital, Washington, DC, USA

Jason R. Pickett, MD Austin/Travis County EMS System, Austin, TX, USA

Douglas M. Pokorny, DO Department of Surgery, Trauma, and Critical Care, University of Texas Health Science Center at San Antonio, San Antonio, TX, USA

Douglas Frederic Powell, MD University of West Virginia, Heart and Vascular Institute, Morgantown, WV, USA

Todd E. Rasmussen, MD Department of Surgery, Walter Reed National Military Medical Center, Bethesda, MD, USA

F. Edward Hebert School of Medicine, Uniformed Services University, Bethesda, MD, USA

Katherine Remick, MD, FAAP, FACEP, FAEMS San Marcos Hays County EMS System, San Marcos, TX, USA

National EMS for Children Innovation and Improvement Center, Houston, TX, USA

Austin-Travis County EMS System, Austin, TX, USA

Dell Medical School at the University of Texas at Austin, Austin, TX, USA

Dell Medical School, Austin, TX, USA

Department of Pediatrics, Dell Children's Medical Center, Austin, TX, USA

Avraham I. Rivkind, MD Department of General Surgery and Trauma, Hadassah Medical Center, Jerusalem, Israel

Douglas A. Romney, MD Harvard Medical School, Boston, MA, USA

Department of Emergency Medicine, Beth Israel Deaconess Medical Center, Boston, MA, USA

Michael Rozenfeld, MA Sheba Medical Center, Gertner Institute for Epidemiology and Health Policy – The Israel National Center For Trauma and Emergency Medicine Research, Chaim Sheba Medical Center, Ramat-Gan, Israel

Greg T. Rule, MSE, BS Applied Research Associates, Inc., Hollywood Park, TX, USA

Valerie G. Sams, MD Division of Trauma, Department of Surgery, Brooke Army Medical Center, San Antonio, TX, USA

Czarina E. Sánchez, MD Emergency Department, Brooke Army Medical Center, Fort Sam Houston, TX, USA

León D. Sánchez, MD, MPH Harvard Medical School, Boston, MA, USA

Department of Emergency Medicine, Beth Israel Deaconess Medical Center, Boston, MA, USA

Ritu R. Sarin, MD, FACEP Department of Emergency Medicine, Beth Israel Deaconess Medical Center, Boston, MA, USA

Richard B. Schwartz, MD Department of Emergency Medicine and Hospitalist Services, Augusta University Medical Center, Augusta, GA, USA

Jansen N. Seheult, MB BCh BAO, MSc, MD, LRCP&SI Department of Pathology, University of Pittsburgh Medical Center, Pittsburgh, PA, USA

Stacy A. Shackelford, MD Joint Trauma System, Defense Health Agency, San Antonio, TX, USA

Geoff Shapiro, EMT-P EMS and Operational Medical Training, Emergency Health Services Program, The George Washington University School of Medicine and Health Sciences, Washington, DC, USA

Brian P. Shreve, MD Department of Emergency Medicine, Division of Operational and Disater Medicine, Carolinas Medical Center, Charlotte, NC, USA

E. Reed Smith Jr., MD, FACEP Arlington County Fire and Police Department, Arlington, VA, USA

The George Washington University School of Medicine and Health Sciences, Washington, DC, USA

Hideaki L. Tanaka, MD Military and Emergency Medicine, Uniformed Services University, Hurlburt Field, FL, USA

Nelson Tang, MD Center for Law Enforcement Medicine, Johns Hopkins Medical Institutions, Baltimore, MD, USA

Bradley W. Thomas, MD, FACS Section of Emergency General Surgery, Carolinas Medical Center, Charlotte, NC, USA

Joshua R. Todd, EMT-P, FP-C City of Austin Emergency Medical Services, Austin, TX, USA

A. Francois Trappey, MD Department of Pediatric Surgery, McGovern Medical School, University of Texas Health Science Center at Houston, Houston, TX, USA

Tim Walilko, PhD Human Effects and Risk Assessment Group, Arlington Division, Applied Research Associates, Inc., Albuquerque, NM, USA

Sage Guerke Weikel, MA, MS Emergency Management, Department of Healthcare Quality, Beth Israel Deaconess Medical Center, Roxbury, MA, USA

Jason P. Welter, DO Department of Orthopaedics, Wright-State University Boonshoft School of Medicine, Dayton, OH, USA

John M. Wightman, MD, MA, FACEP Department of Military and Emergency Medicine, F. Edward Hébert School of Medicine, Uniformed Services University, Bethesda, MD, USA

Mark H. Yazer, MD University of Pittsburgh, Pittsburgh, PA, USA

Avraham Yitzhak, MD, MHA Israel Defense Forces, Department of Surgery, Soroka Medical Center, Beer Sheva, Negev, Israel

Leanne R. Young, BSME, MS, PhD Applied Research Associates, Inc., Albuquerque, NM, USA

Part I

Introduction

Howard R. Champion

This section of this book presents contemporary expertise in the systematic multidisciplinary planning and response to explosion-related events and injuries. The chapters in this section embody the knowledge acquired and lessons learned from explosive events in civilian and in war settings in multiple countries over the past 20 years, together with the structured approach to this type of injury that we have developed through the Department of Defense Committee on Tactical Combat Casualty Care (CoTCCC) and its civilian counterpart, the Committee for Tactical Emergency Casualty Care (C-TECC).

The various chapters identify considerable efforts by multiple government agencies in many countries and provide useful source references to the reader. Taken as a whole they provide a roadmap for communities and providers to optimize the response to, and outcomes of, those injured in such events. There is some redundancy, but this allows for different perspectives and emphasis drawn from expertise in multiple countries and settings, both civilian and military. Variations in statistics are caused by period of study and data source.

The classification of injuries from explosions appears in various forms in multiple chapters. At the request of the US DoD Office of the Secretary of Defense, this was created by myself (Dr. Champion) with the help of Graham Cooper, PhD, one of the world's leading experts in blast biophysics and physiology.

H. R. Champion
Professor of Surgery, Uniformed Services University of Health Sciences, Bethesda, MD, USA

SimQuest. And, Annapolis, MD, USA

DoD Taxonomy of Injuries from Explosive Devices [1]

1. *Primary*. Blast overpressure injury resulting in direct tissue damage from the shock wave coupling into the body.
2. *Secondary*. Injury produced by primary fragments originating from the exploding device (preformed and natural (unformed) casing fragments, and other projectiles deliberately introduced into the device to enhance the fragment threat) and secondary fragments, which are projectiles from the environment (debris, vehicular metal, etc.).
3. *Tertiary*. Displacement of the body or part of body by the blast overpressure causing acceleration/deceleration to the body or its parts, which may subsequently strike hard objects causing typical blunt injury (translational injury), avulsion (separation) of limbs, stripping of soft tissues, skin speckling with explosive product residue and building structural collapse with crush and blunt injuries, and crush syndrome development.
4. *Quaternary*. Other "explosive products" effects – heat (radiant and convective), and toxic, toxidromes from fuel, metals, etc. – causing burn and inhalation injury.
5. *Quinary*. Clinical consequences of "post-detonation environmental contaminants" including bacteria (deliberate and commensal, with or without sepsis), radiation (dirty bombs), tissue reactions to fuel, metals, etc.

In general, the multimechanistic injuries from explosions play out as follows:

DoD Nomenclature for Blast Injury Categories After Explosions [2]

Category	Definition	Typical injuries
Primary	Produced by contact of blast shockwave with body Stress and shear waves occur in tissues Waves reinforced/reflected at tissue density interfaces Gas-filled organs (lungs, ears, etc.) at particular risk	Tympanic membrane rupture Blast lung Eye injuries Concussion
Secondary	Ballistic wounds produced by: Primary fragments (pieces of exploding weapon) Secondary fragments (environmental fragments, e.g., glass) Threat of fragment injury extends further than that from blast wave	Penetrating injuries Traumatic amputations Lacerations Concussion
Tertiary	Blast wave propels individuals onto surfaces/objects or objects onto individuals, causing whole body translocation Crush injuries caused by structural damage and building collapse	Blunt injuries Crush syndrome Compartment syndrome Concussion
Quaternary	Other explosion-related injuries, illnesses, or diseases	Burns Toxic gas and other inhalation injury Injury from environmental contamination
Quinary	Injuries resulting from specific additives such as bacteria and radiation ("dirty bombs")	

Chapter 1 provides a summary of the complexities associated with blast injury and the planning and implementation of a state-of-the-art response. This is followed in Chap. 2 by a review of blast biophysics that explains the mechanistic basis for injuries that occur as a result of explosions. Chapter 3 reviews the state-of-the-art research focus and gaps. Dr. Kobi Peleg's Chap. 4 builds on an understanding of the biophysics of blast and provides a scholarly review of the environmental, mechanistic, and operational threat types that influence wouding epidemiology and thus the outcome of injured patients.

Chapters 5 and 6 deal, respectively, with civilian and military responses and differences in preparedness, and Chap. 7 provides information on the varieties of improvised explosive devices. Chapter 8 gives a state-of-the-art description of the London planning and response system and how it is coordinated through LESLP. In addition, this chapter serves to emphasize the generalizability of response to explosive events and the responses to other mass casualty and major events such as active shooter, earthquake, etc.

The final chapter in this section, a discussion of the Madrid train bombing of 2004, provides an opportunity to analyze and configure an optimal response system based on "lessons learned" in this massive tragedy, which produced over 2000 casualties. Perhaps the most important message in this section is the need for multidisciplinary, multiagency, multi-institutional planning, joint rehearsal, and continued reassessment of the response.

Injures from explosions are becoming more common. David Miliband, Chief Executive of the International Rescue Committee and previously UK Foreign Secretary, has identified the following impacts of explosives:

- 142 Million children are living in high intensity conflict zones.
- More than 20,000 civilians were killed by explosive weapons in 2018.
- 973 Attacks on health facilities and health workers occurred, 167 of whom died.
- Since 2013, there has been 150% increase in landmine-related casualties, 8605 in 2016 alone.

In summary, explosive devices are not just a matter of military declared wars but are increasingly used in civilian conflicts, which are producing healthcare burdens on civilian hospitals and internal displacements involving 41 million people and some 29.5 million refugees. Taken as a whole, this section paves the way for the clinical focus of Part II.

References

1. Department of Defense Directive Medical Research for Prevention, Mitigation, and Treatment of Blast Injuries Department of Defense Directive 6025.21E July 5, 2006, Enclosure 2 online https://www.esd.whs.mil/Portals/54/Documents/DD/issuances/dodd/602521p.pdf?ver=2018-10-24-112151-983.
2. Champion HR, Holcomb JTS, Young LA. Injuries from explosions: physics biophysics pathology and required research forms. J Trauma. 2009,66:1468–1477.

Overview of Blast Injury

1

Scott D. Deitchman, Isaac Ashkenazi, and Henry Falk

Blast incidents and the resulting trauma are an unfortunate and real threat to health. It was first proposed in the late eighteenth century that changes in air pressure from explosions could produce injury or death. More nuanced, modern understandings of blast injury date from observations during the First World War [1]. Blast incidents occur in military conflict from both military and improvised munitions. Acts involving bombings and explosions are by far the most common types of terrorist acts. Blast injuries also result from nonintentional events such as industrial explosions. Although blast incidents are rare outside of areas of military or social conflict, when they occur, the scale in terms of number and types of injuries can range from mild to catastrophic. This chapter briefly reviews the various types of injuries that result from blast trauma, introduces the settings in which blast injuries occur and the epidemiology of blast injuries in different settings, and provides a summary of health preparedness and response strategies for incidents involving blast trauma. These topics will be expanded upon in subsequent chapters.

S. D. Deitchman (✉)
RADM (Ret), US Public Health Service, Duluth, GA, USA

Uniformed Services University of the Health Sciences, National Center for Disaster Medicine and Public Health, Duluth, GA, USA

I. Ashkenazi
Israel Defense Forces, Yehud, Israel

International Expert for Disaster Management & Crisis Leadership, Faculty of Health Sciences, Ben Gurion University of the Negev, Yehud, Israel

Emory University, Rollins School of Public Health, Atlanta, GA, USA

H. Falk
Environmental Health, Emory University, Rollins School of Public Health, Atlanta, GA, USA

D. W. Callaway, J. L. Burstein (eds.), *Operational and Medical Management of Explosive and Blast Incidents*, https://doi.org/10.1007/978-3-030-40655-4_1

Types of Blast Injuries

Blast injuries can be particularly challenging because of the severity of the often-multisystem injuries and also the unique characteristics of blast injuries. A number of excellent review articles provide a broad overview of these issues [2–4].

Blasts and explosions are complex events that can cause injury through multiple mechanisms. Future chapters explore the mechanisms of injury in greater detail; however, the most common way of characterizing blast injuries is mechanistic:

- *Primary* – barotrauma, where striking changes of atmospheric pressure directly resulting from the blast particularly affect air-filled organs or air/fluid interfaces in the body
- *Secondary* – penetrating injuries primarily related to shrapnel, bolts, screws, and other added metallic objects from the blast device
- *Tertiary* – bodily effects from being thrown by the wind or due to injuries sustained from collapsing structures
- *Quaternary* – other direct effects such as burn injuries or inhalation of toxic chemicals
- *Quintenary/Quinary* – some but not all sources add this fifth category, described as a delayed hyperinflammatory response

Blast Injury Scenarios

Blast injuries can result from explosions in a wide range of settings involving diverse types of explosive agents and devices. For this overview, we divide these into three general scenarios: exposure to explosions in military conflicts; exposures related to acts of terrorism using explosive devices; and exposures to accidental explosions, including explosions in industry in which the resulting injuries or fatalities are considered occupational injuries.

Blast Injuries from Military Conflicts

Military conflicts long have involved the use of explosive munitions, originally entailing a hollow metal casing into which was packed explosive powder and a fuse to ignite that powder. This led to the development of specialized exploding military munitions, including bombs, rockets, grenades, and mines. Exploding munitions can be used against materiel, personnel, or both. The injuries resulting from explosive munitions are the consequences of blast effects from the explosive force, thermal effects of the explosion, and ballistic effects of fragments from the detonating munition. Originally, the dispersed fragments were pieces of the munition casing, but starting in the nineteenth century militaries added primary fragments to their munitions to increase the number of projectiles resulting from the explosion [5].

In more recent combat theaters, including the wars in Iraq and Afghanistan, service members increasingly have been exposed to blast injury from improvised explosive devices (IEDs) (Fig. 1.1). IEDs vary in construction, deployment, and types of explosives and shrapnel used in the device [6]. Current IEDs can be divided into three categories: roadside explosives and mines, often constructed from military munitions, usually 122 mm or greater, and sometimes with hardware including ball bearings, nuts or bolts, or nails added (Fig. 1.2); explosively formed projectiles (EFPs), which use an explosive charge to deform a metal plate, usually copper, into a penetrating weapon (Fig. 1.3); and suicide bombings using weapons including human-worn devices (person-borne IEDs, or PBIEDs) and explosives packed in cars or trucks (vehicle-borne IEDs, or VBIEDs) or onto pack animals [7, 8]. IEDs are defined by their components including the casing used, the type of main charge, and the initiating system used to trigger the detonation [8].

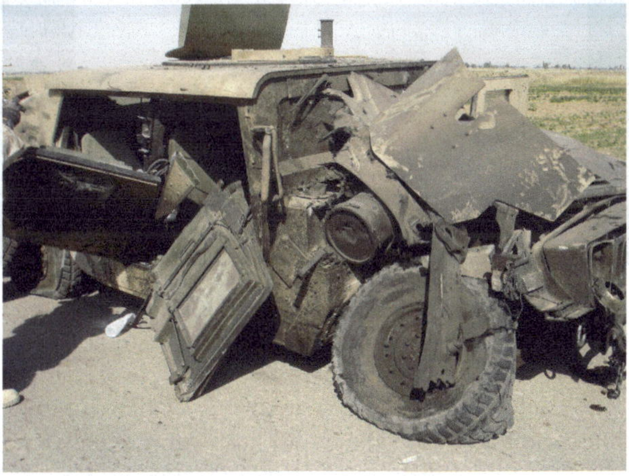

Fig. 1.1 Remains of an armored Humvee military vehicle after being struck on the right side by single man-driven, forward-loaded suicide vehicle–borne improvised explosive device, Iraq, 2005. (Photo: Staff Sgt. John B. Francis, USMC. Courtesy US Department of Defense)

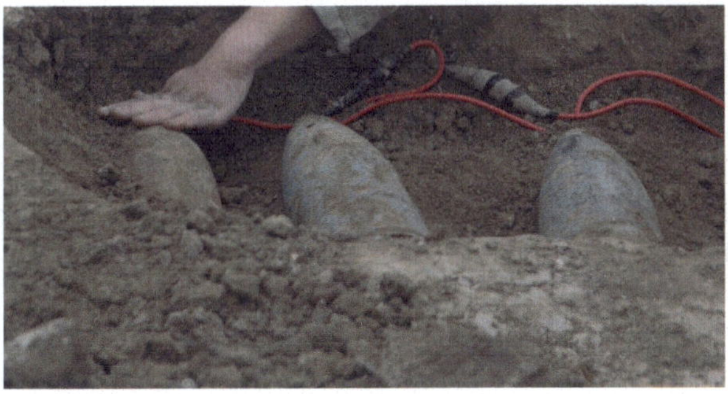

Fig. 1.2 IED detected in Iraq, 2005. Three 124-mm artillery rounds wired together with a single 126-mm round, the total combined payload approximately 400 lbs. of explosives (photo edited to remove personal identifying information). (Photo: Major Arnold Strong, Oregon National Guard. Courtesy US Department of Defense, Oregon National Guard)

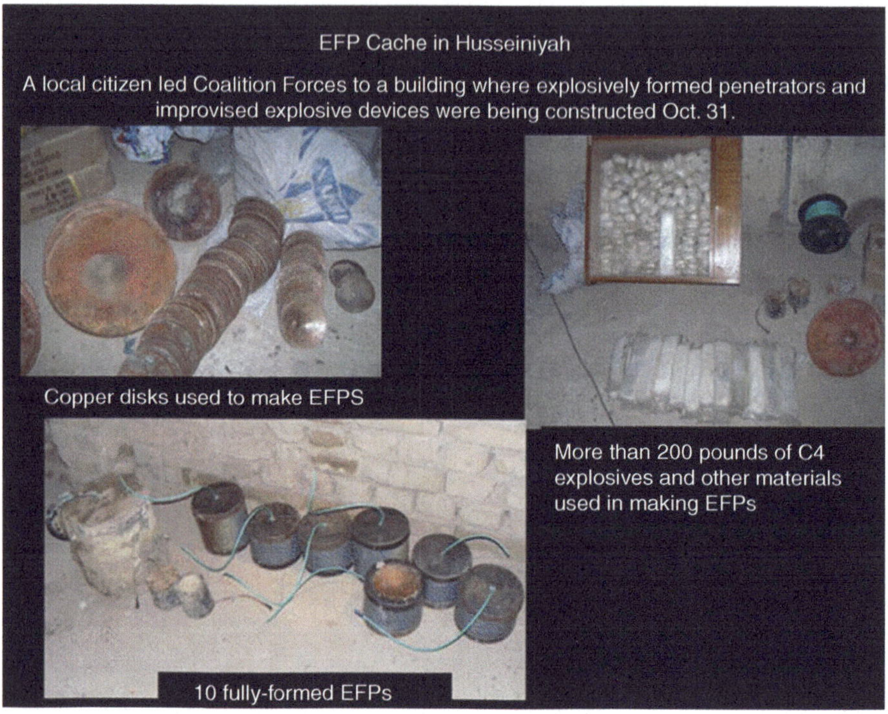

Fig. 1.3 Cache of explosively formed penetrators (EFPs) found in Iraq, 2007. (Courtesy US Department of Defense)

Recent epidemiologic assessments of blast injuries in military combat operations, using US service members as a representative population, were summarized in a literature review of blast injuries among the combat cohorts participating in Operation Enduring Freedom (primarily Afghanistan), Operation Iraqi Freedom (Iraq), and Operation New Dawn (Iraq). Among 1,992,232 soldiers deployed to Afghanistan or Iraq during 2005–2009, there were 5862 injuries from explosive devices. These accounted for a majority (74%) of all injuries at a prevalence rate of 30.5 per 10,000 deployed. Explosion-related musculoskeletal injuries accounted for 82% of musculoskeletal wounds and were experienced by 22.9 per 10,000 deployed. Explosion-related spinal injuries accounted for 75% of spinal casualties and were reported among 3.3 per 10,000 deployed. Major amputations (loss of a limb proximal to the wrist or ankle) caused by IED detonation were reported at a rate of 38.3 per 100,000 troop years in the Iraq theater (Operations Enduring Freedom and New Dawn) and 87.8 per 100,000 troop years in the Afghanistan theater (Operation Enduring Freedom) [9]. These rates are presented as examples, and comparable rates from other militaries may vary as they employ different equipment and tactics against different adversaries in different theaters.

As conventional and unconventional weapons and the tactics of their deployment evolve, so do protective technologies employed against them, resulting in changes to specific rates and patterns of combat-related blast injuries. Different exposure mechanisms may lead to different injuries; for example, combat thoracolumbar burst fractures are a unique pattern of injury that occurs as a result of vertical forces imparted by an explosion beneath an armored vehicle [9]. Protective technologies also alter patterns of injury. In a study of US combatant wounds incurred during Operations Enduring Freedom and Iraqi Freedom from 2001 to 2005, the percentage of thoracic wounds among was 6% (this included wounds from all mechanisms, not limited to blast injuries). Contrasting with a reported 13% in Vietnam, the difference was attributed to the use of personal protective equipment (PPE) such as body armor, in the two recent conflicts [10]. Additionally, though the protection provided by personal gear, including helmets and body armor, has increased survival, a significant proportion of service members who were close to a detonation of high explosives, such as IEDs, developed persistent neurologic and behavioral symptoms despite appearing to be relatively unharmed [6]. Beyond improved PPE, some have suggested that patients with massive blast injuries have survived due to advances in first responder care and forward surgery implemented in these recent conflicts [11].

Military personnel are not the only victims incurring blast injury in conflict zones. Civilians living, working, or transiting the area also are at risk. An injury, death, and disability survey conducted among 900 households in Baghdad, Iraq, found that for the period 2003–2014, injuries from blast or explosion were the most common type of intentional injury in 2008–2011 and in 2013–2014. Although gunshots accounted for more deaths, the majority of disabilities resulted from blasts or explosions. The sources of the blasts and explosions accounting for these injuries (e.g., military use of munitions vs IED) were not reported [12]. A 2015 United Nations report from Afghanistan showed that in the first 6 months of 2015, IEDs resulted in 22% of civilian deaths and injuries related to the conflict. A majority of these (846 of 1108 IED-related deaths and injuries) were civilian casualties of attacks targeting military forces [13].

Additional civilian casualties result from explosions of unexploded ordnance remaining after military forces have departed the area. The threat arises when parties to the conflict depart without marking or clearing unexploded ordnance from the former battlefield. In addition to inadvertently triggering the ordnance, civilians may become casualties when collecting scrap metal, tending to livestock, or farming. The same 2015 United Nations report documented that casualties from exploding remnants of war in Afghanistan accounted for 4% of reported civilian deaths and injuries. Children were put at particular risk by naively playing with recovered devices [13]. The problem extends to most of the globe (Fig. 1.4). In 2016, at least 2089 persons globally were killed and 6491 injured by landmines, cluster submunitions, and other explosive remnants of war. Seventy-eight percent of victims with known status were civilians, 20% were members of the military or security forces, and 2% were deminers. At least 42% of the civilian casualties were children. Rather than declining, the global incidence of such casualties has been increasing in recent years (Fig. 1.5) [14].

The problem is by no means new or recent. Unexploded ordnance from both World Wars still are uncovered in Europe, some causing fatalities upon explosion

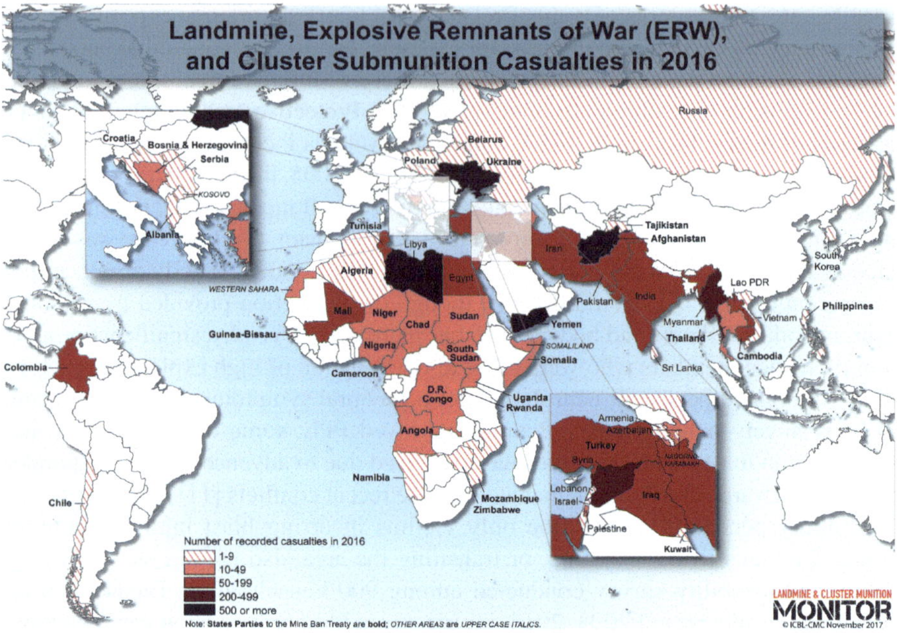

Fig. 1.4 Global reports of casualties from landmines, explosive remnants of war (ERW), and cluster submunitions in 2016. (Source: Landmine Monitor 2017. Courtesy of International Campaign to Ban Landmines – Cluster Munition Coalition)

[15, 16]. In 1988, one of the authors (SD) visited the Palauan island of Peleliu. Residents warned him against picking up unexploded munitions left over from the American invasion of the then Japanese-held island, 44 years earlier, saying that inadvertent detonations of these aging munitions accounted for several recent deaths.

Blast Injuries from Terrorism

Blast incidents are the most frequent type of terrorist attack. The suggested reasons for this preference for blast attacks include: difficulty obtaining the materials and expertise required to implement sophisticated biological, chemical, radiological or nuclear attacks; a contrasting relative ease of construction, materiel availability, and destructive capacity for IEDs; and the success of explosive devices for creating social, economic, and psychological instability in a community [17–19]. The explosives used by terrorists include commercial and homemade explosives in addition to the military explosive IEDs described in the previous section.

Data in the Global Terrorism Database, an open-source database including information on terrorist events around the world from 1970 through 2017, describe that of 181,691 incidents recorded during this time period, there were 88,052 (48.5%) attacks in which a bombing or explosion was the attack type. Explosives, bombs, or

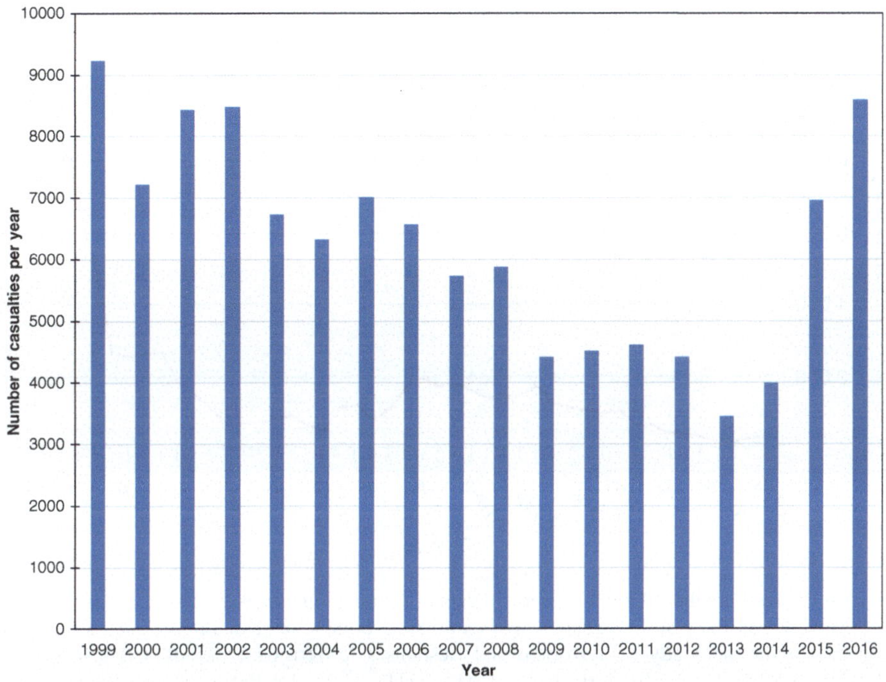

Fig. 1.5 Global number of reported casualties from landmines/explosive remnants of war, 1999–2016. (Source: Landmine Monitor 2017. Courtesy of International Campaign to Ban Landmines – Cluster Munition Coalition)

dynamite were the primary attack weapon. Of these, only 6283 (7.1%) worldwide were suicide attacks. These statistics can vary by region. For example, in the subset of 30,922 attacks occurring in the Middle East and North Africa, 3667 (11.9%) were suicide attacks. Of the global incidents with reported casualties, 36% resulted in one or more fatalities and 45% resulted in one or more nonfatal injuries. The most catastrophic incidents were relatively infrequent, with only 0.1% of incidents resulting in 101 or more fatalities and 0.4% causing 101 or more injuries [20]. Chapter 9 describes one such large event.

Whatever the reason for their selection, terrorist bombs can have truly destructive effects. Blast victims as a group tend to be more severely injured than victims of other types of trauma. Kluger et al. compared injuries among 906 victims of terrorist bombings to injuries of 55,033 individuals injured by nonterrorist trauma during the same period. They found that bombing victims were more likely to be severely injured (injury severity score 16 or higher), have Glasgow Coma Scale scores of 4 or less, be hemodynamically unstable upon arrival to hospital, have injuries in more body regions, require surgical intervention, need intensive care, and require longer hospital stays [21]. Despite this impact, during the period 1970–2017, the worldwide annual incidence of these attacks rose to a peak in 2013, and then, for reasons unclear, through 2017 was gradually declining (Fig. 1.6) [20].

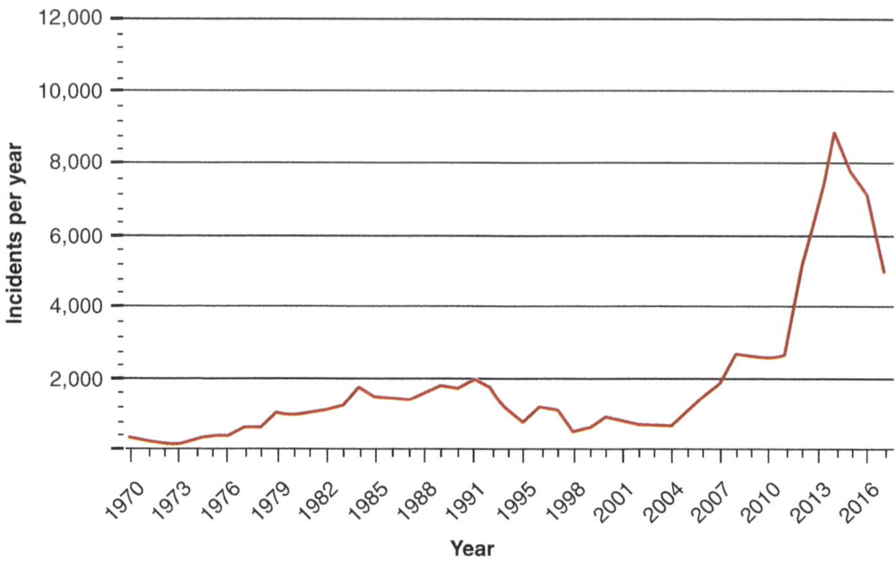

Fig. 1.6 Annual number of global reports of acts of terrorism in which the attack was a bombing or explosion and the primary weapon was explosives, bombs, or dynamite. (Source: National Consortium for the Study of Terrorism and Responses to Terrorism (START), University of Maryland. (2018). The Global Terrorism Database (GTD) [Data file]. Retrieved from https://www.start.umd.edu/gtd)

The nature of injuries from terrorist use of explosives varies with factors such as the size of the device, distance from the detonation, and the materials, including shrapnel, used in device construction. The setting of the detonation also affects the nature and severity of resulting injuries. Outdoor detonations result in different patterns of injury and mortality rates than do detonations in confined spaces. Injuries from indoor detonations are more severe due to the amplifying effect created when blast waves deflect off solid surfaces, and indoor victims additionally risk injury from resulting structural failures [22]. Golan et al. suggested, this confined space effect accounted for the difference in injury patterns seen in bus bombings when comparing persons inside the bus to persons outside of but adjacent to the bus. Victims inside the bus had higher injury severity scores, had more body regions injured, were more likely to require surgery or intensive care, and had higher mortality rates [23].

The nature of terrorism blast injuries also varies by victim age. An Israeli study assessed 837 hospitalized civilian and nonactive military victims injured by terrorist explosions. Children 0–10 years old were more likely than adults 16–45 years old to sustain severe injuries, to have traumatic brain injury, undergo at least one surgery, or require intensive care. These variations may be due to physical or anatomic differences between age groups and also may be affected by differences in medical protocols for different age groups [24].

Multimodal attacks (i.e., combining bombs, small arms attacks, or fire) are increasing in frequency. Attacks may include bombings in one location and concurrent or near-concurrent armed assault in others, as occurred in the attacks in Paris on November 13, 2015 [25]. The assailants in Mumbai attack starting on November 26, 2009 each carried a combination of automatic rifles, handguns and two types of explosives: hand grenades, and IEDs containing the high-grade explosive RDX (cyclotrimethylenetrinitramine) and ball bearings for shrapnel. These terrorists left IEDs with delay timers at some locations, hurled hand grenades at others, and attacked with firearms in still other locations [26]. Combined attacks of this type are regrettably effective. A review of incidents through 2014 found that attacks using both explosives and firearms caused 2.8 times more deaths than those involving only explosives [27].

Other Sources of Blast Exposure

While the previous sections have described blast injuries from devices intended to cause harm, blast injuries also occur in unintended circumstances. These can result from accidental detonations involving explosives used in nonmilitary settings, including mining, building demolition, fireworks, pyrotechnics, etc. In the United States, for example, the Bureau of Alcohol, Tobacco and Firearms (ATF, part of the Department of Justice) received reports of 687 explosions in 2017, of which 180 (26%) were accidental (of the remainder, 335 [49%] were bombings and 157 [23%] were undetermined, while 15 explosions were still under investigation at the time of the report). These resulted in 58 injured victims, seven injured suspects, and two injured fire service personnel or law enforcement officers. The victim injuries primarily were caused by accidental explosions. These explosions also caused 16 victim fatalities and one fatality to a suspect. In these incidents, the most common reported devices were pyrotechnics and fireworks (70 incidents, 31%), flash powder and other pyrotechnic mixtures (44 incidents, 19%), and black powder (nine incidents, 4%).The ATF report does not detail how many casualties, nor which devices, were associated with accidental vs deliberate events [28].

Accidental detonations can involve substances other than explosives. Dust explosions can occur in industrial settings when combustible dust particles are dispersed in sufficient quantity, concentration, and confinement in the presence of an ignition source and atmospheric oxygen. A primary dust explosion may disperse more dust, resulting in a larger secondary explosion. The combustible dusts can be diverse, including flour, sugar, metal dusts, plastics, and, in general, any combustible material reduced to a finely divided state [29]. These can be massive events; a 2009 sugar dust explosion at a sugar refinery killed 14 and injured 36 (Fig. 1.7) [30].

Other potentially explosive substances used in the industry can result in occupational blast exposures. Again using US examples, data collected from the Bureau of Labor statistics indicate that in 2016, there were 680 nonfatal injuries, and 55

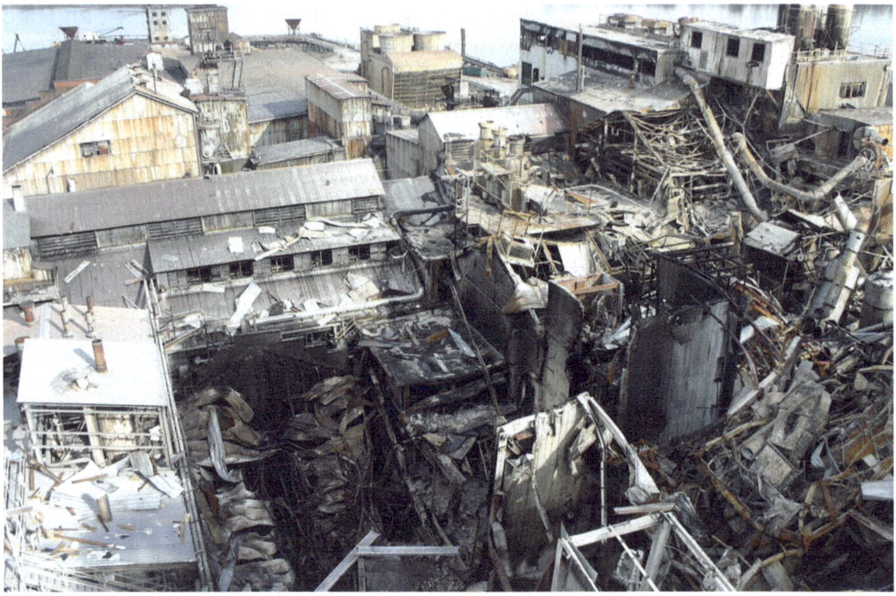

Fig. 1.7 Aftermath of a sugar dust explosion at a sugar refinery, 2008. (Source: Chemical Safety Board, Wikipedia)

fatalities, from explosions reporting in goods-producing industries and service industries combined [31, 32]. Some of these can be catastrophic. A 2013 detonation of fertilizer grade ammonium nitrate at a Texas fertilizer plant injured 252 persons, including members of the public thousands of feet away, and killed 12 emergency responders and 3 members of the public. Most fatalities resulted from fractures, blunt force trauma, or blast force injuries. Among survivors, blast injuries included pneumothorax, blast lung, blast abdomen, fractures, closed head injuries, traumatic brain injuries, and skin burns [33].

Preparing for Blast Events

The response to a blast event with associated injuries, especially a large event with many victims, must be driven by extensive prior planning. The specific elements contributing to preparedness for responses to blast incidents will be described in detail in subsequent chapters and are only summarized here.

Preparedness begins with individual preparation. Prepared persons, whether victims or bystanders, can contribute to their own survival. In the 1996 Khobar Towers bombing, the affected population (victims and bystanders) were military personnel trained to administer immediate first aid and self-treatment. Over 39% of injured persons received such treatment [34]. Individual training programs are available, such as *Stop the Bleed*, a national awareness campaign to encourage bystanders to help in a bleeding emergency [35].

The next level of preparedness is community preparedness to respond to the incident, stabilize the scene, provide prehospital care to victims, and distribute victims for definitive care. These preparations include provisions for interagency communications, on- or near-site triage, ambulance dispatch and staging, casualty distribution, and decontamination as needed [36].

Preparedness in emergency departments and their parent hospitals is likewise essential. Because the organizational system used for daily activities frequently cannot meet the needs of an emergency, hospitals can define emergency roles for personnel in advance [37]. A solution with broader application, preparing for diverse emergencies not limited to blast incidents, is to organize using the Hospital Incident Command System (HICS) [38]. The need for surge planning goes well beyond the emergency and surgical departments and includes other high-demand programs such as nursing, intensive care units, radiology, blood bank, pharmacy, and medical supply [36]. Because surgical specimens may contain valuable forensic evidence, surgical and pathology programs should be prepared to process and store samples in a manner consistent with forensic standards [39].

Staffing surge capacity is critical. A terrorist bombing of a train in Madrid in 2004 happened to occur at one hospital's overlap between shifts, so the hospital had more than usual staff on scene [40]. Health care facilities cannot rely on such a fortuitous coincidence and should have advance plans for summoning additional staff as needed. This planning particularly requires participation of hospital administration, although they support the other functions as well [36]. Other surge activities include: cancelling elective surgeries to free up operating rooms and staff, moving intensive care unit (ICU) patients to lower level care units as appropriate to free up ICU beds, using the recovery room beds as a supplementary ICU, discharging hospitalized patients when possible, designating an area for families, and preparing a designated information center [41].

The health care response to a terrorist bombing can be emotionally and physically difficult. Israeli intensivists experienced in terrorist bombing responses suggest emergency staffing plans should include provisions to relieve nurses and physicians after 8–12 hours [42]. As with any emergency event, having trained behavioral health personnel available to support responders, families, and patients benefits all who may be affected by the event or its response [36].

Conclusion

Blast injuries, both fatal and nonfatal, can result from explosions occurring in diverse settings and involving various explosive materials. Military personnel and nearby civilians can be injured by explosions of military munitions used in combat or of improvised explosive devices. The same devices, when left on former battlefields, can injure civilians who encounter them. Blast incidents also are the most frequent type of terrorist attack, whether using explosives alone or in combination with other weapons. Accidental detonations of explosives can occur in nonmilitary settings, including mining, building demolition, fireworks, and pyrotechnics, while dust explosions and explosions of industrial materials such as fertilizers can occur without conventional explosives. Health care systems must be prepared in advance for the large-scale consequences of some blast incidents.

Pitfalls

- Victims of blast exposure may incur any of a constellation of injuries, some obvious and other subtle. Vigilant clinical assessments are essential.
- Blast injuries outside of combat setting frequently represent failures of prevention: failure to clear unexploded military munitions, failures to prevent accidents involving civilian use of explosives, and failure to control dust concentrations and ignition sources in industrial and agricultural settings.
- Absent explicit preparation for mass casualty incidents, health care systems risk being overwhelmed by casualties from large-scale blast events.

Disclaimer The appearance of US Department of Defense (DoD) visual information does not imply or constitute DoD endorsement.

References

1. Institute of Medicine. Gulf war and health: volume 9: long-term effects of blast exposures [Internet]. National Academies Press; 2014 [cited 2018 Aug 14]. 228 p. Available from: https://www.nap.edu/catalog/18253/gulf-war-and-health-volume-9-long-term-effects-of.
2. DePalma RG, Burris DG, Champion HR, Hodgson MJ. Blast injuries. N Engl J Med. 2005;352(13):1335–42.
3. Wolf SJ, Bebarta VS, Bonnett CJ, Pons PT, Cantrill SV. Blast injuries. Lancet. 2009;374(9687):405–15.
4. Mathews ZR, Koyfman A. Blast Injuries. J Emerg Med. 2015;49(4):573–87.
5. Bellamy R, Zajtchuk R. Chapter 1. The weapons of conventional land warfare. In: Textbooks of military medicine. Conventional warfare: ballistic, blast and burn injuries. [Internet]. Washington, D.C. 20307–5000: Office of the Surgeon General at TMM Publications, Center of Excellence in Medical Research and Education Walter Reed Army Medical Center; 1991. Available from: http://www.cs.amedd.army.mil/borden/bookDetail.aspx?ID=a99f565c-4029-4f74-b57a-2a6747614173&pageTitle=Conventional Warfare: ballistic, blast, and burn Injuries.
6. Perl D. Military TBI: is it the same as civilian TBI? Bridges. 2016;46(1):65–8.
7. Ramasamy A, Hill AM, Clasper JC. Improvised explosive devices: pathophysiology, injury profiles and current medical management. J R Army Med Corps. 2009;155(4):265–72.
8. Improvised explosive device [Internet]. Camp Lejune NC 28542-0042: United States Marine Corps, Field Medical Training Battalion; [cited 2018 Aug 14] p. 17. Report No.: FMSO 211. Available from: https://www.trngcmd.marines.mil/Portals/207/Docs/FMTBE/Student%20Materials/FMSO%20Manual/211.pdf.

9. Greer N, Sayer N, Kramer M, Koeller E, Velasquez T. Prevalence and epidemiology of combat blast injuries from the Military Cohort 2001–2014 [Internet]. Washington (DC): Department of Veterans Affairs (US); 2016 [cited 2018 Jul 25]. (VA Evidence-based Synthesis Program Reports). Available from: http://www.ncbi.nlm.nih.gov/books/NBK447477/.
10. Owens BD, Kragh JF, Wenke JC, Macaitis J, Wade CE, Holcomb JB. Combat wounds in operation Iraqi freedom and operation enduring freedom. J Trauma. 2008;64(2):295–9.
11. Baker MS. Casualties of the global war on terror and their future impact on health care and society: a looming public health crisis. Mil Med. 2014;179(4):348–55.
12. Lafta R, Al-Shatari S, Cherewick M, Galway L, Mock C, Hagopian A, et al. Injuries, death, and disability associated with 11 years of conflict in Baghdad, Iraq: a randomized household cluster survey. Dalal K, editor. PLoS One. 2015;10(8):e0131834.
13. Afghanistan midyear report 2015: protection of civilians in armed conflict [Internet]. Kabul, Afghanistan: United Nations Assistance Mission in Afghanistan; 2015 Aug [cited 2018 Aug 14] p. 95. Available from: https://unama.unmissions.org/sites/default/files/unama_protection_of_civilians_armed_conflict_midyear_report_2015_final_august.pdf.
14. Casualties. In landmine monitor 2017 [Internet]. International Campaign to Ban Land mines – Cluster Munition Coalition; 2017 Dec [cited 2017 Aug 15] p. 51–62. (Landmine Monitor). Available from: http://the-monitor.org/media/2615219/Landmine-Monitor-2017_final.pdf.
15. Leatherdale D. How dangerous are unexploded bombs? [Internet]. BBC News. 2015 [cited 2018 Aug 20]. Available from: https://www.bbc.co.uk/news/uk-england-33861431.
16. Routine disposal goes wrong: three killed in explosion of World War II bomb in Germany [Internet]. Spiegel Online. 2010 [cited 2018 Aug 20]. Available from: http://www.spiegel.de/international/germany/routine-disposal-goes-wrong-three-killed-in-explosion-of-world-war-ii-bomb-in-germany-a-698245.html.
17. Nuclear Threat Initiative. Despite WMD fears, terrorists still focused on conventional attacks | Analysis | NTI [Internet]. 2013 [cited 2018 Aug 15]. Available from: http://www.nti.org/gsn/article/despite-wmd-fears-terrorists-still-focused-conventional-attacks/.
18. Improvised Explosive Devices (IEDs) [Internet]. Department of Homeland Security. 2018 [cited 2018 Aug 15]. Available from: https://www.dhs.gov/topic/explosives.
19. Edwards DS, McMenemy L, Stapley SA, Patel HDL, Clasper JC. 40 years of terrorist bombings - a meta-analysis of the casualty and injury profile. Injury. 2016;47(3):646–52.
20. National Consortium for the Study of Terrorism and Responses to Terrorism (START). (2017). Global terrorism database. [Internet]. Available from: http://www.start.umd.edu/gtd.
21. Kluger Y, Peleg K, Daniel-Aharonson L, Mayo A. Israeli Trauma Group. The special injury pattern in terrorist bombings. J Am Coll Surg. 2004;199(6):875–9.
22. Arnold JL, Halpern P, Tsai M-C, Smithline H. Mass casualty terrorist bombings: a comparison of outcomes by bombing type. Ann Emerg Med. 2004;43(2):263–73.
23. Golan R, Soffer D, Givon A, Israel Trauma Group, Peleg K. The ins and outs of terrorist bus explosions: injury profiles of on-board explosions versus explosions occurring adjacent to a bus. Injury. 2014;45(1):39–43.
24. Jaffe DH, Peleg K. Israel Trauma Group. Terror explosive injuries: a comparison of children, adolescents, and adults. Ann Surg. 2010;251(1):138–43.
25. The Paris Black Friday 13/11/2015 Attacks - What do we know? What should we do? [Internet]. Herzliya, Israel: International Institute for Counter-Terrorism; 2015 Nov [cited 2018 Aug 17] p. 2–3. Available from: https://www.ict.org.il/UserFiles/ICT-The-Black-Friday-Paris-Attacks-Nov15.pdf.
26. Rabasa A, Blackwill RD, Chalk P, Cragin K, Fair C, Jackson B, et al. The lessons of Mumbai [Internet]. Arlington: RAND Corporation; [cited 2018 Aug 17] p. 37. Report No.: OP249. Available from: https://www.rand.org/content/dam/rand/pubs/occasional_papers/2009/RAND_OP249.pdf.
27. Miller E. Mass-fatality, coordinated attacks worldwide, and terrorism in France [Internet]. College Park: National Consortium for the Study of Terrorism and Responses to Terrorism (START); 2015 Nov [cited 2018 Aug 17] p. 1–6. Available from: http://www.start.umd.edu/pubs/START_ParisMassCasualtyCoordinatedAttack_Nov2015.pdf.

28. United States Bomb Data Center (USBDC) Explosives incident report 2017 [Internet]. US Department of Justice, Department of Alcohol, Tobacco and Firearms, US Bomb Data Center; 2017 [cited 2018 Aug 1] p. 19. Available from: https://www.atf.gov/file/128106/download.
29. Combustible dust in industry: preventing and mitigating the effects of fire and explosions [Internet]. Washington DC: US Department of Labor, Occupational Safety and Health Administration, Directorate of Standards and Guidance, Office of Safety Systems; 2005 [cited 2018 Aug 17] p. 9. Report No.: SHIB 07-31-2005. Available from: https://www.osha.gov/dts/shib/shib073105.pdf.
30. Sugar dust explosion and fire, imperial sugar company [Internet]. Chemical Safety Board; [cited 2018 Aug 17] p. 90. Report No.: 2008-05-I-GA. Available from: https://www.csb.gov/assets/1/20/imperial_sugar_report_final_updated.pdf?13902.
31. Bureau of Labor Statistics. Case and demographic characteristics for work-related injuries and illnesses involving days away from work. Table R64, Detailed event or exposure by industry division. [Internet]. [cited 2018 Jul 26]. Available from: https://www.bls.gov/iif/oshcdnew2016.htm.
32. Bureau of Labor Statistics. Census of Fatal Occupational Injuries (CFOI) - Current and Revised Data. Table A-9. Industry by event or exposure, 2016 [Internet]. 2016 [cited 2018 Jul 26]. Available from: https://www.bls.gov/iif/oshcfoi1.htm.
33. A public health report on injuries related to the west (Texas) fertilizer plant explosion, April 2013 [Internet]. Waco-McLennan County Public Health District; 2014 Jun [cited 2018 Aug 17] p. 16. Available from: http://www.waco-texas.com/userfiles/cms-healthdepartment/file/pdf/West-Texas-Report-6-2014.pdf.
34. Thompson D, Brown S, Mallonee S, Sunshine D. Fatal and non-fatal injuries among U.S. Air Force personnel resulting from the terrorist bombing of the Khobar Towers. J Trauma. 2004;57(2):208–15.
35. Know a serious bleed when you see it [Internet]. Stop the bleed. [cited 2018 Aug 17]. Available from: https://stopthebleed.usuhs.edu/.
36. Hunt R, Kapil V, Basavaraju S, Sasser S, McGuire L, Sullivent E. Updated in a moment's notice: surge capacity for terrorist bombings [Internet]. Centers for Disease Control and Prevention, National Center for Injury Prevention and Control, Division of Injury Response; 2010 [cited 2018 Aug 17] p. 60. Available from: https://stacks.cdc.gov/view/cdc/5713/.
37. Kluger Y, Mayo A, Soffer D, Aladgem D, Halperin P. Functions and principles in the management of bombing mass casualty incidents: lessons learned at the Tel-Aviv Souraski Medical Center. Eur J Emerg Med. 2004;11(6):329–34.
38. Hospital incident command system guidebook, 5th ed [Internet]. Rancho Cordova: California Emergency Medi cal Services Authority; 2014 [cited 2018 Jul 26]. Available from: http://hicscenter.org/Shared%20Documents/HICS_Guidebook_2014_7.pdf.
39. Byrne-Dugan CJ, Cederroth TA, Deshpande A, Remick DG. The processing of surgical specimens with forensic evidence: lessons learned from the Boston Marathon bombings. Arch Pathol Lab Med. 2015;139(8):1024–7.
40. de Ceballos JPG, Turégano-Fuentes F, Perez-Diaz D, Sanz-Sanchez M, Martin-Llorente C, Guerrero-Sanz JE. 11 March 2004: the terrorist bomb explosions in Madrid, Spain--an analysis of the logistics, injuries sustained and clinical management of casualties treated at the closest hospital. Crit Care. 2005;9(1):104–11.
41. Gutierrez de Ceballos JP, Turégano Fuentes F, Perez Diaz D, Sanz Sanchez M, Martin Llorente C, Guerrero Sanz JE. Casualties treated at the closest hospital in the Madrid, March 11, terrorist bombings. Crit Care Med. 2005;33(1 Suppl):S107–12.
42. Aschkenasy-Steuer G, Shamir M, Rivkind A, Mosheiff R, Shushan Y, Rosenthal G, et al. Clinical review: the Israeli experience: conventional terrorism and critical care. Crit Care. 2005;9(5):490–9.

Blast Physics and Biophysics

2

Charles E. Needham, Leanne R. Young, and Howard R. Champion

Introduction

Injuries from explosions cover a spectrum from minor to lethal. Those at the severe end of this spectrum can be exceedingly complex. The blast event itself creates energy in a variety of forms – a shock wave, a blast wind, a fireball, and fragmentation, to name the most common. The various components of the blast lead to multiple mechanisms of energy transfer to the human body, often leading to anatomic and physiological impacts to multiple systems in the body. For a robust understanding of blast physics, the reader is directed to a text dedicated to this subject (e.g., *Blast Waves* [1]). This chapter provides only a high-level discussion of the physics of explosions, with a particular emphasis on how energy released in an explosion can cause injury to an individual and how factors such as the detonation environment, device construction, distance from detonation, and blast energy influence the bio-effects of blast.

Formation of a Blast Wave

A blast wave is generated when energy is released or deposited, in a localized region, at a rate that is greater than can be dissipated at the speed of sound. There are many sources of blast waves, including the sudden release of a high-pressure

C. E. Needham
Needham Consulting, LLC, Albuquerque, NM, USA

L. R. Young
Applied Research Associates, Inc., Albuquerque, NM, USA

H. R. Champion (✉)
Professor of Surgery, Uniformed Services University of the Health Sciences, Bethesda, MD, USA

SimQuest. And, Annapolis, MD, USA
e-mail: hchampion@simquest.com

D. W. Callaway, J. L. Burstein (eds.), *Operational and Medical Management of Explosive and Blast Incidents*, https://doi.org/10.1007/978-3-030-40655-4_2

gas, heating by an electrical discharge, an object moving faster than the local speed of sound, and energy deposited by the detonation of an explosive mixture. Herein, we will concentrate on the latter. More specifically, we will concentrate on solid or liquid explosive mixtures, which constitute the vast majority of explosives.

The energy deposited by an explosion is rather restricted and is in the range between about 3.0^{10} and 1.3^{11} ergs per cubic centimeter (ergs/cc^3). To make this more meaningful, ambient air has an energy density of about 2.5^6. The energy deposited by a liquid or solid explosive is therefore a few hundred thousand times that of ambient air. The pressure generated by such energy release ranges from 7.0^{10} to 4.32^{11} dynes/square centimeter (dynes/cm^2) (1 million to 6 million pounds per square inch, psi). This is the pressure that is generated inside the explosive as it is detonating and is *independent of the size of the explosive*. The detonation wave travels through the explosive at a rate between 4 and 10 kilometers per second (km/sec). (13,000 and 32,000 ft/sec). By comparison, the ambient air sound speed is ~0.34 km/sec (1100 feet/sec). Thus, the rate of energy deposition easily surpasses the criteria for the generation of a blast wave.

When the detonation front reaches the outside edge of the explosive, the detonation products rapidly expand, compressing the material surrounding the explosive. For now, we will assume the surrounding medium is air. The blast wave is characterized by a discontinuous jump in overpressure, density, and velocity, followed by an exponential decay in each parameter. Figure 2.1 is a cartoon of a generalized blast wave parameter as a function of range at a fixed time. This curve could represent the overpressure, density, velocity, or dynamic pressure. As the blast wave passes a point fixed in space, a pressure gauge, for example, would record a discontinuous jump at the arrival time to *a peak overpressure*. This is immediately followed by an exponential decay to a minimum pressure in the *negative phase*. The time the pressure crosses ambient pressure marks the end of the *positive phase*. The difference between the arrival time and the end of the positive phase is the positive phase duration. The integral of the overpressure through the positive duration is the *overpressure impulse*. The overpressure impulse is a measure of the energy in the blast wave and is important for target response. The integral of the dynamic pressure through the positive phase is the dynamic pressure impulse. This value, too, is important for target response, because it is correlated to the acceleration and motion of an object.

An important characteristic of *all* explosions is that the peak values of all parameters occur at the shock front. The overpressure, wind velocity, and dynamic

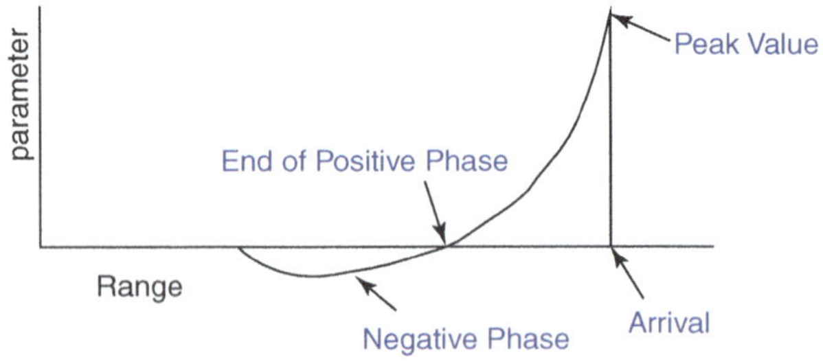

Fig. 2.1 Cartoon of a parameter vs range at a fixed time. (Reprinted from Needham [1], 2010 Mar 17)

pressure peaks all arrive at the same time, at the shock front. The shock front travels supersonically even as the peak pressure decays to a sound wave. In general, each blast parameter has a different decay rate and positive duration.

Many articles have stated that the blast wave is *followed* by the wind gust. This false impression is most likely caused by the fact that although the greatest acceleration of an object is simultaneous with the arrival of the shock front, some time passes before any significant velocity is attained. This gives the impression that the wind velocity increases behind the shock front when, in fact, the wind velocity is decreasing. The acceleration of the object is decreasing while its velocity is increasing.

The expanding detonation products remain behind the expanding shock front and are referred to as the "fireball." Figure 2.2 demonstrates that at early times, the detonation products (fireball) are compressing the surrounding air and are immediately behind the shock front. By a time of just over half a millisecond, the fireball growth slows and the primary shock pulls away. For this example of 1 pound of TNT, the fireball reaches a radius of approximately 3.5 feet (just over 1 meter). The region inside the fireball has an elevated temperature of about 3000 K, but remains hot for only a few milliseconds.

The pressure in the blast wave is decaying with the distance from the charge, and the rate depends directly on the size of the charge. For example, an overpressure of 1 bar (100 kPa) occurs at a distance of 200 meters for a kiloton, but that

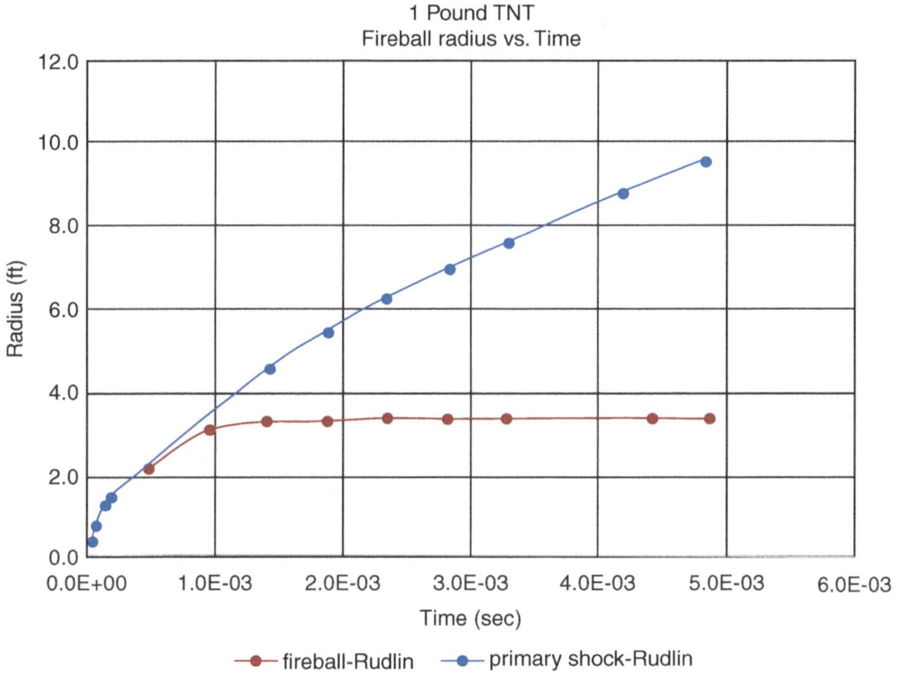

Fig. 2.2 Fireball radius vs time (Rudlin data). (Reprinted from Needham [1] 2010 Mar 17)

same pressure occurs at a distance of 2 meters for a 1-pound charge or a distance of 20 cm from a 0.5 gram charge. To decay by a factor of 2 from the 1 bar pressure, a 1 kiloton blast takes about 100 meters. The peak overpressure from a 1-pound charge requires just 1 meter to decay from 1 bar to 0.5 bar, and the half gram charge takes only 10 cm (4 inches).

Construction of Blast Devices

All munitions and IEDs are held in a case or container. The case of an explosive can range from a few inches of steel for a penetrating bomb to less than a millimeter of plastic for a jug of liquid explosive to about 0.1 mm for a typical soda or beer can. Assuming the container is filled with a high-quality explosive, the case will break into fragments, which will be accelerated to velocities of 0.6–3.6 km/sec (2000–12,000 ft/sec). The actual velocity of the fragments depends on the case thickness and density and on the explosive properties. A beer can filled with TNT will generate fragment velocities of 12,000 feet per second. Generally, the energy required to accelerate the fragments is about half of the energy of detonation, although for light plastic cases only about 25% of the energy is needed.

Figure 2.3 shows the range of blast overpressure and fragments with various munitions. A cursory review of this figure shows that range of fragment throw dramatically exceeds the range of significant (greater than 2 psi) blast overpressure. In addition, the energy and momentum density of solid fragment materials is more than a thousand times that of the air blast. Although the probability of being hit by such debris falls off as the square of the distance from the detonation, the

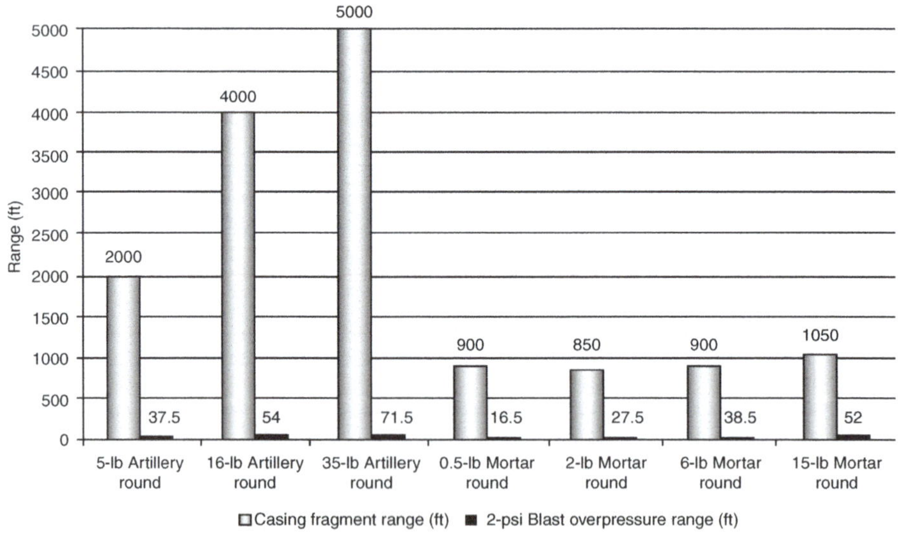

Fig. 2.3 Range of fragment throw and blast overpressure effect. (Reprinted from Champion et al. [7])

energy and momentum of injury causing debris decays very slowly with distance. Thus, the fragments and debris create an additional and possibly greater hazard than the air blast.

Interactions with the Environment

Aboveground Detonations

The position of the explosive relative to its surroundings will change the propagation and the properties of the blast wave. If the detonation occurs above the ground, there will be an incident and a reflected shock. At the reflecting surface, the overpressure at the shock front increases by more than a factor of 2 and can approach a factor of 14 at pressures over 1000 PSI. The overpressure in the reflected shock decays as it travels away from the reflecting surface. The stronger reflected shock travels inside the shock bubble of the primary shock and, therefore, travels faster than the primary shock. At a ground range approximately equal to the height of burst, the two shocks combine to form a Mach stem or Mach shock (Fig. 2.4). The height of the Mach stem increases with distance. The top of the Mach stem is labeled as the triple point, because it is the point where the primary, reflected, and Mach shocks meet. Below the triple point, objects will experience a single blast wave with about twice the overpressure of the primary shock. Above the triple point, an object will experience two shocks with a separation that increases with the height above the triple point. Either of the two shocks may have the higher pressure, again depending on the distance between shock arrivals.

Buried Detonations

When a charge is buried, the propagation of the air blast is more complicated. Generally, the blast is directed upward; the direction of least resistance. A layer of soil with a thickness ranging from a few millimeters to 10 cm covers the explosive

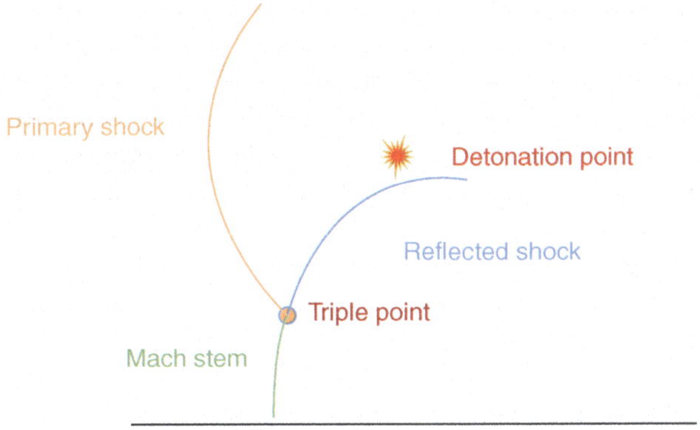

Fig. 2.4 Cartoon showing Mach shock geometry. (Reprinted with permission from Charles Needham)

device. The acceleration of this mass of soil absorbs energy from the air blast, thus reducing its threat. However, a crater is formed by the detonation, and the combined crater ejecta mass and the mass of the cover soil constitute a high energy and momentum threat to nearby objects.

Detonations Near Structures, Objects, or People

Primary damage from air blast is caused by the immediate interaction of an object with the blast wave. When the blast wave strikes an object, the incident overpressure is reflected. Upon reflection, the overpressure increases by at least a factor of 2. The increased pressure is caused by the stagnation of the dynamic pressure when it strikes the object. The reflection factor is a weak function of the angle of incidence for angles from perpendicular to the reflecting surface to about 45°. The largest reflection factor may occur near the 45° angle (where a Mach stem forms) and then decreases to a value of 1 as the shock travels parallel to the surface. The overpressure falls below the incident value as the shock engulfs the object. On the back side of the object, the shocks engulfing the object will collide and cause a brief spike in overpressure that may be greater than that of the incident shock.

The pressure loads on an object are dependent on the geometry of the object and its orientation relative to the incident wave. It is the pressure differential between front and back that causes an object to move. Blast experiments with simple objects have demonstrated a direct relationship between the incident dynamic pressure impulse and the distance an object is moved. This is generally true for most objects and is caused by the stagnation of the dynamic pressure and conversion to overpressure on the upwind side of the object. As an example, consider an object that is 6-feet tall and 2-feet wide or 12 square feet (1728 square inches) in area. An incident blast wave with a 10 psi peak generates a reflected pressure of 25 psi, resulting in a total force of 43,200 pounds on the upstream side of the object. Under such force, a 220 pound (100 kilogram, kg) object would be initially accelerated at more than 190 times gravity (190 g's). If we reduce the incident overpressure to just 1 psi, the acceleration becomes about 15 g's. In general, these forces decay rapidly and exist for only a few milliseconds at the 10 psi level for conventional explosives of a few pounds. By comparison, a person wearing a seat belt and traveling at 30 miles per hour experiences around 30 g's of force in a front-end collision with a fixed object. Being struck by a 10 psi blast wave generates more than 6 times the acceleration resulting from a 30 mph head-on crash. This difference in acceleration is a direct result of the time over which the force is applied. For a blast wave, the load is applied in the time it takes for the blast wave to travel a few centimeters or less than 0.5 millisecond (because the body is not planar). In an automobile crash, the force is applied during the time it takes for the crushing of the front of the car (which absorbs energy) and the tightening of the seat belt (a distance of ~40 cm or so), about 50 milliseconds (ms) or ~100 times as long as a blast wave load.

Interior Detonations

When a detonation occurs inside a room, the primary shock will reflect from the floor, walls, and ceiling. Thus, an object in the room will be subjected to a multitude of shocks coming from many different directions. Mach stems can form on any of the reflecting surfaces. The highest pressure may occur at any of the shock fronts, depending on the geometry of the room, the position of the detonation, and the position and orientation of the object.

Underwater Explosions

In water, the body reacts very differently to pressure waves and is more susceptible to injury. Close to the explosion, there is a very rapid, high-pressure wave front. At greater distances, the waveform more closely approximates the low-frequency, continuous waveform. Water is approximately 800 times denser than air and approximately 10,000 times less compressible. A diver in shallow water or at the surface will receive not only the direct blast wave from the explosion but also the reflected waves from the surface or seabed and any surrounding structures. As a rule of thumb, explosions underwater are roughly three times stronger than their counterparts on land [2–4], and the deeper the subject is immersed, the greater the effect of the blast.

Delivery Systems

In addition to the size of the explosive device, its construction, and whether it is in a closed or open space, another key factor that impacts the effects of an explosion is the delivery system. Other chapters will discuss delivery systems in some detail, but a brief summary is provided herein for the sake of considering the effect of delivery system on associated injuries.

There is a very wide spectrum of delivery systems with extremes used in military combat and terrorist activities, and with increasing frequency, a blending of the two. Military munitions include those with specifically hardened casing to penetrate armor or concrete bunkers before detonating. Mines have been extensively used in all forms of combat to attack dismounted or minimally protected mounted targets. Some of these can be detonated by pressure; others are remotely detonated. Still others are designed to gain a certain vertical velocity before detonating, thus increasing the risk of damage to aboveground targets. The patterns of injury vary considerably with the delivery systems. The "bouncing Betsy" mine will, for example, likely injure the torso, whereas a buried mine will injure the lower limbs and upwards, depending on size. In some conflicts, small explosives, particularly attractive to children, have been used with significant impact on civilian populations.

Explosive weapons used by insurgents and terrorists are predominantly improvised explosive devices (IEDs), a term encompassing the plethora of weaponized explosives (often built around artillery and mortar rounds) that are deployed to achieve tactical objectives. IEDs are the weapon of choice for terrorists and are designed to cause "gross disruption and disintegration of the body" [5]. They include bare charges, booby traps, car and truck bombs, and large culvert bombs directed at vehicles. In contrast to conventional military ordnance, in which the projected primary fragments are created by the breakup of the casing surrounding the explosive, IEDs not only generate fragments of shell casing but also metal objects such as nails, nuts and bolts, or ball bearings packed inside or around the explosive mixture. Precise timing and location are also used to maximize the numbers of injured and dead [6] (e.g., during morning rush hour on a London Tube, in a crowded restaurant in Tel Aviv, on buses, in military convoys, in lines of police force recruits in Iraq) [6].

Under-vehicle explosions produce a range of injury patterns that are a function of both the level of vehicle protection and the power of the device. For example, occupant risk factors were not a design criterion of the original HMVEE, which had very little protective armor, particularly on the underside. Thus, occupants of HMVEEs typically have a higher risk of direct blast injury. In contrast, the MWRAP is specifically designed to deflect under vehicle explosions. While this under-vehicle protection is valuable, occupants can still sustain lower limb, spine, and head injuries from impacting the roof inside the vehicle, as the entire vehicle is lifted or translocated in response to a blast. In the current conflicts in Iraq and Afghanistan, roadside and under-carriage IEDs are frequently used to target vehicles. In their 2008 study of injuries from roadside IEDs, Ramasamy et al. [7, 8] classified IEDs as (1) explosive-formed projectiles, (2) conventional explosive devices formed from munitions, and (3) suicide or vehicle-borne devices. In their subset of patients (100 casualties who were killed in action or admitted to a British field hospital in southeastern Iraq in 2006), only 2 (3.7%) of the 53 IED-related casualties had significant primary blast [8]. These results led the authors to conclude that "the blast component of these devices is not a significant factor in injury causation."

Most explosives used against vehicles detonate outside the vehicle, although a shaped charge munition can enter a vehicle and then explode. When a detonation occurs close to but outside a vehicle, the resulting blast wave diffracts around, reflects off, and, to a much lesser extent, transmits into the interior of the vehicle. The momentum imparted to the vehicle causes acceleration and displacement of both vehicle and occupants, frequently resulting in blunt injury. Because only a small portion of the blast wave is transferred into the vehicle, the risk of blast overpressure injuries to its occupants is substantially reduced relative to personnel in the free field. Test data illustrating this point are provided in Fig. 2.5, with blast overpressure impulse measurements taken from inside an armored vehicle located 10 feet (3 m) from a 38.75 lb (17 kg) bare charge of C-4 explosive. The peak incident overpressure outside the vehicle is 28 times that inside the vehicle, and the impulse (the integral of pressure and time) is three times that inside the vehicle. From an injury perspective, those inside the vehicle would be at some risk of eardrum rupture and well below the threshold for lung injury, but individuals standing outside and adjacent to the vehicle (but protected from fragment injury) would have a ~ 50% risk of death from primary blast injury such as blast lung.

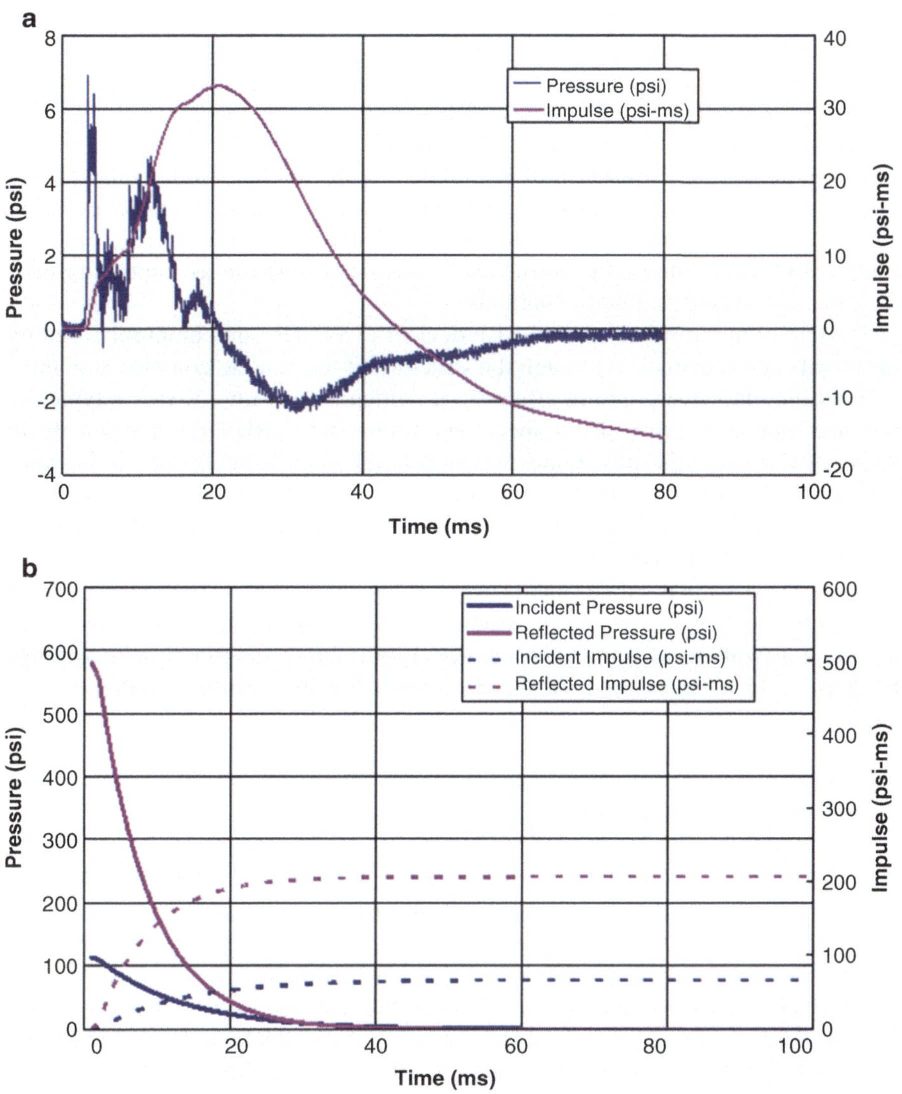

Fig. 2.5 Blast overpressure and impulse inside (**a**) and (**b**) adjacent to a vehicle located 10 feet (3 m) from a 38.75-lb (17 kg) bare charge of C-4 explosive. (Reprinted from Champion et al. [7])

Further, because seatbelts are only intermittently available and infrequently used and airbags are not available in military vehicles, vehicle displacement (with or without flipping or rollover) caused by the overpressure loading can result in significant standard blunt injury to the occupants, often with concussion or blunt traumatic brain injuries (TBIs) of various degrees. These blunt injuries are similar to those seen in civilian motor vehicle crash occupants before the advent of crashworthiness standards. Data from the Joint Theater Trauma

Registry (JTTR), a database of injured combatants from Iraq and Afghanistan who did not die at the scene, document that most TBIs on the battlefield are associated with explosions, and 97% are classified as minor concussions. Of casualties with documented head injuries, 44% had no recorded evidence of anatomic intracranial injury, although there was often a brief, transient loss of consciousness or concussion. Prevention of blunt head injury or standard concussion is a major concern, especially in light of recent research establishing a connection between mild TBI and posttraumatic stress disorder (PTSD) [9, 10]. This has reignited research interest in mitigation strategies as simple as improving padding inside the current combat helmets.

Vehicle-borne improvised explosive devices (VBIEDs) are commonly used by insurgents and terrorists. Although the structure of the vehicle contains and, thus, reduces the blast overpressure effects to the intended victims, VBIEDs typically produce increased injury from secondary fragments. VBIEDs range widely in destructive power and in how much explosive they can hold. In-vehicle delivery systems can be particularly lethal, as shown in the Marine barracks bombing in Lebanon, which caused President Reagan to withdraw troops from that country, and in the Oklahoma bombing in the United States. Use of such vehicles may or may not be associated with a suicide event. When an in-vehicle bomb is detonated near a structure, not only are the traditional blast injuries a concern, but there are often a plethora of minor glass-penetration injuries associated with window breakage, and there may be substantial loss of life in a building collapse (e.g., Oklahoma).

Enhanced Blast Weapons

Although much of this text has been about conventional blast weapons, it is worth noting that a new class of blast weapons, "enhanced blast weapons," is increasingly in use. These weapons are designed specifically to use the primary blast wave to engage the target; secondary fragment effects are minimal. Enhanced blast weapons have been used with devastating effect in military campaigns in Chechnya [11, 12] and Afghanistan [11, 13], and are available on the black market [11, 14]. The enhanced effects of these weapons are due to the use of explosive mixtures that decay more slowly from the peak overpressure, leading to a higher cumulative positive phase impulse. The most common type of enhanced blast weapons is the thermobaric weapon, in which chemically active metals, such as aluminum and magnesium, are added to a condensed explosive mixture. During detonation, these metals do not take part in the detonation reaction but, instead, react with the oxygen in the surrounding air [15]. In general, enhanced blast weapons are most effective in enclosed spaces, where the quasi-static pressure generated by the blast is sustained for longer periods of time, until the enhanced pressure is vented via natural or explosively created openings in the structure.

Blast Energy Coupling to Body Tissue

The term "blast injury" is somewhat of a misnomer, since without protective equipment, the most common injuries resulting from an explosion are typically caused by fragment penetration or blunt trauma from flying debris, rather than the blast overpressure itself. As a result of a lack of uniform knowledge and a common frame of reference for the understanding effects of explosions, blast physicists and physicians collaborated to develop a blast injury classification system, which was codified in 2006 in the Department of Defense (DoD) Directive 6025.21E. The distance from the explosive power, construction of the device, and the environment determine which of the various mechanisms of injury are most prevalent.

As defined in DoD Directive 6025.21E, primary blast injuries are those that can be attributed to the blast overpressure itself – that which is most accurately called a "blast injury." Secondary blast injuries are penetration wounds caused by fragments, typically embedded in the explosive mixture or generated by the disassembly of the casing surrounding the explosive mixture during the early stages of detonation. Tertiary blast injuries are primarily blunt trauma, but may also be penetration wounds, caused either by entrained debris in the blast wave or by whole body translation (i.e., individuals picked up and thrown by the blast "wind"). Quaternary blast injuries are burn injuries. These are usually *assumed* to be caused by the fireball created early in the detonation process but, in fact, the fireball is typically short lived, and burns in a blast event most often occur when a blast in or near a building causes the initiation of a fire and individuals in the vicinity are unable to extricate themselves from the burning vehicle or building. Quinary blast injuries are exceptionally rare and are caused by radiologic or otherwise hazardous *additives* to an explosive mixture.

It should be noted that the terms "primary" through "quinary" are in no way related to the severity or frequency of the injuries nor the distance at which the injuries occur. For example, as shown in Fig. 2.6, closest to a free-field blast source, individuals are at risk of death from both blast overpressure to the lungs (primary) or from fragment penetrations (secondary). Further away, the risk of death drops, but the risk of injury from blast overpressure (primary) remains – this time to the ears – as does the risk of injury from fragment penetrations (secondary). Although tertiary injuries are not included in this graphic, they occur at near to mid-ranges from ground zero. Quaternary blast injuries will typically occur relatively near ground zero, where the fireball has ignited flammable materials in the vicinity and quinary blast injuries can occur from near to far field, depending upon the nature of the hazardous materials added to the explosive mixture.

In general, blast injuries are complex, with multiple mechanisms of injury and multisystem impacts. This complicates therapeutics, but to a large degree, secondary, tertiary, and quaternary injuries are well understood – with respect to both the underlying mechanism of injury and treatment protocols. In contrast, primary blast injuries, particularly those impacting the central nervous system, are poorly understood and present both diagnostic and therapeutic challenges.

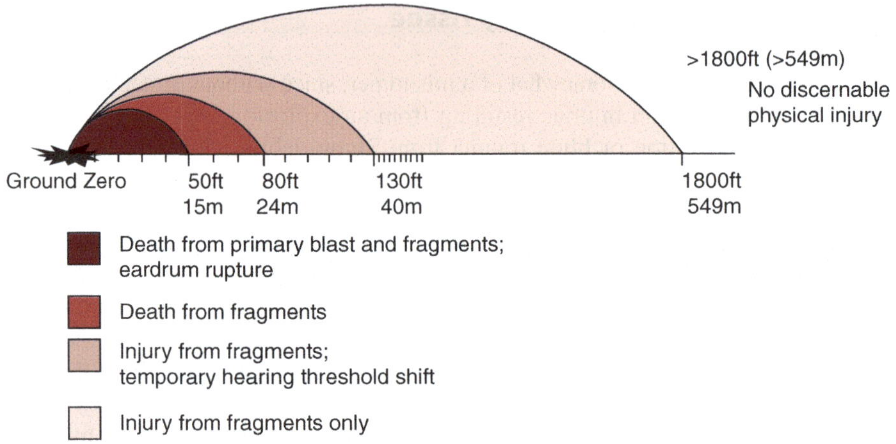

Fig. 2.6 Morbidity and mortality as a function of distance from open-space detonation of a 155-mm (220-lb, ~100-kg) shell. (Reprinted from Champion et al. [7])

Mechanism of Injury

As has been discussed briefly, blast waves have the potential of causing injuries through many different mechanisms. The first mechanism that usually comes to mind is injury caused by overpressure. The arrival of the blast wave causes a sudden increase in the pressure applied to the external parts of the body. The resultant sudden squeezing of internal organs, such as the lungs, bowel, or circulatory system, can cause injury. Ear drums can rupture, lung tissue can be torn, and bowels ruptured. A sudden compression of the thorax can cause a sudden increase in blood pressure throughout the body. This sudden increase in pressure may cause rupture of blood vessels anywhere in the body.

Figure 2.7 indicates that for short duration blast waves, the level of reflected overpressure that causes injury increases as the duration decreases. If the duration is greater than about 20 milliseconds, the injury level is independent of the reflected overpressure. These results are for a single peaked, near ideal blast waveform. The threshold for injury is about 90 kilopascals (kPa). This corresponds to an incident overpressure of 36 kPa or ~5 psi. The 99% lethality reflected overpressure for durations greater than 20 ms is 600 kPa. This corresponds to an incident overpressure of 170 kPa or ~25 psi. Table 2.1 summarizes the relationship between peak overpressure and risk of lung injury or death from blast overpressure.

Injuries caused by the propagation of the blast wave through the body are unique to explosions. As mentioned earlier, a uniform pressure wave will accelerate objects with different densities at different rates, inversely proportional to their density. The lungs, for example, are basically constructed of air-filled alveoli, which have a tissue density that is 1000 times that of the air they contain. This huge density difference results in significant differential velocities, which cause shearing of the tissue.

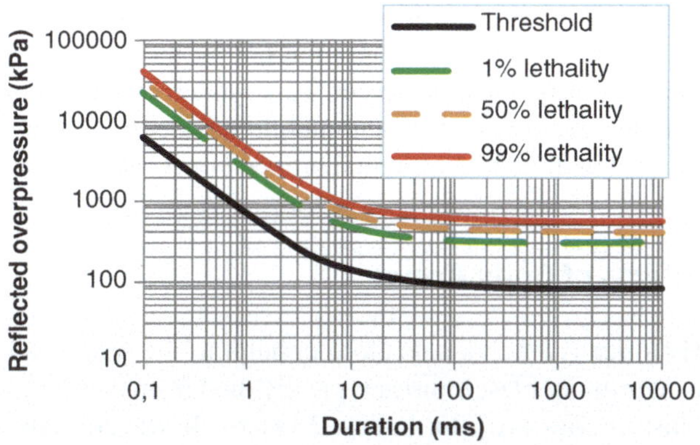

Fig. 2.7 Lethality estimates as a function of reflected overpressure and duration. (Adapted from [18])

Table 2.1 Short-duration primary blast overpressure effects upon unprotected persons [7]

Pressure (psi)	Effect
2	Auditory shift
5	Possible eardrum rupture
15	50% chance of eardrum rupture
30–40	Slight chance of lung injury
80	50% chance of lung injury
100–120	Slight chance of death
130–180	50% chance of death
200–250	Probable death

psi pounds per square inch

In underwater blast events, the longer duration exposures translate to increased impulse, which leads to pulmonary hemorrhage as by far the most frequent injury, followed by injury to the susceptible gas-filled intestines. In contrast, in air-blast events, primary blast abdominal injury is uncommon and reported incompletely in the literature.

Both the mechanism and thresholds for blast injury to the brain are less understood. In the brain, grey matter is a just a few percent more dense than white matter. This leads to the hypothesis that when a blast wave is passing through the brain, the white matter is accelerated more than the grey matter, causing shearing of the connective tissue. Another hypothesis is that the sudden increase in blood pressure caused by thorax compression causes expansion of blood vessels in the brain, resulting in shearing of tissue in the vicinity of the blood vessels. These shearing effects have been documented in postmortem evidence of scarring at shearing interfaces between white and grey matter and at blood vessel interfaces in victims of blast exposure. The resulting scar pattern was unique to blast exposure and was not observed in victims of blunt trauma injury.

The primary injury mechanism for dynamic pressure is the sudden acceleration and resultant translation of the body. The acceleration of different parts of the body is dependent on the density of that body part. For a uniform frontal loading, the thorax will be most rapidly accelerated with the head and extremities experiencing less acceleration because they are more dense. At high pressure loads, this differential acceleration can lead to injury; however, it is more likely that injury will not be caused by the initial acceleration but by the subsequent abrupt deceleration when the body strikes a solid object. This sudden stop upon impact is similar to the accelerations experienced in automobile accidents and causes similar injuries. These injuries include blunt trauma, broken bones, and traumatic brain injury.

Effects of Body Armor

Historically, individuals close enough to the seat of an explosion to suffer significant primary blast injuries typically died from overwhelming penetrating secondary blast injuries [16]. In the last 20 years, however, body armor designed to mitigate the threat from penetrating missile trauma has been highly effective at mitigating the effects of not only secondary blast injuries but also primary blast injuries to the lungs. As a result of both the improvements in body armor and improvements in combat medical care, more individuals have been enabled to survive near-field exposure to a blast, only to subsequently exhibit symptoms of a primary blast injury to the brain [10, 16, 17].

Conclusion

Explosions create a multimechanistic capability of human injury dependent of the size of the explosive element, the casing, the environment, and the distance of the target therefrom. The effects are both macroscopic and microscopic. An understanding of the multiple mechanistic multisystem injury that results from explosions is an essential prerequisite to adequate assessment and treatment.

References

1. Needham CE. Blast waves. New York: Springer; 2010.
2. Champion HR, Baskin T, Holcomb JB. Injuries from explosions. In: PHTLS basic and advanced prehospital trauma life support. Military 8 ed. St. Louis: National Association of Emergency Medical Technicians, Mosby; 2016.
3. Briggs SM, Brinsfeld KH. Advanced disaster medical response. Boston: Harvard Medical International Trauma & Disaster Institute; 2003.
4. Citaulo DL, Frykberg ER. The surgeons and acts of civilian terrorism. J Am Coll Surg. 2006;203(6):942–50.
5. Horrocks CL. Blast injuries: biophysics, pathophysiology and management principles. J R Army Med Corps. 2001;147:28–40.
6. Stein M, Hirshberg A. Medical consequences of terrorism. The conventional weapon threat. Surg Clin North Am. 1999;79:1537–52.
7. Champion HR, Holcomb JB, Young LA. Injuries from explosions: physics, biophysics, pathology, and required research focus. J Trauma. 2009;66:1468–77.
8. Ramasamy A, Harrisson SE, Clasper JC, Stewart MP. Injuries from roadside improvised explosive devices. J Trauma. 2008;65:910–4.

9. Schneiderman AI, Braver ER, Kang HK. Understanding sequelae of injury mechanisms and mild traumatic brain injury incurred during the conflicts in Iraq and Afghanistan: persistent post-concussive symptoms and posttraumatic stress disorder. Am J Epidemiol. 2008;167:1446–52.
10. Hoge CW, McGurk D, Thomas JL, Cox AL, Engel CC, Castro CA. Mild traumatic brain injury in U.S. soldiers returning from Iraq. N Engl J Med. 2008;358:453–63.
11. Owers C, Morgan L, Garner JP. Abdominal trauma in primary blast injury (Br J Surg DOI: 101002/bjs7268). Br J Surg. 2011;98(2):179–80. PubMed PMID: 21104701.
12. Dearden P. New blast weapons. J R Army Med Corps. 2001;147:80–6.
13. WAH-64D Apache attack helicopter. http://www.armedforces-int.com/news/british-military-using-hellfireweapons-in-afghanistan.html. Accessed 1 March 2010.
14. Murray SB, Anderson CJ, Zhang F, Gerrard KB, Hlady S, Yoshinaka A. Force protection against enhanced blast. Ralston: Defence R&D Canada–Suffield; 2006.
15. Trzciński WA, Maiz L. Thermobaric and enhanced blast explosives–properties and testing methods. Propellants Explos Pyrotech. 2015;40(5):632–44.
16. Mellor SG. The relationship of blast loading to death and injury from explosion. World J Surg. 1992;16:893–8.
17. Cripps NP, Cooper GJ. The influence of personal blast protection on the distribution and severity of primary blast gut injury. J Trauma. 1996;40(Suppl):S206–11.
18. Bowen IG, Fletcher ER, Richmond DR. Estimate of man's tolerance to the direct effects of air blast. Albuquerque: Lovelace Foundation for Medical Education and Research; 1968.

State of the Science: Blast Injury Pathophysiology

3

Leanne R. Young, Geoffrey Ling, Tim Walilko, Greg T. Rule, and Howard R. Champion

Introduction

As described in the previous chapter, the nature and severity of blast injuries is largely a function of the charge and device casing, standoff distance, and presence or absence of reflecting surfaces. From an injury perspective, the organs most vulnerable to primary blast injury are those that are gas-containing (ears, lungs, and bowel) or where there are significant tissue density differences. The general risk of injury or death from primary blast overpressure injury is provided in Table 3.1, and mortality rates in Operations Enduring Freedom (OEF) and Iraqi Freedom (OIF) are given in Table 3.2. In these most recent conflicts, protective equipment for the thorax and abdomen had improved markedly, reducing the incidence of secondary (penetrating) wounds to the thorax and abdomen. As a result, injuries to the extremities, particularly traumatic amputations, now compete with traumatic brain injury (TBI) for the ignominious title of "signature injury" of the OEF/OIF conflicts. Unlike thoracic protective gear, which effectively protects against not just

L. R. Young (✉)
Applied Research Associates, Inc., Albuquerque, NM, USA
e-mail: lyoung@ara.com

G. Ling
Division of Neuro Critical Care, The Johns Hopkins Hospital, Baltimore, MD, USA

T. Walilko
Human Effects and Risk Assessment Group, Arlington Division,
Applied Research Associates, Inc., Albuquerque, NM, USA

G. T. Rule
Applied Research Associates, Inc., Hollywood Park, TX, USA

H. R. Champion
Professor of Surgery, Uniformed Services University of the Health Sciences,
Bethesda, MD, USA

SimQuest. And, Annapolis, MD, USA

D. W. Callaway, J. L. Burstein (eds.), *Operational and Medical Management of Explosive and Blast Incidents*, https://doi.org/10.1007/978-3-030-40655-4_3

Table 3.1 Short-duration primary blast overpressure effects upon unprotected persons [1, 2]

Pressure (psi)	Effect
2	Auditory shift
5	Possible eardrum rupture
15	50% chance of eardrum rupture
30–40	Slight chance of lung injury
80	50% chance of lung injury
100–120	Slight chance of death
130–180	50% chance of death
200–250	Probable death

psi pounds per square inch

Table 3.2 Comparison of explosion-related injuries in Iraq: Mar. 2003–Dec. 2004 vs Jan. 2005–Oct. 2006 [3]

Injury type	2003–2004	2005–2006	$p<$
No. patients (*N*)	2588	1935	
Primary blast injury (%)	11.5	14.5	<0.01
Tympanic membrane rupture (%)	8.7	10.3	NS
Blast lung (%)	3.1	4.6	<0.01
Intestinal blast (%)	0.1	0.1	NS
Mortality (%)	1.4	1.5	NS

penetrating wounds but also blunt trauma and overpressure, helmets are designed primarily to protect against ballistic threats and have not been found to have collateral benefits in protecting against blunt trauma or blast. Thus, tertiary (blunt trauma) injuries are also likely a major contributor to the prevalence of closed head wounds in combat. The following pages provide a system-by-system review of the state of the science with respect to injuries to five major physiological systems – auditory, respiratory, digestive, vascular, and neurological – with a bias toward the topic of blast-induced TBI, where the most significant scientific advances have been made in the last 15–18 years.

Auditory System

Blast overpressure to unprotected ears is one of the most common injuries in a combat environment, with 16% of blast-injured individuals suffering from perforation of the tympanic membrane [4]. The wound usually results in some initial loss of hearing, and about half of those victims also suffer from tinnitus. Post healing, whether surgical or spontaneous, about half of the patients continue to suffer from hearing loss. In addition to rupture of the tympanic membrane, blast loading on the ears can also cause sensory cells to be torn from their supporting cell attachments when the basilar membrane is displaced. Where scar tissue forms, the mechanical properties of the basilar membrane can change, negatively impacting the function of the cochlea in regions beyond that which was initially damaged [5].

The thresholds for blast injury to the auditory system are a function of peak overpressure and positive phase impulse. For a short-duration pulse, the threshold for an auditory shift is 2 pounds per square inch (psi), with the threshold for tympanic membrane rupture at 5 psi, and a 50% chance of tympanic membrane rupture at 15 psi [6].

Every person considered to be at risk of explosive blast exposure should undergo an otoscopic examination. The presence of tympanic membrane rupture is a clinical sign that the patient likely was within the blast overpressure shock wave. If so, then there is increased risk of other injuries such as traumatic brain (TBI) or hollow viscera injury. Though an important marker of likely blast overpressure exposure, the lack of tympanic membrane damage *does not rule out* other clinically relevant primary blast injuries.

Respiratory System

Blast overpressure to the respiratory system has received significant research funding over the last 30 years, in recognition of the high mortality rates associated blast injury to the lungs. In spite of this research, the mechanism of blast lung injury remains the subject of some debate. One school of thought is that "blast lung" injury is a low-frequency phenomenon in which the blast induces compression of the thoracic wall over a 2- to 3-millisecond period, producing shear waves that induce strain at locations that are fixed. These shear waves move at different velocities as they pass through tissues of varying densities, causing disruption of the alveolar-capillary interface [7]. Another school of thought argues that blast lung injury is a high-frequency phenomenon in which supersonic stress waves passing through the lungs cause air bubbles to form within the alveoli, leading to alveolar rupture [8].

The threshold for lung injury is a function of both the peak overpressure and the blast impulse. The first injury risk curves were published in 1968 and were known as the "Bowen's Injury Risk Curves" (Fig. 3.1) [9].

While these curves were designed to represent blast *tolerance*, they were widely accepted as indicating the risk of blast injury to the lungs. Unfortunately, although

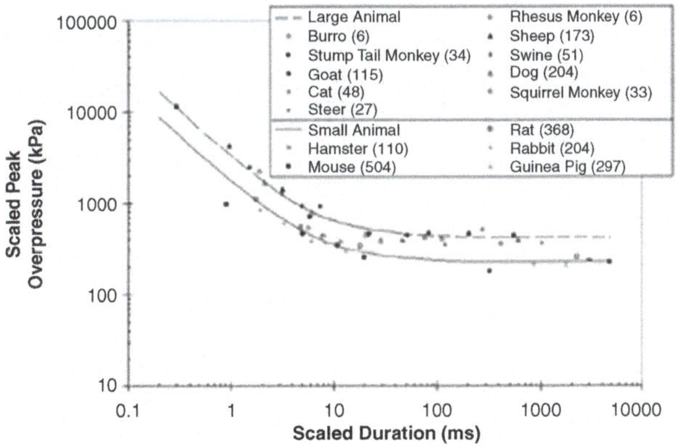

Fig. 3.1 Bowen's injury risk curve. (Reprinted from Bowen et al. [9])

the Bowen curves represented a significant step forward in understanding the risk of blast injury, they fell far short of providing meaningful insights into thresholds for injury, since they assumed a Friedlander blast wave and an unprotected thorax, both of which are rarely operationally relevant conditions. More complex blast lung injury models were developed in the 1990s, but these models typically require input data not available outside of the blast testing environment and still assume an unprotected thorax [10, 11]. In 2012, Bass et al. published data showing updates to the Bowen curves based upon large animal data collected in over 50 experiments since 1968, with adjustments to account for blast wave attenuation through hard (Level IV) armor [12]. The resulting curves are shown in Fig. 3.2. Although these curves still have the limitation of assuming a Friedlander blast wave, the inputs are readily available in most blast situations, and they provide an initial estimate of the effects of protective gear on injury thresholds.

The clinical presentation of explosive blast lung may be subtle and delayed by several hours. This is because explosive blast lung injury is an acute lung injury (ALI) for which inflammation is a prominent cause of clinical deterioration. Presenting signs and symptoms may be shortness of breath, cyanosis, and hemoptysis, and early chest radiography may reveal bilateral peri-hilar infiltrates known as the "butterfly" sign [3, 13]. Close early observation is critical. Patients

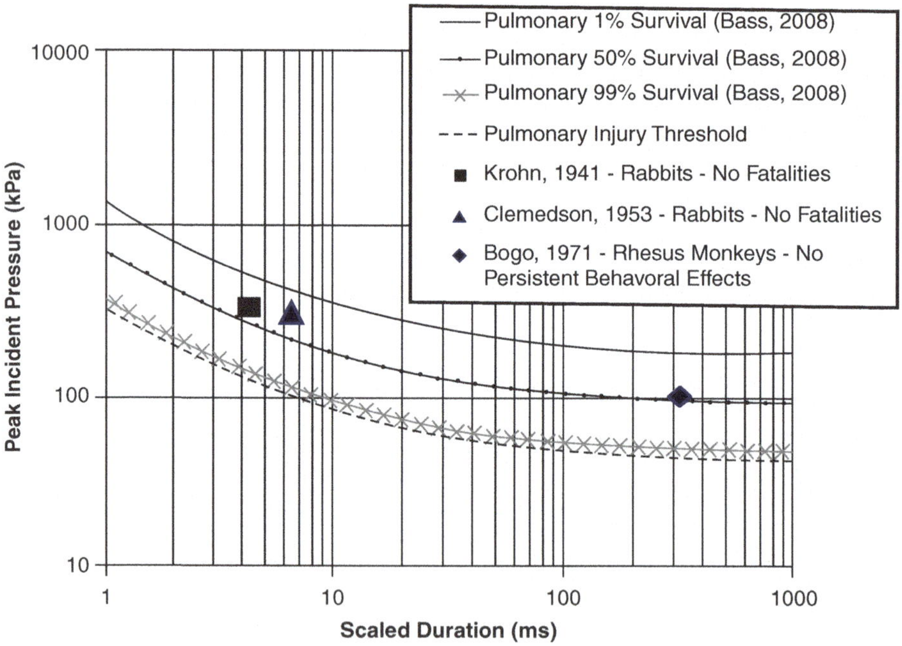

Fig. 3.2 Comparison of pulmonary injury threshold and survival curves with and without the assumption of blast attenuation through thoracic ballistic protective gear. (Reprinted with permission from Springer Nature: Annals of Biomedical Engineering, Bass et al. [12] Copyright 2012)

who are able to adequately ventilate without assistance at 2 hours after injury are unlikely to progress to needing intubation or mechanical ventilation.

Digestive System

A recent comprehensive review found an estimated rate of abdominal primary blast injury (PBI) of 3.0% in hospitalized survivors of blast [14]. The rate of abdominal trauma after primary blast exposure appears only marginally higher in enclosed-space detonations than in open-space detonations, but may be as high as 69% in immersion (underwater) blast [14]. From this limited data we can conclude that abdominal injuries caused by blast are relatively uncommon, but that certain situations, such as blasts in enclosed spaces or under water, can increase the incidence of blast overpressure injury, in general, and abdominal blast injury, in particular. It should be noted that there are "enhanced blast weapons," which may also lead to increased rates of abdominal blast injuries, but the statistics for these newer weapons are still very limited.

In abdominal PBI, the shear wave generates gross body wall and visceral motion and exerts its pathological effect through the tearing of restraining tissues because of differential acceleration [5]. As stated by Owen et al. [1], an abdominal blast injury is caused when the "incident blast wave is coupled across the abdominal wall, generating both a high-velocity, low-amplitude stress wave and a low-velocity, high-amplitude shear wave. The stress wave acts at the microscopic level, causing injury by tissue spalling and implosion. When a compressive stress wave reaches a tissue density interface, such as that between the intestinal wall and the gas-filled lumen, it is partially reflected as a tension wave. Most tissues are weaker in tension than compression and the surface or boundary shreds (spalls), just as the surface of the water is sprayed upwards by an underwater explosion. The passing stress wave compresses pockets of gas, which then re-expand, releasing large amounts of kinetic energy and destroying the restraining tissues; this is implosion."

The threshold for injury to the bowel is higher than that for the lungs. As a result, the frequency of survivors with blast bowel injuries is relatively low (0.6% of military casualties in a 2009 report from Operation Iraqi Freedom [15]). Blast bowel injuries typically include a mural hematoma, which may result in a minor submucosal hemorrhage or a full-thickness perforation. The intramural hematoma can develop hematemesis or melena as a result of the mucosal and submucosal hemorrhage. Shear tears to mesenteric vessels can cause hemoperitoneum. The primary challenge in blast injury to abdominal structures is that they may be difficult to diagnose, and, therefore, may initially go untreated.

Vascular System

Vascular injuries are an important and clinically challenging component of injuries from explosions. They are dealt with comprehensively in Chap. 31, which also identifies the relative frequency of vascular injuries in the limbs and neck and torso. Since the majority of preventable deaths and prehospital deaths occur from bleeding, vascular injuries of any significance are the priority in early care of the injured.

Neurological System

Traumatic brain injuries were dubbed the "signature injury" of Operations Iraqi and Enduring Freedom, with closed head injuries representing the "new" discovery of those conflicts. It has been estimated that between 15% and 20% of returning veterans from Afghanistan and Iraq have traumatic brain injuries (TBI), although these numbers are highly suspect due to the lack of meaningful tools for diagnosing mild TBI [16]. Most of the attention to TBI in the last 15 years has been to *blast-induced* TBI, meaning *primary* blast-induced TBI. The complex nature of blast physics, however, particularly in a combat environment, suggests that many of the blast-induced closed, traumatic brain injuries may have been caused by rapid head acceleration or blunt trauma instead of, or in addition to, direct effects of the shock wave.

Blunt Trauma and Acceleration Injury Mechanism

Blunt trauma and acceleration cause injury via three mechanisms: skull deformation, translational and rotational motion, and intracranial pressure (ICP) [13]. Skull deformation, both elastic and plastic, transmits stress to underlying tissues, leading to contusions at the site of impact. Additionally, when the skull rebounds from initial deformation, the dura mater and skull can be separated, causing epidural hematomas [17].

Translational motion of the skull causes injury because the brain is not rigidly attached to the skull, and its motion lags behind that of the head and skull. This leads to contusions at the site of impact between the inner table of the skull and the brain (*coup* lesions). Subsequently, when the head ceases to move, the brain may continue to move, leading to an impact on the interior of the skull at side opposite of the point of initial impact (*contrecoup* lesions) [18]. There appear to be two mechanisms of injury associated with rotational motion. First, because the brainstem is relatively fixed, rotational motion of the head and skull leads to contusions where the brain is most constrained: around the foramen magnum and ventral frontal compartments [19]. Second, the rotational motion of the brain around the fixed point of the brainstem also leads to shear tearing at interfaces between adjacent tissues moving at different rates as a result of different densities [20]. These tears are most pronounced near the surface of the brain, where motion is the greatest; they are least pronounced near the center of gravity of the brain, where motion is the least. Generally, the more significant the rotational motion, the deeper into the brain structures are found shear tears.

Relative motion of the brain within the skull results in increased intracranial pressure (ICP) [15]. As the brain moves toward the skull in response to head acceleration, the intracranial pressure between the brain and the skull is increased locally, with a corresponding decrease in ICP distally, where the brain is moving away from the skull. Both the ICP pressure gradients and the shearing from brain motion stretch and enlarge axons, causing damage to microtubules and leading to diffuse axonal injuries (DAI).

Blunt Trauma and Acceleration Thresholds for Injury

Thresholds for blunt trauma injury have been a topic of research for over 60 years. The most commonly used metric is the Head Injury Criterion (HIC) [21], which was developed based upon skull fracture in 23 drop-tests of five embalmed cadavers in the 1950s [22]. Prasad and Mertz developed the Head Injury Risk Curve using human cadaver test data and found that an HIC of 1400 is associated with a 50% probability of a life-threatening brain injury and an HIC of 700 is associated with a 5% probability of a life-threatening brain injury [23].

In addition to the Head Injury Criterion, other injury criteria have been developed, although none are in wide use. In recognition that the HIC is insufficient when applied to mild TBI, the principal component score (wPCS) has been proposed as a metric for evaluating the risk of mild TBI [24]. In recognition that the HIC is designed only for translational motion, the Head Injury Power (HIP) criterion [25] has been proposed to account for the rate of change of both translational and rotational kinetic energy, and both Rotational Injury Criterion (RIC) and Power Rotational Head Injury Criterion (PRHIC) are based upon angular acceleration [26]. The existing blunt trauma injury criteria have been useful to the development of protective equipment to reduce the risk of skull fractures and hematomas. However, we continue to lack criteria for the threshold of *mild* TBI. Moreover, the susceptibility of the brain to injury increases with repeated impacts, and a criterion that accounts for this repeated impact effect is still under development [13].

Blast Injury Mechanism

Elucidation of the injury mechanisms of primary blast loading to the brain has been impeded by poor replication of blast loading environments in a laboratory setting [27]. Much of the research has been conducted using shock tubes which can, in fact, produce a highly realistic free-field shock wave. However, these tubes have been misused, placing test specimens outside the tube or using a tube that is too small to avoid substantial artifacts due to a distorted flow pattern around the specimen. As a result of these challenges, the mechanism of brain injury caused by exposure to blast overpressure remains a topic of some debate. Currently, there are several hypotheses under investigation, all without sufficient data to be either definitively discredited or substantially supported. One hypothesis is that energy transferred from the shock wave to the torso causes damage to the brain via (1) the difference between the pressure in the ventral body cavity and the cranial cavity; (2) a pressure wave transmitted via blood vessels to the brain; and (3) a breakdown of small cerebral blood vessels and the blood brain barrier as a result of the sudden increase in perfusion pressure [28]. Another hypothesis is that as the shock wave transmiths through the skull it initiates stress waves in the brain tissues. These stress waves include micro and marco level tearing within the first 2 milliseconds of the blast event, with shear wave amplitudes that are magnified at material boundaries, such as the interfaces between gray and white matter [29]. These same forces are also hypothesized to cause macroscale damage, particularly in the brainstem and white matter of the corpus callosum [30]. Still another hypothesis is that the elastic deformation of the skull ("skull flexure") under blast loading initiates pressure gradients, increases intracranial pressure, initiates cerebrospinal fluid micro-cavitation, and may cause acceleration of the brain within the skull cavity [13, 31].

Due to the large number of variables associated with exposure to blast and confounding factors in human populations, such as previous TBI history, large animal models are now being used to both elucidate physiological and neurological effects of exposure to blast and determine thresholds of injury. Using these models, researchers interpret the response of the brain after exposure to blast by quantifying the relationship between the intensity of the exposure, the number of repetitions, and the timeframe over which the exposures occur. Large animals, such as the Yucatan mini pig, are an appropriate model since they have a brain anatomy similar to humans, making the transformation of the findings from the animal to a human-relevant loading possible. The use of the large animal model has shown that inflammation is present at subthreshold blast levels, suggesting the brain is reacting to blast at low-exposure levels, but the brain may be capable of compensating for those changes such that no behavioral changes are detected. As the blast intensity and the number of exposures increase, markers of neurodegeneration start to express themselves. The expression of neurodegenerative markers seems to be associated with changes in animal behavior 24 hours after exposure. Similar to the human population studies, animal behavioral changes trend to baseline after 24 hours. What animal testing can show us is that while behavior is trending back to preexposure levels, inflammatory, neurodegeneration, and other markers are still showing a measured response 72 hours after exposure.

The pathophysiologic effects from exposure to blast overpressure are diverse and differ from effects observed from other threats, such as blunt impact. For the most severe cases of blast exposure, brain injuries include edema, intracranial hemorrhage, and vasospasm. On the other end of the spectrum, transient neurological effects are observed for up to 24 hours for repeated exposure to heavy weapons fire and breaching during training. The symptoms for in-training repeated blast exposure include memory recall deficits, emotional dysregulation (indicated by increased volatility), loss of sleep, etc. These changes occur with no detectible change in the brain anatomy using standard CT and MR imaging. Other factors that affect the magnitude of the neurological response include the orientation of the body/head to the direction of blast as well as the use of protective equipment.

The most prominent pathophysiologic characterists of blast-inducted TBI are edema, intracranial hemorrhage, and vasospasm. In severe blast TBI, intracranial hypertension is common, with hyperemia and severe edema occurring in the acute post-injury period [28]. Traumatic cerebral vasospasm (TCV) has been observed in swine models [32], nonhuman primates [33], and humans [34]. TCV from blast can last up to 30 days, which is twice as long as the TCV that occurs with conventional TBI. Traumatic cerebral vasospasm is positively correlated to acute subarachnoid hemorrhage and is predicted by the number of injured lobes and the presence of a pseudoaneurysm. The occurrence of a pseudoaneurysm with traumatic cerebral vasospasm is thought to be the result of arterial damage leading to subarachnoid hemorrhaging. Diffuse axonal injury due to sheer strain has been found in white matter tracts arising from the cortex, frontostriatal, frontoparietal, and frontotemporal pathways [35]. Other abnormalities have been observed using Diffusion Tensor Imaging (DTI) in the orbitofrontal white matter, cingulum bundles [36], and uncinate fasciculus [37]. Exposure to blast loads ranging from 11 psi to 29 psi have let to distortion of apical dendrites of pyramidal neurons, with shrunken and condensed soma in the CA3 region of the hippocampus. The CA1 region of the hippocampus also showed a significant reduction in pyramidal neurons [30]. These changes in the hippocampus may be the cause of memory impairments in some blast TBI patients [28].

Blast TBI Injury Thresholds

Efforts to identify blast TBI injury thresholds are, like those of blunt TBI, impeded by the lack of clear diagnostics for *mild* TBI. Historically, blast-induced TBI risk has been estimated using acceleration-loading standards, such as the Head Injury Criterion (HIC). However, because of the extremely short load duration for blast exposure (under 10 milliseconds), acceleration-based criteria are not valid for blast scenarios.

Only a few studies have been conducted that were designed to characterize exposure thresholds for any level of injury. This is due to a variety of reasons, not the least of which is the variability in responses among individuals of the same species as well as the challenge of scaling one species response to human equivalency. For example, Rafaels et al. (2011) performed blast testing on rabbits and ferrets to determine the threshold for single-impact blast injury. Using logistic regression, a 50% probability of lethality curve was generated [38]. This work yielded the interesting result that a 50% risk of fatality from blast exposure to the brain is, in fact, at overpressures well above the level for a 99% risk of fatality from blast exposure to an unprotected thorax (Fig. 3.3a). In fact, at overpressures well above the unprotected pulmonary 99% risk of fatality level (Fig. 3.3a). In contrast, the 50% risk of mild brain injury (defined as bleeding) occurs at levels similar to the unprotected threshold pulmonary injury (Fig. 3.3b) [9].

Most recently, data from the large animal studies are being used to both guide the development of threshold levels and support stand-down and return-to-duty recommendations. Blast thresholds that factor in blast intensity, number of repetitions and timeframe over which the exposures occur are being developed are using combined

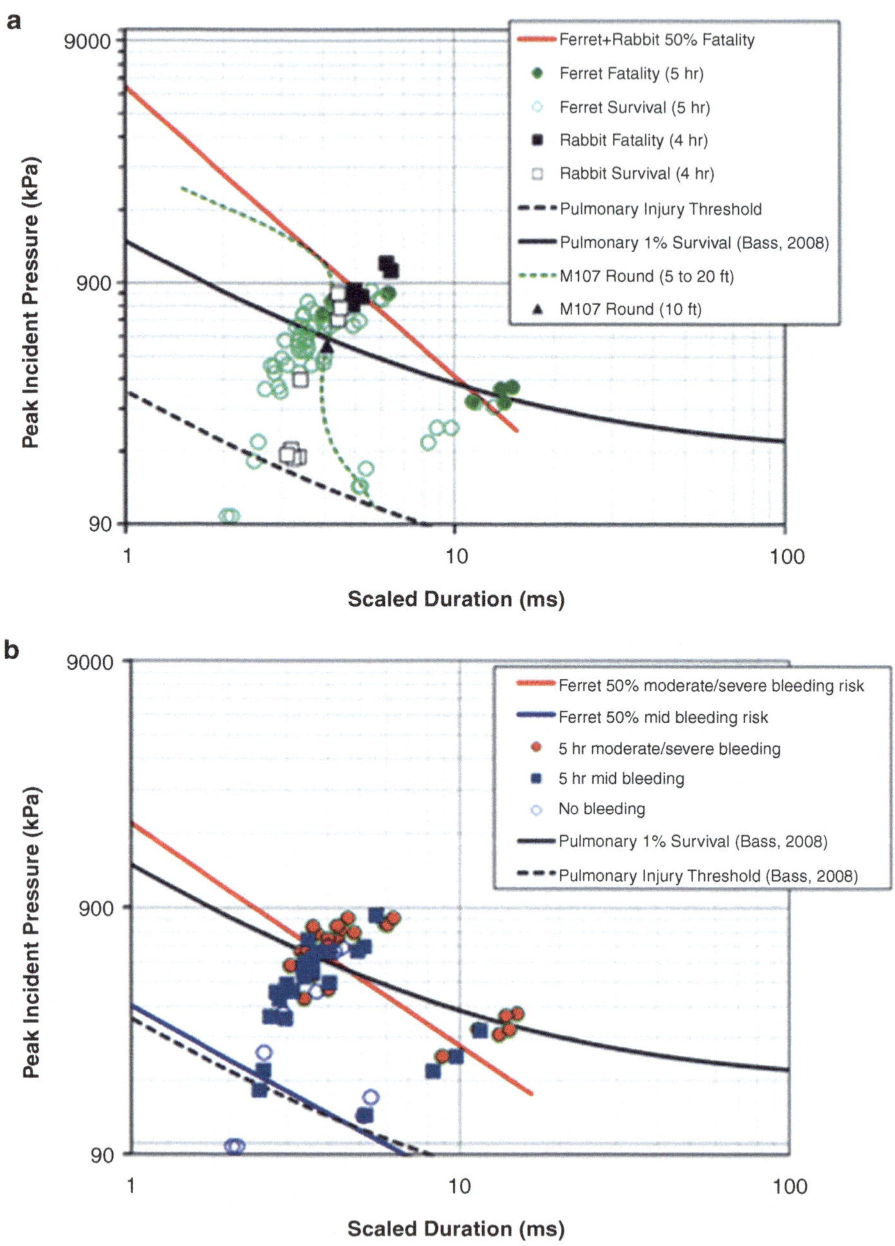

Fig. 3.3 (**a**) Risk function for 50% fatality from primary blast based upon scaled ferret and rabbit data; (**b**) risk function for 50% mild-to-moderate/severe meningeal bleeding based upon scaled ferret data. (Reprinted with permission from Springer Nature: Annals of Biomedical Engineering, Bass et al. [12]. Copyright 2012)

data from animal and human studies [39]. These combined datasets are integrated using the assumptions that energy transmitted through the skull interacts with the brain to cause injury and that both human and pig intracranial tissue will react similarly to pressure once through the human or pig skull. Biomechanical tests have been conducted to measure the energy transmitted through the skull for the human and the animal under shock tube loading conditions. Transfer functions derived from these tests provide a means to determine equivalent incident pressures *outside* the skulls that produce similar pressures *inside* the skull. In this way, researchers are able to develop transfer functions that account for differences in skull anatomy between the human and mini pig. Algorithms based upon integrated data sets indicate that the threshold for a transient neurological effect from a single exposure is below the threshold for respiratory injury. The algorithms also validate that exposure to multiple exposures reduces the magnitude of the exposures that a subject can tolerate. The observed transient neurological effects do not appear to affect the operational readiness of the forces relative to the ability of the soldier to move, shoot, and communicate. However, observations indicate that the level of effort for a blast-exposed soldier to complete the task is greater than that of a nonblast exposed individual. The long-term effect of this observation on the individual and force readiness is unknown. Additionally, blast overpressure alone does not cause severe brain injuries until extremely high pressures, outside reasonable military range, are attained. This observation suggests that neurological injury associated with exposure to blast in the military is likely the result of either a combination of blast *and* impact or the accumulated effects over time from repeated blast exposures. Additional research is required to quantify the combined effects of these factors.

The clinical management of TBI begins with diagnosis. For mild TBI or concussion, symptoms may be subtle. For this reason, any person suspected of having been exposed to explosive blast should be screened for TBI using validated clinical tools, such as the Military Acute Concussion Evaluation (MACE) or Sport Concussion Assessment Tool (SCAT5). The MACE is the military acute concussion evaluation and is intended for use in military settings [40, 41]. The SCAT is the sport concussion assessment tool, 5th edition [42]. Both are clinical tests of cognitive function and balance. If found to be abnormal on either test, the patient is at significant risk of having suffered a mild TBI/concussion and should be evaluated by an appropriate advanced medical provider so that the diagnosis of TBI can be made. Clinical treatment of concussion is conservative with attention toward reducing the risk of subsequent or secondary TBI before the patient has fully recovered. Symptoms such as headache, dizziness, tinnitus, and insomnia should be treated. Patients should not return to regular activity until fully recover, which is when symptoms have resolved and no do they longer require treatment and when provocative testing does cause a symptom recurrence [43, 44].

Patients who have suffered moderate to severe TBI will require advanced medical care. After appropriate attention to immediate life threats, patients need to be evacuated to a Level 1 trauma center with neurosurgical and neurological intensive care. Neuroimaging, typically with beginning with noncontrast CT-head, should be performed [10]. Clinical management should follow the Guidelines for the Management of Severe TBI, focused on intracranial pressure (ICP) control, blood pressure and cerebral perfusion pressure management, airway and ventilatory therapy, early seizure and deep vein thrombosis prophylaxis, and ensuring adequate nutrition. The role of decompressive craniectomy is still being determined. At present, neither steroid use nor induced hypothermia is advocated [45, 46].

Skeletal/Muscular Systems

The limbs are the most frequently injured parts of the body in combat blast events. Because of the need for mobility in the operational setting, limbs are relatively unprotected compared to the head and torso. At the severe end of the spectrum, blast-related limb injuries are characterized by their massive soft tissue damage and often unsalvageable injuries to multiple limbs. The severity and nature of severe combat limb injuries from explosions is rarely replicated in civilian peacetime trauma medicine except in extreme circumstances (e.g., run over by a train).

Limb injuries that are a combination of blast overpressure and fragments (i.e., primary plus secondary blast injury) are common. The exposure of limbs to the device and blast overpressure damage to the tissues produces not only massive soft tissue injuries, resulting in loss of muscle mass, but also microscopic damage to the tissue and microvasculature, adding to a risk of slow healing and infection. In general, blast wounds have a high infection rate, with extensive soft tissue damage, volumetric muscle loss, nerve damage, and complex scarring. Blast-related extremity injuries, in particular, result in significant damage and often multiple amputations [47]. These wounds tend to be colonized by multiple pathogens, and complex soft tissue wounds are particularly susceptible to invasive fungal infections.

Research on primary blast overpressure effect on limbs has produced the counter intuitive finding that major fractures and amputations do not occur at the joints, but above and below these areas, for example, 4–8 inches down the tibia and up the femur. The past 10 years have seen explosion research into prosthesis and soft tissue/muscle regeneration. The result is an increase in the functionality of amputated and seriously damaged limbs [48].

Conclusion

The last 20 years have seen dramatic improvements in our understanding of blast-induced injuries. When Operation Iraqi Freedom began, the general consensus was that the risk of primary blast-induced brain injuries was low, with the working assumption being that blast levels required to damage the brain would result in terminal blast lung injuries. Today, we now recognize that improvements in thoracic protection make these formally lethal blast levels survivable – and individuals now live to experience not only blast-induced traumatic brain injuries, but also catastrophic orthopedic injuries. Of these, the blast-induced traumatic brain injuries are least understood and have received the most significant investments in research. Today, however, we are still struggling to understand the mechanism of blast TBI, and the threshold for injury is elusive. Worse still, making the diagnosis of mild TBI remains difficult, so that individuals exposed to blast may not receive the care they need. Over the coming years, investments in research are needed to provide better materials for protecting limbs, diagnose mild blast TBI, and prevent blast TBI.

References

1. Owen-Smith M. Bomb blast injuries: in an explosive situation. Nurs Mirror. 1979;149(13):35–9.
2. Champion HR, Baskin T, Holcomb JB. Injuries from explosives. PHTLS Prehospital Trauma Life Support: military edition. 6th ed. St. Louis: Mosby; 2007. p. 563–81.
3. Stein M, Hirshberg A. Medical consequences of terrorism: the conventional weapon threat. Surg Clin North Am. 1999;79(6):1537–52.
4. Ritenour AE, Wickley A, Ritenour JS, Kriete BR, Blackbourne LH, Holcomb JB, et al. Tympanic membrane perforation and hearing loss from blast overpressure in operation enduring freedom and operation Iraqi freedom wounded. J Trauma Acute Care Surg. 2008;64(2):S174–8.
5. Patterson JH Jr, Hamernik RP. Blast overpressure induced structural and functional changes in the auditory system. Toxicology. 1997;121(1):29–40.
6. DePalma RG, Burris DG, Champion HR, Hodgson MJ. Blast injuries. N Engl J Med. 2005;352(13):1335–42.
7. Stuhmiller JH, Phillips YY, Richmond DR. The physics and mechanisms of primary blast injury. In: Zajtchuk R, Jenkins DP, Bellamy RF, editors. Conventional warfare: ballistic, blast, and burn injuries. Washington, DC: Office of the Surgeon General of the United States Army; 1991. p. 241–70.
8. Cooper GJ, Townend DJ, Cater SR, Pearce BP. The role of stress waves in thoracic visceral injury from blast loading: modification of stress transmission by foams and high-density materials. J Biomech. 1991;24(5):273–85.
9. Bowen IG, Fletcher ER, Richmond DR. Estimate of man's tolerance to the direct effects of air blast, Technical Progress Report, DASA-2113, Defense Atomic Support Agency, Department of Defense, Washington, DC, October 1968.
10. Axelsson H, Yelverton JT. Chest wall velocity as a predictor of nonauditory blast injury in a complex wave environment. J Trauma. 1996;40:S31–7.
11. Stuhmiller JH. Biological response to blast overpressure: a summary of modeling. Toxicology. 1997;121:91–103.
12. Bass CR, Panzer MB, Rafaels KA, Wood G, Shridharani J, Capehart B. Brain injuries from blast. Ann Biomed Eng. 2012;40(1):185–202.
13. Singh AK, Ditkofsky NG, York JD, Abujudeh HH, Avery LA, Brunner JF, Sodickson AD, Lev MH. Blast injuries: from improvised explosive device blasts to the Boston Marathon bombing. Radiographics. 2016;36(1):295–307. https://doi.org/10.1148/rg.2016150114.
14. Owers C, Morgan JL, Garner JP. Abdominal trauma in primary blast injury. Br J Surg. 2011;98(2):168–79.
15. Plurad DS. Blast injury. Mil Med. 2011;176(3):276–82.
16. Young L, Rule GT, Bocchieri RT, Walilko TJ, Burns JM, Ling G. When physics meets biology: low and high-velocity penetration, blunt impact, and blast injuries to the brain. Front Neurol. 2015;6:89.
17. Post A, Hoshizaki TB. Mechanisms of brain impact injuries and their prediction: a review. Trauma. 2012;14(4):327–49. https://doi.org/10.1177/1460408612446573.
18. Yoganandan N. Frontiers in head and neck trauma: clinical and biomechanical. Amsterdam: IOS Press; 1998.

19. Hardy WN, Khalil TB, King AI. Literature review of head injury biomechanics. Int J Impact Eng. 1994;15(4):561–86. https://doi.org/10.1016/0734-743X(94)80034-7.
20. Ommaya AK, Gennarelli TA. Cerebral concussion and traumatic unconsciousness. Correlation of experimental and clinical observations of blunt head injuries. Brain. 1974;97(4):633–54. https://doi.org/10.1093/brain/97.1.633.
21. Versace J. A review of the severity index. No.710881. SAE Technical Paper 1971.
22. Lissner HR, Lebow M, Evans FG. Experimental studies on the relation between acceleration and intracranial pressure changes in man. Surg Gynecol Obstet. 1960;111:329–38.
23. Prasad P, Mertz HJ, Dalmotas DJ, Augenstein JS, Digges K. Evaluation of the field relevance of several injury risk functions. SAE Technical Paper; 2010 Nov 3.
24. Greenwald RM, Gwin JT, Chu JJ, Crisco JJ. Head impact severity measures for evaluating mild traumatic brain injury risk exposure. Neurosurgery. 2008;62(4):789. https://doi.org/10.1227/01.neu.0000318162.67472.ad.
25. Newman JA, Shewchenko N, Welbourne E. A proposed new biomechanical head injury assessment function-the maximum power index. Stapp Car Crash J. 2000;44:215–47.
26. Kimpara H, Iwamoto M. Mild traumatic brain injury predictors based on angular accelerations during impacts. Ann Biomed Eng. 2012;40(1):114–26. https://doi.org/10.1007/s10439-011-0414-2.
27. Needham CE, Ritzel D, Rule GT, Wiri S, Young L. Blast testing issues and TBI: experimental models that lead to wrong conclusions. Front Neurol. 2015;6:72.
28. Chen Y, Huang W. Non-impact, blast-induced mild TBI and PTSD: concepts and caveats. Brain Inj. 2011;25(7-8):641–50.
29. Taylor PA, Ford CC. Simulation of blast-induced early-time intracranial wave physics leading to traumatic brain injury. J Biomech Eng. 2009;131(6):061007.
30. Chafi MS, Karami G, Ziejewski M. Biomechanical assessment of brain dynamic responses due to blast pressure waves. Ann Biomed Eng. 2010;38(2):490–504.
31. Magnuson J, Leonessa F, Ling GS. Neuropathology of explosive blast traumatic brain injury. Curr Neurol Neurosci Rep. 2012;12(5):570–9.
32. Bauman RA, Ling G, Tong L, Januszkiewicz A, Agoston D, Delanerolle N, et al. An introductory characterization of a combatcasualty-care relevant swine model of closed head injury resulting from exposure to explosive blast. J Neurotrauma. 2009;26(6):841–60. https://doi.org/10.1089/neu.2009-0898.
33. Lu J, Ng KC, Ling G, Wu J, Poon DJ, Kan EM, et al. Effect of blast exposure on the brain structure and cognition in Macaca fascicularis. J Neurotrauma. 2011; https://doi.org/10.1089/neu.2010.1591.
34. Armonda RA, Bell RS, Vo AH, Ling G, DeGraba TJ, Crandall B, et al. Wartime traumatic cerebral vasospasm: recent review of combat casualties. Neurosurgery. 2006;59(6):1215–25. https://doi.org/10.1227/01.neu.0000249190.46033.94.
35. Folmer RL, Billings CJ, Diedesch-Rouse AC, Gallun FJ, Lew HL. Electrophysiological assessments of cognition and sensory processing in TBI: applications for diagnosis, prognosis and rehabilitation. Int J Psychophysiol. 2011;82(1):4–15. https://doi.org/10.1016/j.ijpsycho.2011.03.005.
36. MacDonald CL, Johnson AM, Cooper D, Nelson EC, Werner NJ, Shimony JS, et al. Detection of blast-related traumatic brain injury in U.S. military personnel. N Engl J Med. 2011;364(22):2091–100. https://doi.org/10.1056/NEJMoa1008069.
37. Davenport ND, Lim KO, Armstrong MT, Sponheim SR. Diffuse and spatially variable white matter disruptions are associated with blast-related mild traumatic brain injury. NeuroImage. 2012;59(3):2017–24. https://doi.org/10.1016/j.neuroimage.2011.10.050.
38. Rafaels K, "Dale" Bass CR, Salzar RS, Panzer MB, Woods W, Feldman S, et al. Survival risk assessment for primary blast exposures to the head. J Neurotrauma. 2011;28(11):2319–28.
39. Ongoing Research with the Office of Naval Research, Code 34 under Contract N00014-14-C-0254.
40. French L, McCrea M, Bagget M. The Military Acute Concussion Evaluation (MACE). J Spec Oper Med. 2008;8(1):68–77.

41. Stone ME Jr, Safadjou S, Farber B, Velazco N, Man J, Reddy SH, et al. Utility of the Military Acute Concussion Evaluation as a screening tool for mild traumatic brain injury in a civilian trauma population. J Trauma Acute Care Surg. 2015;79(1):147–51. https://doi.org/10.1097/TA.0000000000000679.
42. Echemendia RJ, Meeuwisse W, McCrory P, Davis GA, Putukian M, Leddy J, et al. The sport concussion assessment tool 5th edition (SCAT5): background and rationale. Br J Sports Med. 2017;51(11):848–50.
43. Management of Concussion/mTBI Working Group1. VA/DoD clinical practice guideline for management of concussion/mild traumatic brain injury. J Rehabil Res Dev. 2009;46(6):CP1–68.
44. Department of Veterans Affairs and Dept of Defense. 2016. https://www.healthquality.va.gov/guidelines/Rehab/mtbi/mTBICPGFullCPG50821816.pdf.
45. Brain Trauma Foundation; American Association of Neurological Surgeons; Congress of Neurological Surgeons. Guidelines for the management of severe traumatic brain injury, third edition. J Neurotrauma. 2007;24(Suppl 1):S1–106.
46. Carney N, Totten AM, O'Reilly C, Ullman JS, Hawryluk GW, Bell MJ, et al. Guidelines for the Management of Severe Traumatic Brain Injury, fourth edition. Neurosurgery. 2017;80(1):6–15. https://doi.org/10.1227/NEU.0000000000001432.
47. Prevention, mitigation, and treatment of blast injuries FY15 report to the executive agent https://blastinjuryresearch.amedd.army.mil/assets/docs/ea_report/FY15_Report_to_the_Executive_Agent.pdf.
48. Patel HD, Dryden S, Gupta A, Ang SC. Pattern and mechanism of traumatic limb amputations after explosive blast: experience from the 07/07/05 London terrorist bombings. J Trauma Acute Care Surg. 2012;73(1):276–81.

Operational Considerations: Review of Contemporary Data

4

Kobi Peleg, Moran Bodas, and Michael Rozenfeld

Introduction

In previous decades, most blast events occurred in the military and industrial arenas, but the current threat shifts more toward terrorism. Indeed, injuries caused by terror-related explosions are of major concern in recent years, with increasing threats of terrorism worldwide. Prime examples are the Oklahoma bombing (1995), September 11th attacks (2001), Madrid train bombings (2004), London underground bombing (2005), Mumbai attacks (2008), Paris attacks (2015), Brussels bombings (2016), the Manchester suicide attacks (2016), and more. What once was presumed to be a concern mainly for countries close to conflict zones, such as Israel, Iraq, Afghanistan, and some regions of India and Pakistan, is now a global threat.

A common misconception is to confuse blast injuries with blast events. The former describes a type of injury mechanism found in the latter. In reality, blast events usually result in combined injuries, of which "blast effect" is only a single kind. Blast events take different shapes and forms, which occur in varying contexts. These events can occur in combat-related scenarios (e.g., war or civil conflicts), criminal acts (e.g., assassinations and mafia-driven incidents), and terrorism.

K. Peleg (✉) · M. Bodas
Sheba Medical Center, Gertner Institute for Epidemiology and Health Policy – The Israel National Center For Trauma and Emergency Medicine Research, Chaim Sheba Medical Center, Ramat-Gan, Israel

The Department of Emergency Management & Disaster Medicine, School of Public Health, Sackler Faculty of Medicine, Tel-Aviv University, Tel-Aviv, Israel
e-mail: kobip@gertner.health.gov.il

M. Rozenfeld
Sheba Medical Center, Gertner Institute for Epidemiology and Health Policy – The Israel National Center For Trauma and Emergency Medicine Research, Chaim Sheba Medical Center, Ramat-Gan, Israel

D. W. Callaway, J. L. Burstein (eds.), *Operational and Medical Management of Explosive and Blast Incidents*, https://doi.org/10.1007/978-3-030-40655-4_4

Terror-related blast events frequently cause multiple casualties, with a risk of overwhelming healthcare services in the case of Mass Casualty Events (MCE), and are associated with immediate and delayed psychological effects, both to the victims present at the scene and on the wider community level. They also produce patterns of injury that are different from prior experience with industrial explosions and military casualties: multiple penetrating injuries from improvised fragment elements combined with other types of blast-related trauma result in injuries of much higher severity in survivors of the immediate blast.

In general, injuries caused by blast are typically divided into five types. Primary blast injuries are direct effects caused by initial overpressure or underpressure associated with the explosive detonation. These include rupture of tympanic membranes, pulmonary damage, and rupture of the hollow viscera. Secondary blast injuries are caused by debris carried by the blast (e.g., small shrapnel), leading to penetrating trauma or fragmentation injuries. Tertiary blast injuries are caused by the physical displacement of the victim, for instance, being thrown by the blast wind or being affected by structural collapse. These include crush injuries, blunt trauma, fractures and traumatic amputations, open or closed brain injuries, and penetrating trauma. Quaternary blast injuries include all other injuries, such as burns, asphyxia, crush injuries, and inhalation of toxic compounds. Quinary blast injury is a relatively new concept. It includes delayed effects such as chronic pain, malnutrition, and immunosuppression [1–4].

The unique characteristics of terror-related explosion events require a thorough review to prepare all levels of medical treatment for casualties of such incidents, from the prehospital setting, through the hospitals, and all the way to rehabilitation and mental health. This chapter will therefore discuss the main operational considerations stemming from the modern trends of terror explosion injuries noted in recent evidence-based research. In particular, the chapter will describe how *explosive device* characteristics interact with *physical location* of the explosion to define the patterns of injury and required clinical resources, as well as the influence of the *general setting of the event* (military/civilian, urban/rural) on scene and medical management.

Epidemiology of Explosion Injuries

Blast casualties are different from explosion casualties (e.g., industrial explosion), and both are different from terror-related explosion casualties. While the first two might demonstrate mostly the classical blast injuries, such as traumatic amputations, blast lung and intestine perforation, accompanied by less severe injuries, such as ruptured tympanic membrane [1, 5], the casualties of terror-related explosions will likely present a more diverse and complex pattern of injury.

For instance, studies from the Second Intifada in Israel (2000–2005) show that about two-thirds of the blast victims presented with penetrating injuries, 48% suffered from blunt injuries, and high-severity burns were presented with 20% of terror explosion victims (Fig. 4.1) [6, 7]. A large proportion of secondary blast injuries will be to the extremities, followed by torso injuries [6]. Tertiary trauma will lead to contusions, bone and skull fractures. Blast trauma per se is also encountered

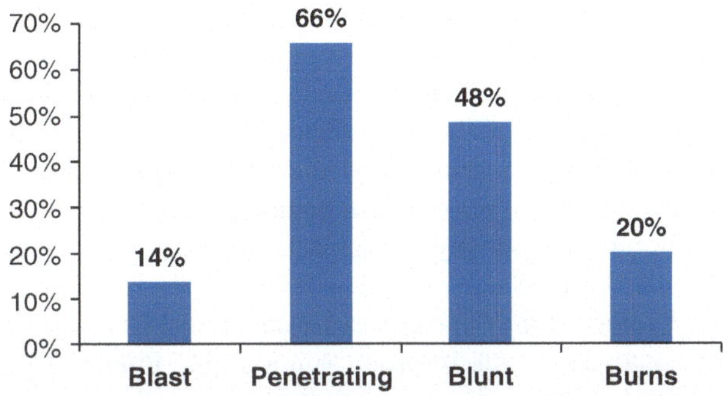

Fig. 4.1 Prevalence of explosion-related trauma mechanisms in the Second Intifada (2000–2005). (Data from the Israeli National Trauma Registry of 823 casualties from 65 terror-related explosion events. Data sums up to more than 100% due to combined injuries (e.g., 19% blast + penetrating))

but on a lower scale than expected: a recent study has found that only 14% of primary blast injuries were present among explosion survivors [7]. A relatively high proportion of casualties (~19%) presented with combined injuries (e.g., blast and penetrating). Similar patterns of injury from explosive incidents were reported from fighting in Iraq and Afghanistan, especially after the conflicts have entered the counter-insurgency phase [8, 9].

Perhaps one of the most important characteristic of terror-related explosion injuries, however, is multidimensional injury pattern (MIP), that is, the manifestation of injuries of different mechanisms in the same patient. MIP contributes to an overall higher injury severity and lower odds of survival [8]. Injuries to multiple body regions are also to be expected.

On the other hand, when reviewing the full spectrum of past explosion events, the first thing to notice is how different all these events are both in their contextual profile and the patterns of casualties they produce. Some of the events, such as criminal assassinations and home accidents, may produce only a single casualty; others, such as most terror attacks, produce significantly more treatable injuries than deaths, whereas explosions resulting in building collapse may cause an appalling death rate on par with the volume of treatable injuries. The patterns of treatable injuries from different explosion events also seem to differ greatly, even when the events themselves belong to a similar category, such as terror attacks or industrial accidents.

The extent to which individuals become affected by explosion events, as well as the severity of injuries, number of casualties, types of injuries, and medical resources needed, varies in accordance with several factors, including type of explosive device, physical location of the detonation, and the setting of the event.

Type of Explosive Devices

The results of a terror-related explosion incident will greatly depend on the type of explosive device and the way it is used to inflict damage. A suicide bomber vest will disperse shrapnel at the torso level in a circular pattern causing upper body injuries to people in the vicinity of the explosion, while an improvised explosive device (IED) left on the ground will mostly injure the lower body parts [6, 10]. A vehicle-based explosive device (VBIED) will contain much more explosives and will therefore cause much more damage than a suicide bomber; however, an explosion at a munitions factory or storage facility is likely to be of incomparably bigger proportions. A small charge implanted in a car for criminal assassination will rarely physically injure someone outside the car. On the other hand, terrorists may use more than one explosive device or even more than one kind of device in the same attack in order to maximize the number of casualties. Finally, a high-explosive aircraft bomb will mostly cause blast and penetrating injuries, whereas a fuel/air bomb dropped by the same aircraft will cause mostly burns.

Another important aspect to consider in type of explosive device is the use of metal fragments in order to maximize injury in terroristic explosions. Often, these elements will cause penetrating injuries that pose a medical challenge on their own merits. Yet, as suggested already above, when it comes to terrorism we can expect everything. For example, when executing the terror attack at Mike's Place Pub in Tel-Aviv on April 30, 2003, in order to get past security guards, the terrorist avoided using any metal components in the explosive device, including shrapnel. While the results of this attack were horrific, the casualties presented with almost no penetrating injuries, rather only blast, blunt, and burns injuries. The only penetrating wounds were caused by glass broken on site as a result of the explosion.

The type of explosive device will also likely influence the way it is used. Perhaps one of the most prominent examples illustrating this is the Boston Marathon bombings on April 15, 2013. The perpetrators of this terror attack used a pressure cooker bomb as an IED. This low-yield IED, given its shape and weight, was left by the terrorists near a building and on the ground. The explosion resulted in predominantly secondary blast injuries (i.e., penetrating wounds caused by ball bearings, nails, screws, and pieces of the pressure cooker housing acting as shrapnel) mostly to the lower limbs. Almost three-quarters (32 out of 43) of patients undergoing radiography in this event retained shrapnel fragments, mostly embedded in the lower extremities [3].

In striking contrast to the Boston marathon bombing, we describe one of the suicide attacks that occurred on a bus to Jerusalem in 1979. As the bus was making its way to Jerusalem, near Ma'ale Edumim, on the outskirts of the city, a bomb exploded inside the bus. The terrorists placed it in the overhead compartments usually used to place small carry-on bags. The resulting casualties suffered mostly from head and chest injuries. In other suicide terror incidents, in which terrorists carried their explosive vest on their torso, the resulting casualties demonstrated scattered injuries to all body parts.

Indeed, no two explosions are the same. This is when dealing with terror-related explosions. The characteristics of these events change greatly depending on a multitude of factors contributing to the outcomes of the event. The examples provided above from Boston and Israel are helpful in demonstrating the difficulty in establishing a unified profile of explosion events. In essence, this means that emergency planners, as well as medical practitioners, should work on principles rather than protocols when preparing for and responding to an explosion event.

Physical Location of the Detonation

To a great extent, the results of an explosion incident depend not only on the explosive, penetrating agents, and resulting fireball but also their interaction with the surrounding space. Depending on the level of confinement of the location and its structural composition, the severity of injuries may differ. For example, confined spaces may enhance the impact on the potential victims through the refraction of the blast wave from the walls and the containment of the fireball, resulting in extremely high temperatures [4, 5, 11]. On the other hand, more open spaces will quickly dissipate the shockwave and fireball, but will provide a noninhibited pathway for the flying debris and shrapnel. While these differences seem highly intuitive, it is worth noting that researchers are still debating whether or not these basic differences are enough to properly explain the resulting variation in the patterns of injuries (Table 4.1).

Thus, it was found that that the injury patterns are different between a simple explosion inside a building and an explosion strong enough to cause the building to *collapse*, as in the latter case the addition of crush injuries heightens the overall injury severity, with the situation further aggravated by the need to extract the victims from under the rubble [11]. Explosions *inside buildings* are characterized by a larger proportion of critical (ISS 25+) injuries, among all due to severe TBI and abdomen injuries and a combination of multiple injuries [7].

Table 4.1 The main characteristics of different explosion locations

Context	Expected medical implications	Additional considerations
Physical space		
Building collapse	High mortality; crush injuries	Need to extract the victims from under the rubble
Inside building	Head and neck, abdomen and extremities injuries Severe TBI; burns Multiple injuries	High in-hospital mortality
Near building	Face and extremities injuries Blast injuries among survivors	Due to lower security measures and high density of crowds, these are presumably more "inviting" targets
Inside bus/ train	Head and neck, face and extremities injuries Serious blast injuries among survivors Multiple injuries	High on-scene mortality
Near bus/ train	Mild head and neck injuries. External injuries, leg fractures. No penetrating injuries	Possibly attacked by VBIEDs, i.e., larger explosive devices
In the open	Extremities and abdomen injuries; mostly penetrating No burns	Injuries highly dependent on device composition

The classification of open versus closed spaces, in the context of explosions, was further developed in light of terror-related explosion incidents. In Israel, for example, vast differences in patterns of injuries were observed between casualties of explosions happening inside a building versus inside a bus, both considered as "closed spaces." It was also found that *buses*, and by association *train cars*, could be considered as a kind of "*hyper-confined*" spaces. This is true because of them being narrow and with lower ceilings, having metal rather than concrete walls, and usually containing a dense crowd of potential victims before the explosion. Buses/train cars are different from inside buildings, as the higher confinement cause greater immediate mortality due to blast and higher proportion of primary blast injuries among survivors [7, 12]. Among survivors of the initial explosion inside a bus, a relatively high proportion (19%) of severe chest injuries could be encountered; almost half of the survivors will sustain injuries to multiple body regions [7]. Despite the differences, in all confined settings an explosion results in increased frequency of burns because even though the effects of a blast wave inside a confined space may vary depending on the context, the containment by four walls will consistently increase the effect of the fireball produced by the explosion [7, 11].

An additional variation regarding explosions involving buses is between explosions inside buses and near them. In cases when the suicide bomber was not allowed to enter or an intentional attack was performed by closing to a bus with a VBIED, it was found that the injuries are much less severe, with most injuries being superficial due to glass fragments. Data also shows an increased volume of lower extremity fractures due to bus walls bending inwards [13].

Lastly, some significant variations in injury profiles were registered regarding so called *semi-confined* or *semi-open* spaces, such as open markets and restaurants, as well as explosions next to a building wall [7, 14]. A somber example of this scenario was the Dolphinarium nightclub explosion in Israel that happened on June 1, 2001. This suicide bombing killed 21 teenagers waiting in line outside next to the concrete wall and injured an additional 100 civilians. After inquiring into the exceptionally high mortality of this incident, it was found that in this scenario the refraction of the blast wave from a single wall may have magnified the blast wave effect and increased both the volume and the severity of casualties [7]. The presence of a large crowd of people next to a building wall in semi-open environments also explains the higher incidence of primary blast injuries in explosions near buildings as compared to those that happened inside buildings, because people already inside a building are not necessarily clustered near the walls and could be more freely distributed through the inner space.

Regarding completely *open* settings, it is important to remember that physical factors at play here are less universal and homogenous. Therefore, the resulting impact is being strongly dependent on the profile of the event (e.g., the number and the composition of explosive devices and the density of the crowd [15]). In an open setting, the blast overpressure and thermal energy dissipate rapidly and penetrate trauma by shrapnel elements predominates [4, 11]. The most frequent injuries expected would be to the abdomen and extremities [7, 11].

In terms of injury severity, the proportion of severe injuries tends to increase almost linearly in relation to the level of enclosure, it being the highest inside buildings (especially if the building collapses), followed by explosions inside buses and train cars, explosions near buildings, and open spaces [7] (Fig. 4.2). The lowest proportion of severe injuries is usually found in explosions near buses, as in this case the metal walls of the bus and sometimes its motor serve to protect people sitting inside. This hierarchy of injury severity is important to comprehend as it affects the requirements for hospital resources following the explosion event. Victims arriving from more enclosed environments require proportionally more surgeries and ICU beds and have higher in-hospital mortality.

Setting of the Event

Whether an explosion will result in fewer or many casualties and/or higher or lower levels of injury severity also depends on circumstantial factors associated with the event's setting. For example, the density of services provided in the vicinity of the event, namely, whether the event takes place in urban or rural setting. Geography is expected to lead to dramatic differences in event management and patient outcomes for given injury patterns.

With the exception of industrial explosions, the majority of explosions, especially terror-related ones, occur in urban settings. This is true in light of the larger pool of high-profile targets and greater chances to find large crowds [16]. On the other hand, security may be perceived as lower in the countryside, inviting a potential attack, perhaps with additional assault measures other than explosives. For example, during a double terror attack at the Utoya Island resort in Norway (2011), the terrorist detonated explosive devices in Oslo, prior to executing a firearms-based murder spree [17]. Israel has abundant experience in multimodal terror attacks, yet

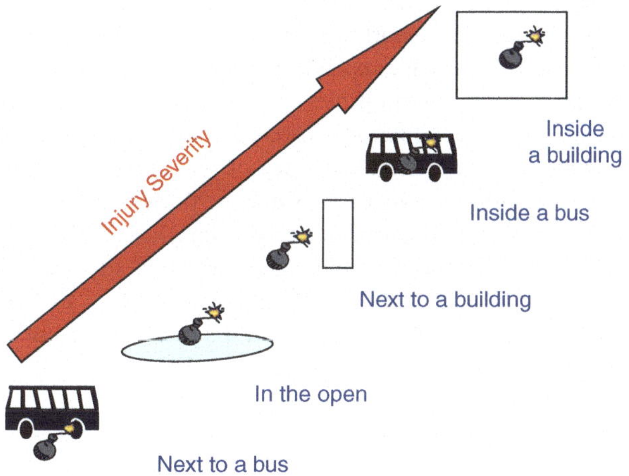

Fig. 4.2 The trend of injury severity of hospitalized patients by type of physical space of the explosion

accounts of such incidents were also recorded in Madrid train bombings, Boston Marathon bombing, London underground bombings, etc. [10, 18, 19].

Urban and rural settings also differ on the kind of explosion we expect to occur in them [16]. For instance, most criminal acts utilizing explosives, such as throwing grenades or planting bombs into cars for assassinations or Mafia-style threatening, tend to happen more frequently in urban environments. In rural places, on the contrary, we can expect more industrial explosions, as industrial zones in developed countries rarely remain within city limits. Domestic explosive incidents (i.e., those happening inside a house) may happen both in urban and rural environments, though their origins are likely to be different, with natural gas explosions more characteristic to cities and agricultural assets, such as fertilizers or grain storage facilities, more of a blast risk in the countryside.

Perhaps the most important aspect highlighting the differences between urban and rural settings is the accessibility to medical resources and services (i.e., "services density"). The number and the quality of hospitals and EMS in the urban area exceed that which exists in a rural setting. With longer transport times to medical treatment, as is the case in most rural settings, there are significantly higher odds of aid arriving too late and patients deteriorating while waiting for definitive treatment. A large number of severe patients may also overwhelm areas with lower health services density and quality of trauma-related healthcare services. In many cases, explosion events in rural areas require utilization of helicopters as a main mean of transportation to and from the scene. In case of MCE, this may lead to evacuation performed by medical priorities, with patients most likely to benefit from immediate evacuation receiving priority over others. However, lack of proper facilities for utilizing ambulance or military/police helicopters may still cause significant delays in patient evacuation, as happened in the Utoya attack [17].

While the potential abundance of healthcare services in urban and especially metropolitan areas is clearly an advantage, the inability to utilize them properly can quickly become a challenge. All attempts to get to the scene or evacuate casualties from it could be thwarted by intensive city traffic, the disturbance of the transport grid due to a serious explosion event, and the need to employ security and safety. While on the scene in urban environment, systematic triage has to be employed in order to guide evacuation efforts to different hospitals based on proximity and level of care, the number and severity of remaining casualties, and available transportation means. Some evacuations may be performed by the police or by the bystanders; however, this uncoordinated effort may lead to crowding of the closest hospitals, while other facilities in the same city used suboptimally [10]. Due to these challenges, in a rural environment, it could be more advisable to "bring the hospital to the event" ("Stay and Play") than to "bring the event to the hospital" ("Scoop and Run"), as practiced in urban scenarios.

Military Versus Civilian Contexts: Explosive Devices, Injuries, and Operational Considerations

Injuries caused by explosions are well documented in the context of combat zones [20]. Explosions represent the most common mechanism of injury (78%) and death (63%) on the modern battlefield [21]. According to [22], nearly three-quarters of all combat injuries over the period from 2005 to 2009 (31 per 10,000 deployed) were due to explosions. In the recent conflicts in Iraq and Afghanistan, the incidence of primary blast injury in US military personnel was 12.2%; however, blast overpressure was the cause of death in only 1.5% [5]. Much of our understanding of blast injuries stems from military-based contexts. Yet, there is a growing threat of blast injury in civilian contexts. This threat spans from terrorism [8], through criminal acts, all the way to industrial accidents [23].

Due to the extensive experience with blast trauma obtained in the recent military conflicts, it is very tempting to rely on knowledge from military medicine in regards to this type of injury event. However, injuries from terror and war are not necessarily comparable [24]. There are vast differences between the military and the civilian contexts of explosion injuries, as well as between the different types of civilian contexts, such as terror-related, industrial/domestic accidents, and criminal activities. These differences concern both the explosive devices and circumstances causing the explosion, the epidemiology of produced injuries, the location of event site, and the balance between vulnerabilities and protective factors important for preparedness and response (Table 4.2). Therefore, extrapolation from military texts, such as the Combat Casualty Care textbook, should be undertaken with caution [2]. According to Reade [2]: "Mistaken preconceptions of the medical consequences of explosion can lead planners and managers to allocate resources incorrectly and clinicians to focus attention away from the most likely pathology."

The differences between military- and civilian-based explosion scenario are ample. It is worthwhile to consider several of the prominent ones in order to highlight the importance in additional research and study into civilian contexts to solidify our understanding of blast injuries in modern times. Perhaps the most obvious difference between the two contexts is demographics. The demographic composition of military and civilian casualty population is very different, with military explosion victims being much younger and mostly male while terror victims have a wider age and gender distribution [24]. This is especially important due to higher incidence of pediatric and geriatric cases among terror victims, with both groups presenting unique challenges for the responders. Blast injuries of children younger than 11 years old present a specifically major challenge, due to their higher rates of traumatic brain injury (TBI), lower rates of injuries to extremities, and overall higher injury severity [25].

Table 4.2 Characteristic of civilian explosion events[a]

	Typical circumstances	Typical number of casualties	Type of explosion	Typical wound pattern
Industrial or domestic accident	Breach of usual safety precautions Domestic accidents in particular are often associated with misuse of drugs or alcohol	1–5	Low explosive, e.g., LPG, gasoline	Burns, including respiratory burns from inhalation of hot gases 1st and 2nd blast injury is rare; 3rd is uncommon except with very large explosions
Terrorist event	High-visibility target with optimized media exposure and recognizable landmarks	50–100	High explosive, particularly ammonium nitrate	Depends on the location of the incident
Homicide/ suicide	Attackers known to victim. Explosion used as a mechanism of inflicting trauma without the need for proximity	1–2	Pipe bomb, usually loaded with low explosive charge	Blast-fragmentation

[a]Reproduced with permission from Reade [2]. https://healthmanagement.org/c/icu/issuearticle/blast-injury

In addition, considering the differences in target populations across the two contexts (i.e., soldiers versus civilians), it is readily understandable why military explosion incidents cause less-severe injuries; soldiers wildly use protective gear, such as helmets and body armor [25, 26]. With the most important body areas protected, injury patterns in military casualties will be very different from civilians. Civilian victims of terror explosions are also worse off in terms of sustained injuries, as a result of a combination of penetrating injuries, with blast, blunt, and burn injuries occurring to the same patient. Aiming to cause more casualties, terrorists equip their bombs with penetrating agents, such as bearing balls, nails, nuts, and bolts, resulting in a large volume of penetrating injuries. This improvised shrapnel may result in multiple injuries of the same patient, while increasing the demand for surgeries for the patients arriving from the event [8].

Reade [2] provides a detailed account of the epidemiology of civilian explosion injuries. According to the author, most survivors of explosion injury do not have clinically significant primary blast trauma. Mainly, civilian victims of terrorism, for example, present with penetrating low-energy transfer blast fragmentation wounds or crush injury in the case of structural collapse. The number of patients and the number of affected body parts is the main difference between blast and non-blast civilian victims. Table 4.2 summarizes the characteristics of civilian explosion incidents [2].

The literature provides additional insights into the unique characteristics and epidemiology of civilian explosion injuries. For instance, Regens, Schultheiss, and Mould [27] surveyed the data of 77,258 successful terrorist MCIs that occurred between 1970 and 2013 that involved the use of explosives, firearms, and/or incendiaries. They reported that explosions cause more complex damage than other conventional weapon types, including traumatic amputation of extremities, ruptured eardrums, mild-to-severe traumatic brain injury, and/or penetrating injuries from shrapnel. Supporting evidence from [28] notes that conventional blunt, penetrating, and thermal trauma are the most common forms of injury following high-explosive detonations. Soft tissue, orthopedic, and head injuries dominate, and severe head injury is a leading cause of death in explosion victims.

In a study published in 2010, Peleg et al. demonstrated the abovementioned differences between civilian and military casualties when comparing injury data of both cohorts in the context of war (Second Lebanon War in 2006) and terrorism (Second Intifada during 2000–2003). According to the study, critical injuries and multiple body regions injuries were more likely in terror scenarios rather than war. Soldiers tended to present with less severe injuries from war than terror incidents. In-hospital mortality was higher in terror scenarios (7%) compared to war (2%), particularly among civilians [24].

Moreover, the mechanism of injury varied for civilians and soldiers according to conflict type. Specifically, the study reported that civilians in terror compared with war presented with less-blunt injuries (36% vs 45%, $p = 0.042$), approximately the same rate of penetrating injuries (~70%) and more burn injuries (10% vs 2%, $p = 0.002$). Civilians and soldiers also differed in injuries caused by multiple mechanisms with a prevalence of ~20% among civilians compared to only 10% among soldiers. Differences were also observed in terms of injury severity. Mild wounds (ISS: 1–8) were reported for 53% of civilians and 67% of soldiers, whereas critical wounds (ISS: 25+) reported for 17% of civilians and 6% of soldiers. Civilians compared with soldiers were twice as likely to present with internal wounds (30% vs 15%, respectively). See also Table 4.3 [24]. Broadly, terror victims were more severely wounded than war casualties.

Other Civilian Considerations of Explosion Events

In the overall context of explosion events, it is imperative to discuss also nonintentional events involving explosives, such as domestic or industrial accidents. These incidents may involve a larger volume of casualties. A domestic explosion scenario may result from gas, gasoline, or boiler explosions and fuel-air mixture explosions, such as sawdust, grain dust, or even pain [29–31]. Electric hardware and fireworks accidents are also common [2]. Industrial explosions mainly result from overpressured gases and liquids, misuse of industrial explosives and faulty machinery. Accidents at ammunition storage facilities and fertilizer plants may be especially destructive, causing vast devastation and significant mortality and morbidity, sometimes measured in the hundreds [29, 30].

In these scenarios, casualties suffering from severe blast trauma would likely be declared as fatalities on-scene, while patients presenting for treatment would suffer mostly from a combination of blunt and penetrating trauma, with burns and

Table 4.3 Body region injured and nature of injury among civilians and soldiers injured in terror and war in Israel from October 2000 through December 2006[a, e]

	Civilians				Soldiers			
	Total	Terror	War		Total	Terror	War	
	$N = 1784$	$N = 1658$	$N = 126$	P^b	$N = 802$	$N = 456$	$N = 346$	P^b
No. body regions injured[c]				<0.001				0.715
1	41.9	40.6	57.9		67.5	66.7	68.5	
2–3	51.6	52.5	39.7		30.8	31.7	29.5	
4+	6.6	6.9	2.4		1.8	1.5	1.8	
Body region								
TBI	16.5	16.6	14.3	0.491	6.1	7.2	4.6	0.126
Other head and neck	43.6	44.3	33.3	0.016	31.0	28.9	33.8	0.140
Spine and back	4.8	4.9	2.4	0.193	3.0	3.5	2.3	0.325
Torso	42.7	42.8	42.1	0.878	23.9	27.9	18.8	0.003
Extremities	58.3	58.0	62.7	0.299	69.2	68.9	69.7	0.809
System-wide/unspecified	33.7	35.6	8.7	<0.001	14.2	12.5	16.5	0.110
Nature of injury[d]								
Open wound	58.3	58.9	50.0	0.050	63.8	65.8	61.3	0.187
Fracture	37.8	38.1	34.1	0.380	31.8	36.6	25.4	0.001
Internal	30.2	31.0	19.0	0.005	14.7	18.0	10.4	0.003
Vascular	8.4	8.5	6.3	0.399	5.9	7.7	3.5	0.012
Burns	10.1	10.7	2.4	0.003	5.9	4.8	7.2	0.152

[a]Civilian casualties included all nonmilitary and nonactive soldiers
[b]χ^2 tests were performed to assess distributional differences between injuries from terror and war
[c]Multiple injuries according to 5 body regions: head and neck, spine and back, torso, extremities, and system-wide/unspecified. Data are missing for civilians: terror $n = 17$ and soldiers: terror $n = 2$
[d]Classified according to Barel Injury Diagnosis Matrix [32]
[e]Reproduced with permission from Peleg et al. [24]

tympanic blast injuries also present in some patients [29, 30]. Entrapment of victims due to building collapse and continuing fires endangering both victims and the first responders are also likely. Additionally, as most industrial facilities are located in a nonurban environment, the evacuation times may be longer, with coordination challenges related to destination protocols and mode of transportation.

Industrial accidents resulting in explosions are widely documented [23, 30]. We can learn about the injury characteristics of such events from the example of the incident in the West Fertilizer Company plant in West, Texas. On April 17, 2013, a fire and subsequent explosion occurred at the factory, causing severe damage to the nearby neighborhood. A total of 252 nonfatal casualties directly related to the explosion were treated. Of those, about half had documented abrasions/contusions and lacerations/penetrating trauma. Other injuries included TBI (21%), tinnitus/hearing problems (14%), eye injuries (12%), inhalational injuries (12%), sprain/strain (11%), fractures/dislocations (8%), tympanic membrane ruptures (5%), and burns (2%). Primary blast injuries, including pneumothorax, blast lung, and blast abdomen injuries, were seen in 5% of patients [29].

Implications for Preparedness and Treatment

The most important aspect of explosion events is how they are different in terms of their geographic location and the parameters of their physical environment, their social context, and the technical characteristics of the explosive mechanism or device behind the explosion. These differences cause significant variation in the volume and profile of casualties, the speed and the complexity of the response, as well as the consequent demand for medical resources. With so many factors influencing the response effort, it is nigh impossible to develop a universal system of preparedness for explosion events, even if we narrow our scope exclusively to MCEs. Because of a multitude of potential scenarios, it is hard to produce a point-by-point response plan that will be robust enough to guide the responders in each specific scenario.

A more optimal approach would be to rely not on protocols but on several universal, yet flexible principles, which will have the potential to be applicable to every scenario. Such an approach will enable quick adaptation to most needs raised by any given situation without unnecessary encumbrance by strict protocols. These principles should concern the basics of scene management, the knowledge on potential challenges and contradictions characteristic to explosion casualties, the priorities and procedures for triage at different stages and for evacuation, the capabilities of available response teams and coordination between them, and the limitations and advantages incurred by different contexts and locations.

Conclusion

No two explosions are the same. This is especially true when dealing with terror-related explosion incidents, which often result in diverse and complex patterns of injuries. The epidemiology of explosion injuries, as learned from decades of experience with terror-related and other explosion incidents, is highly complex and requires careful attention to details if one wishes to tailor the response adequately. In this chapter, we demonstrated the effects of different factors on injury pattern as a result of explosions. We highlighted the importance of the explosive device, the location of the detonation, and the general setting of the incident over the outcomes. Lessons learned from years of experience, as well as carefully crafted research spanning over decades, provide the evidence-based conclusions needed to improve and perfect the medical response to terror-related and other explosion incident.

References

1. DePalma RG, Burris DG, Champion HR, Hodgson MJ. Blast injuries. N Engl J Med. 2005;352(13):1335–42.
2. Reade MC. Blast injury - what to expect in civilian vs military contexts. ICU Manag Pract. 2015;15(4):164–6.

3. Singh AK, Ditkofsky NG, York JD, Abujudeh HH, Avery LA, Brunner JF, et al. Blast injuries: from improvised explosive device blasts to the Boston Marathon bombing. Radiographics. 2016;36(1):295–307.
4. Beaven A, Parker P. Blast injuries: a guide for the civilian surgeon. Surgery. 2018;36(8): 394–401.
5. Champion HR, Holcomb JB, Young LA. Injuries from explosions: physics, biophysics, pathology, and required research focus. J Trauma Acute Care Surg. 2009;66(5):1468–77.
6. Aharonson-Daniel L, Klein Y, Peleg K. Israel Trauma Group. Suicide bombers form a new injury profile. Ann Surg. 2006;244(6):1018–23.
7. Rozenfeld M, Givon A, Shenhar G, Renert L, Peleg K. A new paradigm of injuries from terrorist explosions as a function of explosion setting type. Ann Surg. 2016;263(6):1228–34.
8. Kluger Y, Kashuk J, Mayo A. Terror bombing-mechanisms, consequences and implications. Scand J Surg. 2004;93(1):11–4.
9. Kelly JF, Ritenour AE, McLaughlin DF, Bagg KA, Apodaca AN, Mallak CT, et al. Injury severity and causes of death from operation Iraqi freedom and operation enduring freedom: 2003–2004 versus 2006. J Trauma. 2008;64:S21–7.
10. Kellermann AL, Peleg K. Lessons from Boston. N Engl J Med. 2013;368:1956–7.
11. Arnold JL, Halpern P, Tsai M-C, Smithline H. Mass casualty terrorist bombings: a comparison of outcomes by bombing type. Ann Emerg Med. 2004;43:263–73.
12. Kosashvili Y, Loebenberg MI, Lin G, Peleg K, Feigenberg Z, Kluger Y, et al. Medical consequences of suicide bombing mass casualty incidents: the impact of explosion setting on injury patterns. Injury. 2009;40:698–702.
13. Golan R, Soffer D, Givon A, Israel Trauma Group, Peleg K. The ins and outs of terrorist bus explosions: injury profiles of on-board explosions versus explosions occurring adjacent to a bus. Injury. 2014;45:39–43.
14. Almogy G, Rivkind AI. Terror in the 21st century: milestones and prospects--part I. Curr Probl Surg. 2007;44(8):496–554.
15. Kress M. The effect of crowd density on the expected number of causalities in a suicide attack. Nav Res Logisit. 2005;52:22–9.
16. Stamm BH. Terrorism risks in rural and frontier America. IEEE Eng Med Biol. 2002;21(5):100–11.
17. Sollid SJ, Rimstad R, Rehn M, Nakstad AR, Tomlinson A-E, Strand T, et al. Oslo government district bombing and Utøya island shooting July 22, 2011: the immediate prehospital emergency medical service response. Scand J Trauma Resusc Emerg Med. 2012;20(1):3.
18. Aylwin CJ, König TC, Brennan NW, Shirley PG, Davies G, Walsh MS, et al. Reduction in critical mortality in urban mass casualty incidents: analysis of triage, surge, and resource use after the London bombings on July 7, 2005. Lancet. 2007;368(9554):2219–25.
19. De Ceballos JPG, Turégano-Fuentes F, Perez-Diaz D, Sanz-Sanchez M, Martin-Llorente C, Guerrero-Sanz JE. 11 March 2004: the terrorist bomb explosions in Madrid, Spain--an analysis of the logistics, injuries sustained and clinical management of casualties treated at the closest hospital. Crit Care. 2005;9(1):104–11.
20. McGuire R, Hepper A, Harrison K. From Northern Ireland to Afghanistan: half a century of blast injuries. J R Army Med Corps. 2019;165(1):27–32.
21. Cannon JW, Hofmann LJ, Glasgow SC, Potter BK, Rodriguez CJ, Cancio LC, et al. Dismounted complex blast injuries: a comprehensive review of the modern combat experience. J Am Coll Surg. 2016;223(4):652–64.
22. Greer N, Sayer N, Kramer M, Koeller E, Velasquez T, Wilt TJ. Prevalence and epidemiology of combat blast injuries from the Military Cohort 2001–2014. VA ESP Project #09–009; 2016.
23. Pittman W, Han Z, Harding B, Rosas C, Jiang J, Pineda A, et al. Lessons to be learned from an analysis of ammonium nitrate disasters in the last 100 years. J Hazard Mater. 2014;280:472–7.
24. Peleg K, Jaffe DH. Israel Trauma Group. Are injuries from terror and war similar?: a comparison study of civilians and soldiers. Ann Surg. 2010;252(2):363–9.
25. Jaffe DH, Peleg P, Israel Trauma Group. Explosive injuries: a comparison of children, adolescents, and adults. Ann Surg. 2010;251:138–43.

26. Peleg K, Rivkind A, Aharonson-Daniel L, Israel Trauma Group. Does body armor protect from firearm injuries? J Am Coll Surg. 2006;202:643–8.
27. Regens JL, Schultheiss A, Mould N. Regional variation in causes of injuries among terrorism victims for mass casualty events. Front Public Health. 2015;3:198.
28. Wightman JM, Gladish SL. Explosions and blast injuries. Ann Emerg Med. 2001;37(6):664–78.
29. Metzger K, Akram H, Feldt B, Stone K, Alvey S, Henley S, et al. Epidemiologic investigation of injuries associated with the 2013 fertilizer plant explosion in West, Texas. Disaster Med Public Health Prep. 2016;10(4):583–90.
30. Laboureur DM, Han Z, Harding BZ, Pineda A, Pittman WC, Rosas C, et al. Case study and lessons learned from the ammonium nitrate explosion at the West Fertilizer facility. J Hazard Mater. 2016;308:164–72.
31. Kao H-K, Yung Loh CY, Kou H-W, Kao K-C, Hu H-C, Chang C-M, et al. Optimizing mass casualty burns intensive care organization and treatment using evidence-based outcome predictors. Burns. 2018;44(5:1077–82.
32. Weil YA, Mosheiff R, Liebergall M. Blast and penetrating fragment injuries to the extremities. J Am Acad Orthop Surg. 2006;14:S136–S139.

Civilian Hospital and Healthcare System Preparedness (Location, Preparedness, Epidemiology Review of Data)

5

Paul Biddinger and Sarita Chung

Introduction

Hospitals, emergency medical services (EMS) providers, and other organizations within the civilian healthcare system very rarely, if ever, encounter victims of blast incidents in their normal course of operations. However, when blast incidents do occur due to industrial accidents, acts of violence, or other causes, the local civilian healthcare system must be prepared to respond instantly and meet the specialized demands that are predictable with such incidents. These demands may include the need to anticipate special safety and security threats to first responders and first receivers, the need to expertly specially manage the transport and distribution of injured victims, the need to create immediate trauma and burn surge capacity among receiving hospitals, and the need to ensure that responding clinicians are adequately familiar with the unique injury patterns associated with blasts.

Because blast incidents are unpredictable and unfold so rapidly, there is generally insufficient time to develop optimal response strategies to these events in the minutes after they occur. Therefore, communities and healthcare systems must create detailed and specialized plans to respond to blast incidents prior to the event or risk exposing the injured victims and their responders to further harm and/or preventable mistakes in their medical care. Adequate civilian healthcare system planning for blast incidents requires knowledge of the unique epidemiology of these kinds of incidents and complex coordination across the community and within

P. Biddinger (✉)
Center for Disaster Medicine, Department of Emergency Medicine, Massachusetts General Hospital, Boston, MA, USA
e-mail: pbiddinger@partners.org

S. Chung
Division of Emergency Medicine, Department of Medicine, Boston Childrens Hospital, Boston, MA, USA

D. W. Callaway, J. L. Burstein (eds.), *Operational and Medical Management of Explosive and Blast Incidents*, https://doi.org/10.1007/978-3-030-40655-4_5

hospitals before blast events occur in order to save the greatest number of lives and to minimize morbidity.

Prehospital Care

Public Safety Answering Point (PSAP) Actions

When blast incidents occur, local public safety agencies (i.e., EMS, police and fire departments) are usually the first to be notified, most commonly through the local public safety answering point (PSAP). In most communities in the United States, the local PSAP is reached by calling 911, though sometimes full seven-digit or ten-digit phone numbers are required. The operator answering the initial call for assistance must try to gather as much information as possible in as short a time as possible to assist and protect first responders as they are dispatched. As with all PSAP calls, the operator will try to determine the location of the event, the number of persons affected, and the potential injuries and/or medical complaints. The operator will also try to determine if there are any known safety threats to first responders as they arrive. When a blast event is reported, the PSAP operator should also make special additional queries of the caller(s) in order to help identify if other hazards may be present in the area. These queries may include asking about the presence of violent actors still on scene, about persistent vapor clouds or unusual particulates following the explosion, or whether victims are exhibiting any of the specific symptoms that are associated with chemical hazards. These groups of symptoms, or "toxic syndromes," are sometimes called toxidromes. Common toxidromes associated with chemicals that may be involved in blasts are listed in Table 5.1. The use of scripts in blast events to guide PSAP operators' questions to gather information that will improve the safety and speed of the response has been recommended as a best practice for these rare events [1]. Fire, police, EMS, and medical experts may be helpful in jointly creating these scripts to ensure all hazards and perspectives are appropriately represented.

Initial Scene Response

When the first police, fire department, and EMS units arrive on the scene, many of their initial tasks will be similar to their usual first priorities in responding to other types of incidents. These priorities include assessing the safety of the scene, attempting to identify potential hazards to arriving responders, identifying what has happened at the scene, and estimating what additional resources may be needed to respond. In blast incidents, while these initial tasks remain a priority for the first arriving responders, they may require special modifications.

With respect to surveying the scene for safety, responders should assume that all blast events are intentional events until proven otherwise. This means that that they should assume that there may be additional hazards that further threaten both

Table 5.1 Common toxic syndromes/toxidromes observed in mass chemical exposures (https://chemm.nlm.nih.gov/toxicsyndromes.htm)

Acute Exposure to Solvents, Anesthetics, or Sedatives (SAS) Toxidrome
Central nervous system depression leading to a decreased level of consciousness (progressing to coma in some cases), depressed respirations, and in some cases ataxia (difficulty in balancing and walking)
Anticholinergic Toxidrome
Under stimulation of cholinergic receptors leading to dilated pupils (mydriasis), decreased sweating, elevated temperature, and mental status changes, including characteristic hallucinations
Anticoagulants Toxidrome
Alteration of blood coagulation that results in abnormal bleeding, indicated by excessive bruising, and bleeding from mucous membranes, the stomach, intestines, urinary bladder, and wounds, as well as other internal (e.g., intracranial, retroperitoneal) bleeding.
Cholinergic Toxidrome (Also Called Pesticide or Nerve Agent Syndrome)[a]
Over stimulation of cholinergic receptors leading to first activation, and then fatigue of target organs, leading to pinpoint pupils (miosis), seizing, wheezing, twitching, and excessive output from all secretory cells/organs ("leaking all over" – bronchial secretions, sweat, tears, saliva, vomiting, incontinence)
Convulsant Toxidrome
Central nervous system excitation (GABA antagonism and/or glutamate agonism and/or glycine antagonism) leading to generalized convulsions
Irritant/Corrosive Toxidrome
Immediate effects range from minor irritation of exposed skin, mucous membranes, pulmonary, and gastrointestinal (GI) tract to coughing, wheezing, respiratory distress, and more severe GI symptoms that may progress rapidly to systemic toxicity
Knockdown Toxidrome
Disrupted cellular oxygen delivery to tissues may be caused by simple asphyxia due to oxygen displacement by inert gases, hemoglobinopathies (e.g., carbon monoxide, methemoglobin inducers), impairing oxygen transport by the red blood cell, and/or impairment of the cell's ability to use oxygen (e.g., mitochondrial inhibitors such as cyanide). All of these situations lead to altered states of consciousness, progressing from fatigue and lightheadedness to seizures and/or coma, with cardiac signs and symptoms, including the possibility of cardiac arrest
Opioid Toxidrome
Opioid agonism leading to pinpoint pupils (miosis) and central nervous system and respiratory depression
Stress-Response/Sympathomimetic Toxidrome
Stress- or toxicant-induced catecholamine excess or central nervous system excitation leading to confusion, panic, and increased pulse, respiration, and blood pressure

Source: Report to the Toxic Chemical Syndrome Definitions and Nomenclature Workshop (PDF – 2.01 MB) (May, 2012)

[a]NOTE: *CHEMM-IST* uses "Pesticide Syndrome (also called Cholinergic or Nerve Agent Syndrome)" instead of the document's recommended "Cholinergic Toxidrome" name

victims and responders. They must always be aware of the possible presence of so-called secondary devices, which are additional explosive devices that may be placed around an incident scene and are designed to detonate later and injure or kill bystanders and first responders as they provide aid to the victims. There is persistent controversy about how best to balance the duties and opportunities of first responders to emergently aid injured victims with the responders' right to protect their own lives during the response. In general, modern response focuses on three options:

increased medical and evacuation capabilities for law enforcement, joint law enforcement and medical teams (i.e., escorted care), or creation of "warm corridors." The challenges of operating in high-threat environments are addressed in Chap. 15 on warm zone operations.

First responders must also be alert for clues to the possibility of chemical or radiation hazards that can be associated with blasts, such as vapor clouds, unusual particulate debris, or toxidromes among the first victims they encounter. In general, the presence of excess radiation can easily be ruled in or ruled out with the correct equipment used at the incident scene, while the presence of chemicals at an incident scene may be significantly harder to detect. In some communities, first responders may be trained and equipped use a variety of detection devices to assess for potential chemical or radiation hazards at the scene. In other communities, such surveillance requires the deployment of specialized hazardous materials teams, generally from the fire service. When hazardous substances are detected or suspected, trained personnel must decontaminate patients prior to transporting them to healthcare facilities (see Chap. 42 for more information). Responders must also remain extremely vigilant to note whether there has been physical or structural damage to the environment around the incident that could cause further injuries from falling debris, collapsing structures, ruptured gas lines, or other threats. In some cases, this may require special technical expertise that must be summoned to the scene.

Responders in the field should utilize the incident command system (ICS), or similar incident management structure, to organize and unify their response to blast incidents in the field. The ICS is a management system that allows differing groups of responders to operate within a common organizational structure during emergencies [2]. It is widely used among differing kinds of agencies and allows them to come together under a single command structure with unified efforts in five functional areas: command, operations, planning, logistics, and finance and administration. Use of the ICS allows EMS, police, fire, and other responders from differing departments and jurisdictions to assemble and coordinate their response to the security, medical, safety, and other concerns that arise with complex blast events. As soon as ICS leadership is established on scene, those leaders must quickly determine what additional response assets are needed to safely access, treat, and transport injured victims and immediately mobilize sufficient resources to meet those needs to the greatest extent possible.

Communication with Healthcare Facilities

As early as possible in the response, first responders must make the area's hospitals aware of blast incidents so those hospitals may begin to prepare to receive casualties. Effective hospital response to blast events requires an extremely rapid mobilization of appropriate personnel and resuscitation resources, including medical supplies and treatment rooms that can receive a large surge of complex patients. Unfortunately, it is extremely common for emergency departments (ED), operating rooms, and inpatient units to be overcrowded on a daily basis and lack sufficient "surge" capacity to respond to mass-casualty incidents [3]. The current state of hospitals operating at or near full capacity creates a significant barrier to MCI response and mandates a system-wide, whole-of-community early warning mechanism.

When communicating with hospitals about a blast event, there are details that should be shared in addition to usual estimates about the numbers of patients. The first of these details should be whether the blast occurred in a closed space or open space; closed-space blasts result in significantly different and more severe injury patterns [4].Second, first responders should communicate whether they have identified special populations who have been involved in the blast (e.g., children or the elderly), and whether they are observing special injury patterns. Hospitals' advance knowledge of these special kinds of injuries can help them mobilize additional specialty medical personnel, such as pediatric surgeons, vascular surgeons, burn specialists, and others as early in the response as possible. Third, first responders should communicate with area hospitals as soon as possible about whether they suspect the coincident presence of hazardous substances in the event. Because historical data show that a significant number of patients can arrive at hospitals transported by means other than EMS [5], it is essential that hospitals be alerted to the potential need to decontaminate patients when needed. Performing decontamination at the hospital is challenging, and most hospitals' response requires additional mobilization of area fire department or other specialized hazardous materials teams. Therefore, it is essential to minimize the delay in notifying area hospitals and thus minimize delays in care and resuscitations as contaminated victims arrive at the hospital.

Triage and Patient Care

If the number of patients is greater than the number of ambulances on scene, EMS providers must identify which patients require transport to the hospital first. At present, many different kinds of disaster triage systems are in place in the United States to guide out-of-hospital triage; however, data comparing the effectiveness of the differing available systems is suboptimal. To help to improve the quality of out-of-hospital triage, the Federal Interagency Committee on Emergency Medical Services (FICEMS) recommended in 2013 that state and local EMS providers adopt triage systems that are based on the Model Uniform Core Criteria (MUCC), which form a science and consensus-based national guideline that recommends 24 core criteria for all mass-casualty triage systems [6]. These criteria are listed in Table 5.2. Currently, the SALT (Sort-Assess-Lifesaving Interventions-Treatment) triage system, which is in common use, adheres to the MUCC. The SALT algorithm is shown in Fig. 5.1.

The leading causes of early death after blast incidents are (in decreasing order): multiple trauma, head trauma, thoracic injury, and abdominal injury [7]. Because the resources needed to save the lives of the majority of patients with these critical injuries exist only in the hospital setting, an expert consensus panel consisting of more than 50 national and international experts in the management of blast

Table 5.2 Model Uniform Core Criteria for Mass Casualty (MUCC)[a]

Triage systems and all of their components must apply to all ages and populations of patients
Triage systems must be applicable across the broad range of mass-casualty incidents in which there is a single location with multiple patients
Triage systems must be simple, easy to remember, and amenable to quick memory aids
Triage systems must be rapid to apply and practical for use in an austere environment
Triage systems are resource dependent, and the system must allow for dynamic triage decision based on changes in available resource and patient conditions
The triage system must require that the assigned triage category for each patient be visibly identifiable (i.e., flags, tarps, markers, tags)
Triage is dynamic and reflects patient condition and available resources at the time of assessment. Assessments may be repeated whenever possible and categories adjusted to reflect changes
Sorting of patients:
Simple commands must be used to prioritize victims for individual assessment
The first priority for individual assessment is to identify those who are likely to need a lifesaving intervention (unable to follow commands, no purposeful movements, obvious threat to life)
The second priority for individual assessment is to identify those who are unable to follow the command to ambulate to an assigned place but are able to follow other commands or make purposeful movement
The last priority for individual assessment is to identify those who follow commands by ambulating to an assigned place (or make purposeful movements) and have no obvious life-threatening conditions
All patients must be assessed individually regardless of their initial prioritization during global sorting. This includes the assessment of walking patients as soon as resources are available
Lifesaving interventions (LSI):
LSI are considered for each patient and provided as necessary, before assigning a triage category. Patients must be assigned a triage category according to their condition after any lifesaving interventions
LSI are performed only if the equipment is readily available, the intervention is within the provider's scope of practice, the intervention can be performed quickly (less than 1 minute), and the intervention does not require the provider to stay with the patient
LSI include the following: controlling life-threatening external hemorrhage, opening the airway using basic maneuvers (for an apneic child, consider 2 rescue breaths), +/− performing chest decompression, and providing auto-injector antidotes
Individual assessment:
Each victim must be assigned to 1 of 5 triage categories with an associated color and initial (immediate/red, delayed/yellow, minimal/green, expectant/gray, dead/black)
Assessment must not require counting or timing of vital signs and instead must use yes/no criteria. No diagnostic equipment may be used (pulse ox, BP cuff, EKG monitor, AED)
Capillary refill must not be used as a sole indicator of peripheral perfusion
Patients who are not breathing after 1 attempt to open their airway (in children 2 rescue breaths) must be classified as dead and visually identified as such
Patients are categorized as immediate if they are unable to follow commands or make purposeful movements or they do not have a peripheral pulse, or they are in obvious respiratory distress, or they have a life-threatening external hemorrhage, and they are unlikely to survive given the available resources. These patients should receive resuscitation or comfort care when sufficient resources are available
Patients are categorized as delayed if they are able to follow commands or make purposeful movements, and they have peripheral pulse, and they are not in respiratory distress, and they do not have a life-threatening external hemorrhage, and their injuries are considered minor

Table 5.2 (continued)

Patients are categorized as minimal if they are able to follow commands or make purposeful movements, and they have peripheral pulse, and they are not in respiratory distress, and they do not have a life-threatening external hemorrhage, and their injuries are considered minor Patients categorized as immediate are the first priority for treatment and/or transport followed by patients categorized as delayed and minimal. Patients categorized as expectant should be provided with treatment and/or transport as resources allow. Efficient use of transport assets may include mixing categories of patients and using alternate forms of transport

[a]Reproduced from PLOS Currents online at: https://images.app.goo.gl/bzMD9vBbvjdpV1eXA

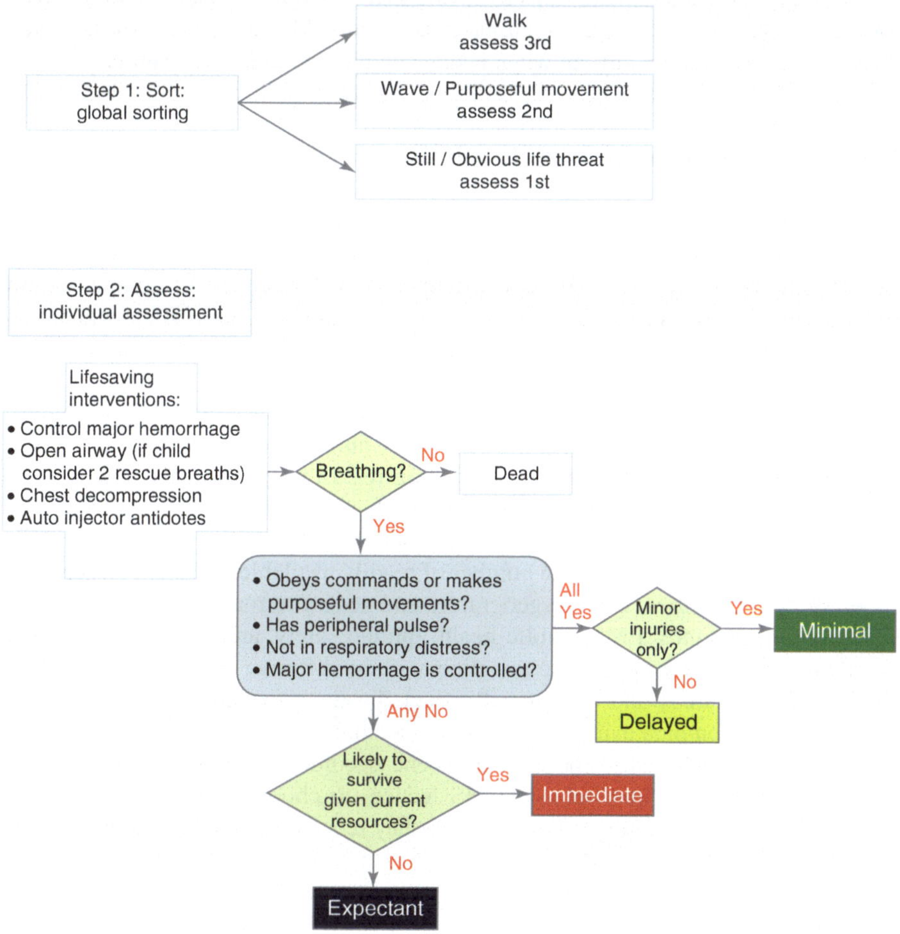

Fig. 5.1 The SALT algorithm. (https://chemm.nlm.nih.gov/salttriage.htm)

casualties recommended that on-scene medical interventions be limited to basic life-support measures for the most seriously injured casualties [8]. Therefore, transport of critically injured victims should not be delayed to provide advanced life support measures on scene. One notable intervention that is indicated in the field, and is strongly recommended by multiple professional organizations (e.g., Committee for Tactical Emergency Casualty Care, the American College of Emergency Physicians, the American College of Surgeons, the Hartford Consensus, etc.), is early hemorrhage control. For example, the Hartford Consensus recommends the broadest possible training of first responders and the public in the use of tourniquets to control life-threatening limb bleeding and the use of wound packing to control junctional bleeding prior to patient transport [9]. Community first-response agencies should take steps to ensure that they have substantial numbers of tourniquets available among responding units in the field and may be used immediately on first responders' arrival when needed and by the public if available.

Patient Distribution Among Hospitals

Historical data demonstrate that the hospitals closest to the incident scene typically receive the greatest number of victims following mass-casualty incidents, and that those hospitals can easily become overwhelmed [5, 10]. Even level 1 trauma centers can become overwhelmed with large numbers of patients, and patient outcomes may suffer when any hospital becomes overloaded [11]. Therefore, EMS must attempt to distribute patients as thoughtfully as possible among the potential first receiver hospitals, taking into account those hospitals' distance from the event and their differing clinical care capabilities [12]. A number of differing models have been proposed to help guide decision-making regarding patient distribution [13–15]. Regardless the model, critical data inputs when constructing the model include demographic details about each community, including the total number of hospitals, the number of trauma centers, the number of readily available ambulances, regional blood bank capabilities, and the geography and access to roads within the region. Therefore, community EMS, public health, public safety, and healthcare partners should all plan jointly in advance to anticipate how differing blast locations within their catchment areas and design will affect the most expeditious and effective patient distribution plan using their resources available.

If the hospital closest to the incident scene becomes severely overwhelmed, it may be advisable for hospital and EMS leaders to choose to transfer groups of patients away from that hospital even before they receive a complete medical evaluation in the emergency department or other care area. Transferring critically injured victims to another facility where they can receive immediate evaluation and resuscitation if the victims cannot otherwise receive those services at the overwhelmed hospital in time may save lives. In addition, transferring groups of minimally injured ("green-triaged") patients away from the overwhelmed hospital may lessen the overall burden of response on the facility and allow them to concentrate their limited resources on treating the critical victims already in their care. The transfer of patients away from the overwhelmed facilities in disasters is permitted under the Emergency Medical Treatment and Active Labor Act (EMTALA) so long as such transfers are anticipated as part of a community disaster plan and are undertaken as a coordinated effort among hospitals, EMS, and public health authorities [16].

Hospital Care

Response to blast events generally requires a "whole-hospital" response that extends well beyond the emergency department and operating theaters. Time is essential in mobilizing hospital resources, and many hospital mass-casualty plans do not adequately anticipate the breadth of response that may be required of them in a very short interval after a blast. Hospitals should utilize detailed, prescripted response protocols that automate the large number of actions immediately required to effectively respond to mass-casualty blast events as well as utilize the ICS to lead their institutions, and scripted planning for blast MCIs can significantly improve coordination of the institution's response [17–19].

Facility Security and Safety

Like first responders, hospitals must first assume that blast events are intentional, until proven otherwise. This means that they must be able to protect their facility and the patients, staff and visitors who are inside the facility when the event occurs. Upon hearing of a blast incident in the area, hospitals should be able to quickly secure all access to the institution and limit arriving patients and visitors to one or two entrances that can be effectively managed by hospital security and medical personnel. It may be advisable to maintain one entrance for arriving victims and one separate entrance for arriving hospital visitors and others in order to minimize crowding and delays in ensuring immediate patient access to the facility. The decision of whether to secure access to the facility should be made immediately by security, emergency medicine, and hospital leadership staff and be based on the best available information from public safety officials on scene.

Though it has fortunately been rare for hospitals to be primarily targeted in blast attacks, hospitals have increasingly been concerned about their vulnerability as secondary targets in blast incidents [20, 21]. Regrettably, most hospitals are ill-equipped to effectively barricade their campus from an oncoming vehicle-borne improvised explosive device (VBIED) or to screen arriving ambulances or patients for the presence of hidden explosives or other weapons during an MCI. Hospital security directors and other leaders should work with the law enforcement and other security experts in their community to discuss the vulnerability of their facility and to discuss how best to mitigate these risks through changes to their physical campus and response protocols.

As mentioned above, it is possible that chemical or radiation hazards may be used in an intentional blast attack or accompany an industrial blast accident. Because as many as 75% to 80% of victims may present to the closest hospitals immediately, bypassing EMS transport, hospitals are significantly vulnerable to potential contamination from arriving contaminated victims. As a matter of regulatory compliance, hospitals must plan for the arrival of potentially contaminated patients, be able to limit the extent of collateral exposure from the presentation of a contaminated patient or patients, and be able to safely provide initial triage and care for arriving victims if they are contaminated [22, 23]. Hospitals must anticipate the potential for chemical or radiation contamination with all blast incidents. However, because there are important differences in the threats of radiation and chemicals to clinicians and to the facility, hospitals must be able to distinguish between chemical hazards and radiation hazards in their response plans and act accordingly. Working with public safety and specialized hazmat team experts, they must also be able to determine when decontamination of patients is not needed following blasts, since the delays caused by patient decontamination can cause excess mortality when decontamination is not required.

Creating Resuscitation Capacity

In blast events, large volumes of patients can present within minutes to nearby hospitals, leaving them little time to prepare to receive incoming victims. Following the Boston Marathon bombing in 2013, the first patients began arriving at area hospitals in less than 10 minutes after notifications, and the entire scene was cleared of critical casualties in just 18 minutes [24]. Fifty percent or more of the total number of patients are likely to arrive in hospital emergency departments within the first hour after the blast [25]. Effective hospital response to blast events requires an extremely rapid mobilization of appropriate personnel and resuscitation resources to meet the needs of the arriving patients. Unfortunately, because of routine emergency departments and hospital crowding, this mobilization is often severely constrained. In order to rapidly create treatment room capacity within the emergency departments, hospitals should include their admitting offices, hospital nursing supervisors, hospitalists, and patient transporters in their blast response protocols and notification systems. These partners can respond immediately to the ED, take over the care of existing patients, identify available destinations for those patients outside of the ED, and transport the stretchers to those locations within minutes.

Of course, emergency physicians, advanced practice providers, nurses, surgeons, anesthesiologists, intensivists, and others are essential to resuscitate the arriving victims. Using automated technology that immediately notifies all of the necessary staff to report to the hospital with one call is strongly preferred over use of manual call trees. Call trees take time and generally only access one phone or pager at a time, whereas automated systems can call, text, page, email, and otherwise notify needed responders within seconds. The automated call systems should be configured to include all of the necessary responders for blast events, including emergency department physicians, surgeons, anesthesiologists, nurses, respiratory therapists, radiologists, radiology technicians, blood bank staff, laboratory staff, hospitalists, admitting representatives, hospital nursing supervisors, security staff, relevant hospital administrators and leaders, and others. Because blast events are extremely rare, hospitals should be there on the side of caution over-notification and over-mobilization of resources in case they are actually all needed for an overwhelming event.

Resuscitation teams in the ED should be created from the groups of mobilized responders and generally assigned to specific rooms to await patient arrivals. This helps to minimize the noise and crowding in the hallways of the ED that frequently accompany large disasters. The resuscitation teams should be created and jointly led by a senior emergency physician who can direct use of the ED resources to where they are most needed and a senior surgeon who can direct the operative decision-making among the resuscitation teams. Together, the emergency physician and surgeon must also make joint decisions regarding the relative priorities for patient access to the x-ray and Computed Tomography (CT) imaging suites, as well as the ICU (intensive care unit) beds when needed. The lead emergency physician and surgeon should also endeavor to keep the anesthesiologist in charge of the Operating Rooms (ORs) apprised of the situation, including the expected numbers of patients, the types of injuries seen, and the anticipated number of patients who will emergently need access to the OR. By communicating frequently with the OR, the ED team is more likely to have the right resources available for their patients who need emergent surgery. Similar to the ED, groups of resuscitation teams should assemble in the operating room and ICUs of the hospital; however, in general, those teams should not report to the ED unless requested in order to minimize crowding.

Triage

In general, triage of arriving patients should occur at the entrance of patients to the emergency department [26]. There is controversy about which clinicians are best utilized to perform triage of the arriving patients. Some authors have suggested utilizing junior clinicians or advanced practice providers (APPs) in order to allow more senior clinicians to perform resuscitations and surgical procedures [27], while others have argued that hospitals should utilize senior providers combined with nurses to perform triage in order to perform the most effective triage [28]. While the most critically injured (typically red-triaged) patients must be taken immediately into resuscitation rooms, it is common in mass-casualty incidents that yellow- and green-triaged patients may be required to wait before receiving care, since there is often a delay between the incident occurring and the mobilization of sufficient clinical space and staff to treat all of the arriving victims. For those patients who are not taken immediately into resuscitation rooms, it must be recognized that initial hospital triage cannot be relied upon to accurately detect all patients with life-threatening injuries, and triage must be repeated [29]. As with triage of blast victims in the field, there is a general lack of quality data about the best method to be used to ensure patients are appropriately triaged.

Patient Registration and Tracking

In many recent mass-casualty incidents, including those caused by blasts, hospitals have experienced significant problems being able to utilize their electronic health record (EHR) systems effectively [30]. Problems include being unable to register arriving patients quickly enough, having difficulty using multiple similar patient ID numbers for unidentified patients, slowing of the system, lack of sufficient devices, and others. While it is often tempting to shift hospital operations to "downtime" (i.e., paper) systems in response to blast mass-casualty incidents, doing so removes the other efficiency, communications, and safety tools that are built into these systems and creates a potential for greater miscommunication of results and data. Hospitals should assemble clinicians, registrars, and Information Systems (IS) leaders to carefully explore ways they can streamline their disaster patient registration process for arriving victims and identify specific barriers to the use of the system in an MCI so that they can be addressed and mitigated.

Patient Care

Because blast incidents are extremely uncommon, physicians will rarely use specialized training about blast injury patterns in their daily practice. Nonetheless, emergency physicians, surgeons, and others who may respond to these events must have a basic familiarity with the unique patterns of injury associated with blast events. More senior clinicians must be presented with updates to older teachings, such as about the relationship between tympanic membrane rupture and severe injury. Older physicians may have been taught that patients with intact tympanic membranes are not likely to have severe injuries, even though more recent data show that 50% of pulmonary blast injury occurs in patients with intact tympanic membranes [31]. All physicians must be aware that the severity of injuries sustained from blasts may not be as immediately apparent as they are in other kinds of traumatic injury. Traumatic brain injuries, blast lung injury, and abdominal blast injuries, in particular, may all have delayed presentation of the signs and symptoms of illness. For example, the symptoms of blast lung injury can be delayed for as long as 48 hours [25]. Periodic refresher trainings regarding blast injury management for clinicians are helpful, but just-in-time resources may also be of use, such as those produced by the National Center for United States Centers for Disease Control and Prevention National Center for Injury Prevention and Control [25].

Blast incidents also tend to create a greater need for selected medical specialists because of the patterns of injury. Numerous authors have described a tremendous demand on x-ray machines, CT scanners, and radiologists to interpret the studies following blasts [32]. Patients also typically have far greater frequency of eye and ear injuries, as well as orthopedic and vascular with blast incidents than with many other types of trauma [33]. Hospitals should have specific and detailed contingency plans to be able to mobilize sufficient numbers of these specialists if possible to support the care needed for these patients in blast events. Blasts may also create associated burn and inhalation injuries, and appropriate burn surgery and pulmonary specialists should be mobilized as soon as these patterns of injury are recognized in the event.

Blood products may be needed in large quantities in the ED, the OR and the ICU following blast events. Because of this reason, a large group from blood bank leadership and staff should also be included in the automated activation of the hospital's mass-casualty protocol and messaging system.

Mental health concerns are extremely prevalent following blast events, especially in the setting of intentional events. This is true for both patients with and without preexisting mental illness as well as for hospital staff and other responders. Hospitals must mobilize their psychiatrists, psychologists, social workers, and other appropriate clinicians to help address these concerns. For staff and patients, the mental health support needs that result from a blast incident can last for months, years, or longer.

Vulnerable Populations

Certain groups, notably older adults, pregnant women, and children, are especially vulnerable to adverse outcomes in blast events. Blasts can create large numbers of pediatric patients, depending on the location of the event, and area hospitals may not initially have sufficient numbers of pediatric-trained clinicians available to treat all of the arriving pediatric victims. In addition, children injured during terrorist events have higher injury severity score (ISS) and longer lengths of stay in the intensive care unit (ICU) and in the hospital than children injured in nonterrorist events [28]. Healthcare systems should anticipate the fact that these vulnerable patients may have even greater medical needs than other victims and preemptively mobilize additional resources to assist them when they are identified as victims.

Other Operational Concerns

Because of the potential for delayed presentations of injury following blasts, hospitals should anticipate the need to monitor many patients who appear otherwise relatively well for longer periods than in other kinds of disaster events. Patients may require prolonged monitoring of their oxygen saturations and perhaps repeated chest imaging to detect pulmonary injury. They may require repeated abdominal examinations to detect abdominal hemorrhage or perforation [34]. Hospitals should anticipate the need to open additional observation unit areas in the hospital that can be staffed by appropriate clinicians and equipped with the necessary monitors to safely observe patients at risk of occult blast injury and identify subtle symptoms and signs as early as possible for intervention.

Coordination Across the Healthcare System and Coalitions

Over the past decade, the United States Department of Health and Human Services' Assistant Secretary for Preparedness and Response (ASPR) has encouraged the development and growth of multidisciplinary coalitions for emergency preparedness and response formed with members of the EMS, hospital, public health, and emergency management communities, among others. In the recently published ASPR document, "2017-2022 Health Care Preparedness and Response Capabilities," the role of coalitions is highlighted as essential for effective community disaster response. The capabilities that are defined in the ASPR document for coalitions are: "ensuring a strong foundation for health care and medical readiness (including strong administrative and financial backing for disaster planning efforts), ensuring health care and medical response coordination by understanding that each of the key participants in the health care coalition has a role to support one another in response, promoting continuity of health care service delivery (recognizing that disruptions in service delivery constitute failure), and planning for medical surge to ensure timely and efficient care to patients even when the demand for health care services exceeds available supply" [35].

Coalitions have at least two extremely important potential roles to play in response to blast incidents. First, because the coalitions are not directly involved in the provision of care, they are able to step back and gather intelligence and other information about the event and process that information and distribute it to coalition members to optimize the region's situational awareness. In some communities, coalition staff may be able to monitor social media, which has been demonstrated to be an early indicator of the severity of events, and disseminate appropriate information [36]. Second, because coalitions are based in the public health and healthcare sectors, they are able to monitor the effectiveness of the response as it is ongoing and assist with addressing emergent resource requests, requests for coordination of actions, and identifying obstacles or gaps in the overall healthcare system response.

Conclusion

Blast incidents are extremely rare, and most civilian hospitals and clinical staff will have little experience in responding to such incidents when they do occur. Because these events unfold extremely quickly with intense needs for a rapid medical response, but also with the potential for additional harm for victims and for responders if they are not aware of potential pitfalls, it is essential that EMS, hospital, and healthcare system managers develop plans that reflect a knowledge of the epidemiology of blast threats and patterns of injury associated with those threats.

Pitfalls

- Failure to create whole of community response plan can result in overwhelmed hospitals and deficient patient care.
- Failure to create dynamic triage systems and expedited flow procedures can create bottlenecks and worsen patient morbidity and mortality.
- Failure to create multidisciplinary integrated response teams that conduct routine exercises to test system vulnerabilities, patient tracking, and care accountability can negatively impact response.

References

1. Donovan CM, Bryczkowski C, McCoy J, Tichauer M, Eisenstein R, Bucher J, et al. Organization and operations management at the explosive incident scene. Ann Emerg Med. 2017;69(1):S10–9.
2. United States Department of Homeland Security Federal Emergency Management Agency: ICS Review Materials. https://training.fema.gov/emiweb/is/icsresource/assets/reviewmaterials.pdf. Accessed 6 July 2018.
3. Committee on the Future of Emergency Care in the United States Health System, Institute of Medicine of the National Academies. Hospital-based emergency care at the breaking point. Washington, DC: National Academies Press; 2006. p. 259–85.
4. Leibovici D, Gofrit ON, Stein M, Shapira SC, Noga Y, Heruti RJ, et al. Blast injuries: bus versus open-air bombings--a comparative study of injuries in survivors of open-air versus confined-space explosions. J Trauma. 1996;41(6):1030–5.
5. Auf der Heide E. The importance of evidence-based disaster planning. Ann Emerg Med. 2006;47(1):34–49.
6. Federal Interagency Committee on Emergency Medical Services (FICEMS). National implementation of the model uniform core criteria for mass casualty incident triage. 2013. https://www.ems.gov/nemsac/dec2013/FICEMS-MUCC-Implementation-Plan.pdf. Accessed 6 July 2018.
7. Lemonick DM. Bombings and blast injuries: a primer for physicians. Am J Clin Med. 2011;8(3):134–40.
8. Lacy C, Ballagh R, Donovan CM, Bucher J. Management of explosive incidents: overview of the project and summary of best practices consensus statements of the expert panel. Ann Emerg Med. 2017;69(1):S1–3.
9. Jacobs LM and the Joint Committee to Create a National Policy to Enhance Survivability from Intentional Mass Shooting Events. Bulletin of the American College of Surgeons. 2015. http://bulletin.facs.org/2015/07/the-hartford-consensus-iii-implementation-of-bleeding-control/#.W0A-xNJKjD4. Accessed 6 July 2018.
10. Radebach M. Healthcare Response to a No-notice Incident: Lessons Learned from Las Vegas Festival Shooting. United States Department of Health and Human Services Assistant Secretary for Preparedness and Response Blog. 2018. https://www.phe.gov/ASPRBlog/Lists/Posts/Post.aspx?List=f59454e5-a08d-4a13-9abe-0d31ef99f1af&ID=308&Web=e1195e40-c916-4c28-aa5a-de2eda4302e4. Accessed 6 July 2018.
11. Hirshberg A, Scott BG, Granchi T, Wall MJ, Mattox KL, Stein M. How does casualty load affect trauma care in urban bombing incidents? A quantitative analysis. J Trauma. 2005;58(4):686–95.

12. Bloch YH, Schwartz D, Pinkert M, Blumenfeld A, Avinoam S, Hevion G, et al. Distribution of casualties in a mass-casualty incident with three local hospitals in the periphery of a densely populated area: lessons learned from the medical management of a terrorist attack. Prehosp Disaster Med. 2007;22(3):186–92.
13. Wang Y, Luangkesorn KL, Shuman L. Modeling emergency medical response to a mass casualty incident using agent based simulation. Socio Econ Plan Sci. 2012;46(4):281–90.
14. Adini B, Aharonson-Daniel L, Israeli A. Load index model: an advanced tool to support decision making during mass-casualty incidents. J Trauma Acute Care Surg. 2015;78(3):622–7.
15. Dean MD, Nair SK. Mass-casualty triage: distribution of victims to multiple hospitals using the SAVE model. Eur J Oper Res. 2014;238(1):363–73.
16. United States Department of Health and Human Services Assistant Secretary for Preparedness and Response Technical Resources, Assistance Center, and Information Exchange (ASPR TRACIE) Fact Sheet: EMTALA and Disasters. http://naemt.org/docs/default-source/ems-preparedness/aspr-tracie-fact-sheet-emtala-and-disasters.pdf. Accessed 6 July 2018.
17. El Sayed M, Chami AF, Hitti E. Developing a hospital disaster preparedness plan for mass casualty incidents: lessons learned from the downtown Beirut bombing. Disaster Med Public Health Prep. 2018;12:379–85.
18. Biddinger PD, Baggish A, Harrington L, D'Hemecourt P, Hooley J, Jones J, et al. Be prepared — the Boston marathon and mass-casualty events. N Engl J Med. 2013;368(21):1958–60.
19. Goralnick E, Gates J. We fight like we train. N Engl J Med. 2013;368(21):1960–1.
20. DeCauwer H, Somville F, Sabbe M, Mortelm LJ. Hospitals: soft target for terrorism? Prehosp Disast Med. 2017;32(1):94–100.
21. Finucane DJ. Unhealthy complacency: the vulnerability of US hospitals to direct terrorist attacks. J Healthcare Risk Manag. 2018;37(3):8–12.
22. United States Occupational Safety and Health Administration (OSHA). OSHA best practices for hospital-based first receivers of victims. 2005. https://www.osha.gov/dts/osta/bestpractices/html/hospital_firstreceivers.html. Accessed 6 July 2018 from Mass Casualty Incidents Involving the Release of Hazardous Substances.
23. The Joint Commission. Environment of Care (EC) and Life Safety (LS) chapter revisions for the life safety code update. 2016. https://www.jointcommission.org/assets/1/6/PrePub_LifeSafetyCode_Disposition_HAP_v2.pdf. Accessed 6 July 2018.
24. Biddinger PD, Baggish A, Harrington L, D'Hemecourt P, Hooley J, Jones J, Kue R, Troyanos C, Dyer KS. Be prepared — the Boston marathon and mass-casualty events. N Engl J Med. 2013;368(21):1958–60.
25. United States Centers for Disease Control and Prevention National Center for Injury Prevention and Control Division of Injury Response. Blast Injuries Fact Sheet. https://www.naemt.org/docs/default-source/education-documents/phtls/trauma-resources/articles-from-other-organizations/Blast_Injuries_Fact_Sheets_for_Professionals.pdf. Accessed 6 July 2018.
26. Halpern P, Tsai MC, Arnold JL, Stok E, Ersoy G. Mass-casualty, terrorist bombings: implications for emergency department and hospital emergency response. Prehospital Disaster Med. 2003;18:235–41.
27. DePalma RG, Burris DG, Champion HR, Hodgson MJ. Blast injuries. New Engl J Med. 2005;352(13):1335–42.
28. Gale SC, Shiroff AM, Donovan CM, Rhodes SC, Rhodes JS, Gracias VH. Medical management at the health care facility. Ann Emerg Med. 2017;69(1):S36–45.
29. Kleber C, Cwojdzinski D, Strehl M, Poloczek S, Haas NP. Results of in-hospital triage in 17 mass casualty trainings: underestimation of life-threatening injuries and need for re-triage. Am J Disaster Med. 2013;8(1):5–11.
30. Landman A, Pruitt P, Moore SE, Theriault J, Dorsica E, Harris S, Crim H, Lurie N, Goralnick E. The Boston Marathon bombings mass casualty incident: one emergency department's information systems challenges and opportunities. Ann Emerg Med. 2015;66(1):51–9.
31. Peters P. Primary blast injury: an intact tympanic membrane does not indicate the lack of a pulmonary blast injury. Mil Med. 2011;176(1):110–4.

32. Brunner J, Rocha TC, Chudgar AA, Goralnick E, Havens JM, Raja AS, Sodickson A. The Boston Marathon bombing: after-action review of the Brigham and Women's Hospital emergency radiology response. Radiology. 2014;273(1):78–87.
33. Tobert D, von Keudell A, Rodriguez EK. Lessons from the Boston Marathon bombing: an orthopaedic perspective on preparing for high-volume trauma in an urban academic center. J Orthop Trauma. 2015;29 Suppl 10:S7–10.
34. https://www.naemt.org/docs/default-source/education-documents/phtls/trauma-resources/articles-from-other-organizations/Blast_Injuries_Fact_Sheets_for_Professionals.pdf. Accessed 6 July 2018.
35. Harvey M, Hunt R, Hick J, Hanfling D. The role that health care coalitions play in support of mass casualty response. Ann Emerg Med. 2017;70(1):106–7.
36. Callcut RA, Moore S, Wakam G, Hubbard AE, Cohen MJ. Finding the signal in the noise: could social media be utilized for early hospital notification of multiple casualty events? PLoS One. 2017;12(10):e0186118.

6 Military Trauma System Response to Blast MCI

Robert W. DesPain, William J. Parker, Matthew J. Bradley, and Todd E. Rasmussen

Introduction

Blast injuries have the potential to rapidly create large numbers of casualties with multiple complex wounds. A single blast can quickly overwhelm a medical response system due to the number and severity of casualties. Terrorist attacks, such as the 2013 Boston Marathon Bombing, the 2006 Mumbai Train Bombing, and the 2004 Madrid Train Bombing, demonstrate the magnitude and lethality of blast injuries. These events and the likelihood of further intentional acts of violence underscore the need for a prepared medical response to these and other types of mass casualty incidents. The United States military experience with wartime trauma in the most recent conflicts has matured into a global trauma system designed to ensure optimal care of wounded casualties. The success of our military trauma system did not happen overnight and the lessons learned from experience with blast injury and mass casualty incidents can be applied to civilian trauma systems [1, 2].

R. W. DesPain · W. J. Parker (✉)
Department of General Surgery, Walter Reed National Military Medical Center, Bethesda, MD, USA
e-mail: William.j.parker70.mil@mail.mil

M. J. Bradley
Department of Surgery, Walter Reed National Military Medical Center, Bethesda, MD, USA

T. E. Rasmussen
Department of Surgery, Walter Reed National Military Medical Center, Bethesda, MD, USA

F. Edward Hebert School of Medicine, Uniformed Services University, Bethesda, MD, USA

D. W. Callaway, J. L. Burstein (eds.), *Operational and Medical Management of Explosive and Blast Incidents*, https://doi.org/10.1007/978-3-030-40655-4_6

Mass Casualty Incident

A mass casualty incident (MCI) overwhelms available medical capacity and capability, including personnel, supplies, equipment, and space [3]. The absolute number of casualties does not define an MCI, as patient volume surge capacity is facility dependent and even affected by the time of day. For instance, five casualties may inundate one receiving facility, but not another. Similarly, those five casualties could overrun the same facility depending on when they are received, that is, accepting patients during the peak hours of the day versus overnight, when staffing is typically lower. Fifty burn patients will overwhelm a region. Thus, an MCI depends not only on the number and type of casualties that occur but also the setting in which they are treated.

Challenges of Blast Injuries and Mass Casualty Incidents

During Operation Enduring Freedom (OEF) and Operation Iraqi Freedom (OIF), explosive injury was the most common cause of trauma leading to multiple fragment wounds at multiple anatomical sites [4]. Blasts can be categorized into five distinct mechanisms that result in injury: primary, secondary tertiary, quaternary, and quinary (Table 6.1). Of these five mechanisms only primary is unique to blast [5–7].

The degree of injury and mortality depends on the energy of the blast, if the blast occurred in an open or confined space, and the patient's proximity to the blast. Casualties closest to the source of the explosion often die immediately or very soon after. If they survive, they are often the most severely injured [7, 8]. In the open air, the intensity of the blast wave decreases rapidly as the wave propagates. The radius of effect of the blast wave is often smaller than the radius of the effect of

Table 6.1 There are five possible categories of blast injury

Type of blast injury	Description	Examples of injury
Primary	Interaction of the blast wave with the body. Gas-filled structures are most susceptible	Blast lung, tympanic membrane rupture, hollow viscous perforation
Secondary	Results from flying debris such as bomb fragments or other projectiles energized by the explosion	Penetrating or blunt injuries
Tertiary	Results from displacement of the body by the blast	Fractures, traumatic amputation, closed and open head injury
Quaternary	Miscellaneous collection of remaining injuries not caused by previous three mechanisms to include burns and exacerbation of existing comorbidities	Burns, asthma, COPD, angina
Quinary	Illnesses or injuries caused by the addition of chemical, biological, or radiological substances to the bomb	Radiation illness

The injuries are not exclusive and each one can occur in a single patient airborne fragments. Primary blast injuries that occur in open air are limited to the origin of the blast. Patients who are close enough to sustain serious primary blast injury usually have lethal secondary or tertiary injuries. The likelihood of a primary blast injury increases when the blast occurs in an enclosed area, when the patient is wearing body armor and when the explosion is large [5]. This is a result of increased pressures the blast generates as the wave is reflected. This reflected wave can be magnified eight to nine times in a closed space in comparison to open air and can cause both increased lethality and more devastating injuries [5, 9].

The medical care of blast-injured casualties should follow the same standard trauma management as applies to their specific injuries. The complexity in their care arises from the fact that a single blast patient can suffer from all five categories at once. These complex patients can quickly overwhelm even the most well-prepared health system. If not mindful of the situation, multiple simultaneously injured patients can immediately absorb all available medical capabilities and capacity of a system. Effective management of such an incident depends on triage and an already established and rehearsed system to deal with both the complexity and volume of casualties.

Security Considerations with Mass Casualty Incident

Security of not only the blast scene but also the medical treatment facility is paramount for effective response to a mass casualty incident. Terrorist attacks often occur in public areas, where access is largely open. The point of injury (POI) needs to be secured to prevent further casualties and injuries to arriving medical personnel. After one explosion, there is always the concern for follow-on coordinated blasts attacking first responders. Providers at any level becoming casualties dooms the medical response. In addition to scene security, medical treatment facilities also must be protected. A secure medical treatment facility governs the flow of patients and access to the medical treatment facility. In this way, the triage process can be tightly controlled and prevent any bystander interference. In the military environment, most patients are armed. All weapons need to be identified and secured prior to entry to a medical facility. In addition, providers care for all wounded, including injured enemy combatants. As a result, there is a genuine threat of nonwounded enemy combatants being included with casualties entering the treatment facilities without proper screening. Therefore, vigilance to the screening process is imperative, especially with the "walking wounded" to avoid further attacks within the treatment facility [3, 10].

Triage During Mass Casualty Incident

Effective triage is the first step in a medical facility's ability to manage an MCI. The underlying role of triage is to do the greatest good for the greatest number of people. This triage differs significantly from traditional emergency department triage.

Most civilian providers in the United States rarely practice true triage. Hospitals are resource rich, and for the majority of patients the maximum amount of resources can be applied. Usually when a patient arrives in the emergency department, they are triaged to determine what level of resources they will require. The goal of treatment is to provide the greatest good for that *individual* patient [9, 11]. Thus, it is a drastic shift to provide the greatest good for the greatest number of patients. The first step is to determine if there is a need for medical intervention and then determine if that intervention is possible given the current situation. During an MCI, triage should be a fluid and continual process, keeping in mind that a patient's status and the overall situation can change.

Triage categories are immediate, delayed, minimal, and expectant (Table 6.2). The minimal category is best applied to patients who, when asked, can "stand up," don't have occult life-threatening injuries, and can be treated in a delayed fashion with minimal emergency resources [10]. Injuries that are "minimal" consist of minor lacerations, small burns, and small bone fractures. Patients in the "minimal" category may be able to assist in the care of other patients. Depending on the location of the MCI, these patients may arrive first for medical treatment as they simply can walk to medical treatment and even bypass the established triage process. If not managed effectively, casualties can threaten the effective triage process by their early arrival and use of medical personnel and equipment. Patients in the minimal category reinforce the importance of controlling access to medical care as discussed in the "Security" section.

Expectant patients are not expected to survive. The expectant category would include patients who arrive without vital signs [3]. Outside of an MCI, the identification of a patient without vital signs would initiate advanced cardiac life support (ACLS) protocols and cardiopulmonary resuscitation (CPR). Due to the nature of an MCI, there is rarely an indication for CPR, especially in the early phases of response [12]. Identifying a patient as expectant and not performing CPR is extremely difficult for medical providers, but it is necessary to sustain the MCI response. Expectant patients should not be abandoned. Instead, they should be isolated away from other treatment areas and be kept comfortable. If, after all other patients have been treated and the situation allows, expectant patients can be retriaged, which could potentially lead to receiving heroic treatment.

Table 6.2 There are four categories of triage: delayed, immediate, minimal, and expectant

Category	Tag color	Criteria
Delayed		Operative intervention required, but condition allows time before intervention without loss of life, limb, or eyesight
Immediate	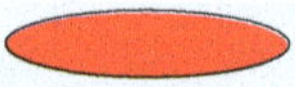	Operative intervention, with a good chance of success, required within minutes to 2 hours to prevent loss of life, limb, or eyesight
Minimal	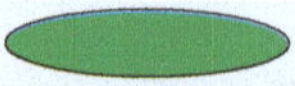	Ambulatory, minor injuries that can wait for definitive attention
Expectant	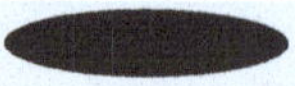	Survival is unlikely, whether due to nature of injuries or the limited nature of resources

For easy identification, a color-coded tag is often applied to each casualty during a mass casualty incident

The last, and often unmentioned, category of triage is the deceased (often labeled "black"). The deceased should be respectfully placed in a clearly identified morgue that is isolated from the ongoing emergent medical care. If possible, the morgue should even be physically separate and kept at a cool temperature [3, 10].

Considerations Related to Unexploded Ordnance(s)

A special mention should be made of the extreme circumstance of an unexploded ordnance (UXO) embedded within a patient. The ordnances are usually rockets, grenades, or mortar rounds that can be triggered in a variety of ways, including direct impact and electromagnetism. These patients should be triaged as delayed, isolated from other patients, and moved to a safe area. Unexploded ordnances have also been found in patients in the morgue, highlighting the need for careful screening of all patients [13]. Upon discovery, an explosive ordnance team should be notified and present prior to invasive interventions. The patient should be operated on last in a protected area away from the main operating room. While plain radiographs may be appropriate, potential explosive-triggering stimuli such as CT scan, ultrasound, or monopolar electrosurgery should be avoided. The removal should be accomplished in the most efficient manner possible with the fewest number of people involved. If possible, anesthesia should be regional or local. When the situation is ready for operative removal of the ordnance, the surgeon should be alone with the patient. The selection of the surgeon is a difficult process. Should it be an unmarried person without children? Should it be the oldest person? Ideally it is a volunteer, but what if there are multiple volunteers? There is no right answer, but a discussion should be had beforehand regarding selection for such a high-risk operation. With that being said, in a review of the United States military experience with unexploded ordnance, 32 out of 32 patients as well as the treatment teams survived the removal [14].

Triage Officer for Mass Casualty Incident

The decision-making surrounding triage should be done at the expert level. The triage officer not only has to have the experience of trauma situations but also be comfortable making life and death decisions. The triage officer should be the system's most experienced trauma surgeon or emergency physician. For the military, this position falls to the most veteran combat surgeon. A surgeon has the skillset to identify wounds, understand the impact, and determine the requirement for the operating room as well as the resources needed [10, 12]. While there may be the tendency to think that the triage officer should be someone who will not be needed in the operating room, such as a dentist or a primary care provider, this is incorrect. It is because of the knowledge of surgical care that a trauma surgeon is most useful as the triage officer during a blast MCI. During a trauma-related MCI, the triage officer should be a trauma surgeon or emergency physician. However, if the MCI is a result of a biological exposure, such as anthrax or smallpox, or a chemical exposure, such as Sarin nerve agent, the triage officer should be an expert in those fields, such as an infectious disease physician or an emergency physician.

The importance of the triage officer is magnified by the results of inappropriate triage. There are two categories of inappropriate triage: undertriage and overtriage. Undertriage occurs when a casualty has injuries that should place him/her in the immediate category, but instead is identified as delayed. This obviously can lead to treatment delay and the resulting morbidity and possible mortality. Overtriage occurs when patients with non-life-threatening injuries are identified as immediate and evacuated to a medical facility or receive operative care at the current location. Under normal circumstances, overtriage can be considered a budgetary or administrative issue, and medical facilities would rather overtriage than undertriage. It does not cause any patient harm. However, during an MCI, overtriage can increase the mortality of the MCI as resources are inappropriately allocated and potentially salvageable lives are lost [15].

The triage officer must also be aware of both internal and external factors that influence the response to the MCI. This often requires coordination with the medical facility's logistics, bed manager, operating room director, and, in the military, the command structure and nonmedical line officers. Although the triage officer has limited control of these factors, effective triage will depend on his knowledge and awareness of them.

External factors in a theater of combat include the tactical mission, weather, operational and medical facility security, and the specifics of the event that is causing the MCI. The ultimate role of military medicine is to support the warfighter to complete the mission [16]. This may mean medical attention is first directed to those who can return to the fight as soon as possible. The fight may be far forward or it may be defending against an attack on the base where the medical treatment facility is located. Ultimately, the medical treatment facility needs to be secure and safe to allow for effective triage and medical care. In addition, the current operation or security may limit the ability for resupply or evacuation. The weather may also prevent the use of rotary wing or fixed wing aircraft for which resupply and evacuation depend. If patients are unable to be moved to the next level of care, resources can diminish quickly and prevent the capability of caring for new patients.

The triage officer must also be aware of internal factors, including medical supplies, operating room space, bed space, available personnel, and provider stress. Knowledge of the cause of the MCI can help anticipate the level of strain that will be put on the system. The answers to questions such as: (i) Was it a blast or small arms fire? (ii) Did the blast originate from military grade explosives or was it homemade? (iii) Did the blast occur in a building or in the open air? (iv) Did it occur in an isolated area or was it a populous area? help to predict the number of injured, the severity of injuries, and the classification of injuries.

Anticipation of Resource Needs for Mass Casualty Incident

Medical resources during an MCI include surgical instruments and the ability to sterilize, ventilators, medications, dressings, sutures, and blood and blood storage capabilities. Blood products may be quickly utilized in an MCI, and access to further blood products may be limited. Based on the most recent conflicts in Afghanistan and Iraq, roughly 20% of combat casualties will require blood transfusions and roughly 7% of casualties will require massive transfusions, defined as greater than ten units of packed red blood cells transfused in 24 hours [17]. Furthermore, blast injury patients are more likely to require massive transfusions compared to casualties from small arms fire. In a review of mass casualty incidents between December 2003 and December 2004 treated at a military treatment facility during Operation Iraqi Freedom, 4% of patients injured in firefights required a massive transfusion protocol, compared with 9% injured during a blast [17]. Transfusion requirements are greatest in the first 24 hours of an MCI, but the requirements remain elevated for the days following an MCI [2]. Adequate response to an MCI carries the understanding the blood bank will be stressed not only during the immediate response but also in the days after.

The military has a unique ability to surge the availability of blood products with a walking blood bank, which can be used for the emergency collection and transfusion of fresh whole blood. Fresh whole blood can be used when the current blood supply is depleted or when other blood products cannot be delivered at an acceptable rate to maintain resuscitation. The risks of whole blood are numerous even in a controlled population like the military. The risks include HIV, hepatitis C, syphilis, and endemic diseases such as malaria or dengue [3]. These risks can be mitigated and fresh whole blood is lifesaving in the appropriate setting [18]. The process by which the walking blood bank is activated and utilized should be developed, planned, and rehearsed long before it is needed. It is a complicated process that requires coordination of multiple parts and people. In the best of circumstances, it takes approximately 45 minutes from request to transfusion [3]. Early knowledge of the mechanism of injury, such as blast, allows for early activation of the walking blood bank, which can decrease the time to transfusion [19].

Within this military experience, there are examples of resource utilization that may not be possible during all MCIs. In one instance, following a vehicle-born explosion that caused 24 casualties, two patients required massive transfusion and laparotomy. One patient received 27 PRBC, 4 FFP, and 2 units of fresh whole blood. The other patient received 41 PRBC, 14 FFP, and 5 units fresh whole blood. These two patients accounted for 89% of all blood products transfused during this MCI. Both patients ultimately died from their injuries in the operating room [2]. This level of resource utilization was possible during this particular MCI, but it may not be possible in all MCIs. It may be difficult to justify this amount of resources during an MCI depending on the facility's capability, capacity, and resources. MCI response teams need to be mindful of other resources besides blood products, such as operating room utilization. An incident like this may be an example in other situations where a surgeon needs to retriage a patient on the operating room table.

In addition to blood products, two other resources often create a choke point in the care and flow of patients: the operating room and mechanical ventilation support. In one review of the clinical resource utilization during the 72 hours following three separate blast-related MCI in 2008 in Iraq, 50 patients were treated, with 76% requiring an immediate operation upon presentation. In total, 75 operations, consisting of 191 procedures, were performed. Nearly 50% of patients required ICU-level care, and 50% required mechanical ventilation outside of the operating room [2]. This example underscores the resources needed in the immediate and short-term period to sustain patients. Even if the initial response is adequate, something as seemingly minor as a ventilator will likely be required to continue to care for patients and needs to be planned for.

Roles of Care During Mass Casualty Incident

The current military trauma system is built upon the distribution of manpower and resources to levels of care or roles. There are four roles through which patients are cared for following injury (Table 6.3). Each role has the capabilities of the role before it and then adds to that role. There are slight differences amongst the branches of services (i.e., Army vs Navy) regarding the specific makeup and organization, but the overall fundamentals are the same.

Role I care occurs at the point of injury. This care includes self-aid, buddy-aid, or a combat lifesaver, including Army medics, Navy corpsman, and Air Force pararescuemen. Overall, care involves triage, immediate life-saving interventions, and evacuation. There are no surgical capabilities and, for the majority, no blood products. Patients cannot be held for any extended period. The outcome of care is either evacuation to a higher level of care or return to duty [3]. The care delivered at Role I is driven by the Tactical Combat Casualty Care (TCCC) guidelines. The development of TCCC began in the 1990s with the Naval Special Warfare Command and

Table 6.3 The United States Military distributes medical resources and capabilities to four separate levels or roles of care

Role	Capabilities	Example
1	Injury point of care. No blood products or surgical capabilities	Combat medic on the battlefield
2	Damage control surgery Limited blood products Limited ICU-level care	Forward surgical team
3	Sustained operative, ICU, and blood product capabilities on par with most trauma facilities	Combat Support Hospital, USNS Comfort
4	Full resources and capabilities of any civilian medical center	Walter Reed National Military Medical Center

Each role has the capabilities of the role before it and then expands on those capabilities spurred out of the necessity to care for combat casualties in the field while managing the tactical requirements of the mission [20]. TCCC has since undergone several iterations with the goal of reducing preventable deaths on the battlefield. The survivability of casualties from the current conflicts speaks to the success of TCCC. The basic guidelines of TCCC are as follows: (1) take cover and return fire; (2) direct casualty to cover and apply self-aid; (3) prevent casualty from sustaining further wounds; and (4) stop life-threatening hemorrhage; if extremity, apply tourniquet. All combatants are trained to complete these steps. The Special Operations medics undergo extensive training in order to provide additional levels of care, such as surgical airways, needle decompression, pelvic binder placement, and administration of TXA [21].

Role II care includes basic primary care, laboratory, radiographic, and damage control surgical capabilities. An example of a Role II is a Forward Surgical Team (FST), with a mission to provide lifesaving resuscitative surgery. Traditionally, the FST performs damage control surgery on patients too critically injured to evacuate over long distances without further stabilization. Team members typically include general surgeon, orthopedic surgeon, nurse anesthetist, critical care nurse, and technicians. The operating capabilities are usually two tables that can do a total of 30 operations in 72 hours. Postoperative capabilities include ICU-level care for up to 8 patients for up to 6 hours. There is a limited supply of stored blood products. Further operations at the FST must be supplemented and augmented by a Role III [3].

A well-established Role III functions similar to a trauma center in the United States. A Role III is capable of providing initial triage, resuscitation, definitive surgery, and sustained postoperative care. Typically, there are multiple operating rooms and hospital beds potentially capable of caring for a few hundred patients. There is a blood bank, advanced imaging to include CT scan, and an ICU ward. In theater, the ultimate destination of the critically wounded is a Role III. The Navy hospital ships, USNS Mercy, and USNS Comfort function as a Role III with massive care capabilities deployable throughout the world [3]. Role IV medical care includes the long-standing established facilities such as Walter Reed National Military Medical Center.

The benefit of these roles of care is the ability for triage at each role and the control of casualty flow. The most severely injured are rapidly identified and evacuated to an appropriate level of care. If the evacuation is anticipated to be too stressful, damage control surgery is performed. Patients are stabilized before each evacuation to ensure survivability.

Patient Evacuation from a Mass Casualty Incident

The military model of medical treatment throughout the continuum of care depends on a reliable evacuation process. There are three categories of evacuation precedence: Urgent/Category A, Priority/Category B, and Routine/Category C. Examples of injuries that would necessitate urgent evacuation include penetrating torso injuries, airway or respiratory difficulty, an unconscious state, the presence of shock, severe traumatic brain injury, and burns greater than 20% total body surface area. Traditionally, Urgent evacuation requires evacuation ideally within 2 hours. However, following the implementation of the "Golden Hour" rule, casualties identified as Urgent mandated evacuation to a military treatment facility with surgical capability within 60 minutes from the time evacuation mission was approved. For Priority casualties, evacuation should occur within 4 hours. Injuries meeting Priority classification include extremity hemorrhage controlled with a tourniquet, open extremity fracture, and burns between 10% and 20% total body surface area. Routine evacuations should occur within 24 hours. Injuries in this category include mild traumatic brain injury, penetrating extremity injury with bleeding controlled without tourniquet, and burns less than 10% of total body surface area [21].

The request for medical evacuation from the point of injury is a standardized protocol known as the "9-Line Medevac Request" (Table 6.4). Through ideally secure

Table 6.4 9-Line Medevac Request

Line	Item	Explanation
1	Location of pickup site	
2	Call sign and frequency of radio at the pickup site	
3	Number of patients by precedence	A – urgent casualties B – priority casualties C – routine casualties
4	Special equipment required	A – none B – hoist C – extraction equipment D – ventilator
5	Number of patients by type	L – litter casualties A – ambulatory casualties E – escorts
6	Security of pickup site	N – no enemy P – possible enemy E – enemy in area X – armed escort required
7	Pickup site marking	A – panels B – pyrotechnics C – smoke signal (with color) D – none E – other
8	Casualties by nationality and status	A – US/Coalition military B – US/Coalition civilian C – Noncoalition D – Noncoalition civilian E – Opposing forces/detainee F – Child
9	Pickup site terrain, obstacles, and contamination	Description of any obstacles to approach or presence of chemical, biological, radiological, or nuclear contamination

The 9-line Medevac Request is a standardized process by which the point-of-injury team details their casualty evacuation needs communications, the team at the point of injury communicates with their command, the need for evacuation of injured soldiers. The "9-Line Medevac Request" provides a format to relay information regarding the location of the injured, the number of casualties and their evacuation precedence, whether special equipment is required, the number of casualties in a stretcher, the security at the location, how the location is marked, the nationality of casualties, the type of terrain at the location, and any obstacles at the location. Following receipt of this information, command can request additional information in conjunction with consultation with medical providers. The goal of this request is to provide a standardized format for communication to allow rapid and effective evacuation to the necessary role of care [21, 22].

Command and Control During a Mass Casualty Incident

During a mass casualty incident, establishment of command and control is the first step in the systemic response. Part of command and control is an effective communication system [23]. The military operates under a well-established command and control system. There is a set hierarchy and communication platform that exists during every mission. Similar to the Incident Command System, every Role III facility has a command center to coordinate the medical response to casualties. Together, the tactical operations commander (TOC) and patient administrator (PAD) assist in the evacuation of casualties and the mobilization of resources at the Role III facility. The Director of Trauma at a Role III assists with the coordination of medical care.

Simulation and Rehearsal for Mass Casualty Incidents

The military's dedication to simulation is unparalleled. From flight simulators to a mockup of Osama bin Laden's compound, simulation has helped operators prepare for the real event. Mass casualty incident response is no different. Predeployment and deployment training and exercises help to prepare treatment facilities for an MCI. Training not only needs to prepare medical personnel to deal with multiple complex injuries but also to do so in a resource limited environment. This austere training is typically completely opposite to what physicians face in a nondeployed setting. In a simulation of a MCI, even an experienced forward surgical team was found to have 20% preventable deaths in the care it delivered. Poor communication, including medical documentation, and inappropriate triage leading to ineffective resource utilization were the main sources of preventable deaths [24]. Thus, even a combat-hardened forward surgical team had room for improvement identified on simulation. The implications for a civilian mass casualty incident are clear. Training and simulation can improve communication, clearly define provider roles, and impart confidence for a real mass casualty incident [25].

Conclusion

The principles of mass casualty incident management are the same whether the source of injury is a terrorist bomb, an industrial accident, or a school shooter. The terrifying nature of a blast injury arises not only from the number of potential casualties but also the nature of possible injuries. Medical resources can be overwhelmed by both. Lessons from the United States military experience with mass casualties and blast injuries can apply to the civilian medical system. The goal in a mass casualty incident is to provide the greatest good for the highest number of patients. An effective response starts with appropriate triage, a dynamic and ongoing process. Providers should have defined roles of care established, and participating providers should be well-identified and well-practiced. An effect response also includes the ability to immediately activate personnel and sequester materials and supplies while also being prepared to sustain the response. Finally, while the hope is mass casualties are rare, each event should be used to prepare for the next.

Pitfalls

- *Triage officer*. The importance of the triage officer cannot be understated. This position should be held by someone with the most trauma experience and ideally previous mass casualty events. This person should be identified well in advance. The triage officer should be comfortable not only stating that a patient needs the operating room immediately but also determining that expectant care is necessary in a patient that may have benefitted from an operation if not injured during a mass casualty incident.
- *Patient identification and record keeping*. The ability to consistently and accurately identify patients from initial injury to definitive medical care is crucial to delivering safe and effective care. Nowhere more important and basic does this come into play in the administration of blood products. There must be a system by which the medical care a patient receives is documented and follows that patient to the next level of care.
- *Simulation*. The most well-defined and well-thought-out response to a possible mass casualty incident will fail during a real incident if the response has not been well-rehearsed. A medical treatment facility should regularly engage in mass casualty simulations to include the entire system: security teams, hospital communications, medical providers at all levels, blood bank, sterile processing, pharmacy, and pastoral care.

References

1. Elster EA, Butler FK, Rasmussen TE. Implications of combat casualty care for mass casualty events. JAMA. 2013;310(5):475–6.
2. Propper BW, Rasmussen TE, Davidson SB, Vandenberg SL, Clouse WD, Burkhardt GE, et al. Surgical response to multiple casualty incidents following single explosive events. Ann Surg. 2009;250(2):311–5.
3. Cubano MA, editor. Emergency war surgery. 4th ed. Fort Sam Houston: Office of the Surgeon General, Borden Institute; 2013.
4. Belmont PJ Jr, McCriskin BJ, Sieg RN, Burks R, Schoenfeld AJ. Combat wounds in Iraq and Afghanistan from 2005 to 2009. J Trauma Acute Care Surg. 2012;73(1):3–12.
5. Horrocks CL. Blast injuries: biophysics, pathophysiology and management principles. J R Army Med Corps. 2001;147(1):28–40.
6. Champion HR, Holcomb JB, Young LA. Injuries from explosions: physics, biophysics, pathology, and required research focus. J Trauma. 2009;66(5):1468–77; discussion 77.
7. Prevention, Mitigation, and Treatment of Blast Injuries: FY14 Report to the Executive Agent. US Department of Defense Blast Injury Research Program Coordinating Office. 2014.
8. Balazs GC, Blais MB, Bluman EM, Andersen RC, Potter BK. Blurred front lines: triage and initial management of blast injuries. Curr Rev Musculoskelet Med. 2015;8(3):304–11.
9. Born CT, Briggs SM, Ciraulo DL, Frykberg ER, Hammond JS, Hirshberg A, et al. Disasters and mass casualties: II. Explosive, biologic, chemical, and nuclear agents. J Am Acad Orthop Surg. 2007;15(8):461–73.
10. Aydelotte JD, Lammie JJ, Kotora JG, Riesberg JC, Beekley AC. Combat triage and mass casualty management. In: Martin MJ, Beekley AC, Eckert MJ, editors. Front line surgery: a practical approach. New York: Springer; 2017. p. 17–37.
11. Born CT, Briggs SM, Ciraulo DL, Frykberg ER, Hammond JS, Hirshberg A, et al. Disasters and mass casualties: I. General principles of response and management. J Am Acad Orthop Surg. 2007;15(7):388–96.
12. Baker MS. Creating order from chaos: part I: triage, initial care, and tactical considerations in mass casualty and disaster response. Mil Med. 2007;172(3):232–6.
13. Howell CM, Sontgerath JS, Simonet LB. Unexploded ordnance in an expectant patient: a case report. Mil Med. 2016;181(3):e302–5.
14. Lein B, Holcomb J, Brill S, Hetz S, McCrorey T. Removal of unexploded ordnance from patients: a 50-year military experience and current recommendations. Mil Med. 1999;164(3):163–5.
15. Frykberg ER. Medical management of disasters and mass casualties from terrorist bombings: how can we cope? J Trauma. 2002;53(2):201–12.
16. Remick KN, Shackelford S, Oh JS, Seery JM, Grabo D, Chovanes J, et al. Surgeon preparedness for mass casualty events: adapting essential military surgical lessons for the home front. Am J Disaster Med. 2016;11(2):77–87.
17. Beekley AC, Martin MJ, Spinella PC, Telian SP, Holcomb JB. Predicting resource needs for multiple and mass casualty events in combat: lessons learned from combat support hospital experience in Operation Iraqi Freedom. J Trauma. 2009;66(4 Suppl):S129–37.
18. Nessen SC, Eastridge BJ, Cronk D, Craig RM, Berseus O, Ellison R, et al. Fresh whole blood use by forward surgical teams in Afghanistan is associated with improved survival compared to component therapy without platelets. Transfusion. 2013;53(Suppl 1):107S–13S.
19. Bassett AK, Auten JD, Zieber TJ, Lunceford NL. Early, prehospital activation of the walking blood bank based on mechanism of injury improves time to fresh whole blood transfusion. J Spec Oper Med. 2016;16(2):5–8.
20. Butler FK Jr. Tactical medicine training for SEAL mission commanders. Mil Med. 2001;166(7):625–31.

21. TCCC Guidelines for Medical Personnel – cotccc.com [Internet]. Tactical Combat Casualty Care. 2016 [cited 2018 Jul 23]. Available from: http://www.cotccc.com.
22. Medical Evacuation. Department of the Army. Army Techniques Publication: ATP 4-02.2. 2016.
23. Frykberg ER, Armstrong J, Weireter LJ, editors. Disaster management and emergency preparedness course. Disaster Subcommittee, Committee on Trauma, American College of Surgeons; 2010. https://www.facs.org/quality-programs/trauma/education/dmep.
24. King DR, Patel MB, Feinstein AJ, Earle SA, Topp RF, Proctor KG. Simulation training for a mass casualty incident: two-year experience at the Army Trauma Training Center. J Trauma. 2006;61(4):943–8.
25. Pereira BM, Ryan ML, Ogilvie MP, Gomez-Rodriguez JC, McAndrew P, Garcia GD, et al. Predeployment mass casualty and clinical trauma training for US Army forward surgical teams. J Craniofac Surg. 2010;21(4):982–6.

The Modern Explosive Threat: Improvised Explosive Devices

7

Brian P. Shreve

Introduction

Since the beginning of United States combat operations in October 2001 in response to the 9/11 terror attacks, improvised explosive devices (IEDs) have been the most common cause of battlefield fatalities and further account for 38–64% of US and coalition combat injuries sustained [1–4]. One may assume that the use of IEDs is currently confined to the two combat theaters where the United States is currently engaged and is not representative of a what medical providers face worldwide. However, data from 2012 indicates that excluding Iraq and Afghanistan, there were a reported 500 IED detonations per month worldwide [1]. This data does not reflect a large number of events localized to one or two countries, but, rather, over half of United Nations (UN)-recognized countries have been impacted by IEDs [5]. This increase in IED use has led to a significant burden of disease, with approximately 105,000 deaths worldwide from 2011 to 2015 [5]. Of these 105,000 casualties, over 80% of them were civilians representing not only a topic important to those conducting military and anti-terrorism operations but to local governments and worldwide organizations such as the UN [5].

Background

IEDs are weapons born from necessity. A quick glance at the conflict in Afghanistan highlights the contrast between the two sides; a large, industrial nation, with immense resources and a large conventional army versus a group of tribes without state support, with limited resources, using a guerrilla force. The IED is an attempt

B. P. Shreve (✉)
Department of Emergency Medicine, Division of Operational and Disater Medicine, Carolinas Medical Center, Charlotte, NC, USA
e-mail: brian.shreve@atriumhealth.org

D. W. Callaway, J. L. Burstein (eds.), *Operational and Medical Management of Explosive and Blast Incidents*, https://doi.org/10.1007/978-3-030-40655-4_7

by one side to level the playing field. Bomb makers can use simple components to create the detonator and containers for IEDs, adulterate the explosives with a variety of materials (e.g., nails, ball bearing, human waste), and can use a variety of easily accessible delivery mechanisms (e.g., automobiles, backpacks, carcasses).

Many may think that IEDs are a new phenomenon due to the recent proliferation of these devices and increased awareness, thanks to constant media reports. According to the Oxford dictionaries, however, the first use of the term IED was in the 1970s, and combatants have used IEDs since long before the term was coined [6]. The concept of an improvised device started to be recorded in the 1940s military manuals, which described a process by which one could modify or construct an explosive device if the situation arose where conventional explosives were unavailable or if conducting asymmetric warfare [7]. These tactics and techniques eventually spilled into the civilian sector with the publication of texts such as *The Anarchist's Cookbook*. While this may seem innocuous, the codification of how to produce homemade explosives plays a part in the proliferation of IEDs. Recently, the expanded and loosely regulated Internet has allowed criminals to develop and quickly disseminate plans for explosives and IEDs at the click of a mouse. Increased bandwidth capabilities and streaming services allow videos demonstrating how to build and test IEDs to spread with near impunity. Now more than ever, it is easier to get a hold of plans for an explosive device.

The use of IEDs has become so advanced that now an organization will implement an "IED campaign." The IED campaign will have an overarching goal that will often aid the insurgency, terror group, or criminal organization. For example, a campaign may be introduced with the goal of impacting a local election or to intimidate a local police force. Just like a political campaign, an IED campaign has a very complex support system that can be broken down into three components: *organization, resources and operations*. The *organization* must have secure communications, a public affairs apparatus typically with access to social media to spread propaganda, and a supportive populace. *Resources* will encompass a broad number of elements to include people, money, intelligence, bomb-making materials, and facilities where devices can be produced. *Operations* will be comprised of the building of the device itself, the storage of the device, the training associated with the deployment of the device, and then execution of the operation itself [8]. As one can see, the manufacture and deployment of IEDs has now become a sophisticated operation with many moving parts. Given the large number of people involved in the creation of IEDs, this provides many opportunities to disrupt and counter the effectiveness of IED campaigns.

IED Basics

The United States Department of Defense currently defines an IED as "A weapon that is fabricated or emplaced in an unconventional manner incorporating destructive, lethal, noxious, pyrotechnic, or incendiary chemicals," which incorporates a large variety of devices with varying degrees of lethality, targets, and mechanisms of detonation [9]. With such a wide definition, the number of potential devices is limitless, from the basic pipe bomb to an explosively formed penetrator (EFP) triggered by radar as the target approaches. Regardless of the complexity of a device, it will consist of five parts: a power source, a switch, an initiator, a main charge, and a container [10]. It is important to know these different parts of an IED as they can all be addressed and potentially used in countermeasures to decrease the effectiveness of the device.

IEDs are categorized by the method by which they are delivered, with the two most common being vehicle-borne IED (VBIED) and person-borne IED (PBIED). Both VBIED and PBIED are commonly carried out as suicide bombing. Each of these methods of delivering the ordnance to the target comes with its advantages and disadvantages from the standpoint of those using the devices. The VBIEDs, which came to prominence in Iraq, are able to deliver a large amount of explosives to the target. However, given the size of the delivery vehicle, it can be difficult to reach the intended target, and countermeasures such as roadblocks can be effective in hindering the effectiveness of VBIEDs. VBIEDs are usually comprised of explosives, and the vehicle itself serves as the source of shrapnel. An example of the massive amount of damage caused by VBIEDs is the Oklahoma City Bombing in 1995, which resulted in 168 deaths, numerous injuries, and damage to 300 surrounding buildings [11]. The PBIEDs' effectiveness lies in the portability of the device. Typically, PBIED can be delivered to the desired target with ease and little risk for detection. The biggest limiting factor for these devices is the personnel themselves, as the device weight cannot be too heavy to be transported. As suicide bombings have become more common, the devices have become more refined. Originally, the devices were mostly explosives and were ineffective. But over time, IEDs have become a 50/50 mix of explosives and shrapnel in an attempt to increase lethality [7]. The Moscow Metro Bombings are an example of the effectiveness of PBIEDs; 40 people were killed and over 100 were injured in multiple coordinated attacks.

An alternate way to classify IEDs is by the intended target, antipersonnel and anti-vehicle being the most common. A common example of an anti-vehicle IED widely used in Iraq is the explosively formed penetrator (EFPs) [12]. The EFP concept was invented in 1910 in Germany but has seen increased and widespread use in the war in Iraq [13]. These devices are different than many of the other devices classified as IEDs in that this weapon is a projectile more than it is an explosive. The concept behind EFPs is similar to that of shaped charges like those used in antitank rounds. An explosive is placed in a container with a "liner" which can consist of many materials but is usually steel or copper [13]. When the device is detonated, this causes the liner to deform and be propelled in the direction the device is aimed. This fast-moving, hot piece of metal is now able to penetrate armor. As one can surmise, the impact of this device will differ from more traditional IEDs, which draw their effectiveness from the amount of ordnance or shrapnel contained in the device. EFP attacks result in higher percentages of blunt and thermal trauma compared to traditional "blast" incidents.

IEDs demonstrate the largest degree of variability in the explosive used and in the triggering method. Explosives can be procured from ordnance made for military use, such as 155-mm artillery shells to homemade explosives (HME) that are made from a "recipe" pulled from the Internet or from a sympathetic organization. Triggering methods offer the same variability as the explosive content device does. Triggers can be "dumb" requiring no presence of an individual; for example, a pressure-switch-activated IED similar to a landmine. Or, the trigger may be highly sophisticated, such as a radiofrequency signal that is timed and initiated by an individual observing the target. The possibilities for IED design are endless. This basic truth makes it difficult to develop effective countermeasures. For those interested in exploring the full variability of devices, the *Improvised Explosive Device Lexicon* produced by the United Nations Mine Action service is a good resource [10]. A brief look at that document demonstrates the wide variety of potential devices and classification systems relating to IEDs.

Regardless of the explosive or trigger used, there are some general techniques that amplify the lethality of IEDs. The first technique is called *coupling* and is the linking of two devices together. The first device is unfused and the second contains the fuse. When the vehicle passes over the second device, it triggers and detonates both devices simultaneously, taking advantage of the first device, which is typically positioned to be directly under the triggering vehicle [14]. *Coupling* is especially effective when used against route-clearing vehicles. *Boosting* is another method employed in which devices are stacked upon one another, with the top explosives contained in nonmetal containers. This technique helps to avoid detection and causes a bigger blast when the device is detonated [14]. *Shaped charges* (i.e., EFPs) are the next enhancement used in an attempt to defeat the increased vehicle armor that is used as a countermeasure against IEDs. The last and possibly the most relevant to the prehospital provider is a "*daisy chain*," in which multiple devices are strung together so that when one device is triggered, all of the devices detonate. The *daisy chain* spread devices across a geographic area in a way that attempts to mimic the spacing of the vehicles in a convoy, thus causing maximum damage to multiple vehicles simultaneously in one event.

Medical Management Implications of IEDS

Blast injuries have traditionally been categorized by the mechanism by which the injury is caused: primary, secondary, tertiary, and quaternary. Primary blast injuries are the result of overpressurization or underpressurization and damage structures such as tympanic membranes, the pulmonary system, and hollow viscera, the most worrisome of these injuries being those to the pulmonary system. Typically, injuries involving the lungs will have immediate respiratory failure and require immediate intervention; in rare cases, significant pulmonary injury can be delayed but will be heralded by signs such as dyspnea and hemoptysis [15]. While pulmonary injury carries a grave diagnosis, remarkably, data from the conflict in Iraq showed that less than 4% of casualties from IEDs, despite close proximity to the blast, suffered pulmonary injury, and all of those injured were fatalities [2]. While data from the conflict in Iraq does not show a high incidence of primary blast injuries, civilian bombings commonly demonstrate this wounding pattern. One study comparing injuries from bombings occurring on buses to those in an open-air environment shows an increase in primary blast injury from those involved in bombings in confined spaces, with associated higher morbidity related to lung injury, burns, and overall increased mortality [16, 17]. This finding is an important distinction in the comparison of combat and civilian IED victims, as the civilian setting may see an increased frequency of enclosed-space PBIED attacks and higher levels of primary blast injury. For medical providers, these observations also highlight the importance of obtaining details of the event as it can help to identify potential pathology.

Of most concern to the first responder is secondary blast injury caused by fragments that are propelled by the explosion. Secondary blast injuries account for the highest burden of death and injury from blasts and, in particular, IED attacks [15]. The wounds caused by secondary blast injuries have evolved over time, mirroring the increased frequency and sophistication of IED use. Data indicates that in casualties of a blast incident, 70–87% suffer trauma to the extremities, 20–25% to the head and neck, and less than 10% sustain injuries to the torso [2, 18]. Ocular injuries are frequently associated with IEDs in civilian events. However, in one study from Iraq, few casualties experienced ocular injuries; this is likely due to the fact that ballistic eye protection is now in standard use among troops in the Iraqi theater [2]. Increased ballistic protection, Kevlar and ceramic plates that cover most of the torso, is likely to account for the distribution of injuries that is currently being seen from combat theaters as there has been an overall increased percentage of extremity injuries and a decrease in torso injuries [18]. When compared to traditional landmines, IEDs are more likely to cause traumatic amputations, have higher rates of multiple traumatic amputations, and associated significant injuries to the perineal and gluteal regions [19]. One specific injury pattern that prehospital providers should be aware of is the association of pelvic fractures with bilateral amputations, with data from one sample indicating that 100% of casualties suffering pelvic fractures had bilateral traumatic amputations [19]. Management of these highly morbid injuries comprises a major focus in the prehospital treatment of IED blasts.

The last two categories are seen even less on the battlefield: tertiary blast injuries, which are due to the effects of wind created by the explosion, and quaternary injuries, which encompasses a wide variety of injuries ranging from burns to exposure to toxic inhalants. One may assume that burns would represent a significant burden of disease in combat operations as many IEDs are detonated in close proximity to vehicles with a potential fuel source but only 15% of casualties sustained burns and none were greater than 5% body surface area [2].

One clinically important quaternary injury that cannot be overlooked is infection. IEDs have a propensity for causing severe contamination by pathogens as the device is typically buried and the blast is directed upwards at the target, forcing soil along soft tissue plains far above the site of injury [19]. Acinetobacter infection has been one of the most commonly associated infections, seen in up to 30% of casualties, and complicates treatment as it has been associated with multi-drug resistance [20]. Contaminants are not limited to organisms living in the soil. A study examining the rates of infection after a suicide bombing in a marketplace showed an increased rate of candidemia [21]. Analysis of the market afterwards showed a high prevalence of *Candida*, and it was hypothesized that the *Candida* became airborne during the blast and thus increased the exposure of victims to the pathogen.

While the Department of Defense currently has a broad definition of what constitutes an IED, these devices are primarily used in two capacities as previously discussed (i.e., anti-vehicle device or antipersonnel). With such heterogeneity in devices, the wounding patterns can be unpredictable. However, some generalizations can be made. Devices that are directed at mounted patrols are associated with death secondary to head trauma, followed by hemorrhage while those directed at personnel (e.g., dismounted patrols, open space crowds) result in more extremity and junctional injuries [1]. Casualties in confined spaces or vehicles experience different patterns and increased severity of injuries. When looking at EFPs specifically they present an interesting pattern of "all or nothing" injuries, where personnel will either suffer immediate catastrophic injuries or be relatively unharmed by the projectile [2]. In contrast, a study looking at the injury profile of those involved in suicide bombings casualties have more severe injuries with increased hypotension, decreased LOC, multiple body areas injured, resulting in more surgical interventions, time in ICU and hospital mortality when compared to nonterror explosions [22]. As a medical provider, it is important to be aware of this fact: just the mechanism of being involved in a suicide bombing is a herald of significant morbidity and mortality.

The number of casualties sustained in an explosive event can vary widely depending on the type of target. Data from the conflict in Iraq indicated an average of 2.3 casualties per event, with a range from 1 to 5 [2]. While attacks in combat zones are more frequent, individual civilian terror attacks often have higher numbers of casualties. This observation highlights the importance of employing systems that allow first responders and first receiving facilities to quickly perform triage and immediate lifesaving interventions. Not only can the sheer number of casualties overwhelm the first responder, but frequently these casualties will have sustained multiple injuries; one study reported 2.61 body areas being affected per casualty [2]. Despite the improvement of evacuation times during the recent US conflict, with some as low as 75 minutes from time of injury in Afghanistan as compared to 6 hours at the beginning of the Iraqi conflict, the data indicating increased number of casualties per event and number of body areas injured highlights one of the medic's most important job on the battlefield: education and preparation of all of those on the battlefield prior to deployment [1]. This principle has been best demonstrated by the 75th Ranger Regiment, who at the direction of then Col. Stanley McChrystal required all Rangers, not just medics, to be trained in basic lifesaving maneuvers, which include, management of extremity hemorrhage, tension pneumothorax, and airway obstruction, known as the Ranger First Responder (RFR) program [23]. Despite continual deployment of the 75th Ranger Regiment since the beginning of US combat operations, they have a preventable death incidence of 3%, as compared to 24% for the overall US combat force. This amazing result is a testament to the value of education of all nonmedical personnel. This is an idea that has caught on with many military units, and it is now standard practice for all personnel to carry their own medical kit. While the content of these kits may differ (e.g., hemostatic agent, tourniquet, chest seal, needle-for-needle thoracostomy), the principle is that the contents of that kit are to be used on that individual and they have the ability to perform these interventions on themselves. The principles of the RFR program are not constrained to military operations. Just like in combat, civilian medical personnel are limited in their access to the patient during an active event, with law enforcement arriving first in 60–80% of cases [24]. However, casualties can typically be immediately accessed by bystanders or law enforcement as best exemplified by the 2013 Boston Marathon bombing, where the interventions of "bystanders" may have saved multiple lives [25]. As with the RFR program, the key is a whole of community approach that includes hospitals, EMS and fire agencies, law enforcement and individual community members [26].

Future of IEDS

One of the hallmarks of IED use is the ability of the enemy to develop new devices and tactics that undermine the current countermeasures. Typically, the development of new IED tactics is shorter than the time needed to develop, deploy, and implement IED countermeasures. This results in a battlefield that is constantly changing [8]. Just since the beginning of the conflict in Iraq and Afghanistan, IEDs have become more sophisticated, evolving from old military hardware requiring little skill to assemble to more complex devices such as EFPs with intricate triggering mechanisms. It is hard to predict the future of IEDs as it is a continual game of cat and mouse. However, the conflict in Syria may offer a clue as to the direction of the changes. In January of 2018, there was a report about drones being used to fly explosive devices into Russian outposts [27]. Another threat that has been constant but has not yet been implemented is the coupling of IEDs with other materials such as toxic chemicals, biological toxins, or radiological material [14]. Unfortunately, as the nature of conflict evolves, the IED tactics developed and honed on the battlefields of Iraq, Afghanistan and Syria will metastasize to the civilian settings. It is vital that the medical and first responder community is prepared.

Conclusion

IEDs are not new to conflicts but are seeing increased use not only against military targets but with increasingly frequent use against civilian targets. With the advent of the Internet, there has been a proliferation in IED technology, innovation and sharing resulting in increasingly sophisticated devices despite a basic template for these devices. A plethora of devices can be categorized as IEDs depending on the target, delivery method, explosives, or triggering mechanism. This results in a wide range of potential injury patterns. Many injury patterns are similar to those from traditional explosions with higher frequencies of secondary injuries. IEDs result in higher morbidity and mortality when used in confined spaces, result in higher rates of traumatic amputations, and are associated with clinically significant pathogenic contamination. As demonstrated by the rapid sophistication of IEDs over the past 20 years, the future will hold the same with readily available technology, such as drones being employed to increase the lethality of devices. Regardless, medical providers should constantly be alert to the changes in IED use and change in injury patterns if one hopes to provide optimal care to the victims of IEDs.

Pitfalls
- Failure to understand the difference between IEDs directed at military vs civilian targets and their corresponding wounding patterns
- Neglecting to teach basic lifesaving treatments to nonmedical personnel
- Unawareness of the current IED tactics being implemented in your area of operations and how to best counteract these tactics

References

1. Singleton JA, Gibb IE, Hunt NC, Bull AM, Clasper JC. Identifying future "unexpected" survivors: a retrospective cohort study of fatal injury patterns in victims of improvised explosive devices. BMJ Open. 2013;3(8):e003130.
2. Ramasamy A, Harrisson SE, Clasper JC, Stewart MP. Injuries from roadside improvised explosive devices. J Trauma Acute Care Surg. 2008;65(4):910–4.
3. Holcomb JB, McMullin NR, Pearse L, Caruso J, Wade CE, Oetjen-Gerdes L, et al. Causes of death in US Special Operations Forces in the global war on terrorism: 2001–2004. Ann Surg. 2007;245(6):986.
4. Fox CJ, Gillespie DL, O'Donnell SD, Rasmussen TE, Goff JM, Johnson CA, et al. Contemporary management of wartime vascular trauma. J Vasc Surg. 2005;41(4):638–44.
5. IEDs – a growing threat – UNODA [Internet]. United Nations. United Nations [cited 2018 Oct 11]. Available from: https://www.un.org/disarmament/convarms/ieds-a-growing-threat/.
6. IED | Definition of IED in English by Oxford Dictionaries [Internet]. Oxford Dictionaries | English. Oxford Dictionaries [cited 2018 Sept 30]. Available from: https://en.oxforddictionaries.com/definition/ied.
7. Farazmand A. Crisis and emergency management: theory and practice. Boca Raton: CRC Press; 2014. p. 25–34.
8. Read "Countering the Threat of Improvised Explosive Devices: Basic Research Opportunities: Abbreviated Version" at NAP.edu [Internet]. National Academies Press: OpenBook [cited 2018 Sept 30]. Available from: https://www.nap.edu/read/11953/chapter/2#2.
9. DOD Dictionary of Military and Associated Terms [Internet]. Department of Defense [cited 2018 Sept 25]. Available from: http://www.jcs.mil/Portals/36/Documents/Doctrine/pubs/dictionary.pdf.
10. United Nations Mine Action Service. Improvised Explosive Device Lexicon [Internet]. United Nations [cited 2018 Oct 1]. Available from: http://www.mineaction.org/sites/default/files/publications/UNMAS%20IED%20Lexicon.pdf.
11. FBI. Oklahoma City Bombing [Internet]. FBI; 2016 [cited 2018 Oct 9]. Available from: https://www.fbi.gov/history/famous-cases/oklahoma-city-bombing.
12. Zukas JA, Walters W, Walters WP, editors. Explosive effects and applications. New York: Springer Science & Business Media; 2002.

13. Morrison JJ, Mahoney PF, Hodgetts T. Shaped charges and explosively formed penetrators: background for clinicians. J R Army Med Corps. 2007;153(3):184–7.
14. Wilson C. Improvised explosive devices in Iraq: effects and countermeasures. Washington, DC: Congressional Research Service Report for Congress, Library of Congress; 2007.
15. DePalma RG, Burris DG, Champion HR, Hodgson MJ. Blast injuries. N Engl J Med. 2005;352(13):1335–42.
16. Leibovici D, Gofrit ON, Stein M, Shapira SC, Noga Y, Heruti RJ, et al. Blast injuries: bus versus open-air bombings--a comparative study of injuries in survivors of open-air versus confined-space explosions. J Trauma Acute Care Surg. 1996;41(6):1030–5.
17. Kosashvili Y, Loebenberg MI, Lin G, Peleg K, Zvi F, Kluger Y, et al. Medical consequences of suicide bombing mass casualty incidents: the impact of explosion setting on injury patterns. Injury. 2009;40(7):698–702.
18. Ramasamy A, Hill AM, Clasper JC. Improvised explosive devices: pathophysiology, injury profiles and current medical management. J R Army Med Corps. 2009;155(4):265–72.
19. Smith S, Devine M, Taddeo J, McAlister VC. Injury profile suffered by targets of antipersonnel improvised explosive devices: prospective cohort study. BMJ Open. 2017;7(7):e014697.
20. Godfrey BW, Martin A, Chestovich PJ, Lee GH, Ingalls NK, Saldanha V. Patients with multiple traumatic amputations: an analysis of operation enduring freedom joint theatre trauma registry data. Injury. 2017;48(1):75–9.
21. Wolf DG, Polacheck I, Block C, Sprung CL, Muggia-Sullam M, Wolf YG, et al. High rate of candidemia in patients sustaining injuries in a bomb blast at a marketplace: a possible environmental source. Clin Infect Dis. 2000;31:712–6.
22. Aharonson-Daniel L, Klein Y, Peleg K. Suicide bombers form a new injury profile. Ann Surg. 2006;244(6):1018.
23. Kotwal RS, Montgomery HR, Kotwal BM, Champion HR, Butler FK, Mabry RL, et al. Eliminating preventable death on the battlefield. Arch Surg. 2011;146(12):1350–8.
24. Alonso-Serra HM, Delbridge TR, Auble TE, Mosesso VN, Davis EA. Law enforcement agencies and out-of-hospital emergency care. Ann Emerg Med. 1997;29(4):497–503.
25. Bobko JP, Kamin R. Changing the paradigm of emergency response: the need for first-care providers. J Bus Contin Emer Plan. 2015;9(1):18–24.
26. Fisher AD, Callaway DW, Robertson JN, Hardwick SA, Bobko JP, Kotwal RS. The ranger first responder program and tactical emergency casualty care implementation: a whole-community approach to reducing mortality from active violent incidents. J Spec Oper Med. 2015;15(3):46–53.
27. Reid D. A swarm of armed drones attacked a Russian military base in Syria [Internet]. CNBC. CNBC; 2018 [cited 2018 Sept 30]. Available from: https://www.cnbc.com/2018/01/11/swarm-of-armed-diy-drones-attacks-russian-military-base-in-syria.html.

Interagency Collaboration and Maturation – The UK Experience

8

Robert (Bob) Dobson and Howard R. Champion

Introducton

Emergency medical services around the world have varying degrees of cooperation with colleagues from other agencies, such as police, fire and rescue and military. In some countries the connection is very good, whereas in others it is completely broken or non-existent. One of the classic system challenges is agency rivalries. There is often a lack of trust or understanding of the different roles being played by each agency. Command and control is often compromised by arguments between agencies regarding who is in charge of the incident. The time to discuss such issues is obviously not when the incident happens or when people's lives are in the balance.

For some countries, it has taken a large incident to shake up the views of interagency working, whereas others have looked at the problem from the outside and started to develop their systems by observing best practice elsewhere. Some countries do not have a fully functioning emergency medical service and therefore have no interagency working, and other countries simply ignore the problem and hope it never happens to them.

In most modern countries, the interface between emergency medical services and the police and security staff has been developing and improving over recent years. There is a better understanding of each other's roles and responsibilities.

This chapter has had major input from a senior UK official who wishes to remain anonymous for security reasons.

R. (B.) Dobson
Emergency Services London, London, UK

H. R. Champion (✉)
Professor of Surgery, Uniformed Services University of the Health Sciences, Bethesda, MD, USA

SimQuest. And, Annapolis, MD, USA
e-mail: hchampion@simquest.com

D. W. Callaway, J. L. Burstein (eds.), *Operational and Medical Management of Explosive and Blast Incidents*, https://doi.org/10.1007/978-3-030-40655-4_8

All agencies involved agree that the preservation of life takes precedence, but understanding the current terrorist trends and capabilities has a significant effect on how this can be achieved. For example, a mobile terrorist with a gun or edged weapons, as in the incidents in Mumbai, Paris, or London, may result in the police having to "win the fight" or secure the scene before they can assist the emergency medical services. Fire and rescue services may need to establish safety of structures or buildings, such as occurred in New York on 9/11, or the absence or presence of chemicals, such as the Sarin attack in Tokyo or the underground system in London during the multiple attacks in July 2007.

A structured response system senses not only bomb attacks but also the other "major events" listed above, including "active shooter."

Lessons learned from the above incidents make it essential that the medical response and the security forces understand each other's role, rehearse their interaction, and interface so that security needs can be taken care of and patient care is not delayed. The challenge of expediting patient care in the presence of a security requirement and continued potential or actual risk can be particularly difficult.

In the United Kingdom, the police take the lead role in terrorist-related incidents, and this enables the medical and rescue services to focus on the clinical issues of saving people's lives. That said, safety is everyone's responsibility, and rescue services should not assume that everything is completely safe.

Emergency medical service personnel need to be aware of secondary threats/risks, i.e., one explosion to attract a large emergency response and then a second bomb, people carrying second bombs, multiple locations (e.g., the last London bombing), hostages, high-value targets, etc.

The role of the police and security forces is to

- Secure the scene to control ingress and egress
- Identify and secure any continuing additional threats at the scene
- Apprehend perpetrators
- Ensure safe passage of EMS personnel to patients and patient egress
- Develop forensic analysis and crime scene analyses

United Kingdom

The United Kingdom suffered 30 years of Irish Republican Army (IRA) attacks in both Northern Ireland and England. London was particularly badly hit, with nearly 500 incidents of bombs and hoax devices that were designed to complicate, confuse, and generally give the emergency services the "run around." Trends around the world today are slightly different than the IRA years in London in the 1970s and 1980s.The IRA tactic was to place hoax bombs and then warn the emergency services via newspaper agencies by giving the so-called "coded messages." On occasions, the police were given time to evacuate areas, and on some occasions, there was no warning and bombs would go off, killing innocent people. Bombs and hoax bombs were the norm for London, and it was not unusual to see ambulances, fire engines, and police cars racing in banks of vehicles from one site to another. It was an uncoordinated mess, creating a wall of sirens. Something needed to change.

Led by the Metropolitan Police, the London Emergency Service Liaison Panel (LESLP) was established in 1973 to coordinate London's response to major incidents. Extensive consultation took place between the police, fire and ambulance services, along with the voluntary agencies of St. John Ambulance and the Red Cross and also the military. The forward thinking of the Metropolitan Police Counter Terror Command (now known as SO15) established the early plans and the interagency links that have developed and improved to this day. The many different intelligence departments within the police and that of the UK Security Service (MI5) and the Secret Intelligence Service (MI6) can now be channelled via the police to the LESLP group, thus giving the other emergency services the up-to-date intelligence regarding trends and capabilities of the terrorists. The police will share only what needs to be shared and therefore protect the official secrets of the intelligence agencies.

London has many other large incidents such as fires, train/bus crashes, and floods. LESLP now includes plans to deal with all of these. Some of the main agencies operating within the LESLP are as follows:

- Metropolitan Police
- London Fire Brigade
- London Ambulance Service
- City of London Police
- British Transport Police
- London Councils
- Port of London Authority
- Maritime and Coastguard Agency

LESLP defines a major incident, the functions of the emergency services and other agencies, command and control safety zones, and media liaison. It also gives instructions for incidents that include chemical, biological, radiological, and nuclear devices (CBRN), railway, aircraft, River Thames incidents, or flooding. Due to the wide diversity within the London population, there is also a multi-faith plan that includes involving leaders from the various religions, especially in the care of casualties.

The Therapeutic Vacuum/Armed Police

In terrorist incidents, whether the mechanism is explosive, active shooter, CBRN, or other, there is always a delay from incident to first treatment. In the United Kingdom, responders have coined the term "therapeutic vacuum" to describe the time from first point of injury (POI) until first medical intervention. From the first few seconds after a casualty is injured, up to more than 2 hours in some incidents, armed police and bystanders are often the only people present in the Hot zone able to provide life-saving treatment. This observation contributed to the development of police medics who are able to work in the Hot zone and a specialized ambulance and fire services response comprised of trained and protected personnel to enter the Warm zone under the protection of armed police officers.

Armed police are critical to Hot/Warm zone operations. They can initiate early life-saving treatment, directly evacuate casualties, or facilitate rapid evacuation of casualties via armed police corridors (warm corridors) while the threat is being neutralized or isolated. The overarching principle driving actions in these high-threat scenarios is the European Convention on Human Rights (ECHR), Article 2 "Right to Life," that states that the threat to life from injuries must be addressed as soon as physically possible.

Command and Control

UK command and control is organized into Gold, Silver, and Bronze levels.

Gold	Strategic
Silver	Tactical
Bronze	Operational

The Bronze ambulance service will communicate with the Bronze fire and police levels in geographic specific areas. All services report to a Silver who has an area-wide (e.g., Central London) perspective and picture. Gold in turn reports to government level and would brief the prime minister as required. Gold is often the chief or deputy chief of fire and ambulance services.

Safety Zones

An essential element of any incident is the establishment of safety or work zones (Fig. 8.1).

Within the inner cordon of an incident there are two areas:

1. *Hot zone*. Hot zone is the most dangerous area of the incident, and only essential personnel, such as armed police or fire fighters, will go to this area. They will require the appropriate level of PPE (personal protective equipment).
2. *Warm zone*. Warm zone is less dangerous and where the medical and other support teams can function. It is the link between the Hot and Cold zones, and is a protected area in which rescues workers and support staff can work.

Within the outer cordon of an incident is the following zone:

3. *Cold zone*. Cold zone is the safe zone and is normally where the control and command vehicles are located.

Outside the outer cordon, which is protected by police, would be press and bystanders.

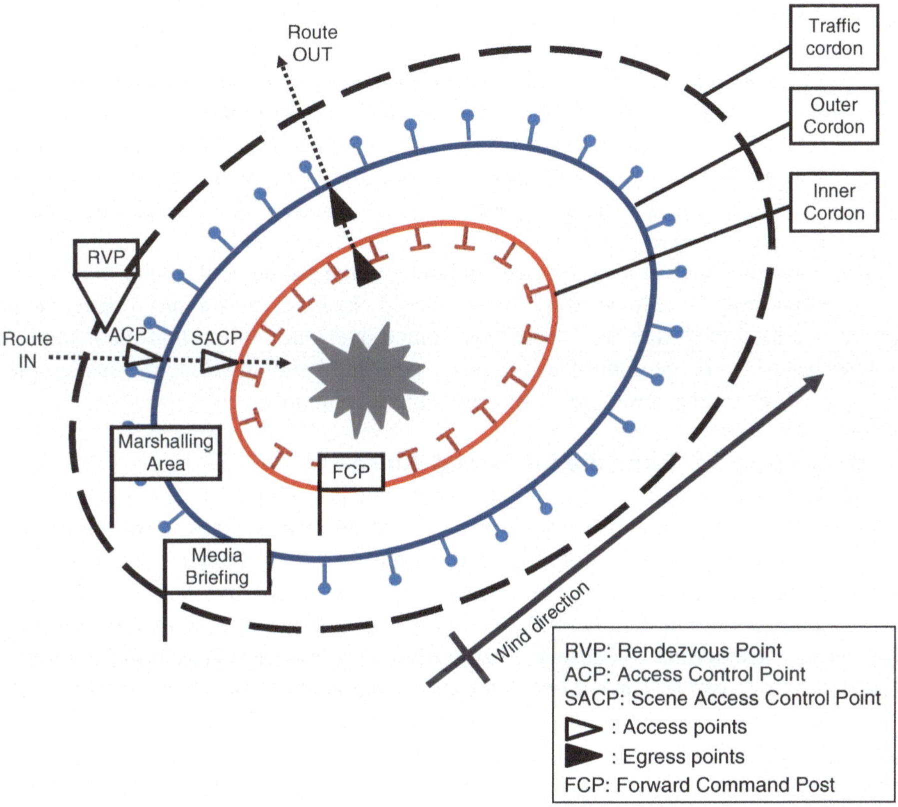

Fig. 8.1 Scene management – standard response to a declared major incident. This diagram uses the Civil Protection Common Map Symbology (Cabinet Office, 2012) (Source: https://www.london.gov.uk/sites/default/files/leslp_mi_procedure_manual_2019_version_10.1.pdf)

The Hot and Warm zone responses in the United Kingdom are coordinated at the forward command point, which focuses on bringing commanders of the three emergency services – security (police), emergency medical services, and fire – together for joint situational awareness and decision-making.

Hot Zone Response

Bystanders and armed police are the only people who will be present initially in the Hot zone of a terrorist attack, and so any immediate life-saving treatment must be carried out by one of these two groups. The UK is unusual in that not all of the police officers are armed, and so this has an impact on which officers will deploy into this area.

Bystanders

It is important to highlight that in the first few moments after injury, it will be bystanders (whether off-duty medical or other emergency service personnel or not) who have the best opportunity to save the life of those injured. Public training programs for immediate care of trauma patients are important to empower bystanders to make a difference, as there are for cardiac arrests from a medical event (typically a heart attack). Public training schemes based on the Committee for Tactical Emergency Casualty Care (CTECC) guidelines [1, 2] along with availability of trauma kits for bystander to use (e.g., in a red or green box next to the public defibrillator boxes) are an excellent way to achieve this. In the United States, a community engagement program called the "Stop the Bleed" has trained over one million non-medical personnel in haemorrhage control. All security personnel should be taught this simple set of routines such as pressure on bleeding and tourniquets.

"Care Under Fire" Principle for Armed Police

Although neutralizing the threat is important, and stopping the killing is a priority in these events to prevent further casualties, stopping the dying of those injured is equally important. Some simple maneuvers can be employed by any responder in the direct threat (or Hot zone) area that can be life-saving and can be performed while continuing to look to neutralize the threat. TECC provides guidelines for first responders with a duty to act (e.g., on-duty law enforcement personnel) for simple maneuvers that can be carried out in the direct threat area [4]. After mitigating the threat and moving to a safer position, this predominately focuses on two main interventions: placing tourniquets and positional airway management by ensuring unconscious casualties or those with airway injuries are in a prone or semiprone position. Bystanders can be directed to help.

Rapid Evacuation of Casualties to Definitive Treatment

Armed police movement of casualties out of the Hot zone is also important if the Hot zone cannot be accessed by advanced medical care. In addition, some casualties from penetrating trauma with internal bleeding can only be saved by definitive haemorrhage control by surgical interventions that requires a surgical team in an operating room and transfusion of blood products. This time is significantly delayed when casualties are not assessed or moved rapidly out of the Hot zone to hospital.

Warm Zone Response

A Warm zone or indirect threat area can be either a delineated area away from the Hot zone or a protected corridor/bubble, provided by armed police. The current UK Joint Emergency Services Interoperability Principles (JESIP) doctrine [3] that focuses on a joint command point and interagency working is a step ahead of many international responses in this respect. It has also been updated in April 2019 to include the option of deploying non-specialist multi-agency responders into the

Warm zone depending on the assessed threat. There are key lessons learned from previous events (e.g., the Manchester arena attack) where the fire response was delayed, that highlight the importance of these joint operations [4].

Armed Police

Armed police are also present in the Warm zone, and this is where a more thorough assessment of casualties can take place and further interventions carried out. Casualties must still be protected by their own PPE if present and so assessment at this point should not include removal of all clothes and PPE without the ability to rapidly be replaced.

Ambulance

The UK ambulance Warm zone response consists of ambulance intervention teams (AITs) specifically trained to work in ballistic PPE in the Warm zone under the protection of armed police. Their training is to perform basic life-saving interventions for penetrating chest injuries and catastrophic external hemorrhage. Despite having more skills than police medics, they only currently take tourniquets, blast bandages, and chest seals as interventions into the Warm zone, rather than their full range of paramedic skills. Their training focuses on triaging the casualties for evacuation to the casualty clearing station in the Cold zone. The triage is kept simple to alive or dead for teams in London, under the assumption that all Priority 3 (P3 – Green) will have walked out under direction and so the remaining casualties will be all Priority 1 (P1 – Red) urgent, Priority 2 (P2 – Yellow) emergent, or dead. Other country teams differentiate between P1 and P2 in the Warm zone.

The deployment into the Warm zone is under the command of a specifically trained ambulance officer from the joint Forward Command Point (FCP) with police and fire at the edge of the Warm zone. The ground Tactical Firearms Commander (TFC) will control the limits of exploitation of these teams. In London these teams are from both the Hazardous Area Response Teams (HART) and the Tactical Response Unit (TRU). TRU usually work as a single responder on a car and can be replaced with a patient within 10 minutes if required in order to be available for a Warm zone response. The HART response also has CBRN and remote rescue capability. TRU does not exist in the rest of the country and so AITs in other areas are all from HART or upskilled standard technicians and paramedics.

Fire Service

Specialist operations teams of fire officers include a Warm zone response in ballistic PPE to work alongside the ambulance response as part of the AIT and specifically to evacuate casualties from the Warm zone.

Cold Zone Response

Unarmed police and standard fire major incident response will be present in this area in addition to the health assets as detailed below.

Health

This is the standard healthcare response as per any major incident. In general, the health response includes a casualty clearing station (CCS) and the full spectrum of ambulance roles.

Physicians/Senior Clinicians

The Cold zone is currently the only place where advanced prehospital medical teams and any physician able to provide medical advice to commanders will be located. In London, London's Air Ambulance (LAA), otherwise known as London Helicopter Emergency Medical Services (HEMS), has a major incident predetermined response of a minimum of four doctor/paramedic teams that should be deployed to the CCS. In addition, there is a London Ambulance Service Medical Adviser who will be deployed to the Cold zone command point.

Scene Evidence

When someone has a road accident, paramedics have a tendency to pick up and bring all the patients belongings with them. In a terrorist incident, everything should stay on scene and only the patient be brought to the hospital. The possibility of bringing something into the hospital from scene is a real threat. One system to prevent this happening is in Israel, where a security check and a triage point are set up outside the hospital. This can be very challenging for the medical staff waiting at the door of the hospital who know that minutes matter. But they also have a flag system. As the doors of the ambulance open, they raise a flag indicating to the doctors waiting at the door the priority of the patient. When a red flag is raised, it is an absolute priority, and the red medical team gets ready to receive the patient. If a green flag is raised, they know from a distance that it is not life-threatening and the green team prepares. Not only does it stop the frustration of not knowing how the patient is, but it also prepares the relevant team.

Develop Forensic Analysis and Crime Scene Analyses

In the case of a bomb explosion, the police need to develop forensic evidence both at scene and also from patients and their clothing at the hospital. In London on April 30, 1999, a bomb went off in Soho and a woman closest to the blast had tiny fragments of wires embedded in her body. Forensic examination of the bomb-maker's hotel where he made the bomb revealed fragments of the same as in the victim's body, and this forensic evidence secured his conviction.

Lessons were also learned at the Clapham Rail Crash in London on December 12, 1988, when 35 people were tragically killed. Some of the victims were moved by paramedics into over 100 body bags. It was a forensic disaster because the forensic teams took years to establish which body part belonged to which victim and then not only to work out cause of death but it also delayed returning the bodies to the relatives so that funerals could take place. One of the key lessons learned and still used to this day is that the dead stay where they are unless they are preventing access or removal of live patients.

Hospital Involvement

At 3.53 pm on November 2, 1991, the Provisional IRA exploded a bomb in Musgrave Park Hospital in Belfast, killing 2 soldiers and injuring 11 people, among them were a 5-year-old girl and a baby that was 4 months old. The bomb was planted in a tunnel between the orthopaedic and children's wards. The bomb was estimated to have contained 20 lb. of Semtex. It caused severe damage to the children's ward to the cost of £250.000. Some of the children on the ward were in traction after operations.

This is one example of terrorist attacks on a hospital within the United Kingdom. Worldwide the story is much different. Approximately 100 terrorist attacks have been perpetrated at hospitals worldwide, in 43 countries on every continent, killing approximately 775 people and wounding 1217 others [5]. The need for hospital interagency work is essential. Hospitals are no longer a safe haven. There have been incidents where they have locked their emergency room doors in reaction to an incident.

Bystander Response

The American system seems to advocate Run, Hide, Fight, whereas the European countries prefer Run, Hide, Tell.

Run, Hide, Tell enables the police to gain intelligence about the incident and also allows the police to know where pockets of "friendlies" can be found. It also gives the police the chance to advise the caller. Fight is the last resort. This can be especially useful in a shopping mall or hotel. The Croatia Special Police have produced a video showing Run, Hide, Tell during a course called Medical Response to Major Incidents [6].

Special Forces Integration

Military assistance to major incidents in London is always done at the request of the civilian authorities and must be approved by the Defence Minister. Military assistance can come in the form of unarmed soldiers from regular units such as Royal Engineers assisting with the recent floods in South West England. In terrorist incidents, UK Special Forces from the Special Air Service (SAS) and Special Boat Service (SBS) can be activated. In 1980, terrorists took over the Iranian Embassy in London. The siege lasted 6 days. The terrorist had threatened to kill a hostage every 30 minutes. The SAS were activated and immediately devised a deliberate action plan in the event that the police should hand the rescue over to them. The capabilities of the SAS and equipment and technology are within the top-secret bracket. After a terrorist killed one hostage, the Metropolitan Police formally signed the rescue over to the Special Forces. All other hostages were successfully rescued.

Recent Lessons Learned

Since the Iranian Embassy siege (Operation Nimrod) in 1980, clear guidelines on what the expectations, role, and responsibility of the civilian emergency services, such as the ambulance and medical services, have been devised in the event of Special Forces being deployed. Currently in London (2019), the firearms department of the Metropolitan Police (SCO19), which includes Special Firearms Officers (SFOs), is highly trained for such incidents. SCO19 Firearms Officers attend any potentially lethal weapons on a regular basis as well as at incidents such as the London Bridge attack on June 3, 2017, where the three terrorists were shot dead by City of London and SCO19 Officers. Only when the scene was safe, were the medical services allowed to move forward to treat the patients. For all of the above incidents, clear instructions needed to be developed because all terrorist incidents in the first instance are fast-moving, and it is the job of the emergency and intelligence services to catch up and understand the potential ever-changing threat. Take, for example, the Charlie Hebdo attack on a French magazine in Paris on January 7, 2015. When the attack happened and random shootings occurred, resulting in 12 people being killed and 11 injured, the terrorist simply disappeared in a getaway car before hijacking a vehicle and making his escape, resulting in French police having to understand what had happened and then having to search for the attackers, very similar to what happened at the Boston Marathon in 2013.

Both incidents at Westminster Bridge and London Bridge started with a motor-vehicle crash. The emergency services were aware of this form of copycat attack, as previously on the evening of July 14, 2016 (Bastille Day), a 16-tonne truck drove along the Promenade Des Anglaise in Nice, France, killing 86 people and injuring 458. More recently, a similar attack happened in Finsbury Park, London, on June 19, 2019, when a hire van driven by a 51-year-old father of four children deliberately drove into Muslim worshippers outside their mosque.

Emergency services are aware that in a terrorist multimodal attack anything can happen at any time by any person or persons from *ANY* background. But there is no time for any big discussions when the incidents occur. Management structures on scene are crucial, and speaking a common language is essential. A good example of this was a recent exercise where the emergency services were confused about where the threat was. One service counted the floors of an office building starting ground (0), 1, 2, 3, 4, 5, whereas the other services counted the floors 1, 2, 3, 4, 5, and 6. So when told that the incident was now on level 6, the other services said that the building only goes up to 5 levels. This was a simple mistake that could have led to lives being lost. The lessons of 9/11 in New York in 2001 had been missed. The American's used the term "Ground Zero," and now it is a key teaching of major incidents involving buildings to establish a common understanding of the scene. Lessons learned from the Madrid train station bombing are detailed in Chap. 9.

Active Issues

Development of Police Medics

One of the newest developments is that of the Specialist Police Medics, and this has borne fruit from the interagency work. In the past, firefighters did not train on defibrillators for fear that they were encroaching on the role of the paramedics. Police officers were given basic first aid skills. As the understanding and respect of each agency has developed so have the benefits. In the United Kingdom, there were some concerns with paramedics being so close to the violence of rioters during civil disorder. Often the violence moved at the speed of the fastest runner and the paramedics would be caught up within a Hot zone with no police protection. The police civil disorder teams now have specialist medics who are trained to treat not only injured police officers but also injured civilians. They also have another unique role of understanding when *immediate* paramedic or doctor assistance is required. They are trained to make a decision of either dragging the patient back to safety or calling the paramedics/doctors forward. They understand that in trauma, time is critical if you want to save lives.

Interagency Response of Hospitals

Interagency response of hospitals is another crucial function in the response to blast incidents. Either the hospital is part of the response or in some cases the hospital has been the target. When hospitals are part of the response, they could either inadvertently become a target or be a planned second target.

High-Value Targets

Special circumstances such as high-value targets and the need for advanced medical care close to the scene also require special plans and procedures for the medical services. The UK Royalty and Diplomatic Protection Department is a unit of the Metropolitan Police and regularly train with paramedics and medical services. Selection for Royalty and Diplomatic Protection Department and SCO19 is from within the Metropolitan Police Service, and so as regular police officers, they are used to working with paramedics regularly on a daily basis on the streets of London. It is because the interagency liaison is working at every level that UK paramedics get involved with Special Operations with the police. But it is a fine line between being successful and being cancelled. The main area of concern has been the security clearance of the paramedics and medical staff. Knowing about ongoing operations or the capabilities of Police Officers is CONFIDENTIAL. Medics have proved they are very good at patient confidentiality but when it comes to the tactics police may use or seeing secret or confidential documents, they are yet to prove they can be trusted. It is one of the biggest challenges, but imagine you are part of an event involving the Queen; the information you receive is not your information to share. Things like rendezvous points or access or egress to palaces are shared with the other emergency services but are not to be given out freely to public or press.

A prime reason for the interagency working is that of the police who may wish to seek evidence and information from the casualties about what has happened. But what if the patient is a terrorist? Imagine how many agencies from police or security services will want to speak with him/her? For both the police and security service, they are dealing with the ongoing incident and have a requirement to find out as quickly as possible who else is involved or if further incidents are likely to occur. And what if one of the injured is from one of the secret agencies where his/her identity must remain secret? At every major incident, the press will not only be at the scene but will also be outside the hospital taking photographs. Any extra or unusual activity will raise suspicion to a level that something unusual might be going on.

Some of the countries doing particularly well with interagency cooperation include the following:

- United Kingdom
- Israel
- Sweden
- Norway
- Croatia
- Slovenia

Why are the above countries doing so well with their interagency cooperation? It is mainly down to the positive attitude of the three main emergency services: police, fire, and ambulance service. One other common theme that makes it easier is that the above countries are dealing with mainly one police service, one fire brigade, and one ambulance service. Most countries appear to have a one fire brigade system but most countries have multiple ambulance services, and in the case of the United States they have multiple police services.

The Future

Currently the focus is on new technologies and equipment. For example, we will know the capabilities of each responder on scene and tracking systems will enable commanders on-site to know where everyone is and relocate staff to meet their skill levels needed. It is technology that will assist in getting the right people to the right place.

It is clear that the work of the Emergency Services will always develop and hopefully improve. The goal will always be the same and that is to save life, no matter what the incident, in the safest possible way to those who have the privilege to be given such a task. The responders on scene will only have their patients for a snapshot of that patient's chain of treatment. It is vital therefore that that short interaction is to the best of everyone's ability. Their families, in addition to the ongoing medical care from Surgeons, Nurses, Physiotherapists, family Doctors and a score and a score of other health professionals as well as their families, may have to care for the patient for the rest of their lives.

Key elements:

- Interdisciplinary communication and planning
- Interdisciplinary training/rehearsal
- Annual reviews

Conclusion

Constant interdisciplinary and institutional communication, review, and rehearsal on an annual basis are essential prerequisites to an effective major event response, particularly those involving explosions. Only then can a strong command and control and understanding of roles in relationships of responders be understood and respected for the benefit of those injured. The London System coordinated by LESLP is a fine example of this and has been tested multiple times and continues to improve, providing a robust template for other systems.

References

1. Committee for Tactical Emergency Casualty Care. http://www.c-tecc.org. Accessed July 2019.
2. Committee for Tactical Emergency Casualty Care. http://www.c-tecc.org/images/4-2019_TECC_Guidelines_for FR_with_a_duty _to_act.pdf. Accessed July 2019.
3. Joint Emergency Services Interoperability Principles (JESIP). https://www.jesip.org.uk/doctrine. Accessed July 2019.
4. The Kerslake Report. https://www.kerslakearenareview.co.uk/media/1022/kerslake_arena_review_printed_final.pdf. Accessed July 2019.
5. International Institute for Counter-Terrorism. https://www.ict.org.il/Article/77/Terrorist-Attacks-against-Hospitals-Case-Studies. Accessed July 2019.
6. https://www.youtube.com/watch?v=t-4wmmC1urM. Accessed July 2019.

Case Study: The Madrid Train Bombing of March 11, 2004

9

Isaac Ashkenazi, Scott D. Deitchman, and Henry Falk

Madrid, the capital of Spain, is a highly Westernized metropolis with a well-developed and modern emergency system that has had extensive experience responding to terror attacks. Nevertheless, the March 11, 2004 (M-11), train bombings resulted in a mass casualty incident (MCI) that produced a casualty load of 2062 victims, almost immediately overwhelming the medical emergency response system [1]. Local ambulance services and hospitals were severely challenged by the multiple casualties, cadavers, inrush of both families and media representatives, etc.

In an era saturated with extremism, it is entirely reasonable to expect future terrorist attacks, including those generating catastrophic levels of casualties. The M-11 train bombing stands as an important marker to prepare for similar catastrophic events and to prevent systemic failures in the response. This case study briefly presents the main lessons learned of this event and provides recommendations for improving emergency system readiness. One of the authors (IA) participated in

I. Ashkenazi
Israel Defense Forces, Yehud, Israel

International Expert for Disaster Management & Crisis Leadership, Faculty of Health Sciences, Ben Gurion University of the Negev, Yehud, Israel

Emory University, Rollins School of Public Health, Atlanta, GA, USA

S. D. Deitchman (✉)
RADM (Ret), US Public Health Service, Duluth, GA, USA

Uniformed Services University of the Health Sciences, National Center for Disaster Medicine and Public Health, Duluth, GA, USA

H. Falk
Environmental Health, Emory University, Rollins School of Public Health, Atlanta, GA, USA

D. W. Callaway, J. L. Burstein (eds.), *Operational and Medical Management of Explosive and Blast Incidents*, https://doi.org/10.1007/978-3-030-40655-4_9

post-event assessments of the response; the case study includes his personal observations as well as those of published post-incident reviews [2–4].

Anatomy of Madrid's Emergency Medical System Prior to M-11

Madrid's medical emergency response system consisted of five main emergency medical systems (EMS) available to assist within the city: Madrid 1-1-2, Servicio de Urgencias Médicas de Madrid (SUMMA), Servicio de Asistencia Municipal de Urgencia y Rescate-Protección Civil (SAMUR-PC), Servicio de Emergencias de la Comunidad de Madrid3 (SERCAM), and Cruz Roja (Spanish Red Cross). A full description of the five EMS role and structure is presented elsewhere [4]. The after-action reviews noted above all acknowledge the competent and critical efforts and actions of the many individual responders in this catastrophic event; the case study below highlights key features of the systemic response that provide lessons learned for future events.

Acute pre-hospital care is carried out by SUMMA 112 and SAMUR-PC. Responsibilities of these two systems are clear during routine operations but less defined during MCI. The division of responsibility between the two on the grounds of whether an incident occurs at private accommodation or at a public place generates difficulties during real a crisis.

SAMUR-PC and SUMMA 112 are among the best ambulance services in the world, in terms of qualified and trained personnel, advanced technology, command and control, and response time (personal observation, IA). Incoming emergency calls are received and assessed by the call center – Madrid 112 and the operators have the responsibility to distribute the tasks among the different emergency entities (i.e., police, rescue service, or medical care).

In Madrid, there are 24 hospitals with emergency rooms and over 10,000 beds.

Description of the Attack

The M-11 attack was directed by an al-Qaeda terrorist cell in Madrid. Fourteen IEDs in sports bags had been placed in different train carriages at Alcalá de Henares station. These trains were traveling toward Atocha station in Madrid. Each bag contained about 10 kg of explosives and a large amount of metal fragments to maximize the number of victims and the severity of injuries.

Ten of the 14 IEDs exploded almost simultaneously aboard four commuter trains during the peak of the Madrid rush hour on a Thursday morning (Fig. 9.1). Four IEDs failed to explode because of technical problems. The detonations resulted in 2062 casualties, 177 (8.6%) of whom were killed immediately (deaths at the scene) and 14 subsequent deaths that occurred in hospital (in-hospital deaths), bringing the total death toll to 191 [4, 5].

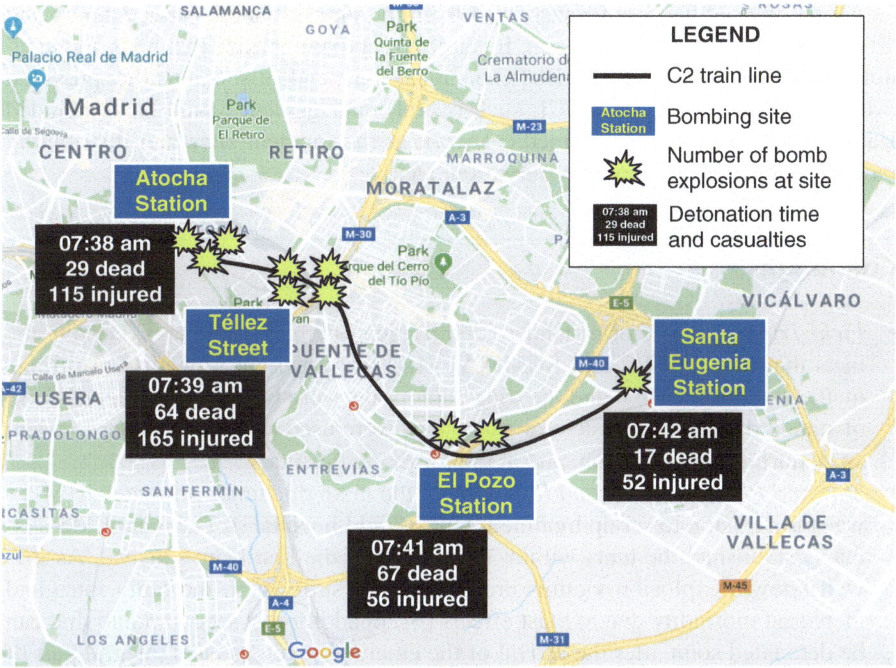
LEGEND
C2 train line
Atocha Station
Bombing site
Number of bomb explosions at site
07:38 am 29 dead 115 injured
Detonation time and casualties
Atocha Station
07:38 am
29 dead
115 injured
Téllez Street
07:39 am
64 dead
165 injured
El Pozo Station
07:41 am
67 dead
56 injured
Santa Eugenia Station
07:42 am
17 dead
52 injured
Madrid
CENTRO
RETIRO
MORATALAZ
VICÁLVARO
USERA
VILLA DE VALLECAS
Google

Fig. 9.1 Locations of bomb detonations in Madrid, Spain, on March 11, 2004. (Map data: Google, Inst. Geogr. Nacional)

Local Emergency Response

The first call reporting explosions in Atocha station was received by Madrid 1-1-2 on 11 March at 07:39 am. SUMMA 1-1-2 and SAMUR-PC were immediately activated. SUMMA 11-2 alerted the hospitals at 07:50 am, while SAMUR-PC immediately sent all available personnel and equipment to the reported sites.

Madrid's emergency services were forced to open four different response sites simultaneously: Atocha station, Tellez Street, El Pozo station, and Santa Eugenia station. The magnitude and unusual nature of the event strained all available resources. The resources mobilized to care for the wounded and their families were unprecedented, involving over 70,000 health personnel, 291 ambulances for transport, 200 firefighters, 13 groups of psychologists, 500 volunteers, thousands of donations of blood at hospitals and in 10 mobile units, and 1725 blood donors from other regions of the country. The 112 emergency communication centers that were set up to handle calls from concerned citizens received more than 20,000 phone calls during the morning of the blasts [5].

All the injured had been transported from the incident sites within 2 hours and 40 minutes after the first explosion. It is important to emphasize that both organizations SUMMA 11-2 and SAMUR-PC operated independently, and neither provided overall management of this MCI; such overall management would have included leading and coordinating the medical work at the incident sites and distributing victims to hospitals (personal observation, IA).

Challenges

- *Field Triage*: No use of a standardized triage system or triage tags. Despite the facts that SAMUR-PC and SUMMA 1-1-2 personnel are trained to use triage methods during a MCI, and the triage color tags were readily available, no form of standardized triage system or triage tags were used at the four major incident sites, during transportation, and at the receiving hospitals.
- *Stay and Play Vs. Scoop and Run*: One of the main dilemmas presented in M-11 was the decision to set up treatment tents ("field hospital"). The local EMS systems established the tents within 30 minutes of the first team's arrival. As it is well known, explosion victims are reported to suffer high mortality rates and increased morbidity due to blast effects [6]. In addition, a second bomb that can be detonated soon after the arrival of the emergency forces is an integral part of the terrorism plans. The "stay and play" approach is based on advanced and prolonged field treatment, whereas the "scoop and run" approach brings the patient almost immediately to a definitive treatment at hospitals [7]. In a situation such as Madrid, with very large numbers of available ambulances and hospitals, only with a fully coordinated response of all available resources could "scoop and run" have been a more feasible or desirable approach.
- *Patient Transportation and Distribution*: Casualties were distributed irregularly to the local medical facilities. A central distribution system was never implemented. Each triage site distributed its casualties to local hospitals according to the site commander's instructions. Nearly 35–45% of the victims were self-referred or self-transported to hospitals in the immediate vicinity of the event by bystanders using cabs and private vehicles and by police. These victims who bypassed the pre-hospital system approached those hospitals in the first minutes without notice, generating primary chaos in the emergency rooms.
- *Victims Tracking*: Soon after the attack, many hundreds of relatives rushed into receiving hospitals to look for their missing family members. The absence of a victim-tracking system worsened the chaos at these facilities. Hospitals in Madrid were not ready for such a scenario. The absence of a victim-tracking system caused deep suffering to families and a huge distraction to hospitals. (The leadership in Gregorio Marañón hospital developed an innovative way to assist families by inviting them to a large assembly hall where a list of injured patients was read out every 30–60 minutes.)
- *Surge Capacity of Hospitals*: There was no updated information on the surge capacity status of receiving hospitals during the first 24 hours. Two hospitals,

Gregorio Marañón and 12 de Octubre, received more than 50% of hospitalized patients, 312 and 255, respectively.

Soon after the first alarm, leaders at Gregorio Marañón, one of the largest hospitals in Madrid, addressed surge challenges with ad hoc decisions to postpone all scheduled ambulatory operations and prepare 22 operating rooms for emergency procedures. By discharging patients, over 400 beds were made available in 5 hours. The hospital later opened a triage area at the ambulance entrance, where patients were categorized and taken accordingly to the appropriate site.

Nevertheless, the hospitals lacked an appropriate surge capacity and capability system that would have facilitated a more reasonable distribution of patients including the large numbers of simultaneously injured persons, enhanced emergency operations, and assured appropriate allocation of needed resources to those hospitals. The Hospital Central de la Defensa Gómez Ulla (Military Central Hospital) received only 5% of the casualty load, even though it constantly maintained the largest surge capacity assets for disasters [4, 8].

- *Psychological Support*: Hospitals were not prepared and trained to provide a psychological support to victims, relatives, and personnel during an MCI. Psychiatric departments had to develop a variety of ad hoc solutions to deal with the "new" psychological challenges. To their credit, departments developed these solutions in less than 5 hours.
- *Communication*: Each EMS agency had its own radio frequency. The respective EMS agency radios were incompatible with one another, and there were no tactical channels for responders in the field [4]. Landline and mobile phone systems became overwhelmed and information sharing between all emergency entities was almost impossible.
- The hospital administrative and medical leaders received no information directly from the incident sites other than through the victims, bystanders, and ambulance personnel.
- *"Siloization"*: With the exception of the Military Central Hospital, none of the hospitals had developed interagency emergency planning to a major incident, and none conducted drills with the local emergency system [4, 8]. Emergency entities in Madrid exercised vertical crisis management within their own organizational continuums. This prevented them from collaborating with and seeking support from one another to improve their overall response efficacy. In addition, each of the organizations established its own command center. The absence of a unified command center and a designated incident commander resulted in contradictory orders from different response managers, which exacerbated the initial chaos.

Lessons Learned

- *Coordinate Three Critical Areas of Casualty Care*: The successful medical response to an MCI depends on effectively coordinating three critical areas of patient care: (1) pre-hospital care, (2) casualty distribution, and (3) hospital care.

Critical steps must be taken throughout the response flow to ensure rapid and efficient patient triage, effective and appropriate distribution of patients to available hospitals and health care facilities, and proper management of the surge of patients at receiving hospitals [9].

- *Active Bystanders*: Educating and training people on preparedness and response tactics can save lives, decrease morbidity, and increase resilience. The immediate responders have a direct impact on the preservation of health care resources and the protection of limited surge capacity assets [10, 11].
- *Patient Transport and Distribution*: Most planning scenarios adequately address pre-hospital and hospital care. Very few consider the potential problems of casualty distribution. As in any emergency, distribution involves matching the medical needs of casualties to available transportation and medical facilities. Because of the unusual nature of injuries found in bombing casualties, a coordinated plan for distributing casualties must be a key component of preparedness plans [9].
- *Hospitals Will Confront Four Mass Events*: Terrorist use of explosives often creates four distinct types of mass events in hospitals: (1) mass casualty event, (2) mass fatality event, (3) mass anxiety event, and (4) mass onlooker events (e.g., families, media, curiosity seekers, volunteers, politicians, public officials). Hospital emergency leaders should consider these events and be prepared for their simultaneous occurrence [9].
- *Hospital Decompression*: Large numbers of casualties commonly self-refer or self-transport to hospitals in the immediate vicinity of the incident. Three main approaches enable hospital facilities to prevent system collapse through decompression: outside diversion, secondary relocation, and triage hospital [9].
- *Victims Tracking*: In an MCI, hospitals are overwhelmed with a sudden influx of casualties and fatalities. Using a victim-tracking data system coordinated across all medical facilities is essential. The system should be capable of registering, documenting, and tracking victims to help make families' searches for missing relatives as efficient as possible. Through this system, citizens can call any hospital throughout the region to locate family members. The system could include digital photographs of each incoming victim and descriptions of victims and their personal belongings.
- *Public Information*: A strategy for clear, reliable, and contiguous messages should be established to inform the public continuously about the progress of the incident. Leaders have a great deal of influence over the expectations, understanding, responses, and resilience of both individuals and communities to an MCI.
- *Exercises and Drills*: Mandatory regular exercises involving all relevant agencies should be conducted, including both annual exercises and unannounced limited-scale exercises. These drills should include the use of smart casualties (people posing as casualties). Four levels of drills are recommended: focal (vertical) exercise; table-top (horizontal) exercises; functional exercises, and full-scale real-time drills [9]. Performance in drills should be methodically evaluated with input from other response agencies. Identified concerns should be addressed prior to the next exercise.

Conclusion

The 2004 Madrid train bombings had all the elements of a "predictable surprise" [12]. Terrorists struck a major transportation system where there was a densely contained, highly vulnerable population at risk, virtually guaranteeing a high-impact, high-visibility mass casualty incident. Because trains are closed environments, the explosions guaranteed blast overpressure, exacerbating the impact of the attack. The resulting injuries encompassed the range that has been described for blast injuries.

The attacks followed the pattern of multifocal, simultaneous, highly aggressive events that are the hallmark of terrorists, severely complicating response to the point of overwhelming and collapse. In Madrid, the emergency response was limited in important ways by deficiencies in experience, training, equipment and coordination of resources. Despite the heroic, competent, and timely actions by many pre-hospital and hospital staff, it is evident that the full range of a systemic response would have been enhanced by the preparedness, planning, and response approaches noted above. In this attack, all of the purposeful cascades that terrorists planned for were achieved. Railway systems will continue to represent one of the more singularly attractive soft targets for future terrorist attacks.

Surge capacity planning and training at a system-wide level are thus critically important for everything related to a national mass casualty incident. Individual technical competencies and institutional capacities in caring for blast injuries are necessary but not sufficient, as institution- and system-wide preparations are needed to prepare for large-scale events. Even for developed nations, in the event of a terrorist MCI or other large blast incident, there will be insufficient resources to support the affected population if pre-event deliberate planning has not been done to address surge. The ability of public health and health care systems to respond to catastrophic MCIs and save as many lives as possible will remain the single most important measure of national resiliency.

References

1. Gutierrez de Ceballos JP, Turégano Fuentes F, Perez Diaz D, Sanz Sanchez M, Martin Llorente C, Guerrero Sanz JE. Casualties treated at the closest hospital in the Madrid, March 11, terrorist bombings. Crit Care Med. 2005;33(1 Suppl):S107–12.
2. Bolling R, Ehrlin Y, Forsberg R, Rüter A, Soest V, Vikström T, et al. KAMEDO Report 90: terrorist attacks in Madrid, Spain, 2004. Prehospital Disaster Med. 2007;22(3):252–7.
3. Gómez AM, Domínguez CJ, Pedrueza CI, Calvente RR, Lillo VM, Canas JM. Management and analysis of out-of-hospital health-related responses to simultaneous railway explosions in Madrid, Spain. Eur J Emerg Med. 2007;14(5):247–55.
4. Carresi AL. The 2004 Madrid train bombings: an analysis of pre-hospital management. Disasters. 2008;32(1):41–65.
5. de Ceballos JPG, Turégano-Fuentes F, Perez-Diaz D, Sanz-Sanchez M, Martin-Llorente C, Guerrero-Sanz JE. 11 March 2004: The terrorist bomb explosions in Madrid, Spain – an analysis of the logistics, injuries sustained and clinical management of casualties treated at the closest hospital. Crit Care. 2005;9(1):104–11.
6. Kluger Y, Kashuk J, Mayo A. Terror bombing-mechanisms, consequences and implications. Scand J Surg. 2004;93(1):11–4.

7. Agiv-Berland A, Ashkenazi I, Aharonson-Daniel L. The cross-national adaptability of EMS protocols for mass casualty incidents. J Homel Secur Emerg Manag. 2012;9(2):1–15.
8. Marghella P, Ashkenazi I. The lessons of tragedy: the 2004 Madrid train bombings. In: Landesman L, Weisfuse I, editors. Case studies in public health preparedness and response to disasters. Burlington, MA: Jones & Bartlett Learning; 2014. p. 134–48.
9. Ashkenazi I, Hunt R, Sasser S, Basavaraju S, Sullivent E, Kapil V, et al. Interim planning guidance for preparedness and response to a mass casualty event resulting from terrorist use of explosives [Internet]. Atlanta GA: US Department of Health and Human Services, Centers for Disease Control and Prevention; 2010 [cited 2018 Aug 20]. Available from: https://stacks.cdc.gov/view/cdc/5705.
10. Hunt R, Ashkenazi I, Falk H. A tale of cities. Disaster Med Public Health Prep. 2011;5 Suppl 2:S185–8.
11. Ashkenazi I, McNulty E, Marcus L, Dorn B. The role of bystanders in mass casualty events: lessons from the 2010 Haiti earthquake. J Def Stud Resour Manag [Internet]. 2012 [cited 2018 Aug 22];01(02). Available from: http://www.scitechnol.com/2324-9315/2324-9315-1-103.php.
12. Bazerman M, Watkins M. Predictable surprises: the disasters you should have seen coming, vol. 317. Cambridge, MA: Harvard University Press; 2004. p. 54.

Part II

Prehospital Management

Prehospital Management of Explosions: Scope of the Problem and Operational Considerations

10

Yevgeniy Maksimenko and Ricky C. Kue

Introduction

In the recent decades, the increased and continued threat of terrorism has forced a paradigm shift in the prehospital response to incidents involving potential terrorist incidents. Responding agencies have had to evolve response plans to train and prepare their providers for this hybrid threat. Explosives and incendiary devices, typically seen on the battlefield, have become increasingly common as terrorist weapons in the civilian setting as the execution of terrorist acts has spread worldwide. In particular, the rise in the use of improvised explosive devices (IEDs) – non-standard explosive devices made from common materials with potential for being contaminated with chemical, biological, or radiological (CBR) agents – has contributed to the need for increased awareness from prehospital providers when responding to such incidents. In the United States, for example, the number of deaths related to terrorist incidents since 1995 have steadily increased, with 2017 being the deadliest year (excluding the 2001 World Trade Center attack) [1]. Furthermore, the readily available instructional videos found on the internet and distributed in print are making IEDs simpler to manufacture.

Over the past two decades, military providers have gained an enormous amount of experience in dealing with blast incidents and injuries [2, 3]. However, the non-military medical establishment has had minimal exposure and thus lack experience

Y. Maksimenko
United States Air Force, Medical Corps, Brookline, MA, USA

Department of Emergency Medicine, Boston Medical Center, Boston, MA, USA

R. C. Kue (✉)
Medical Corps, Vermont Army National Guard, Colchester, VT, USA

Boston University School of Medicine, Boston, MA, USA

D. W. Callaway, J. L. Burstein (eds.), *Operational and Medical Management of Explosive and Blast Incidents*, https://doi.org/10.1007/978-3-030-40655-4_10

in dealing with these incidents. The development of local and regional emergency response plans since the September 11, 2001, attacks on the World Trade Center has led to a more formalized approach to major disaster and incident response and management [4, 5]. Major challenges remain, as proper recognition, adherence to protocol and safety tenets, and the use of good decision-making in the early stages of patient care of a blast incident continue to be inconsistent during actual incidents.

Prehospital response to blast incidents poses a unique challenge from an operational perspective. Many components of a successful prehospital system are stressed during such an event. The ability to accurately dispatch the appropriate resources becomes extremely difficult during a flood of 911 calls that may provide information of conflicting nature. Available resources may quickly be overwhelmed in smaller communities, and mutual aid response may not always be possible in a time-sensitive manner. The loss of infrastructure, such as roads or radio towers, may make it more difficult for emergency responders to actually reach and communicate on the scene. Furthermore, the concept of scene safety during a potential blast incident can become a complex, multidimensional, active process that providers may not recognize early and anticipate the frequent changes. Few prehospital providers are regularly trained to consider the operational and tactical considerations of terrorists, such as target selection or the potential for secondary devices aimed at harming rescuers. This can lead to underestimation of the security of a scene and potential for increased casualties and disruption of the prehospital response to the incident. With increased exposure and improved training, prehospital providers will appreciate that medical treatment becomes secondary to the potential for further loss of life when security/safety is not established. The approach to these incidents needs to continue to evolve, as individual prehospital systems develop plans that match their resources.

Multiple challenges present themselves for each prehospital response to a potential blast incident. These challenges are multifactorial and unique to each incident. Here, we explore some of the potential barriers to a safe and efficient response that minimize actual and potential harm to both the affected victims and the first responders. By looking at individual components of a typical prehospital operations model [6], we aim to describe the specific challenges faced at each step (Table 10.1).

Table 10.1 Individual components of an EMS response

Emergency response system activation
Response and arrival on scene
Scene safety and security (protective measures, exposure prevention)
Scene size-up (recognition of potential blast incident)
Establishment of command
Notification/additional resources
Product identification/evidence preservation
Rescue/medical care
Control, recovery and termination

Emergency Response System Activation

One of the pillars of proper EMS system functionality is the ability of the public to activate the emergency response system by contacting a dispatcher. The most common way this happens is by calling 911. While this number covers nearly 100% of the US population, not all areas have access to 911, and localization of 911 calls from mobile phones is limited [7]. This is often overcome by local phone numbers being available for emergency response, but it still underlines the point that EMS activation should not always be taken for granted.

In situations involving blast incidents, additional barriers to proper prehospital system activation may occur. Disruption of infrastructure – in particular, cell phone towers – can make reaching the proper authorities impossible. Even with intact infrastructure, call volumes can overload the cell phone network and "gridlock" the telecommunication system, creating an additional delay in EMS notification. Confusion and mass hysteria from the people affected by an event can lead to an overwhelming call volume and frequently conflicting information being relayed to the authorities. This introduces an extra difficulty for the dispatcher to activate an organized response to such events.

Dispatcher Role in Potential Bomb Threats

The dispatcher plays an essential role in helping providers get to the right location and notify them of any changes to the scene as they become available. In particular, when dealing with potential terrorist attacks or bomb threats, the dispatcher should follow specific questionnaires to obtain as much information as possible. Questions regarding the location, timing of explosion, and potential identification of the person calling may help prevent the incident before it occurs (Table 10.2).

It is important for dispatchers to consider the volume and specialization required for a large-scale blast incident response. Ready availability of appropriately trained responders can mitigate the morbidity and mortality of victims during blast incidents, as demonstrated by the response to the Boston Marathon bombings in 2013 [8]. However, specialized teams, such as a bomb squad or other equivalent unit, are also critical to mitigate threats on scene during periods when situational information

Table 10.2 Dispatcher-specific questions for a bomb threat phone call

Where is the bomb located?
What does the bomb look like?
What kind of bomb is it?
What will cause it to explode?
When is the bomb going to explode?
Did you place the bomb?
Why did you place the bomb?
What is your name or the name of your group?

is limited. In situations when an incident occurs during regular operations of a municipality, this large pool of resources is often not available and may create an operational constraint for the dispatchers. Establishment of mutual aid agreements, development of regional disaster/major event response plans, and standardized processes for recall of off-duty responders are all essential components for anticipating and minimizing panic during responses to blast incidents.

Response and Arrival on Scene

Once an incident has been identified and a dispatcher has been notified, the next phase of the prehospital response is the actual response to the scene of the incident. Blast incidents present some additional unique challenges to the already potentially difficult environment faced during a prehospital response. Depending on the severity of an incident, the identification of the scene of the incident may not always be obvious to the dispatcher. This ambiguity can lead to imprecise dispatch information and make the scene arrival less straightforward. Particularly, if the blast incident involves any destruction of infrastructure, first responders may have to find a secondary route or method of accessing casualties. Instability of the scene, due to impending building collapse or further safety hazards, can significantly inhibit the ability of the prehospital providers to reach the scene. Situational awareness, adherence to training and validated standard operating procedures (SOPs), and establishment and maintenance of a reasonable degree of personal and scene safety and security can mitigate some of the challenges faced at this stage of the response.

Scene Safety and Security

Scene safety is a critical aspect of any response to an incident. While in traditional EMS and fire training, scene safety was aimed at minimizing injury to providers from violence and traffic, blast incidents create a unique source of potential injury and harm [9]. Amplified by lack of specific training and experience with such events, many prehospital providers may not realize the danger they may be facing and, as a result, compromise the safety of both responders and their patients. This is a common theme for responders involved not only in blast incidents but also in any environment that poses hazard to their safety. Because of this, most EMS agencies have standing protocols preventing their providers from entering any scene deemed unsafe. However, based on the experiences from recent terrorist attacks and mass-casualty incidents (MCIs), the mentality regarding how medical rescue in these situations are approached has begun to change [10]. Seeking cover and waiting for a scene to be established safe may not be a sustainable strategy for more complicated situations, particularly those involving explosives.

In general, any scene involving a threat to safety or health can be broken down into three areas, based on the actual or perceived threat level to a prehospital provider.

Tactical terminology, as well as the National Incident Management System (NIMS), utilizes specific verbiage when describing such zones of operation: Hot, Warm, and Cold [11]. The Hot zone involves an active or direct threat, such as the presence of an unexploded or partially exploded device, fire, or a hazardous materials (HAZMAT) contamination. The Warm zone is a designated area that is separated from the Hot zone by a barrier or distance, but where a potential threat still exists. An example would include a prehospital provider being 100 yards away from a secondary blast device, taking care of a patient behind a cement barrier. The Cold zone is considered the "safe" zone, as no specific threat is yet present in this area. Based on traditional teaching, EMS providers would only function in the Cold zone, where the threat was minimal. Programs such as Tactical Emergency Casualty Care (TECC), adopted from military practices, advocate for the transition of EMS operations away from solely the Cold zone and toward the operationally crucial Warm zone [12–14]. Despite this shifting paradigm, safety is still paramount. Some question the existence of a true Cold zone in the response to blast events given the potential for secondary attacks and or explosions. Well-trained and experienced prehospital providers learn to recognize and mitigate threats to them and their patient's safety before they arise.

All emergency personnel responding to a blast incident must be vigilant in assessing the scene. Aside from the usual environmental and urban dangers, providers should be aware of additional threats unique to a blast, similar to how a potential HAZMAT incident is approached. Specifically, providers should be on high alert for unusual objects, packages, and containers; substances, fumes, and odors; and suspicious persons who may be potential perpetrators. Furthermore, damage from an explosion can create secondary hazards, such as structural instability, gas leak, electrical malfunction, or fires. Situations involving "dirty bombs" (i.e., ones that have a device contaminated with CBR substances) can complicate a scene by making it a dual blast and HAZMAT incident.

An important safety concern for any responding prehospital provider, especially for those first on scene, is the potential for a secondary blast if the explosive device has ot detonated all of its explosive material. Paying attention to some of the four components required for successful detonation (i.e., combustible material, oxidizer to support the rapid burning process, igniting component, and confinement of the ingredients) can help maintain proper safety procedures and establish standoff distances and perimeters for scene organization (see Chap. 12) in order to mitigate some of the threat from unexploded primary or secondary devices.

One additional potential threat faced by prehospital providers at a blast incident scene is the presence of "secondary" devices aimed specifically at the arriving emergency responders. An example of this was the second IED placed at a near distance away from the first IED during the 2013 Boston Marathon bombings possibly meant to injure first responders at the scene of the first blast [8]. This is also a potential "distraction technique" that misdirects initial responders into a false sense of safety and can potentially create difficulty in establishing a safe area for EMS operations. Due to these unique dangers, special operational considerations must be employed. For example, radio/cell phone communication should be cut off immediately if there is potential for an unexploded explosive device that could be remotely activated, until a safe perimeter has been established and cleared. Similar to initial response to HAZMAT incidents, safe distances should be determined and followed based on current best practice guidelines. Depending on the size and potential lethality of an explosive device and its potential for secondary damage, establishing isolation perimeter distances by EMS will vary. As mentioned later, early activation of appropriate resources is essential. Establishing command, minimizing the likelihood of new harm, and maximizing survival from existing injuries are keys to successful incident management.

Protective Measures

Major components of scene safety taught in EMS courses are proper personal protective equipment (PPE) and body substance isolation (BSI). Whereas in routine prehospital responses the uniform of the provider and basic medical gloves may be the only protection necessary, in more complex incidents involving hazardous materials, explosive devices and/or fire and additional protection may be required. Based on the National Fire Protection Association (NFPA) Standards, four levels of HAZMAT protective equipment exist, as shown below [9].

- Level A = SCBA with maximal vapor protection and flash protection
- Level B = Self-contained breathing apparatus (SCBA)
- Level C = Air-purifying respirators (APR) with increased splash protection
- Level D = General duty or work uniform

Although this equipment is stocked by most fire departments and some other response agencies, it is not often easily accessible at the moment of a response, especially for non-fire-department-based first responders. This makes PPE the most important consideration, as it is the only barrier from a responder becoming potentially contaminated or harmed by a hazardous threat on scene. (Of course, it does not provide protection from a secondary device's blast.) Failure to have proper protection for equipment can lead to contamination, causing a potentially damaging depletion of resources and material during a response. Proper stockpiling, maintenance, and ease of accessibility and deployment of appropriate specialized resources can help mitigate the threat to both providers and patients on scene.

Scene Size-Up

Once the immediate scene safety and security issues have been addressed, an evaluation of the scope of the incident becomes necessary. Part of this process begins prior to arrival on scene. In particular, it is important for first responders to always consider, even during regular operations, whether there is a potential for a terrorist attack or blast incident based on the characteristics of the dispatch. This includes the location of the call, some examples of which include a symbolic or historic site, a public event, a controversial event or rally, critical infrastructures, or other

Table 10.3 Physical features of a potential IED

Abandoned container out of place with the surroundings
Obvious/classic-appearing devices with blasting caps, timers, booster charged, etc.
Unusual devices attached to compressed gas cylinders, flammable liquid containers, bulk storage fixtures, other containers
Abandoned vehicles that do not fit the current environment (gasoline tanker in front of a government building)
Entrance thresholds with wires or hardware that appears out of place
Strong chemical odors
Trip wires
Written or verbal threats
Partially exploded devices

vulnerable facilities (e.g., nuclear facility and weapons depot). Also, responders should consider the date and time of the event, which could correspond to important dates or anniversaries of events. Furthermore, the time of day or timing during an event could also be a clue, as a potential terrorist attack could be targeted to maximize casualties at peak hours, such as the attack in Nice, France, during Bastille Day celebrations in 2016 [15]. Additional and more obvious clues from the dispatcher may assist in evaluation of risk. These might include a known bomb threat, reports of an explosion, evidence of blast damage at the scene, a wide area of destruction, large numbers of casualties in a relatively small space, or large unexplained fires. On scene, it is crucial for EMS providers to obtain a reasonable, but not necessarily exact, number of casualties early in the scene size-up process, as this will allow for earlier communication with dispatch and a more efficient coordinated response to the incident.

As the process of patient assessment and triage begins, it is important to ensure that providers and responders continue to maintain vigilance in looking for potential unidentified and/or partially unexploded devices. Characteristics would include obvious wires, blasting caps, chemicals, cans of gasoline or other flammable liquids, compressed gasses, timing devices, etc. (Table 10.3). It is important not only to recognize devices that were planted purposefully but also to remember that certain explosive materials can unintentionally become a secondary hazard during the rescue operations.

Establishment of Incident Command

Once the scene has been assessed and secured, and the number of patients has been estimated to exceed the current medical capabilities, the first responders on scene should declare an MCI and establish an incident command (IC) structure organized around the Incident Command System (ICS) principles [5]. This is a crucial step in coordinating an appropriate response to the incident. However, operational barriers, especially during a scene involving an unknown amount of casualties in an unstable structure with potential secondary hazards, can make this step difficult to accomplish. In particular, if an undetonated device is found, radio operations should be ceased immediately due to the possibility that the IED could be command-detonated via radio; this will likely delay the ability to establish a proper IC structure.

The IC structure should function to coordinate the response by establishing strategic and tactical goals. Strategic goals are the broad aims for the incident response. To accomplish these for a large, complex, or geographically dispersed incident, divisions of labor need to be organized and resourced. For example, assigning roles to the Operations Section, as well as a Medical Operations Branch with the objective of triaging and medically stabilizing patients, would fall in line with the strategic goal of expeditious and effective casualty management. Tactical goals would include specific steps that collectively support achieving each strategic goal. For example, assigning specific personnel to Treatment Teams A and B, with the tactical objective of triaging the first 30 patients on the south side of Building 1, would support a tactical goal of identifying medical resources needed in that location.

Ultimately, the responsibility for managing the incident should be assigned to the most qualified person on scene, though leadership might change hands once the full scale of the incident is realized and appropriate resources are made available. For large-scale incidents, this usually requires the involvement of law enforcement, fire service, and EMS working through a joint command.

Notification and Additional Resources

Following establishment of command, it is important to activate the necessary resources for successful management of the incident. Depending on whether a blast incident involves any unexploded devices or other ongoing threats, including secondary ones aimed at first responders or "dirty bombs" involving CBR or other hazardous materials, specialized response teams may need to be involved as early as possible for proper containment and to minimize secondary harm. Almost any explosive incident will involve the local police department or sheriff's office. Active or anticipated criminal threats may require a tactical law-enforcement response necessitating medical support in the Hot zone (see Chap. 15). Explosive ordinance disposal (EOD) or "bomb squad" teams may be necessary to investigate suspicious items and render them harmless if considered a potential threat. Hazardous materials are usually handled by HAZMAT teams from fire services. Occasionally, some CBR responses might require a more specialized team, often from the federal law enforcement agencies or the military. In particular, during MCIs where resources are insufficient for number of patients, appropriately trained personnel may need to be able to function in all three of the various zones of operations (i.e., Hot, Warm, and Cold zones). Immediate notification of local hospitals and trauma centers will assist in minimizing delays for patient care once patients begin arriving at the hospital (see Chap. 13). Depending on the number of patients involved, activation of additional medical resources may become necessary. Employing local, regional, and state resources to deploy field hospitals and medical providers is yet another possibility. It would also be mistake to overlook the state resources such as the Army or Air National Guards, particularly for extended incidents.

The development of multiple national guidelines and recommendations since early 2000 for improving the response to major disasters and incidents, multiple federal resources have become available for deployment based on the nature and scope of a given incident. These include the US Department of Transportation (DoT), US Department of Defense (DoD), Army Corps of Engineers, Federal Emergency Management Agency (FEMA), Urban Search and Rescue (US&R), Public Health Service (PHS from the US Department of Health and Human Services (DHHS), Environmental Protection Agency (EPA), US Department of Agriculture (USDA), US Department of Homeland Security (DHS), and US Department of Justice (DoJ) – all of which serve a specific function based on the scale and type of incident. Available federal medical resources also available include the National Disaster Medical System (NDMS) which coordinate the readiness and response of deployable Disaster Medical Assistance Teams (DMATs), coordinated through DHHS, as well as the American Red Cross [6].

Product Identification and Evidence Preservation

While identification of the explosive and evidence management will often not be in the forefront of medical responders' minds during an active incident, this information can be crucial in the investigation into potential criminal or terrorist activity that may have caused the incident. First responders rely on the *Emergency Response Guidebook* [16] for identification of unknown and potentially hazardous substances during regular operations. This tool can also be useful during potential blast or terrorist events, as it can help identify those potential secondary threats present on scene and help mitigate the dangers caused by those substances, in case they were ignited or exploded. Additionally, identifying IEDs that are constructed using existing canisters, cylinders, and other containers meant for chemical transport, particularly those labeled appropriately and accurately, can help establish security perimeters and mitigate risk to the public prior to any initial or subsequent explosion.

Evidence preservation on scene is important, though often overlooked by the need to assess and rescue casualties on scene. Effort should be taken to minimize disruption to the scene, in particular if a partially unexploded device or if debris of a potential source explosive is found. This also applies to potential suicidal bombing situations, where the bomber's body should not be moved or handled unnecessarily.

Rescue and Medical Care

While these topics will be covered in more detail in Chap. 13, it is important to consider some of the challenges faced by prehospital providers on the scene of a blast incident. When considered as part of Warm zone treatment algorithms such as those covered in TECC [12] or the THREAT (Threat suppression, Hemorrhage control, Rapid Extrication to safety, Assessment by medical providers, and Transport to definitive care) algorithm described in the Hartford Consensus [13, 14], medical care often comes relatively late when dealing with dangerous incidents. Such situations are often initially MCIs, which create a large but not unique barrier to patient assessment and treatment. Some unique challenges faced by medical providers during blast incidents include physical barriers to patient assessment, such as hearing damage as a result of a blast, difficulty of triage due to unique pattern of injuries and unstable environment, and unique life threats that may not be quickly recognized during patient assessment due to limited clinical experience with such injuries.

Control, Recovery, and Termination

As the last part of major incident management, recovery operations often involve restoring the community and infrastructure back to normal. This process is not always straightforward, particularly when involving terrorism or large number of casualties. In part, this process depends on the resilience and "immunity" of a community to the violence experienced. Community recovery is defined by the US Centers for Disease Control and Prevention (CDC) as the "ability to collaborate with community partners to plan and advocate for the rebuilding of public health, medical, and mental/behavioral health systems" [17]. Returning the physical structure of a community back to what it was prior may not fully compensate for the potential harm done by the event psychologically or emotionally. Debriefing, in particular for those directly involved with the incident, is a crucial step for recovery of prehospital providers and all first responders [18, 19]. As most of these incidents are infrequent, their effect can be potent and proper care for those affected should not be ignored. In communities with no prior or very limited experience, it would be remiss not to reach out to entities trained to deal with recovery from such events, such as FEMA or the CDC. Furthermore, larger communities with potential prior experience of such incidents can benefit from national or international collaborations to improve their debriefing techniques.

Conclusion

EMS providers face unique challenges when responding to potential blast and terrorist incidents. The situational circumstances, particularly those involving massive disruptions of infrastructure, can create exceptional barriers to effective EMS operations. Prehospital providers can follow several guiding principles when dealing with a potential incident. By focusing on three concepts, including active operational risk management, effective recognition of secondary and hazardous materials devices, and efficient activation of appropriate resources and establishment of incident command, a prehospital provider can ensure a potentially uncontrollable situation that becomes manageable and safe.

The principles of operational risk management, which include proper maintenance of scene safety and situational awareness, can help minimize potential harm to first responders at blast injury incidents. Awareness and early recognition of secondary and contaminated explosives devices are essential components of situational awareness that all prehospital providers should exercise when responding to potential blast incidents. Given the complexity of a response to blast incidents, activation of specialized resources and the use of incident command will help with making an otherwise chaotic scene into one that can be managed effectively. Finally, consideration of patient care while a blast threat is actively being mitigated should be undertaken by the prehospital providers. EMS systems should train their providers to not hide behind the dogma of scene safety, in order to provide time-sensitive medical care. With the implementation of Warm-zone medical response strategies, casualty survival can be maximized (see Chap. 15). Following the resolution of an incident, all prehospital personnel should undergo a formal debrief and seek additional help as needed. Through application of the lessons learned by the military and EMS systems around the country, prehospital response to such incidents will continue to improve.

Key Points

- Operational risk management – active maintenance of scene safety and situational awareness
- Awareness and early recognition of secondary and contaminated explosives devices
- Implementation of Warm-zone medical response strategies

Pitfalls

- Lack of situational awareness = not recognizing an event as a potential terrorist attack or blast incident, including potential "dirty bombs" and secondary devices.
- Delay in activation of appropriate resources (including personnel trained for Warm-zone operations) can lead to increased casualty mortality and morbidity.
- Not taking care of rescuers in prolonged incidents = fatigue and accidents related to fatigue.

Pearls

- Prehospital providers must maintain situational awareness to avoid becoming a victim. Assume there remin secondary threats in all operational zones.
- Prehospital training for a response to blast and terrorist incidents is essential for ensuring a coordinated and safe response to an actual incident.
- A formalized debrief should take place for every blast or terrorist incident that prehospital providers are involved in.

References

1. Miller E, Jensen M. American deaths in terrorist attacks, 1995–2017. START: College Park, MD [Internet]. 2018 [cited 5 February 2019] Available from: https://www.start.umd.edu/pubs/START_AmericanTerrorismDeaths_FactSheet_Sept2018.pdf.
2. Ritenour A, Blackbourne L, Kelly J, McLaughlin D, Pearse L, Holcomb J, et al. Incidence of primary blast injury in US military overseas contingency operations. Ann Surg. 2010;251(6):1140–4.
3. Cannon J, Hofmann L, Glasgow S, Potter B, Rodriguez C, Cancio L, et al. Dismounted complex blast injuries: a comprehensive review of the modern combat experience. J Am Coll Surg. 2016;223(4):652–664.e8.
4. Greene J. Post 9/11 federal disaster funds: where did the $7 billion trickle down? Ann Emerg Med. 2008;52(3):263–5.
5. Jensen J, Thompson S. The incident command system: a literature review. Disasters. 2015;40(1):158–82.
6. Department of Homeland Security. Emergency Response to Terrorism: Tactical Considerations: Emergency Medical Services. 2000.
7. US Department of Transportation. 2017 National 911 Progress Report. 2017.
8. Biddinger P, Baggish A, Harrington L, d'Hemecourt P, Hooley J, Jones J, et al. Be prepared — the Boston marathon and mass-casualty events. N Engl J Med. 2013;368(21):1958–60.
9. American Academy of Orthopaedic Surgeons Staff. Emergency care and transportation of the sick and injured. Burlington, MA: Jones & Bartlett Learning, LLC; 2016.
10. Hick J, Hanfling D, Evans B, Greenberg S, Alson R, McKinney S et al. Health and medical response to active shooter and bombing events. NAM Perspectives. 2016;6(6).
11. Pennardt A, Schwartz R. Hot, warm, and cold zones: applying existing national incident management system terminology to enhance tactical emergency medical support interoperability. J Spec Oper Med. 2014;14(3):78–9.
12. Smith R. C-TECC update. J Spec Oper Med. 2014;14(1):118.
13. Callaway D. Translating tactical combat casualty care lessons learned to the high-threat civilian setting: tactical emergency casualty care and the Hartford consensus. Wilderness Environ Med. 2017;28(2):S140–5.
14. Jacobs L, McSwain N, Rotondo M, Wade D, Fabbri W, Eastman A, et al. Improving survival from active shooter events. J Trauma Acute Care Surg. 2013;74(6):1399–400.
15. Solla F, Carboni J, Bréaud J, Babe P, Brézac G, Chivoret N, et al. July 14, 2016, terror attack in Nice, France. Acad Pediatr. 2018;18(4):361–3.
16. 2016 emergency response guidebook. Washington, DC: Department of Transportation, Pipeline and Hazardous Materials Safety Administration; 2016.
17. Center for Disease Control. Public Health Preparedness Capabilities: National Standards for State and Local Planning March 2011. 2011.
18. Hawker D, Durkin J, Hawker D. To debrief or not to debrief our heroes: that is the question. Clin Psychol Psychother. 2010;18(6):453–63.
19. Hunt P. Lessons identified from the 2017 Manchester and London terrorism incidents. Part 3: the postincident and recovery phase. J R Army Med Corps. 2018. pii: jramc-2018-000936. doi: https://doi.org/10.1136/jramc-2018-000936. [Epub ahead of print].

Lessons in Prehospital Trauma Management During Combat

11

Andrew David Fisher and Ethan A. Miles

Introduction

A tragedy of war is failure to implement the hard lessons encountered from previous conflicts. Over the past 19 years of combat, prehospital military medicine has experienced more change than most other areas of the military, including military treatment facilities (MTFs) representing hospitals and clinics. These changes occurred not only as new lessons were learned but also as a result of relearning lessons from previous conflicts. In the current conflicts in Iraq and Afghanistan, the use of improvised explosive devices (IEDs) produced more blast injuries than in any other war [1, 2]. As a result of the significant increase in IED use along with improved torso protection from newer body armor, unique injury survival patterns emerged with large numbers of complex extremity injuries. Seven prehospital lessons have had the largest impact on survival from combat-related blast injuries: formal development and rigorous evaluation of Tactical Combat Casualty Care (TCCC) guidelines, use of tourniquets for extremity hemorrhage, employment of nonmedical personnel to deliver life-saving care at the point of injury, better documentation of care provided in the prehospital setting, evacuation within "the Golden Hour" timeframe, administration of blood products in the field, and the prehospital management of traumatic brain injury (TBI) have all been instrumental in saving lives on the battlefield.

A. D. Fisher (✉)
Texas Medical Command, Texas Army National Guard, Austin, TX, USA

E. A. Miles
Maneuver Center of Excellence, Fort Benning, GA, USA

D. W. Callaway, J. L. Burstein (eds.), *Operational and Medical Management of Explosive and Blast Incidents*, https://doi.org/10.1007/978-3-030-40655-4_11

Tactical Combat Casualty Care

At the onset of hostilities in Afghanistan in October 2001, the majority of battlefield trauma care was based on the prevailing prehospital trauma care concepts in the civilian sector at that time. These concepts were not designed for the prehospital combat setting and included such concepts as follows:

1. Combat medical personnel being trained *not* to use tourniquets because of the unvalidated belief that even short-duration tourniquet application would cause ischemic damage to extremities
2. No allowance or use of hemostatic dressings to stop external hemorrhage from locations not amenable to tourniquet use
3. Treatment of hemorrhagic shock with large-volume crystalloid fluid resuscitation to restore normal blood pressure
4. Intramuscular morphine for battlefield analgesia [3, 4]

The formalization and adoption of TCCC guidelines provided the medical community with a framework to rapidly adopt and implement life-saving tactics at the point of injury (POI), through the evacuation chain, and onto higher echelons of medical care. The "new" concepts of TCCC had been introduced by Butler and colleagues in the original TCCC paper published as a special supplement in *Military Medicine* in August of 1996 [5]. Among other things, TCCC discussed three phases of care – Care Under Fire, Tactical Field Care, and Casualty Evacuation Care – to ensure that medical care rendered was appropriate to the prevailing tactical situation.

Tactical Combat Casualty Care focused on reducing "potentially preventable combat death," defined as mortality that resulted from injuries which were not inevitably fatal had optimal care been provided to the casualty quickly enough [2, 6]. The primary metric chosen for TCCC in the original 1996 paper was to eliminate all deaths on the battlefield that were the result of conditions that could be easily treated in the prehospital environment, such as extremity bleeding, other sources of external hemorrhage, tension pneumothorax, and airway obstruction [5]. The TCCC guidelines articulated three overarching goals as pertinent to success in battlefield medicine: (1) treat the casualty, (2) prevent additional casualties, and (3) complete the mission [5, 7].

The early use of limb tourniquets was strongly recommended to obtain initial control of life-threatening extremity hemorrhage. Intravenous (IV) fluid resuscitation was recommended only when shock had resulted from hemorrhage and then only when bleeding had been controlled. Initially, instead of an isotonic crystalloid fluid such as lactated Ringer's solution or 0.9% sodium chloride (normal saline), 6% hetastarch with a longer intravascular dwell time was recommended. The use of spinal motion restriction was recommended only for casualties who had sustained blunt trauma, not those whose injuries were limited to penetrating trauma. Intravenous morphine was recommended rather than the previously used intramuscular morphine, both to provide faster onset of analgesia and to reduce the likelihood of opioid overdose resulting from the delayed onset of analgesia associated with intramuscular morphine deposition [3].

The recommendations found in the first TCCC guidelines were not in line with mainstream concepts in prehospital trauma care at the time. As a result, very few US military units used TCCC at the start of the recent conflicts. As experience was gained and evidence obtained over the next two decades, TCCC concepts were found to dramatically reduce potentially preventable death on the battlefield [2, 8–11].

Units that adopted TCCC as their standard for battlefield trauma care demonstrated success in decreasing potentially preventable deaths during the campaigns in Iraq and Afghanistan. For instance, during the first 25 days of the Iraq invasion, Task Force 1–15 suffered 32 wounded in action (WIA) and no potentially preventable deaths or casualties who later died of wounds (DOW) [9]. Kelly et al. described casualties from March 2003 to April 2004 and from June 2006 to December 2006 during a similar practice change, with a shift in potentially preventable death rate to 19% vs. 28% [12].

TCCC was recommended as the standard of care for combat first-aid training in member nations by the American, British, Canadian, Australian, and New Zealand armies [13] and by the NATO Special-Operations-convened Human Factor and Medicine Expert Panel 224 in 2011 [14]. In 2018, 17 years after the initiation of combat operations, TCCC was mandated as the US Department of Defense (DoD) standard for battlefield trauma care [7]. TCCC concepts have now also been adopted by civilian law enforcement agencies [15, 16], civilian EMS systems [17, 18], and many other nations.

The authors of the original 1996 TCCC paper realized that TCCC would need to be updated on an ongoing basis as new evidence and new technologies became available, so it called for the establishment of a standing Committee on TCCC (CoTCCC). The CoTCCC was founded in 2001 through a joint effort of the US Special Operations Command and the US Navy Operational Medicine Command [19].

As of 2020, the CoTCCC has 42 voting members, all of whom have deployed in support of US military combat operations. In addition to trauma surgeons, emergency physicians, and operational medicine physicians and physician assistants (PAs), the CoTCCC also has members who are combat medics, corpsmen, and pararescuemen (PJs), so that all TCCC recommendations have considerable input from the individuals who will actually be using TCCC to save lives on the battlefield [19].

The evolution of the CoTCCC and the widespread acceptance of TCCC concepts have facilitated the rapid sharing of battlefield trauma care lessons learned, enabled the rapid evaluation and fielding of cutting-edge techniques and technologies, and focused expert opinion on critical issues in trauma care in order to rapidly come to consensus on best practices and openly share this knowledge globally.

As a result, TCCC has saved countless lives by accelerating the development of new standards for battlefield trauma care by championing the passage of this new medical knowledge directly to those providing medical care in the prehospital setting of care, where 87% of potentially preventable deaths occur [2].

Tourniquets and Pelvic Binding

The majority of combat deaths occur in the prehospital setting and most are non-survivable [2]. The vast majority of casualties who survive the initial wounding often require little prehospital life-saving intervention. It is a small percentage of casualties that require immediate care in order to survive, but these are the patients who benefit the most from prehospital care. Hemorrhage control is the leading intervention to prevent death, and extremity hemorrhage is a leading cause of potentially preventable death in combat [6, 12, 19].

Given their relative low cost and simplicity of construction, IEDs quickly became the weapon of choice in Iraq and Afghanistan [20, 21] and the leading cause of death in Iraq [22]. From 2001 to 2005, of the 6609 wounds in Iraq and Afghanistan, 3575 (54.1%) were extremity wounds [21]. Explosions caused 79% of the wounds in the early years [21], and this number would remain steady for years. In the early years of the Global War on Terror, the use of tourniquets was still discouraged and they were only to be used after all other treatments had failed. Prior to 2006, despite the CoTCCC recommending tourniquets for hemorrhage control, most of the pre-hospital tourniquets were improvised and units were still being advised to use them as a last resort. During the same time, members of the 75th Ranger Regiment were effectively using a ratchet style tourniquet (Fig. 11.1).

After 2006, documented benefits of early hemorrhage control via tourniquet use were recognized. Consequently, distribution and employment of tourniquets slowly became widespread in the US military. In Iraq and Afghanistan when tourniquets were just starting to be used, extremity hemorrhage caused 7.8% of total fatalities [19]. After the greater adoption of prehospital tourniquets from 2006 to 2011, deaths from extremity hemorrhage dropped to 2.6% of total fatalities – a 67% decrease in fatalities from extremity hemorrhage [19].

The commercially made Combat Application Tourniquet® (C-A-T) (C-A-T Resources, LLC, Rock Hill, SC) (Fig. 11.2) and SOF Tactical Tourniquet® (SOFT-T) (Tactical Medical Solutions, Anderson, SC) (Fig. 11.3) were the two

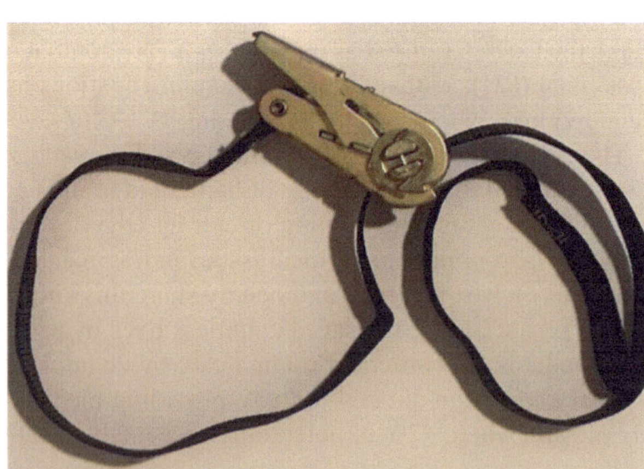

Fig. 11.1 The "Ranger Ratchet" tourniquet. (Photograph courtesy of Harold R. Montgomery)

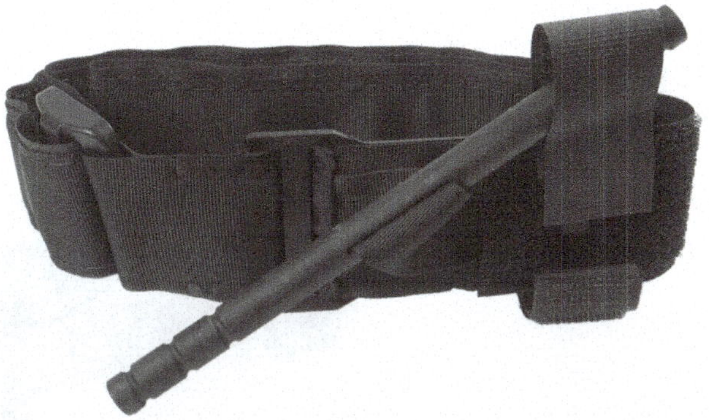

Fig. 11.2 Generation 3 Combat Application Tourniquet® (C-A-T®). (Photograph courtesy of North American Rescue®)

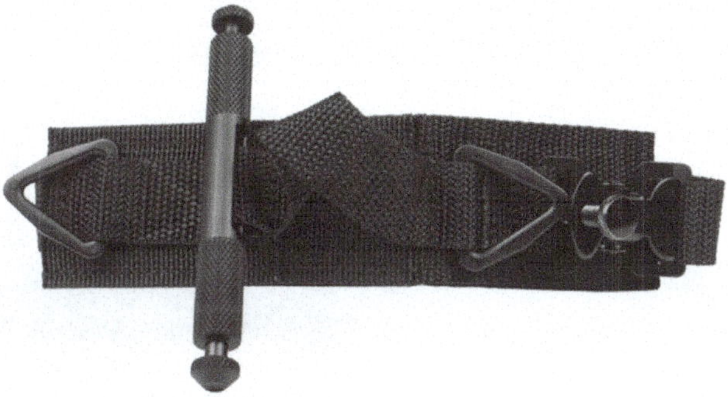

Fig. 11.3 SOF® Tactical Tourniquet. (Photograph courtesy of Tactical Medical Solutions®)

tourniquets tested and evaluated at the US Army Institute of Surgical Research (USAISR) and subsequently recommended by the CoTCCC for use at the POI [23]. The Emergency and Military Tourniquet (EMT) (Delfi Medical Innovations Inc., Vancouver, BC) was recommended for use in medical facilities, given its larger size and reliance on an air bladder.

The C-A-T and SOFT-T would go through many changes and improvements and changes over the years up to the C-A-T® GEN7 (Fig. 11.4) and SOFTT-W® (Fig. 11.5). For many years, tourniquets were considered dangerous due to risk of limb loss from ischemia. Currently, tourniquets are considered safe and effective as thousands of tourniquets have been applied without loss of limb when applied for less than 2 hours [10]. A more recent review by the CoTCCC expanded the tourniquet recommendations to include eight non-pneumatic and two pneumatic tourniquets [24].

If an IED blast injury is significant enough to cause lower-extremity amputation, then there is a relatively high probability of pelvic fracture and pelvic ring disruption. In a 2014 study, Cross et al. showed that, in blast injuries, 10% of unilateral amputations, 30% of bilateral amputations, and 39% of bilateral transfemoral amputations had concurrent pelvic fractures [25]. This discovery led to the common practice of applying a pelvic binder to any casualty with a lower-extremity

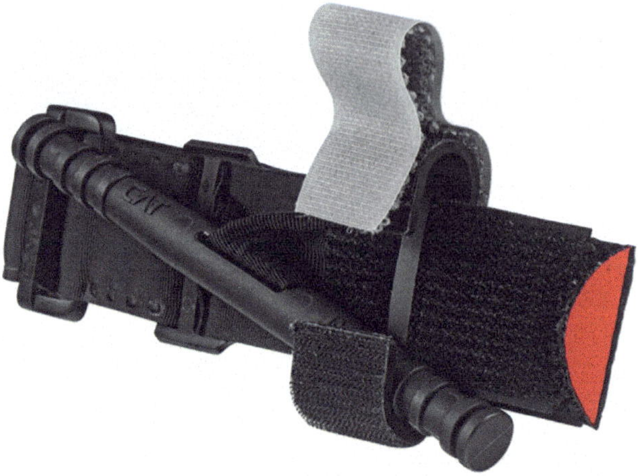

Fig. 11.4 Combat Application Tourniquet® (C-A-T® Gen7). (Photograph courtesy of North American Rescue®)

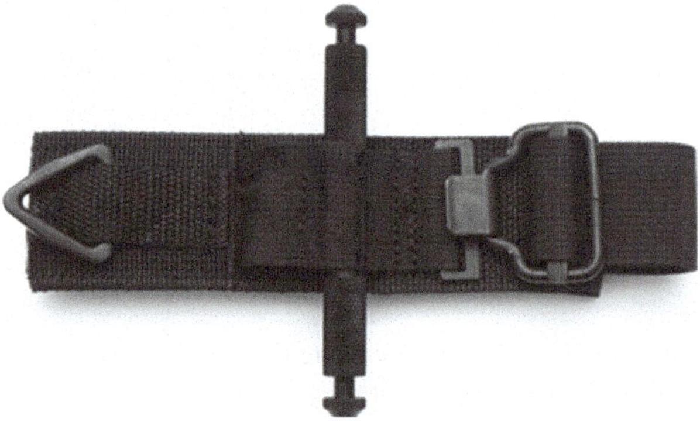

Fig. 11.5 SOFTT-W ® Tactical Tourniquet – Wide. (Photograph courtesy of Tactical Medical Solutions®)

amputation from an IED blast mechanism. Increasing emphasis on pelvic fracture management in blast-injured casualties to decrease noncompressible hemorrhage is an ongoing research effort area for device manufacturers.

Use of Nonmedical Personnel

Military units have seen time and time again that the individual closest to the injured casualty is the most important caregiver, regardless of their designation as a medical provider. This holds true across the spectrum of injuries seen on the battlefield, but particularly so in a mass-casualty (MASCAL) event.

A MASCAL incident is when the number of patients requiring immediate attention overwhelms the medical personnel or equipment required to adequately treat all patients to an expected standard of care. Explosive blasts often cause MASCAL situations as military units typically have only one combat medic on a mission, and adversary tactics employing IEDs are typically designed to inflict maximum damage on the maximum number of individuals. The US Army long ago recognized the issue of limited medical resources on the battlefield, so Colonel (Retired) Robert H. Mosebar created the Combat Lifesaver (CLS) Course in the 1980s [26]. The CLS concept cross-trained nonmedical personnel to provide life-saving medical care on the battlefield in the event the medic is separated, overwhelmed with casualties, or physically unable to respond to the situation. Nevertheless, as of 2017, the US Army only required one CLS per squad of 9–11 people, thus limiting the potential for having a higher percentage of medically trained individuals to deliver immediate care at the POI.

Even before the invasions of Iraq and Afghanistan, the 75th Ranger Regiment recognized the power of numbers in medical response. In 1997, then Regimental Commander Colonel Stanley A. McChrystal and Command Sergeant Major Michael T. Hall outlined their top four priorities (termed "Big Four"): marksmanship, physical training, small-unit tactics, and medical training [27]. This required all soldiers assigned to the 75th Ranger Regiment to be trained in TCCC, which had only been introduced the year prior. The Regiment branded their version of TCCC "Ranger First Responder" (RFR). The RFR program enabled the 75th Ranger Regiment to achieve the goal of zero preventable deaths in the prehospital setting [11]. This effect was noted to be such a success, that US Central Command required all troops deploying to its Area of Responsibility (AOR) to be trained in TCCC [28]. TCCC training is now the standard training for all its military members following curriculum set by the CoTCCC.

In 2016, the National Academies of Science, Engineering and Medicine (NASEM) estimated that up to 20% of civilian trauma deaths are potentially preventable [29]. The concept of training nonmedical personnel in essential life-saving procedures like hemorrhage control has the potential to reduce this unacceptably high rate and is particularly relevant in civilian MASCAL events. The NASEM report, buoyed by professional society endorsement strengthened grass root efforts to teach bystanders and non-military health care professionals how to control hemorrhage with tourniquets and hemostatic dressings. President Barack Obama's administration supported this policy directive for national preparedness, leading the Departments of Homeland Security and Defense to create a structure for public-private partnerships and scaling of the "Stop the Bleed" campaign [30]. Since then, a majority of relevant professional societies have signed on to support the "Stop the Bleed" campaign, build hemorrhage control programmatic, and translate this combat lessons learned to the general population.

Prehospital Documentation

Prior to the current wars in Iraq and Afghanistan, there were no formal means to track prehospital care and outcomes. The lack of documentation left the US military with a significant knowledge gap in prehospital medical care, as roughly 87% of casualties died before reaching the hospital [2]. Recognizing the need to formally capture prehospital medical intervention data, the 75th Ranger Regiment in partnership with Texas A&M Health Science Center Rural and Community Health Institute

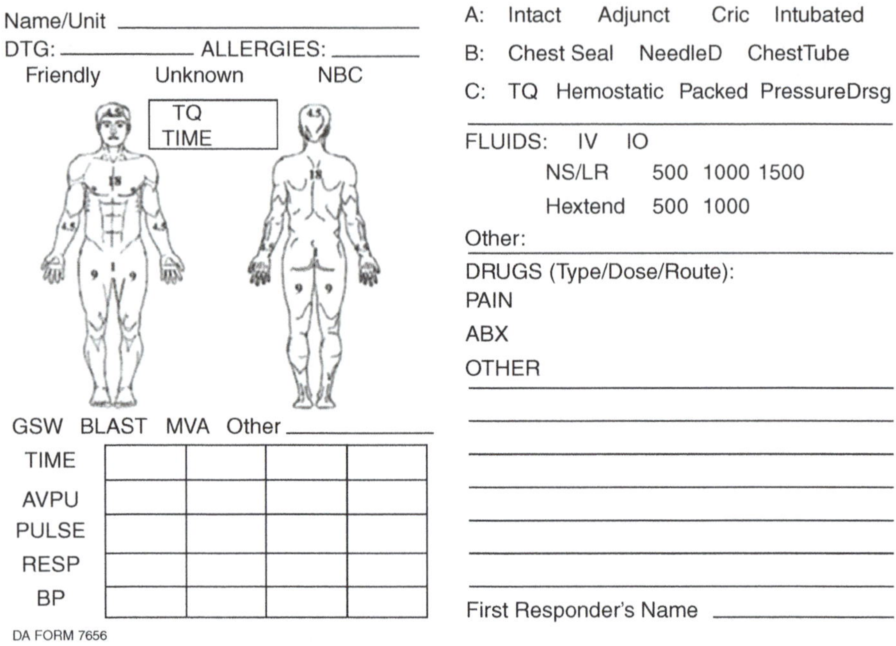
Name/Unit
DTG: ALLERGIES:
Friendly Unknown NBC
TQ TIME
GSW BLAST MVA Other

TIME				
AVPU				
PULSE				
RESP				
BP				

DA FORM 7656

A: Intact Adjunct Cric Intubated
B: Chest Seal NeedleD ChestTube
C: TQ Hemostatic Packed PressureDrsg
FLUIDS: IV IO
NS/LR 500 1000 1500
Hextend 500 1000
Other:
DRUGS (Type/Dose/Route):
PAIN
ABX
OTHER
First Responder's Name

Fig. 11.6 Casualty card, circa 2007

and consulting with the USAISR developed the Prehospital Trauma Registry (PHTR) in 2005 [31]. To capture critical data from the POI, the 75th Ranger Regiment utilized a casualty card with the necessary information (Fig. 11.6). The PHTR was modeled after existing trauma registries and was vital to the 75th Ranger Regiment's success in eliminating preventable death in combat.

There were five goals for the PHTR: (1) augment the commander's decision-making process, (2) reduce morbidity and mortality through force protection modifications and directed procurement, (3) validate and refine the commander's casualty response system, (4) evaluate current TCCC treatment strategies, and (5) guide needed modifications to unit medical and nonmedical personnel.

Kotwal and colleagues showed that 42% of tourniquets were applied by nonmedical personnel and, overall, 25% of all hemorrhages were controlled by individuals who were not medical providers [11]. The 75th Ranger Regiment's prehospital documentation system helped other units and the DoD recognize the importance of using prehospital data to improve combat casualty care, and it has been used a model for several areas of research interest. The casualty card became the standard for the DoD and has now been transformed into an updated DD Form 1380 (Fig. 11.7). The Joint Trauma System (JTS) adopted the PHTR and implemented it in January 2013 as part of the larger DoD Trauma Registry (DoDTR) – "a web-based data collection tool which supports US military performance improvement initiatives with global-wide collection and aggregation of combat casualty care epidemiology, treatments and outcomes" [32].

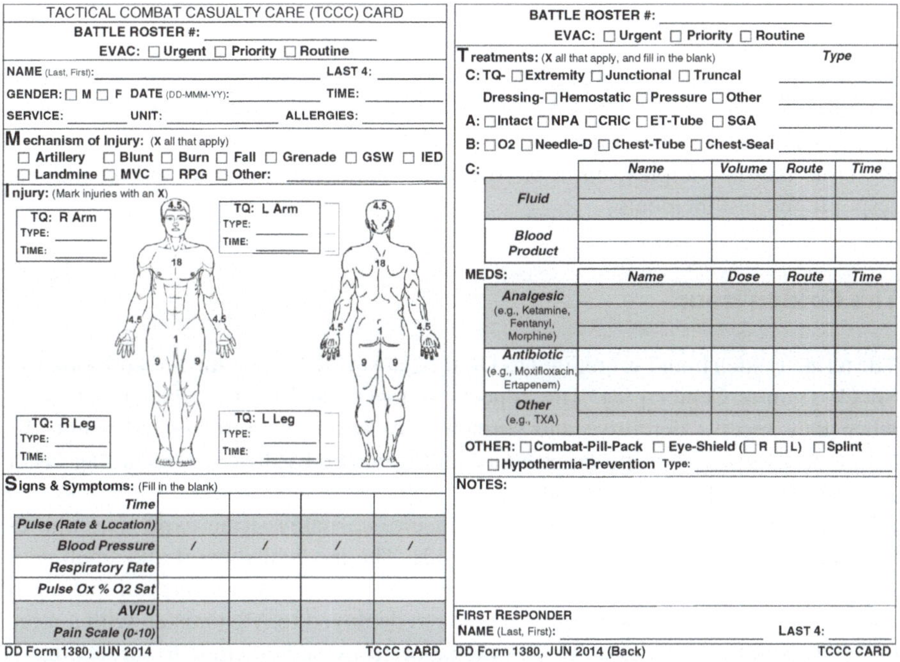
TACTICAL COMBAT CASUALTY CARE (TCCC) CARD

BATTLE ROSTER #: ____

EVAC: ☐ Urgent ☐ Priority ☐ Routine

NAME (Last, First): ____ LAST 4: ____

GENDER: ☐ M ☐ F DATE (DD-MMM-YY): ____ TIME: ____

SERVICE: ____ UNIT: ____ ALLERGIES: ____

Mechanism of Injury: (X all that apply)

☐ Artillery ☐ Blunt ☐ Burn ☐ Fall ☐ Grenade ☐ GSW ☐ IED ☐ Landmine ☐ MVC ☐ RPG ☐ Other: ____

Injury: (Mark injuries with an X)

Signs & Symptoms: (Fill in the blank)

Time				
Pulse (Rate & Location)				
Blood Pressure	/	/	/	/
Respiratory Rate				
Pulse Ox % O2 Sat				
AVPU				
Pain Scale (0-10)				

DD Form 1380, JUN 2014 TCCC CARD

BATTLE ROSTER #: ____

EVAC: ☐ Urgent ☐ Priority ☐ Routine

Treatments: (X all that apply, and fill in the blank) Type

C: TQ- ☐ Extremity ☐ Junctional ☐ Truncal ____

Dressing- ☐ Hemostatic ☐ Pressure ☐ Other ____

A: ☐ Intact ☐ NPA ☐ CRIC ☐ ET-Tube ☐ SGA ____

B: ☐ O2 ☐ Needle-D ☐ Chest-Tube ☐ Chest-Seal ____

C:

	Name	Volume	Route	Time
Fluid				
Blood Product				

MEDS:

	Name	Dose	Route	Time
Analgesic (e.g., Ketamine, Fentanyl, Morphine)				
Antibiotic (e.g., Moxifloxacin, Ertapenem)				
Other (e.g., TXA)				

OTHER: ☐ Combat-Pill-Pack ☐ Eye-Shield (☐ R ☐ L) ☐ Splint ☐ Hypothermia-Prevention Type: ____

NOTES:

FIRST RESPONDER NAME (Last, First): ____ LAST 4: ____

DD Form 1380, JUN 2014 (Back) TCCC CARD

Fig. 11.7 Department of Defense DD Form 1380

By collecting prehospital medical data in a centralized data registry, the medical community has the ability to learn, in near-real time, lessons from an ongoing conflict. The registry can be mined for specifics on interventions, levels of medical training, medical equipment, injury types, and wound patterns in order to rapidly recommend life-saving procedures for the prehospital environment. Thus, the DoDTR not only functions as a database for ongoing research and direction of medical equipment procurement but also serves to collect and distribute lessons learned.

As an example, the DoDTR has shown that a large percentage of potentially preventable wounds resulting in death are from junctional hemorrhage [33, 34], and the efficacy of junctional tourniquets in combat is still limited [35]. Junctional hemorrhage can be defined as bleeding from a site too close to the hips or shoulders to place a proximal tourniquet. Given this information, multiple agencies are directing research efforts to develop effective means of controlling junctional hemorrhage in the prehospital environment. The data on junctional wounds led to the rapid invention and distribution of multiple devices to prehospital providers in both the civilian and military settings. By collecting and sharing real-time data on prehospital injuries and treatments, a community can rapidly respond to and mitigate emerging medical threats in both civilian and military sectors.

Despite the recognized benefit of prehospital documentation, there is still a significant portion of data that goes uncollected. This gap was recognized early on and spurred the creation of the PHTR [36]. A recent study noted that, while 94.8% of patients had data from TCCC AARs ($N = 705$), only 27% of patients could be linked to the DoDTR due to missing identifiers [37]. Data capture and integrity is an ongoing issue that is complex, but it is critical for improving medical and operational response to blast incidents.

The Golden Hour

The term "golden hour" is credited to Dr. R Adams Cowley and the famed Baltimore Shock Trauma Center [38]. The concept is that casualties have better outcomes when they receive definitive and surgical care within 60 minutes. Although the "hour" itself was not proposed as a measure validated by data, it is clear that faster evacuation to definite care is associated with increased survival. Both Iraq and Afghanistan operations had a preponderance of casualties from explosive injuries with varying times to definitive care [39–42]. The medical support and small geographical area of Iraq enabled most casualties to be treated in a surgical facility in an hour or less. The fewer number of soldiers deployed to Afghanistan with a more difficult terrain caused delays in the evacuation from the battlefield to surgical facilities. The case fatality rate (CFR) had been decreasing slowly over the course of the conflict, but as the surge was implemented in 2009, there was a small increase in CFR [43]. Subsequently, Secretary of Defense Robert M. Gates implemented the Golden Hour Policy (GHP) mandating all military operations would be within a 60-minute evacuation time to surgical care. At the time of implementation, the CFR was 13.7 and decreased to 7.6 after the GHP was implemented [43]. This policy implementation with accompanying scientific study and publication in the medical literature further solidified the need to push surgical support as close to the POI as possible in order to reduce mortality. The findings of Kotwal et al. were reexamined, and similar outcomes were observed, so their conclusions remained unaltered [44]. More recent data from the USAISR would suggest that achieving even faster transportation times could further reduce potentially preventable deaths [45].

Blood Far Forward

Once again in warfare, the US military has learned the benefits of using blood transfusions far forward. Despite the clear knowledge of the primacy of blood products for treatment of hemorrhagic shock, the US military entered the War on Terror armed with crystalloids for resuscitation, despite evidence that crystalloids were inadequate and possibly dangerous. As a result, hetastarch colloid fluids were recommended and carried as a primary treatment for hemorrhagic shock. Early on, blood use was limited to medical facilities with rare transfusions in the field or en-route during evacuation to a medical facility. In 2014, the CoTCCC changed the

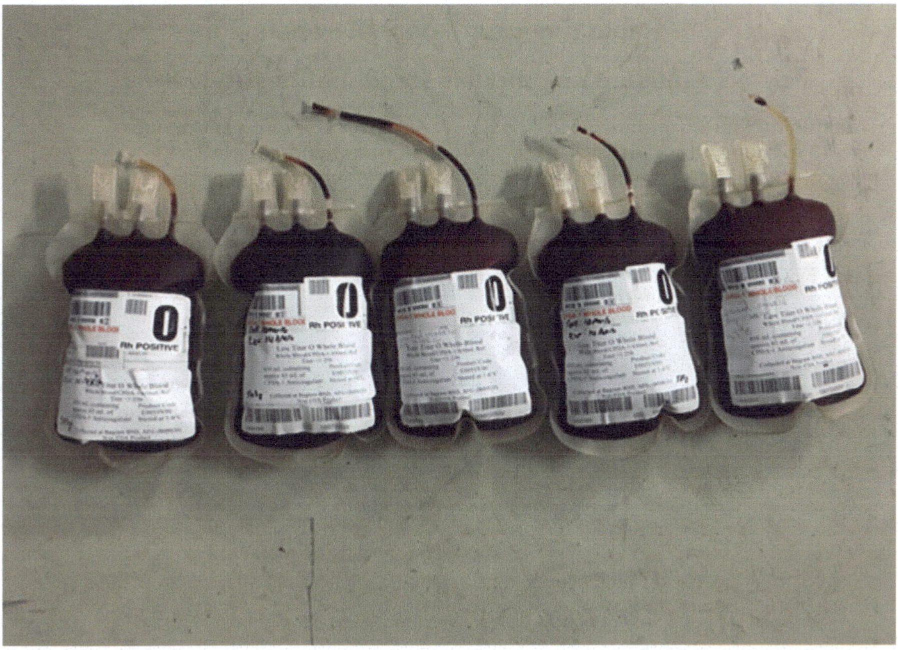

Fig. 11.8 Low-titer group-O whole blood collected at Bagram Airfield, Afghanistan, from the 75th Ranger Regiment's "ROLO" program. (Photograph courtesy of Andrew D. Fisher)

guidelines to recommend whole blood at the POI [46]. As the war progressed, adaptive units realized the clear benefit of blood products for hemorrhagic shock and developed methods to deliver blood to the POI [47].

In 2016, the 75th Ranger Regiment implemented an "O low titer" universal donor program and began carrying low-titer group-O whole blood (LTOWB). Ranger support personnel serve as donors for pre-mission blood collection and prescreened donors are identified within the operational teams to be available for a "walking blood bank" at the POI (Fig. 11.8). During the writing of this chapter, approximately 20 transfusions of LTOWB had been given at the POI with 17 surviving to surgical care (unpublished data). LTOWB does not have a strict definition; however, for the US military, it is defined as blood group O with anti-A and anti-B IgM titers <1:256. The titer limits are based on data from World War II [48]. The use of blood far forward was further reinforced in Shackelford's study where it was observed that providing blood within 13 minutes of medical evacuation (MEDEVAC) take off provided a 20-fold survival benefit (Fig. 11.9) [42]. The success of using blood products, particularly whole blood, for resuscitation of critical trauma patients in the out of hospital setting has spread to multiple civilian trauma systems as they look for ways to increase survivability in patients with hemorrhagic shock [49–51].

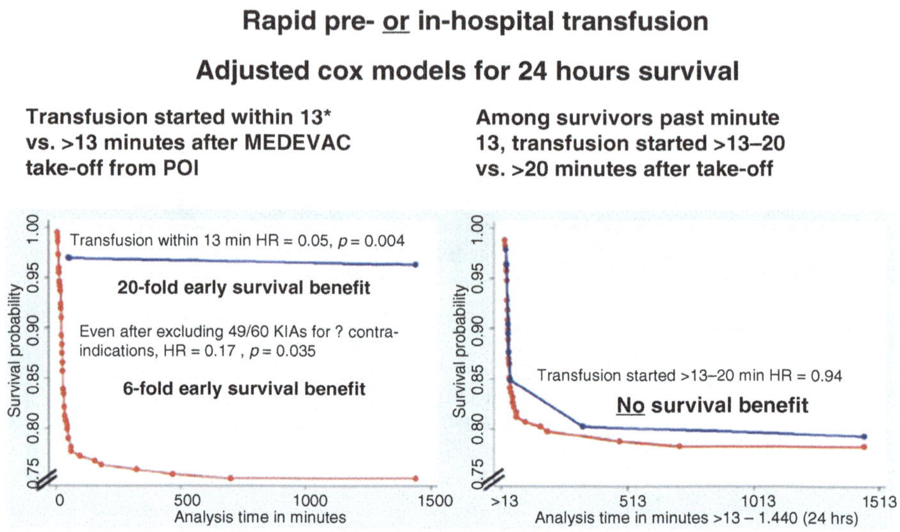

Fig. 11.9 Impact of prehospital blood transfusions on mortality. (Adapted from Shackelford, et al. JTS 2016. Courtesy of Col. Andre Cap)

Traumatic Brain Injury

IED use in the current conflict has led to large numbers of patients suffering traumatic brain injury (TBI). TBI is particularly devastating in the setting of blast injury, as it is commonly seen in conjunction with moderate to severe injury severity scores [2, 39, 52–54] and creates the deadly combination of TBI and hemorrhagic shock. Blood pressure goals for resuscitation from hemorrhagic shock are typically quite low in order to minimize additional bleeding and to facilitate clot formation in noncompressible hemorrhage [47, 55, 56]. This presents a quandary when combined with TBI as the goal is to keep perfusion to the brain as normal as possible. One method to deal with this predicament is to use whole blood for resuscitation, where target blood pressures can be increased due to the hemostatic functionality of whole blood [57].

Overall goals in patients with blast-induced TBI are to avoid “second hit” events of hypoxia by maintaining or supplementing oxygenation and hypotension by keeping a goal systolic blood pressure above 110 mmHg to maintain cerebral perfusion pressure, and to maintain the end-tidal CO_2 ($ETCO_2$) near 40 torr [58]. Although casualties with hemorrhagic shock and TBI present a significantly complex predicament, utilization of whole blood for resuscitation, avoidance of intubation (if possible) while still avoiding hypoxia, and monitoring $ETCO_2$ with a portable device can significantly assist the provider at the point of injury.

Conclusion

The past 17 years of combat have rapidly led to an ever-increasing body of knowledge in the medical treatment of combat casualties in the prehospital setting. The rapid increase in blast injuries secondary to IED use in combat has served to further amplify these lessons. Although the military combat setting is unique in many aspects, the seven best practices in this chapter can be applied across the civilian setting as well. Creating a body of knowledge with expert input and timely sharing of information enables a responsive, learning trauma system that readily adapts to emerging injury patterns in order to save lives and decrease morbidity.

Blast injuries typically produce devastating trauma. Early aggressive use of tourniquets, management of junctional hemorrhage, and pelvic binding when the lower extremities are involved can have a significant impact on survival. Recording and analyzing data from the prehospital environment produces rapid and meaningful results in research, equipment, and techniques for saving lives in the setting where the most preventable and potentially preventable death occurs.

Medical training for nonmedical personnel increased survivability by placing life-saving interventions closest to the point of injury with the greatest effect. Time to definitive surgical care in blast patients is paramount, so any trauma system should continually strive to reduce the "time to steel." Blood, especially whole blood, is by far the resuscitation fluid of choice in patients with hemorrhagic shock. Blast injuries produce a significant amount of TBI and treatment must be geared toward preventing hypoxia, preventing hypotension, and maintaining adequate $ETCO_2$ levels.

Key Points

- Blast injuries typically produce devastating soft tissue and extremity trauma.
- Aggressive use of tourniquets and hemostatic dressings and devices can help decease mortality in blast wounds.
- Nonmedical personnel can have the biggest impact with simple life-saving skills.
- Documentation not only provides real- to near-time changes that help save lives but also maintains a record for future conflicts.
- Since casualties hemorrhage blood, whole blood should be used for resuscitation.
- The goals of TBI should be to prevent hypoxia and hypotension and to maintain adequate $ETCO_2$ levels.
- Quick access to surgical care for the severely injured and wounded should always be paramount.

Pitfalls

- Failure to document medical interventions and lessons learned. Adequate documentation is essential for patient management in the continuum of care and future improvements in trauma management and the overall trauma system.
- Failure to train and integrate nonmedical providers into MASCAL plans. The duration of severe hemorrhage correlates with mortality. Faster hemorrhage control saves lives. Bystanders are always first on scene in blast events; they must be trained and empowered to act.
- Failure to institutionalize early and liberal application of tourniquets for hemorrhage. Tourniquets are fast to apply and save lives in arterial extremity hemorrhage. They should be a core component of the hemorrhage control strategy for routine operations and MASCALs.

Pearls

- Development and implementation of a fresh whole blood transfusion program, such that the ideal resuscitation fluid for hemorrhagic shock can be as far forward as possible.
- Mandating that all assigned personnel are trained in TCCC and ready to deliver life-saving care at or near the POI. Sustainment and just-in-time training are also essential, as many skills are perishable if not used routinely.
- Maintaining an assessment and validation process for all assigned medics to ensure that all assigned medics are qualified to serve and provide care at the highest level possible and to help identify those who may need additional training before deployment.

References

1. Penn-Barwell JG, Roberts SA, Midwinter MJ, Bishop JR. Improved survival in UK combat casualties from Iraq and Afghanistan: 2003–2012. J Trauma Acute Care Surg. 2015;78(5):1014–20.
2. Eastridge BJ, Mabry RL, Seguin P, Cantrell J, Tops T, Uribe P, et al. Death on the battlefield (2001–2011): implications for the future of combat casualty care. J Trauma. 2012;73(6, Supplement 5):S431–S7.
3. Butler FK. Tactical combat casualty care: beginnings. Wilderness Environ Med. 2017;28(2S):S12–S7.
4. Butler FK, Bennett B, Wedmore CI. Tactical combat casualty care and wilderness medicine: advancing trauma care in austere environments. Emerg Med Clin North Am. 2017;35(2):391–407.

5. Butler FK, Haymann J, Butler EG. Tactical combat casualty care in special operations. Mil Med. 1996;161(Suppl 3)
6. Holcomb JB, McMullin NR, Pearse L, Caruso J, Wade CE, Oetjen-Gerdes L, et al. Causes of death in U.S. Special Operations Forces in the global war on terrorism: 2001–2004. Ann Surg. 2007;245(6):986–91.
7. Office of the Under Secretary of Defense for Personnel and Readiness. DoD instruction 1322.24, Medical Readiness Training (MRT). In: The pentagon. Washington, DC: The Pentagon. p. 2018.
8. Savage E, Forestier C, Withers N, Tien H, Pannell D. Tactical combat casualty care in the Canadian Forces: lessons learned from the Afghan war. Can J Surg. 2011;54(6):S118–23.
9. Butler FK Jr, Holcomb JB, Giebner SD, McSwain NE, Bagian J. Tactical combat casualty care 2007: evolving concepts and battlefield experience. Mil Med. 2007;172(11 Suppl):1–19.
10. Kragh JF Jr, Walters TJ, Baer DG, Fox CJ, Wade CE, Salinas J, et al. Survival with emergency tourniquet use to stop bleeding in major limb trauma. Ann Surg. 2009;249(1):1–7.
11. Kotwal RS, Montgomery HR, Kotwal BM, Champion HR, Butler FK Jr, Mabry RL, et al. Eliminating preventable death on the battlefield. Arch Surg. 2011;146(12):1350–8.
12. Kelly JF, Ritenour AE, McLaughlin DF, Bagg KA, Apodaca AN, Mallak CT, et al. Injury severity and causes of death from Operation Iraqi Freedom and Operation Enduring Freedom: 2003–2004 versus 2006. J Trauma. 2008;64(2 Suppl):S21–6.
13. Butler FK Jr, Blackbourne LH. Battlefield trauma care then and now: a decade of Tactical Combat Casualty Care. J Trauma Acute Care Surg. 2012;73(6 Suppl 5):S395–402.
14. Irizzary D. Training NATO Special Forces Medical Personnel: opportunities in technology-enabled training systems for skill acquisition and maintenance. J Spec Oper Med. 2013; supplement https://www.jsomonline.org/NATOSupp/mobile/index.html#p=2.
15. Jacobs LM, McSwain NE Jr, Rotondo MF, Wade D, Fabbri W, Eastman AL, et al. Improving survival from active shooter events: the Hartford consensus. J Trauma Acute Care Surg. 2013;74(6):1399–400.
16. Pons PT, Jerome J, McMullen J, Manson J, Robinson J, Chapleau W. The Hartford consensus on active shooters: implementing the continuum of prehospital trauma response. J Emerg Med. 2015;49(6):878–85.
17. Scerbo MH, Mumm JP, Gates K, Love JD, Wade CE, Holcomb JB, et al. Safety and appropriateness of tourniquets in 105 civilians. Prehosp Emerg Care. 2016;20(6):712–22.
18. Zietlow JM, Zietlow SP, Morris DS, Berns KS, Jenkins DH. Prehospital use of hemostatic bandages and tourniquets: translation from military experience to implementation in civilian trauma care. J Spec Oper Med. 2015;15(2):48–53.
19. Butler FK. Two Decades of saving lives on the battlefield: Tactical Combat Casualty Care turns 20. Mil Med. 2017;182(3):e1563–e8.
20. Ramasamy A, Harrisson SE, Clasper JC, Stewart MP. Injuries from roadside improvised explosive devices. J Trauma. 2008;65(4):910–4.
21. Owens BD, Kragh JF Jr, Wenke JC, Macaitis J, Wade CE, Holcomb JB. Combat wounds in Operation Iraqi Freedom and Operation Enduring Freedom. J Trauma. 2008;64(2):295–9.
22. DeBruyne NF. American war and military operations casualties: lists and statistics, September 14, 2018. Washington, DC: Congressional Research Service, Library of Congress; 2018.
23. Kragh JF Jr, Walters TJ, Westmoreland T, Miller RM, Mabry RL, Kotwal RS, et al. Tragedy into drama: an american history of tourniquet use in the current war. J Spec Oper Med. 2013;13(3):5–25.
24. Montgomery HR, Hammesfahr R, Fisher AD, et al. 2019 Recommended limb tourniquets in tactical combat casualty care. J Spec Oper Med. 2019;19(4):27–50.
25. Cross AM, Davis C, Penn-Barwell J, Taylor DM, De Mello WF, Matthews JJ. The incidence of pelvic fractures with traumatic lower limb amputation in modern warfare due to improvised explosive devices. J R Nav Med Serv. 2014;100(2):152–6.
26. Ampula RL. Origins of the combat lifesaver. AMEDD Historian. 2015;9(Spring 2015):11–3.

27. Kotwal RS, Montgomery HR, Miles EA, Conklin CC, Hall MT, McChrystal SA. Leadership and a casualty response system for eliminating preventable death. J Trauma Acute Care Surg. 2017;82(Supp 1):S9–S15.
28. Votel JL. Killed in Action (KIA) reduction initiative. In: United States Central Command. 2017. https://www.jsomonline.org/TCCC/06%20TCCC%20Reference%20Documents/Gen%20Votel%20Letter%20171106%20-%20TCCC%20Training.pdf. Accessed 10 Aug 2019.
29. National Academies of Sciences, Engineering, Medicine. A National Trauma Care System: Integrating Military and Civilian Trauma Systems to Achieve Zero Preventable Deaths After Injury. Berwick D, Downey A, Cornett E, editors. Washington, DC: The National Academies Press; 2016.
30. Fisher AD, Carius BM, Lacroix J, Dodge PM, Dodd J, Soderlund E, et al. National Stop the Bleed Day: the impact of a social media campaign on the Stop the Bleed program. J Trauma Acute Care Surg. 2019;87(1):S40–S3.
31. Kotwal RS, Montgomery HR, Mechler KK. A prehospital trauma registry for Tactical Combat Casualty Care. US Army Med Dep J. 2011:15–7.
32. Joint Trauma System: The Department of Defense Center of Excellence for Trauma. Registries. http://jts.amedd.army.mil/index.cfm/data/registries. Published 2018. Accessed 13 Nov 2018.
33. Kotwal RS, Butler FK, Gross KR, Kheirabadi BS, Baer DG, Dubick MA, et al. Management of junctional hemorrhage in Tactical Combat Casualty Care: TCCC Guidelines? Proposed Change 13-03. J Spec Oper Med. 2013;13(4):85–93.
34. Kotwal RS, Butler FK Jr. Junctional hemorrhage control for Tactical Combat Casualty Care. Wilderness Environ Med. 2017;28(2S):S33–S8.
35. Schauer SG, April MD, Fisher AD, Cunningham CW, Gurney J. Junctional Tourniquet Use During Combat Operations in Afghanistan: The Prehospital Trauma Registry Experience. J Spec Oper Med. 2018;18(2):71–4.
36. Eastridge BJ, Mabry RL, Blackbourne LH, Butler FK. We don't know what we don't know: prehospital data in combat casualty care. US Army Med Dep J. 2011:11–4.
37. Schauer SG, April MD, Naylor JF, Oliver JJ, Cunningham CW, Fisher AD, et al. A descriptive analysis of data from the Department of Defense Joint Trauma System Prehospital Trauma Registry. US Army Med Dep J. 2017;3–17(Oct–Dec):92–7.
38. Lerner EB, Moscati RM. The Golden Hour: scientific fact or medical "urban legend"? Acad Emerg Med. 2001;8(7):758–60.
39. Eskridge SL, Macera CA, Galarneau MR, Holbrook TL, Woodruff SI, MacGregor AJ, et al. Injuries from combat explosions in Iraq: injury type, location, and severity. Injury. 2012;43(10):1678–82.
40. Stannard A, Morrison JJ, Scott DJ, Ivatury RA, Ross JD, Rasmussen TE. The epidemiology of noncompressible torso hemorrhage in the wars in Iraq and Afghanistan. J Trauma Acute Care Surg. 2013;74(3):830–4.
41. Howard JT, Kotwal RS, Stern CA, Janak JC, Mazuchowski EL, Butler FK, et al. Use of combat casualty care data to assess the US military trauma system during the Afghanistan and Iraq conflicts, 2001–2017. JAMA Surg. 2019;154(7):600–8.
42. Shackelford SA, Del Junco DJ, Powell-Dunford N, Mazuchowski EL, Howard JT, Kotwal RS, et al. Association of prehospital blood product transfusion during medical evacuation of combat casualties in Afghanistan with acute and 30-day survival. JAMA. 2017;318(16):1581–91.
43. Kotwal RS, Howard JT, Orman JA, Tarpey BW, Bailey JA, Champion HR, et al. The effect of a Golden Hour Policy on the morbidity and mortality of combat casualties. JAMA Surg. 2016;151(1):15–24.
44. Howard JT, Kotwal RS, Santos-Lazada AR, Martin MJ, Stockinger ZT. Reexamination of a battlefield trauma Golden Hour Policy. J Trauma Acute Care Surg. 2018;84(1):11–8.
45. Kotwal RS, Scott LLF, Janak JC, Tarpey BW, Howard JT, Mazuchowski EL, et al. The effect of prehospital transport time, injury severity, and blood transfusion on survival of US military casualties in Iraq. J Trauma Acute Care Surg. 2018;85(1S Suppl 2):S112–S21.

46. Butler FK, Holcomb JB, Schreiber MA, Kotwal RS, Jenkins DA, Champion HR, et al. Fluid Resuscitation for hemorrhagic shock in Tactical Combat Casualty Care: TCCC Guidelines Change 14-01 – 2 June 2014. J Spec Oper Med. 2014;14(3):30–55.
47. Fisher AD, Miles EA, Cap AP, Strandenes G, Kane SF. Tactical damage control resuscitation. Mil Med. 2015;180(8):869–75.
48. Berseus O, Boman K, Nessen SC, Westerberg LA. Risks of hemolysis due to anti-A and anti-B caused by the transfusion of blood or blood components containing ABO-incompatible plasma. Transfusion. 2013;53 Suppl 1:114S–23S.
49. McGinity AC, Zhu CS, Greebon L, Xenakis E, Waltman E, Epley E, et al. Pre-hospital low titer cold stored whole blood: philosophy for ubiquitous utilization of O positive product for emergency use in hemorrhage due to injury. J Trauma Acute Care Surg. 2018;84(6S Suppl 1):S115–S9.
50. Dodge M, Thompson D, Bank EA, Nealy W, Fisher AD. Whole blood in EMS may save lives. J Emerg Med Serv. 2018:50–5.
51. Arefieva CAL, Chen B, Redman TT, Fisher AD. The use of low titer group O whole blood in emergency medicine. EM Resident. 2018;45(5):32–3.
52. Schoenfeld AJ, Dunn JC, Bader JO, Belmont PJ Jr. The nature and extent of war injuries sustained by combat specialty personnel killed and wounded in Afghanistan and Iraq, 2003–2011. J Trauma Acute Care Surg. 2013;75(2):287–91.
53. Eastridge BJ, Hardin M, Cantrell J, Oetjen-Gerdes L, Zubko T, Mallak C, et al. Died of wounds on the battlefield: causation and implications for improving combat casualty care. J Trauma. 2011;71(1 Suppl):S4–8.
54. Eastridge BJ, Owsley J, Sebesta J, Beekley A, Wade C, Wildzunas R, et al. Admission physiology criteria after injury on the battlefield predict medical resource utilization and patient mortality. J Trauma. 2006;61(4):820–3.
55. Fisher AD, Washbum G, Powell D, Callaway DW, Miles EA, Brown J, et al. Damage control resuscitation in prolonged field care. J Spec Oper Med. 2018;18(3):109–19.
56. Cap AP, Pidcoke HF, Spinella P, Strandenes G, Borgman MA, Schreiber M, et al. Damage control resuscitation. Mil Med. 2018;183(suppl 2):36–43.
57. Butler F, Holcomb JB, Shackelford S, Barbabella S, Bailey J, Baker J, et al. Advanced Resuscitative Care in Tactical Combat Casualty Care: TCCC Guidelines Change 18-01. J Spec Oper Med. 2019;18(4):37–55.
58. Spaite DW, Bobrow BJ, Keim SM, Barnhart B, Chikani V, Gaither JB, et al. Association of Statewide Implementation of the prehospital traumatic brain injury treatment guidelines with patient survival following traumatic brain injury: the Excellence in Prehospital Injury Care (EPIC) study. JAMA Surg. 2019;154(7):e191152.

First Responders: Clinical Care of Blast Trauma in the Prehospital Setting

12

Jason R. Pickett, Joshua R. Todd, and Ricky C. Kue

Introduction

The clinical care of blast injuries poses a challenge for prehospital Emergency Medical Services (EMS) providers. The complexities of blast trauma arise from both the mechanisms of injury and resultant pathophysiology. For nearly two decades, the United States and coalition partners have engaged in combat operations in the Middle East and Southwest Asia in response to the World Trade Center and Pentagon attacks in 2001. Lessons from the wars in Iraq and Afghanistan provide significant understanding and insight into the traumatic injuries resulting from explosive effects. The Joint Theater Trauma Registry reports that from 2001 to 2005, explosive mechanisms resulted in nearly 80% of documented injuries, the highest rate documented in US combat history [1]. Although explosive blast trauma has typically been thought of as occurring only in combat, blast injuries can occur in civilian settings in the form of intentional terrorist attacks and accidental home and industrial explosions.

Lessons described from civilian terrorist bombing incidents, such as those in Madrid, London, and Boston, have provided insights into the common challenges faced in dealing with these situations that have parallels to the military experience [2–4]. Common issues arising in the civilian response, such as mass-casualty planning

J. R. Pickett (✉)
Austin/Travis County EMS System, Austin, TX, USA
e-mail: jason.pickett@austintexas.gov

J. R. Todd
City of Austin Emergency Medical Services, Austin, TX, USA

R. C. Kue
Medical Corps, Vermont Army National Guard, Colchester, VT, USA

Boston University School of Medicine, Boston, MA, USA

D. W. Callaway, J. L. Burstein (eds.), *Operational and Medical Management of Explosive and Blast Incidents*, https://doi.org/10.1007/978-3-030-40655-4_12

and preparation, appropriate use of personal protective equipment (PPE), limitations in the ability to perform triage, and the rapid scene clearance of critically ill patients to definitive care, are valuable lessons for future planning and best practices.

Patterns of Injuries and Causes of Death

Although blast incidents create significant tactical and operational considerations for EMS first responders, the clinical consequences of the blast incident itself pose a unique medical problem, which requires specific considerations during patient care. Bombing incidents produce unique patterns of injury that, if not recognized by prehospital medical personnel, could result in increased patient morbidity and mortality.

The ways in which the human body interacts with an explosion are highly complex. Explosive injuries have traditionally been classified into: (1) primary blast injuries, which are injuries due solely to the overpressure of the blast wave; (2) secondary blast injuries, which comprise ballistic trauma from device fragmentation, added shrapnel, or debris from the environment; (3) tertiary blast injuries as a result of displacement of the victim; and (4) quaternary explosive injuries due to nonpressure effects that include burns, inhalations, and toxins [5, 6]. Collateral injuries can occur from motor vehicle crashes, building collapse, structural fires, and exacerbation of chronic illnesses.

High-explosive detonations generate a shock wave formed by the instantaneous expansion of gas. As the wave travels through distance and time, it rapidly loses its pressure and velocity. The physics of a blast wave as it interacts with the surface of a human body results in specific injury patterns due to the two effects of energy translated internally: stress waves and shear waves. Stress waves result in disruption of air-tissue interfaces when moving through water-density tissues in various directions around air spaces, thereby stretching and tearing structures at those boundaries [7]. Shear waves are typically developed as a result of the stress wave, traveling perpendicular to stress waves and resulting in sudden, tangential stretching forces on displaced subsurface body tissues [8]. The pathophysiologic effects on the body result from the consequences of extreme pressure differentials developed at body surfaces.

The most common anatomical location of primary blast injury is the tympanic membrane, requiring as little as 5 psi above atmospheric pressure for rupture. The second most common site of primary blast injury is the lungs and occurs at much higher overpressures. Blast lung injury (BLI) can be highly lethal. In published data, evidence of primary BLI was present in 17–47% of those who died from explosions and up to 44% of hospitalized patients; nearly 71% of critically ill patients show evidence of pulmonary injury [9, 10]. Lung injuries occurring from primary blast mechanisms include pulmonary contusions, pneumothorax, and air embolism. Onset of clinically detectable pulmonary damage can be delayed from time of exposure. Rapid onset of symptoms such as dyspnea, hypoxia, and need for ventilatory support tends to predict poor outcomes [5].

When determining the likelihood of significant primary blast injuries, prehospital providers should consider a few factors related to the incident. The likelihood of increasing injury severity with closed-space detonations is due the ability for blast waves to "bounce" and reflect off walls increasing in pressure at surfaces resulting in additive effects. When evaluating the patient, the presence of traumatic amputation should serve as a marker to look for occult explosive injuries to the central nervous system, thorax, and abdomen [5].

In the absence of obvious external trauma, triage is more difficult. Though frequently discussed, the presence of a ruptured tympanic membrane does not accurately predict whether other primary blast injuries are present or likely to develop [11]. Accordingly, prehospital providers should not perform otoscopic examination to conditionally exclude the presence of occult BLI in the absence of other symptoms such as respiratory distress, dyspnea, or chest pain.

An analysis of injuries among patients presenting to the closest hospital to the 2004 Madrid Train Bombings showed that 28.5% of patients were hospitalized for >24 hours—12% of all casualties (32.5% of those hospitalized) were in critical condition. Two died within minutes of arrival and 3 more died during hospitalization, bringing the critical mortality rate to just over 17%. Of the 243 patients with moderate-to-severe trauma, 40% had chest injuries, 36% had "shrapnel" wounds, 18% had fractures, 18% had eye injuries, 12% had head injuries, and 5% had abdominal trauma [12].

Scene Safety and Secondary Attacks

Scene safety is a paramount concern for rescuers in a bombing incident. Attackers may place secondary devices intended to injure first responders, as was done in the Atlanta Northside Family Planning Services Clinic bombing of 1996. Blasts may cause fire directly or may disrupt gas lines, posing additional fire and explosion risks. Explosions may destabilize structures, thus risking collapse and increasing risk to first responders. For example, a nurse who responded to the Murrah Federal Building bombing in Oklahoma City was killed by falling debris [13].

Secondary devices are a frequent concern among responders to bombing incidents [3, 14]. While use of explosives in civilian settings has increased markedly over the past few decades, with a fourfold increase worldwide between 1999 and 2006, the number of civilian bombings with secondary devices remains small [10]. Of the 36,110 bombing incidents in the United States between 1983 and 2002, no more than five involved a secondary device [15].

Staging to await clearance by other responders such as police is one tactic used by many responding organizations. However, this delays potentially life-saving interventions for victims that require care and may directly increase mortality [16]. Due to the complexities of explosive incident response, it is highly unlikely that law enforcement will be able to rapidly clear a blast site and determine if it is safe for additional responders within a meaningful time frame. Explosive detection

K-9 teams remain the most effective means of rapidly locating potential explosive devices, but they have their own limitations such as availability and scene complexity.

In the event of a risk of scene hazardous-material or radioactive contamination, time, distance, and shielding must be used to minimize risk to responders and victims alike. Responders should minimize time spent in the incident area, maximizing staging and operational distance from the impact area, and utilize shielding in the form of terrain features, hard buildings, and personal protective equipment. Clinical interventions must be balanced against the risk to providers and casualties from additional explosions or consequences of explosions (e.g., building collapse). Risks of prehospital operations in the hot, warm, and cold zones are discussed in Chap. 15.

Decontamination

Chemical, biological, and radiological (CBR) dispersal threats are, fortunately, rare in bombing incidents but must be considered. In 1995, members of a cult perpetrated five coordinated attacks on the Tokyo subway system with a nerve agent known as sarin [17]. Chlorine gas was reportedly used by Islamic State militants against Iraqi security forces [18]. The combination of chemical and explosive events is technically challenging for intentional attacks, but more commonplace in industrial accidents.

CBR contamination complicates response to and care for victims of bombing events significantly. First, responders must recognize a CBR event. This may occur through observation of a release of material, receipt of a specific threat, or recognition of a cluster of effects among victims [19]. To prevent secondary contamination and exposure of healthcare personnel, victims require decontamination, which is a procedure that, under the best of conditions, is laborious and time-consuming. This is discussed in greater detail in Chap. 42.

Triage

No triage system has demonstrated superiority over another in the literature, and many valid systems exist to include START, JumpSTART, SALT, and others. Chapter 13 details more thoroughly prehospital scene management and triage. Several mass-casualty incidents and training exercises have demonstrated the limitations of existing triage systems in real-world events [20]. In some cases, patients in disasters who arrive at a nearby hospital do so by means other than EMS transportation and bypass field triage Schemes [21, 22]. Casualties may be transported to the hospital by law enforcement or by other citizens present at the incident [23, 24].

Creating casualty collection points (CCPs) may delay transport to definitive care [25]. Delays in transport are potentially harmful to trauma patients who require surgical intervention and expose rescuers to the potential of secondary attack intended to harm responders to the incident. Concentrating on detailed sorting and tracking of patients takes additional time at the scene and may not significantly help their care, unless robust field-treatment capabilities can be rapidly established. One successful example of aggressive prehospital care occurred after the simultaneous bombings of four commuter trains in Madrid in 2004. The coordinated actions enabled evaluation, treatment, and discharge of victims with minor injuries away from overwhelmed nearby hospitals. After the Madrid train bombings of 2004, the closest facility received over 270 patients in the first 2.5 hours following the blast [26].

Some prehospital systems—notably Israel—defer full triage of casualties at mass-casualty incidents and employ basic "primary triage" schemes in order to minimize time spent on scene at an incident [27]. What is important in any triage scheme is that it be performed rapidly and that limited life-saving interventions such as hemorrhage control, airway management, and decompression of tension pneumothorax be performed immediately upon encountering the casualty and not deferred for rescuers to perform at higher echelons of care.

Clinical Management

Rapid transportation to a capable receiving hospital is a priority of prehospital care, but doing so prior to or without performing certain life-saving interventions could result in a poorer outcome than for a patient who had correctable life-threatening injuries addressed in the field.

The Committee for Tactical Emergency Casualty Care (C-TECC) has created standards for immediate management of trauma casualties for providers ranging from the layperson to professional rescuers and receiving hospital personnel [28]. C-TECC has adopted "MARCHE" as a memory aid for priorities of tasks in dealing with severely injured patients. The acronym stands for massive bleeding, airway, respirations, circulation, hypothermia, and everything else. United States Air Force Pararescue Technicians, have expanded this as a checklist with the mnemonic "MARCH-PAWS" which includes massive bleeding, airway, respirations, circulation, hypothermia, pain, antibiotics, wounds, and splinting [29].

Hemorrhage Control

Massive hemorrhage is the leading cause of preventable death in battlefield trauma [30]. Serious bleeding can render the casualty unconscious in less than a minute, with shock resulting quickly and irreversible shock occurring before arrival of professional responders. Tissue damage from blast trauma can be extensive with large wounds, wide areas of exposed soft tissue, and partial or complete amputations of extremities. A study published by Ashkenazi et al. of blast injured patients in a terrorist attack, described 9 of 66 patients that suffered extremity wounds as a sole cause of hemorrhagic shock and required a mean of 10 units of packed red blood cell transfusion in the first 24 hours of care [31]. A study by Heldenberg et al. of victims of terror-related explosions found that patients with vascular trauma had higher injury severity scores, longer admissions, and a mortality rate five times that of their counterparts without vascular trauma [32]. Kauvar et al. showed that isolated lower-extremity vascular trauma carries a 10% mortality rate [33]. Management of external hemorrhage is a key "life skill" for which medical first responders should possess expertise and all community members should possess competence [34–36].

Extremity Injuries

Significant extremity hemorrhage should be managed with immediate application of direct pressure. If direct pressure is insufficient to control hemorrhage, or if there is an amputation or near-amputation, a tourniquet should be applied to the most proximal area of the extremity [37]. EMS providers should remove the contents of pockets or tactical equipment to prevent interference with the tourniquet. However, generally, in the immediate phase, time should not be taken to remove clothing prior to tourniquet application. A rescuer should never delay application of a tourniquet over concerns about tissue damage or ischemia being caused by the tourniquet. Significant tourniquet complications such as limb loss are exceedingly rare, whereas external hemorrhage may kill a patient in minutes [38, 39].

Several commercial tourniquets are available that have been independently validated by the Committee on Tactical Combat Casualty Care (CoTCCC) and have seen successful use in combat theaters. These tourniquets have been found to be reliable, effective, and easy to use [40, 41]. Commercial tourniquets have advantages over improvised tourniquets due to their ease of use, rapid application, and general reliability when applied properly [42]. If no commercial tourniquet is available, one may be fashioned from suitably wide fabric (2 inches is an ideal width), a rigid windlass to increase tension around the tourniquet to occlude proximal vessels, and a locking mechanism [43].

Junctional Hemorrhage

Wounds to the neck, groin, and axilla (i.e., at the junctions with the torso) are often not amenable to tourniquet application. These injuries should be managed by application of direct pressure and then packing of the wound with dressing material. If sterile gauze is not immediately available, then any fabric can be substituted to gain control of bleeding. Infection or additional contamination of the wound with non-sterile dressing material are distant concerns to the immediate priority of hemorrhage control. Dressings impregnated with hemostatic agents may assist in clot formation; however, wound packing should not be delayed if hemostatic agents are not immediately available [44]. Several commercially available junctional tourniquets now exist that can help with control of hemorrhage that is too proximal for application of a tourniquet. These devices are relatively new to the market and comparative data are still forthcoming.

Noncompressible Hemorrhage

Internal hemorrhage requires immediate surgical management, which is typically unavailable in the field setting. For these patients, adequate volume resuscitation with blood products, reversal of shock physiology, and rapid transport to an appropriate surgical facility are key. Detection of those patients with uncontrolled hemorrhage in the field may expedite triage to surgical management. Point-of-care ultrasonography may be useful to identify intra-abdominal hemorrhage, estimate fluid status, and detect other potentially life-threatening issues such as cardiac tamponade or tension pneumothorax [45, 46].

Emergent thoracotomy and cross-clamping of the aorta may, in rare cases, buy time for the casualty in the field; however, scant literature supports this in the prehospital setting outside of individual case reports [47–49].

Resuscitative endovascular balloon occlusion of the aorta (REBOA) is a percutaneous procedure whereby a balloon is placed through the femoral artery into the proximal or distal aorta, limiting blood flow to the lower part of the body and slowing the rate of hemorrhage. A study by Henry et al. showed that 10% of trauma patients who presented with cardiac arrest could have benefitted from REBOA [50]. Brede et al. showed that a training program for prehospital providers was effective in developing competence in the procedure [51]. Pasley et al. demonstrated that a training program of independent duty medical technicians could bring REBOA closer to the point of injury in the prehospital setting [52]. Despite some promise, REBOA is contraindicated in concomitant chest injury and has little indication in traditional pre-hospital management of blast injuries.

Airway Management

Airway obstruction in the prehospital setting can rapidly lead to brain damage and death, often before arrival of professional rescuers. While endotracheal intubation provides greater protection from aspiration and facilitates positive-pressure ventilation, other devices such as nasopharyngeal airways and supraglottic airways (SGA) can be rapidly placed with minimal preparation. Scant evidence exists to recommend one SGA over another in the emergency prehospital environment [53]. Further, in the trauma setting, SGAs did not result in better outcomes than surgical cricothyroidotomy [54].

A surgical airway is a little-used tool in emergency airway management in the civilian prehospital setting. It does have certain advantages in the field when the airway must be secured quickly and with little preparation or assistance. Studies have demonstrated the rapidity with which an endotracheal tube can be placed through the cricothyroid membrane by paramedics using a simple open surgical approach [55, 56]. Several commercial devices exist to assist in placement of a surgical airway, though they vary in cost, complexity, and success of insertion [57–59].

Patients who are not breathing after airway obstruction has been addressed by positioning, nasal airway, SGA device, intubation, or surgical cricothyroidotomy have little to no chance of meaningful recovery. These casualties should be considered potentially unsalvageable without additional resources and managed accordingly.

Inhalational Injuries

Explosions are often accompanied by fire and potential inhalational injury from smoke or poisonous gases. Inhalation of hot gases and particulates can injure the upper, middle, and lower airways. Products of combustion such as carbon monoxide (CO) and cyanide can asphyxiate casualties even after the exposure has ceased. Supplemental oxygen should be administered to maintain oxygen saturations above 92% in order to accelerate the dissipation of carbon monoxide from the system.

A casualty who has inhaled hot gas may suffer rapid airway compromise due to airway edema [60]. It is important to consider early invasive airway management in patients who are exhibiting hoarseness, soot or edema in the oropharynx or nares, or worsening difficulty of breathing or a sensation that the throat is closing. At least one study suggests a decrease in mortality if the airway is secured prior to frank respiratory compromise [61].

Smoke inhalation may also cause bronchospasm, which should be treated with bronchodilators such as albuterol, ipratropium bromide, metaproterenol, or epinephrine [62–65].

CO can be detected rapidly by CO-oximetry. Hyperbaric oxygen (HBO) treatment may be considered in any patient who has been exposed to CO and exhibits neurological effects such as altered mental status, though most studies have failed to show improved outcomes with HBO in patients poisoned with CO [66, 67]. However, victims of explosions may have traumatic injuries that take precedence over the need for HBO treatment. If given a choice between transporting to an appropriate trauma center without hyperbaric capability and a hospital with a hyperbaric chamber but no trauma designation, the patient should be taken to the trauma center.

Cyanide is a frequent by-product of combustion of many modern building materials. In prehospital cyanide toxicity cases, hydroxocobalamin (Cyanokit®) is the preferred antidote. Hydroxocobalamin should be considered early in patients who have significant smoke exposure and cyanosis that does not resolve with oxygen administration. Although the significance of cyanide toxicity in smoke inhalation victims is uncertain, hydroxocobalamin is generally regarded as safe [68]. Older, multiagent cyanide antidotes may be considered; however, sodium thiosulfate will create a methemoglobinemia that will further impair oxygen delivery in patients who have also been exposed to CO and result in potent vasodilation. Both sequelae are detrimental to hypovolemic patients.

Open Chest Injuries

Tension pneumothorax in the blast casualty can be difficult to detect as it is often bilateral and unequal breath sounds are therefore not present. Rapid decompression of one or both sides of the chest should be considered in any blast casualty with absent or deteriorating vital signs, particularly if positive-pressure ventilations are being provided. To quote one report [69]: "In ventilated patients, (tension pneumothorax) presents rapidly with consistent signs of respiratory and cardiac compromise. In contrast, awake patients show a greater variability of presentations, which are generally more progressive, with slower decompensation."

Needle chest decompression (NDC) thoracentesis is currently the only procedure available to many prehospital providers in the United States. The 68–87% success rate for NDC in pneumothorax [70] may belie the fact that the procedure frequently fails to evacuate an active, ongoing air leak. NDC failed to effectively decompress the thorax in 50% of patients with physiologic evidence of tension pneumothorax despite adequate catheter length [71]. This failure rate is unacceptable in a disease process that is rapidly fatal without successful intervention, particularly when a simple and highly effective alternative exists.

One animal study showed a failure rate of NDC of 58% and NDC failed to restore perfusion in 64% of models [72]. A 2017 review showed lack of objective clinical improvement in 90% and missed pneumothorax or ineffective drainage rate of 25–50% [72]. Other complications include failure to completely penetrate the chest wall, intrathoracic organ injury, cardiac tamponade, and serious bleeding from intercostal or pulmonary vessel injury. In an observational study of 25 emergency physicians, only 60% identified the second intercostal space correctly [73]. Misplacement of a 4.5-cm needle in the anterior chest can easily injure mediastinal structures [74, 75]. This has led to many experts to recommend a lateral insertion along the midaxillary line in the 4th or 5th intercostal space [76, 77].

An observational study of severely injured trauma patients showed NDC successfully relieved tension pneumothorax in only 18% of patients [70, 78]. Longer needles have been recommended by several studies of NDC, but this carries an increased risk of iatrogenic injury to great vessels, lung hilum, and the heart [77–82].

Simple thoracostomy (ST) is a rapid procedure for decompression of a tension pneumothorax, which takes less than 1 minute to perform and has a 97% success rate [83]. The blunt dissection technique carries a low risk of damage to intrathoracic organs and large blood vessels [84]. Unlike NDC, ST maintains an open channel for continuous venting of excess pressure from the pleural cavity. A 2018 study by Dickson et al. described their experience in an urban/suburban ground EMS system, where they found the procedure could be performed safely and effectively by paramedics [85].

Volume Resuscitation

Damage control resuscitation (DCR) principles apply in prehospital management of blast victims in shock. Previous recommendations for resuscitation included large volumes of isotonic crystalloid solutions, usually in the form of 0.9% sodium chloride (normal saline, or NS) or lactated Ringer's (LR) solution. This resuscitation strategy has long been recognized to be inadequate in the setting of blood loss and potentially harmful. Several studies in the past few decades have demonstrated the harm caused with liberal use of crystalloids in the trauma patient [86]. A doctrine of "permissive hypotension" was adopted by most institutions in response to this research, whereby crystalloid solutions were withheld from the trauma patient, even if hypotensive, unless in frank shock [87]. This research, however, compared the use of limited crystalloids versus large-volume crystalloid infusions, but did not examine use of blood for resuscitation to keep the patient normotensive. In effect, crystalloids were shown to be harmful, but the studies did not show that hypotension was helpful [88].

NS and LR are acidic when compared to blood (pH 5.5 and 6.5, respectively). Balanced crystalloid solutions such as Normosol-R, Plasmalyte-A, and Isolyte® have a physiological pH of 7.4. These solutions and LR also have much lower chloride concentrations than NS. The high chloride level in NS leads to impairment of the kidneys' ability to reclaim bicarbonate and, consequently, the bicarbonate buffer system essential to maintaining a normal pH [89]. Balanced solutions are preferable to NS in the resuscitation of injured patients if crystalloid is to be used at all [90–92].

Over-resuscitation with crystalloid IV fluid has several harmful effects [93–95]. No crystalloids have oxygen-carrying capacity or clotting factors and have the net effect of diluting the blood. The lack of protein results in these fluids quickly redistributing to the interstitial space, limiting their effectiveness at increasing blood volume for any significant period of time [96]. Patients during the Vietnam War who received crystalloid resuscitation often developed non-cardiogenic pulmonary edema which was colloquially referred to as "Da Nang lung" [97]. This threshold of harm is lower than previously thought, with increased rates of acute kidney injury, multiorgan system failure, intensive care unit (ICU) length of stay, hospital length of stay, and death once a trauma patient has received in excess of 1.5 L of crystalloids [98]. Poor perfusion may be evidenced by lack of peripheral pulses, skin mottling, and altered mental status, as well as tachycardia and hypotension. If crystalloids are to be administered, these should be limited to small volumes and only that amount needed to reverse frank shock. Balanced crystalloids are preferred to NS, and the recommendation from the CoTCCC is that NS be avoided altogether in trauma.

Damage Control Resuscitation

Urgent surgical management is the mainstay of care for the critically injured trauma patient. The tyranny of distance and an overwhelming number of casualties may prolong evacuation to a surgical asset, leading to irreversible shock and death. It is during this prehospital and presurgical interval that appropriate resuscitation can prolong the patient's life, prevent further deterioration, and optimize the patient's condition in preparation for surgery. In the setting of severe hemorrhage, a cascade of physiological changes known as the lethal triad of hemorrhage (acidosis, coagulopathy, and hypothermia) occurs, which can potentially worsen bleeding and lead to organ failure from prolonged hypoperfusion and inflammation. Major exsanguination can cause death within minutes, well before any significant alteration in body chemistry can take place. Most fatally injured patients, however, die 2.5 hours after the initial injury, after a time when the effects of hypoperfusion have damaged many body systems [99].

In the prehospital setting, the goals of damage control resuscitation (DCR) are mechanical control of hemorrhage, maintenance of the physiologic clotting cascade (i.e., limit dilution and hypothermia while considering tranexamic acid), and supporting perfusion by restoring circulating blood volume [100]. While these interventions usually occur in the hospital setting, it may be appropriate for some prehospital care systems to implement aspects of DCR if time to definitive care is anticipated to be high and allowable within local jurisdictions.

Prehospital Blood Products

There is currently no adequate substitute for lost blood other than blood transfusion. In most institutions, patients receive blood in components of packed red blood cells, plasma, and platelets. Current recommendations are that these should be given in equal ratios to best reconstitute the blood that the patient has lost. Cryoprecipitate may be added for additional fibrinogen and clotting factors. These components have limited shelf life and stringent storage requirements that require significant measures to maintain in a field environment.

Some institutions have begun transfusing whole blood (WB) to trauma patients. And several EMS agencies are now carrying WB or fractionated blood products in the field for resuscitation. Blood products in the civilian EMS setting were previously limited to critical-care interfacility transport services. The logistics required to maintain blood products within a tight temperature range and change them out frequently as they expire had made them seem impractical for EMS. With increasing literature highlighting the dangers of crystalloids in trauma and the recognition of the value of early trauma resuscitation, some EMS systems have started carrying blood products such as packed red blood cells, liquid plasma, or cold-stored whole blood [101].

Whole blood has a relatively short shelf life (21–35 days, depending on the preservative), but has the added advantage of carrying platelets, fibrinogen, and clotting factors. Whole blood has been shown to be at least equivalent to components and may be superior [102, 103]. During the Vietnam War, over one million units of whole blood were transfused [104]. Whole blood has one-third the amount of preservative as an equivalent amount of fractionated products.

In remote environments, US military special operations teams have implemented a "walking blood bank" protocol, whereby ideal donors with type O blood and low levels of antibody titers are identified prior to deployment [105]. When a casualty needs whole blood for survival, a donor on the team will immediately have a unit of whole blood drawn and delivered to the casualty. This enables medics to resuscitate the patient with blood without the logistical concerns of carrying blood products in a combat environment. Additionally, the donor has been found to remain combat effective with minimal noticeable performance decrement after donation of up to 500 mL of whole blood [106]. The Texas Ranger Division of the Texas Department of Public Safety has adopted this transfusion program for rural law enforcement operations in Texas as they often perform high-risk missions far from trauma centers.

Freeze-dried plasma (FDP) has been in use in France since the mid-1990s. This pooled plasma product is shelf-stable at room temperature. The powder can be quickly reconstituted with water in the field and provides advantages over other blood products in that it has a longer shelf life and tolerates field conditions better [107]. Several FDP products are now or soon to be on the market, and these may provide a viable option for trauma resuscitation in prehospital systems that cannot manage cold-stored whole blood, packed red blood cells, or liquid plasma.

Tranexamic Acid

Tranexamic acid (TXA) is an antithrombolytic drug that can be administered via either intravenous or intraosseous routes. There is some data that it can be administered intramuscularly as well [108]. A large randomized controlled trial of TXA showed improved survival in a broad cohort of trauma patients [109]. Subsequent study showed the benefits of TXA are greatest when given inside 1 hour after injury and nonexistent if given outside 3 hours after injury and that the benefit of TXA drops 10% for every 15 minutes that administration is delayed [110].

Administration of TXA in the prehospital setting decreases time to administration [111] and reduces blood product usage [112, 113]. TXA also appears to benefit patients with severe injury scores or evidence of shock [112]. Along with blood products, TXA shows independent survival benefit in hemorrhagic shock and when administered with cryoprecipitate [114]. TXA is often recommended at a dose of 1 g IV over 10 minutes once vascular access has been obtained. However, the ideal dose for trauma has yet to be identified. TXA has been given safely at higher doses in cardiothoracic, orthopedic, and obstetrical surgery.

TXA has shown some benefit in patients with head injury. A large, pragmatic multicenter trial showed that TXA improved survival in patients with mild-to-moderate traumatic brain injury and did not increase the number of patients surviving with poor neurological outcomes [115]. Other studies showed less impressive improvement but did not demonstrate harm from administration of TXA to patients with traumatic brain injury [116, 117]. Recent evidence indicates that a higher initial dose of 2 g intravenously may benefit patients without significant adverse effects. One study showed decreased mortality in these patients with a nonsignificant trend toward slowing progression of the hemorrhage [118]. Another study of military casualties showed lower mortality and an increased number of casualties improving to a Glasgow Coma Scale (GCS) score of 14 or 15 [119].

Hypothermia Management

Decreased perfusion of tissues from shock will decrease oxygen delivery. Anaerobic metabolism is far less efficient at producing heat compared to the electron transport chain that is used when oxygen is plentiful. This can result in hypothermia, which impairs the body's clotting mechanisms. Other pathways for heat loss include moisture evaporation from wounds, convection into the air, conduction via direct contact with the ground, and decreased mobility resulting in decreased heat production. The patient may, therefore, become hypothermic, even in warm ambient temperatures. Additional risk factors for hypothermia in trauma patients arriving by EMS include endotracheal intubation, comorbidities, and increased injury severity [120, 121].

Once the patient has been examined and injuries stabilized, aggressive measures to insulate the patient and provide active warming should be initiated. Several commercially available warming blankets and reflective wraps will serve this purpose. A technique used by the Norwegian Special Operations Commando includes wrapping the patient in clear plastic bubble wrap, which enables the medic to insulate the patient but monitor for unexpected blood loss [122].

It is advisable to utilize fluid warmers, if any intravenous fluids are to be given, to reduce the cooling effect these fluids have when given at storage (room) temperature [123]. The use of inline fluid warmers is paramount if blood products are to be given, because these are often stored at relatively cold temperatures (2–6 °C).

Head Injuries

Blast trauma can lead to a wide spectrum of traumatic brain injuries that range from occult to potentially severe and fatal outcomes. Traumatic brain injuries (TBIs) result in a significant societal burden and financial cost [123, 124]. Aggressive prevention of hypoxia and hypotension has been shown to significantly improve outcomes in moderate and severe head injuries by reducing the incidence of secondary brain injury [125].Severe TBIs, including both blunt impacts and those resulting from penetration of the cranial vault, have significant mortality rates. Cessation of respiratory effort in the trauma casualty is an extremely poor prognostic sign, as it often portends severe and irreversible damage to the central nervous system. Impact brain apnea (IBA) is an underrecognized but significant and preventable contributor to death resulting from TBI [126]. If not rapidly self-terminated or corrected by artificial means, IBA will lead to hypoxia-induced cardiac arrest.

Hypotension, even if only a single episode, dramatically increases mortality rates. In the setting of TBI, there is no identifiable threshold for a safe decrease in blood pressure below that of normalized hemodynamics [127]. Aggressive efforts should be made to optimize hemodynamics, oxygenation, and ventilation in this patient population to prevent secondary brain injury. If other injuries allow, the patient should be maintained in a 30-degree head-elevated position in an effort to lower the intracranial pressure [128]. With evidence of impending or active herniation, such as unilateral dilation of one pupil with decreasing level of consciousness, it may be advantageous to administer 250 mL of a 3% or 5% hypertonic saline solution. Modest hyperventilation targeted to an end-tidal carbon dioxide level of 30–35 mmHg is appropriate in the setting of active herniation as well. Even mild traumatic brain injury (mTBI) can result in significant and persistent symptoms such as headache, nausea, vomiting, vertigo, balance problems, fatigue, sleep disturbances, drowsiness, sensitivity to light or noise, blurred vision, difficulty remembering, or difficulty concentrating [129]. One of the more challenging aspects of managing mild and occult traumatic brain injuries is screening potential patients and reliably identifying mTBI. The Military Acute Concussion Evaluation, a common TBI screening tool based on the Standardized Assessment of Concussion, may have limited application in the civilian setting as a standalone tool [130, 131].

Pain Control

Management of pain at the point of wounding has been shown to reduce posttraumatic stress disorder (PTSD) in combat casualties [132, 133]. Several options exist that are appropriate to the prehospital setting.

For severe pain, transmucosal fentanyl citrate 800 mcg can be used as a lozenge against the buccal mucosa [131]. Intravenous, intramuscular, and intranasal fentanyl at doses of 1–2 mcg/kg causes less histamine release and hypotension than morphine and is relatively short acting [134, 135]. For casualties in shock or in whom there is a concern for loss of airway control, the dissociative anesthetic ketamine can provide analgesia without significant drop in blood pressure or loss of protective airway reflexes [136]. Ketamine is administered intravenously or intramuscularly in doses of 0.1–0.3 mg/kg for pain management [137]. Intravenous acetaminophen is another option recently available in the United States, which can help manage pain without affecting platelet function [138]. Oral pain medication should be deferred unless there are expected significant delays to care. In these cases, responders may use oral acetaminophen or meloxicam for mild-to-moderate pain [139].

Antibiotic Administration

Blasts carry particulate matter in the form of soil, clothing, and other fragments deep into the body, and complex polymicrobial wound infections are common [140]. During Operation GOTHIC SERPENT (aka the Battle of Mogadishu) in 1993, casualties experienced a nearly 30% wound infection rate, although none reached definitive care (and presumably antibiotic administration) for more than 18 hours after the battle started. Early antibiotic therapy is therefore important and may reduce combat infection rates [141, 142].

Antibiotics are rarely given in the civilian EMS setting due to relatively short transport times and lack of perceived benefit. In austere environments with prolonged evacuation times, antibiotics are more practical. Antibiotic therapy for the prehospital setting must meet several operational requirements: They must be simple to administer, must be shelf stable across wide temperature ranges, have broad antimicrobial spectra, and should have relatively long dosing intervals since medical personnel are typically limited and will have multiple tasks to accomplish. Ertapenem, meropenem, ceftriaxone, cefepime, moxifloxacin, and aztreonam are some antibiotics that meet these goals. They have the added advantage that several can be safely administered intramuscularly, if IV and IO access is not obtainable.

Wound Care

Blast injuries are unique from other types of penetrating and blunt trauma in the sheer number of wounds that can be suffered by each casualty. After life-threatening hemorrhage has been addressed, medics should dress other wounds to prevent further blood and insensible fluid loss, protect from contamination, and preserve body heat. This may require a substantial amount of bandage material. Wounds must be monitored for increasing bleeding. Securing dressings with clear cellophane wrap may enable the medic to observe these wounds and preserve body heat. This is also appropriate for abdominal eviscerations where organs must be protected from drying out.

Burn wounds can be severe depending on a casualty's proximity to the blast site. Burn wounds should be addressed appropriately, with focus on stopping the burn process, dressing open wounds with sterile dressings, protection from further heat loss through disrupted skin, and transport to a capable burn or trauma center for definitive care.

It has been estimated that up to 40–50% of the relatively minor wounds affecting the soft tissues and bones can be safely treated with appropriate first-aid measures alone, thus easing the burden on hospital facilities and saving scarce resources and operating time [143].

Splinting

Blasts frequently induce extremity injuries. Fractures and amputations were extremely common at the Boston Marathon Bombing in 2013 and were universal in the Austin bombing incidents in 2018 [144, 145]. A variety of splint materials are available for prehospital use, but padded malleable aluminum splints are versatile, compact, and lightweight. As a general rule, civilian EMS personnel will splint fractures and dislocations in the position found, but will reduce these fractures in the field, if absent distal pulses or sensation indicate vascular compromise [146]. In a prolonged field care scenario, it is prudent to reduce fractures in order to reduce pain, control bleeding, and prevent ischemia.

Conclusion

Management of casualties from blast trauma can quickly tax EMS personnel due to injury burden and the propensity for multiple casualties at a scene. Limiting risk to prehospital providers by minimizing time in the blast zone, utilizing personal protective equipment, quickly extracting victims, and utilizing cover from terrain are the first steps in ensuring adequate prehospital care. Life-threatening hemorrhage should be addressed immediately when found and should not be deferred for other providers or for extraction. Airway management, decompression of pneumothorax, judicial volume resuscitation, and prevention of hypothermia follow hemorrhage control in the immediate period following blast injury. Additional priorities such as pain management, antibiotic administration, wound care, and splinting of fractures and dislocations should be addressed as time and circumstances allow. Casualties must be brought to definitive surgical care as rapidly as possible but actions in the prehospital setting will ensure patients arrive in the best possible condition to survive surgical management.

Key Points

- Blast injuries produce complex, multisystem trauma due to the presence of overpressure, penetrating, blunt, and thermal trauma. EMS trauma care should follow a standardized approach based on TECC that emphasizes immediate hemorrhage control.
- Exsanguinating external hemorrhage must be immediately controlled with direct pressure, tourniquet, wound packing, or junctional hemorrhage device. Casualties with suspected internal hemorrhage must be expeditiously transported to a hospital or other facility capable of performing emergent surgery.
- Tension pneumothorax is often bilateral and therefore more difficult to detect with asymmetric lung sounds. Consider chest decompression in patients with difficulty breathing, unexplained tachycardia, or worsening shock. Needle decompression has a relatively high failure rate due to incorrect placement or high-volume air leak into pleural spaces secondary to bronchopleural fistulae.
- Whole blood or component therapy is the trauma resuscitation fluid of choice.
- Aggressively prevent hypothermia. Blast victims are at high risk for hypothermia, which can result in coagulopathy and increased mortality.

Pitfalls

- Not maintaining a high index of suspicion for secondary threats. EMS and other first responders are at high personal risk during the response to a blast incident. Scene safety is paramount.
- Not placing a tourniquet proximal to a severe extremity injury, regardless of whether or not it is actively bleeding.
- Not fully examining casualties for posterior or hidden wounds.
- Allowing even transient hypoxia or hypotension to occur may initiate or exacerbate secondary brain injury caused by increased intracranial pressure.
- Overuse of IV crystalloid fluids can cause harm without significant benefit in casualties with uncontrolled hemorrhage. Even a relatively small amount, 1.5 L in the adult, increases morbidity and mortality.

Pearls

- Primary blast injuries carry a high mortality and may not be readily apparent during initial examinations by EMS personnel. Providers should consider factors that increase the likelihood of the presence or subsequent development of primary blast injuries (e.g., vicinity of victim to blast site, open- versus closed-space blast, magnitude of explosive device, etc.).
- TXA administered in the prehospital phase of care can reduce bleeding and mortality. Since the benefits of TXA drop rapidly as administration is delayed, it should be administered as soon as feasible.
- Unusual hemodynamic or neurological presentations could be explained by inhalation of poisonous gases or arterial air embolism secondary to lung injury.
- When transportation to a hospital is significantly delayed, antibiotics are essential to prevent infection. The treater must also pay continued attention to pain management, positioning, comfort, and prevention of hypothermia.
- Clear plastic wrapping can be used to bandage penetrating wounds, eviscerations, and burns. It has advantages over fabric dressings, because it is extremely lightweight, compact, and self-adhesive, allows the medic to monitor for continued bleeding, and serves as an occlusive dressing to maintain moisture in wounds and prevent air entry.

References

1. Owens B, Kragh J, Wenke J, Macaitis J, Wade C, Holcomb J. Combat wounds in operation Iraqi freedom and operation enduring freedom. J Trauma. 2008;64(2):295–9.
2. Biddinger P, Baggish A, Harrington L, d'Hemecourt P, Hooley J, Jones J, et al. Be prepared – the Boston Marathon and mass casualty events. N Engl J Med. 2013;368(21):1958–9.
3. Lockey D, MacKenzie R, Redhead J, Wise D, Harris T, Weaver A, et al. London bombings July 2005: the immediate pre-hospital medical response. Resuscitation. 2005;66:ix–xii.
4. Carresi AL. The 2004 Madrid train bombings: an analysis of pre-hospital management. Disasters. 2008 Mar;32(1):41–65.
5. Ritenour A, Baskin T. Primary blast injury: update on diagnosis and treatment. Crit Care Med. 2008;36(Suppl):S311–7.
6. Stuhmiller JH. Blast injury: translating research into operational medicine. In: Lenhart MK, Friedl K, Santee WR, editors. Military quantitative physiology: problems and concepts in operational medicine. Falls Church: Office of the Surgeon General of the United States Army; 2012. p. 267–302.
7. Burns GD, Wightman JM. Explosive events. In: Koenig KL, Schultz CH, editors. Koenig and Schultz's disaster medicine: comprehensive principles and practice. 2nd ed. Cambridge, UK: Cambridge University Press; 2016. p. 463–85.
8. Wightman JM, Gladish SL. Explosions and blast injuries. Ann Emerg Med. 2001;37:664–78.
9. DePalma R, Burris D, Champion H, Hodgson M. Blast injuries. N Engl J Med. 2005;352(13):1335–42.
10. Wolf SJ, Bebarta VS, Bonnett CJ, Bonnett CJ, Pons PT, Cantrill SV, et al. Blast injuries. Lancet. 2009;374:405–15.
11. Leibovici D, Gofrit ON, Shapira SC. Eardrum perforation in explosion survivors: is it a marker of pulmonary blast injury? Ann Emerg Med. 1999;34:168–72.
12. Gutierrez de Ceballos JP, Turégano Fuentes F, Perez Diaz D, Sanz Sanchez M, Martin Llorente C, Guerrero Sanz JE. Casualties treated at the closest hospital in the Madrid, March 11, terrorist bombings. Crit Care Med. 2005;33(1 Suppl):S107–12.
13. Sanger L-B. Nurse dies of injury suffered in rescue mission. The Oklahoman; 24 April 1995. https://newsok.com/article/2499885/nurse-dies-of-injury-suffered-in-rescue-mission. Accessed 5 Mar 2019.
14. Vernon A. Explosive devices what every responder should know about IEDs. JEMS. 2010;35(5):42–7.
15. Kapur G, Hutson H, Davis M, Rice P. The United States twenty-year experience with bombing incidents: implications for terrorism preparedness and medical response. J Trauma. 2005;59(6):1436–44.
16. Gratton M, Garza A, Salomone J, McElroy J, Shearer J. Ambulance staging for potentially dangerous scenes: another hidden component of response time. Prehosp Emerg Care. 2010;14(3):340–4.
17. Olson K. Overview: recent events and responder implications. Proceedings of the seminar on responding to the consequences of chemical and biological terrorism. 1996. 2(36):2–93.
18. Morris L. Islamic State militants allegedly used chlorine gas against Iraqi security forces. Washington Post. 23 Oct 2014.
19. US Department of Health and Human Services, Chemical Hazards Emergency Medical Management. https://chemm.nlm.nih.gov/detailedinfo.htm. Accessed 18 Nov 2019.
20. Ryan K, George D, Liu J, Mitchell P, Nelson K, Kue R. The use of field triage in disaster and mass casualty incidents: a survey of current practices by EMS personnel. Prehosp Emerg Care. 2018;22(4):520–6.
21. Bloch YH, Schwartz D, Pinkert M, Blumenfeld A, Avinoam S, Hevion G, et al. Distribution of casualties in a mass-casualty incident with three local hospitals in the periphery of a densely populated area: lessons learned from the medical management of a terrorist attack. Prehosp Disaster Med. 2007;22(3):186–92.

22. Pinkert M, Lehavi O, Goren OB, Raiter Y, Shamis A, Priel Z, et al. Primary triage, evacuation priorities, and rapid primary distribution between adjacent hospitals—lessons learned from a suicide bomber attack in downtown Tel-Aviv. Prehosp Disaster Med. 2008;23(4):337–41.
23. Aurora century 16 theater shooting after action report for the city of Aurora. http://www.policefoundation.org/wp-content/uploads/2016/08/Aurora-Century-16-Theater-Shooting_AAR.pdf. Accessed 18 Nov 2019.
24. Shartar SE, Moore BL, Wood LM. Developing a mass casualty surge capacity protocol for emergency medical services to use for patient distribution. South Med J. 2017;110(12):792–5.
25. Clumpner M. Analysis of records that represent an active shooter response model utilizing 32 large-scale exercises. Prescott Valley: Northcentral University; 2015.
26. Gutierrez de Ceballos JP, Turégano Fuentes F, Perez Diaz D, Sanz Sanchez M, Martin Llorente C, Guerrero Sanz JE. Casualties treated at the closest hospital in the Madrid, March 11, terrorist bombings. Crit Care Med. 2005;33(1 Suppl):S107–12.
27. Aharonson-Daniel L, Almogy G, Bahouth H, et al. Mass casualty events—suicide bombing: the Israeli perspective. In: Elsayed NM, Atkins JL, Gorbunov NV, editors. Explosion and blast-related injuries: effects of explosions and blast from military operations and acts of terrorism. London: Elsevier Academic Press; 2008. p. 307–35.
28. Callaway DW, Smith ER, Cain J, Shapiro G, Burnett WT, McKay SD, et al. Tactical emergency casualty care (TECC): guidelines for the provision of prehospital trauma care in high threat environments. J Spec Oper Med. 2011 Summer-Fall;11(3):104–22.
29. Kosequat J, Rush SC, Simonsen I, Gallo I, Scott A, Swats K, et al. Efficacy of the mnemonic device "MARCH PAWS" as a checklist for pararescuemen during tactical field care and tactical evacuation. J Spec Oper Med. Winter 2017;17(4):80–4.
30. Eastridge BJ, Mabry RL, Seguin P, Cantrell J, Tops T, Uribe P, et al. Death on the battlefield (2001–2011): implications for the future of combat casualty care. J Trauma Acute Care Surg. 2012;73(6 Suppl 5):S431–7. https://doi.org/10.1097/TA.0b013e3182755dcc. Erratum in: J Trauma Acute Care Surg. 2013 Feb;74(2):706.
31. Ashkenazi I, Sevi R, Turégano-Fuentes F, Walsh MS, Olsha O, Schecter WP, et al. Hemodynamic consequences of extremity injuries following a terrorist bombing attack: retrospective cohort study. Eur J Trauma Emerg Surg. 2018;45:865. https://doi.org/10.1007/s00068-018-1017-5.
32. Heldenberg E, Givon A, Simon D, Bass A, Almogy G, Peleg K, Israeli Trauma Group. Civilian casualties of terror-related explosions: the impact of vascular trauma on treatment and prognosis. J Trauma Acute Care Surg. 2016;81(3):435–40.
33. Kauvar DS, Sarfati MR, Kraiss LW. National trauma databank analysis of mortality and limb loss in isolated lower extremity vascular trauma. J Vasc Surg. 2011;53(6):1598–603.
34. Fisher AD, Callaway DW, Robertson JN, Hardwick SA, Bobko JP, Kotwal RS. The ranger first responder program and tactical emergency casualty care implementation: a whole-community approach to reducing mortality from active violent incidents. J Spec Oper Med. 2015 Fall;15(3):46–53.
35. Levy MJ, Jacobs LM. A call to action to develop programs for bystanders to control severe bleeding. JAMA Surg. 2016;151(12):1103–4.
36. Goolsby C, Rojas L, Moore K, Kretz E, Singletary E, Klimczak V, Charlton N. Layperson ability and willingness to use hemostatic dressings: a randomized, controlled trial. Prehosp Emerg Care. 2019;15:1–7.
37. Bulger EM, Snyder D, Schoelles K, Gotschall C, Dawson D, Lang E, et al. An evidence-based prehospital guideline for external hemorrhage control: American College of Surgeons Committee on Trauma. Prehosp Emerg Care. 2014;18(2):163–73.
38. Kauvar DS, Miller D, Walters TJ. Tourniquet use is not associated with limb loss following military lower extremity arterial trauma. J Trauma Acute Care Surg. 2018;85(3):495–9.
39. Blackbourne LH, Baer DG, Eastridge BJ, Kheirabadi B, Bagley S, Kragh JF Jr, et al. Military medical revolution: prehospital combat casualty care [published corrections appear in J Trauma Acute Care. 2013;74(1):347 and J Trauma Acute Care. 2013;74(2):705]. J Trauma Acute Care Surg. 2012;73(6 Suppl 5):S372–7.

40. Galante JM. Using tourniquets to stop bleeding. JAMA. 2017;317(14):1490.
41. Committee on Tactical Combat Casualty Care. Recommended devices and adjuncts. 2019. Published online. https://books.allogy.com/web/tenant/8/books/f94aad5b-78f3-42be-b3de-8e8d63343866/. Accessed 18 Nov 2019.
42. Lyles WE, Kragh JF, Aden JK, Dubick MA. Testing tourniquet use in a manikin model: two improvised techniques. J Spec Oper Med. 2015;15(4):21–6.
43. King DR, Larentzakis A, Ramly EP, Boston Trauma Collaborative. Tourniquet use at the Boston Marathon bombing: lost in translation. J Trauma Acute Care Surg. 2015;78(3):594–9.
44. Bennett BL, Littlejohn LF, Kheirabadi BS, Butler FK, Kotwal RS, Dubick MA, et al. Management of external hemorrhage in tactical combat casualty care: Chitosan-based hemostatic gauze dressings--TCCC guidelines-change 13-05. J Spec Oper Med. 2014 Fall;14(3):40–57.
45. Wydo SM, Seamon MJ, Melanson SW, Thomas P, Bahner DP, Stawicki SP. Portable ultrasound in disaster triage: a focused review. Eur J Trauma Emerg Surg. 2016;42(2):151–9.
46. Shokoohi H, Pourmand A, Boniface K, Allen R, Petinaux B, Sarani B, et al. The utility of point-of-care ultrasound in targeted automobile ramming mass casualty (TARMAC) attacks. Am J Emerg Med. 2018;36(8):1467–71.
47. Davies GE, Lockey DJ. Thirteen survivors of prehospital thoracotomy for penetrating trauma: a prehospital physician-performed resuscitation procedure that can yield good results. J Trauma. 2011;70(5):E75–8.
48. Van Vledder MG, Van Waes OJF, Kooij FO, Peters JH, Van Lieshout E, Verhofstad M. Out of hospital thoracotomy for cardiac arrest after penetrating thoracic trauma. Injury. 2017;48(9):1865–9.
49. Darocha T, Kosinski S, Serednicki W, Derkowski T, Podsiadlo P, Szpor J, et al. Prehospital emergency thoracotomy performed by helicopter emergency medical service team: a case report. Ulus Travma Acil Cerrahi Derg. 2019;25(3):303–6.
50. Henry R, Matsushima K, Henry RN, Wong V, Warriner Z, Strumwasser A, et al. Who would have benefitted from the prehospital use of resuscitative endovascular balloon occlusion of the aorta (REBOA)? An autopsy study. J Am Coll Surg. 2019. https://doi.org/10.1016/j.jamcollsurg.2019.05.025.
51. Brede JR, Lafrenz T, Krüger A, Søvik E, Steffensen T, Kriesi C, et al. Resuscitative endovascular balloon occlusion of the aorta (REBOA) in non-traumatic out-of-hospital cardiac arrest: evaluation of an educational programme. BMJ Open. 2019;9(5):e027980.
52. Pasley JD, Teeter WA, Gamble WB, Wasick P, Romagnoli AN, Pasley AM, et al. Bringing resuscitative endovascular balloon occlusion of the aorta (REBOA) closer to the point of injury. J Spec Oper Med. 2018 Spring;18(1):33–6.
53. Hardy GB, Maddry JK, Ng PC, Savell SC, Arana AA, Kester A, et al. Impact of prehospital airway management on combat mortality. Am J Emerg Med. 2018;36(6):1032–5.
54. Schauer SG, Naylor JF, Chow AL, Maddry J, Cunningham CW, Blackburn MB, et al. Survival of casualties undergoing prehospital supraglottic airway placement versus cricothyrotomy. J Spec Oper Med. 2019 Summer;19(2):91–4.
55. Barnard EB, Ervin AT, Mabry RL, Bebarta VS. Prehospital and en route cricothyrotomy performed in the combat setting: a prospective, multicenter, observational study. J Spec Oper Med. 2014 Winter;14(4):35–9.
56. Jacobson LE, Gomez GA, Sobieray RJ, Rodman GH, Solotkin KC, Misinski ME. Surgical cricothyroidotomy in trauma patients: analysis of its use by paramedics in the field. J Trauma. 1996;41(1):15–20.
57. Schober P, Hegemann MC, Schwarte LA, Loer SA, Noetges P. Emergency cricothyrotomy-a comparative study of different techniques in human cadavers. Resuscitation. 2009;80(2):204–9.
58. Schauer SG, D Fernandez JR, L Roper J, Brown D, L Jeffers K, Srichandra J, et al. A randomized cross-over study comparing surgical cricothyrotomy techniques by combat medics using a synthetic cadaver model. Am J Emerg Med. 2018;36(4):651–6.
59. Heymans F, Feigl G, Graber S, Courvoisier DS, Weber KM, Dulguerov P. Emergency cricothyrotomy performed by surgical airway-naive medical personnel: a randomized crossover study in cadavers comparing three commonly used techniques. Anesthesiology. 2016;125(2):295–303.

60. Mlcak RP, Suman OE, Herndon DN. Respiratory management of inhalation injury. Burns. 2007;33:2–13. https://doi.org/10.1016/j.burns.2006.07.007.
61. Venus B, Matsuda T, Copiozo JB, Mathru M. Prophylactic intubation and continuous positive airway pressure in the management of inhalation injury in burn victims. Crit Care Med. 1981;9:519–23.
62. Jonkam C, Zhu Y, Jacob S, Rehberg S, Traber LD, Herndon DN, et al. Assessment of combined muscarinic antagonist and fibrinolytic therapy for inhalation injury. J Burn Care Res. 2012;33:524–31.
63. Palmieri TL, Enkhbaatar P, Bayliss R, Traber LD, Cox RA, Hawkins HK, et al. Continuous nebulized albuterol attenuates acute lung injury in an ovine model of combined burn and smoke inhalation. Crit Care Med. 2006;34:1719–24. https://doi.org/10.1097/01.ccm.0000217215.82821.c5.
64. Lange M, Hamahata A, Traber DL, Cox RA, Kulp GA, Nakano Y, et al. Preclinical evaluation of epinephrine nebulization to reduce airway hyperemia and improve oxygenation after smoke inhalation injury. Crit Care Med. 2011;39:718–24. https://doi.org/10.1097/CCM.0b013e318207ec52.
65. Otterness K, Ahn C. Emergency department management of smoke inhalation injury in adults. Emerg Med Pract. 2018;20(3):1–24.
66. Weaver LK. Hyperbaric oxygen therapy for carbon monoxide poisoning. Undersea Hyperb Med. 2014;41:339–54.
67. Buckley NA, Juurlink DN, Isbister G, Bennett MH, Lavonas EJ. Hyperbaric oxygen for carbon monoxide poisoning. Cochrane Database Syst Rev. 2011;(4):Cd002041. https://doi.org/10.1002/14651858.CD002041.pub3.
68. Walker PF, Buehner MF, Wood LA, Boyer NL, Driscoll IR, Lundy JB, et al. Diagnosis and management of inhalation injury: an updated review. Crit Care. 2015;19:351. https://doi.org/10.1186/s13054-015-1077-4.
69. Leigh-Smith S, Harris T. Tension pneumothorax—time for a re-think? Emerg Med J. 2005;22:8–16.
70. Laan DV, Vu TD, Thiels CA, Pandian TK, Schiller HJ, Murad MH, et al. Chest wall thickness and decompression failure: a systematic review and meta-analysis comparing anatomic locations in needle thoracostomy. Injury. 2016;47(4):797–804. https://doi.org/10.1016/j.injury.2015.11.045. Epub 2015 Dec 13.
71. Martin M, Satterly S, Inaba K, Blair K. Does needle thoracostomy provide adequate and effective decompression of tension pneumothorax? J Trauma Acute Care Surg. 2012;73(6):1412–7. https://doi.org/10.1097/TA.0b013e31825ac511.
72. Kaserer A, Stein P, Simmen HP, Spahn DR, Neuhaus V. Failure rate of prehospital chest decompression after severe thoracic trauma. Am J Emerg Med. 2017;35(3):469–74.
73. Ferrie EP, Collum N, McGovern S. The right place in the right space? Awareness of site for needle thoracocentesis. Emerg Med J. 2005;22:788–9.
74. Wernick B, Hon H, Mubang R, Cipriano A, Hughes R, Rankin D, et al. Complications of needle thoracostomy: a comprehensive clinical review. Int J Crit Ill Inj Sci. 2015;5(3):160–9.
75. Lesperance RN, Carroll CM, Aden JK, Young JB, Nunez TC. Failure rate of prehospital needle decompression for tension pneumothorax in trauma patients. Am Surg. 2018;84(11):1750–5.
76. Dickey N. Needle decompression of tension pneumothorax—Tactical Combat Casualty Care recommendations 2012–5. Defense Health Board Memorandum dated 7 July 2012. http://health.mil/dhb/recommendations/2012/2012-05.pdf. Accessed 13 June 2013.
77. American College of Surgeons. Advanced Trauma Life Support: 10th edition changes. http://www.emdocs.net/ready-atls-10thedition-updates/. Accessed 1 Mar 2018.
78. Chen J, Nadler R, Schwartz D, Tien H, Cap AP, Glassberg E. Needle thoracostomy for tension pneumothorax: the Israeli Defense Forces experience. Can J Surg. 2015;58(3 Suppl 3):S118–24.
79. Ball CG, Wyrzykowski AD, Kirkpartick AW, Dente CJ, Nicholas JM, Salomone JP, et al. Thoracic needle decompression for tension pneumothorax: clinical correlation with catheter length. Can J Surg. 2010;53(3):184–8.

80. Inaba K, Ives C, McClure K, Branco BC, Eckstein M, Shatz D, et al. Radiologic evaluation of alternate sites for needle decompression of tension pneumothorax. Arch Surg. 2012;147(9):813–8.
81. Laan DV, Vu TD, Thiels CA, Pandian TK, Schiller HJ, Murad MH, et al. Chest wall thickness and decompression failure: a systematic review and meta-analysis comparing anatomic locations in needle thoracostomy. Injury. 2016;47(4):797–804.
82. Stevens RL, Rochester AA, Busko J, Blackwell T, Schwartz D, Argenta A, et al. Needle thoracostomy for tension pneumothorax: failure predicted by chest computed tomography. Prehosp Emerg Care. 2009;13(1):14–7.
83. Schmidt U, Stalp M, Gerich T, Blauth M, Maull KI, Tscherne H. Chest tube decompression of blunt chest injuries by physicians in the field: effectiveness and complications. J Trauma. 1998;44(1):98–101.
84. Millikan JS, Moore EE, Steiner E, Aragon GE, Van Way CW 3rd, et al. Complications of tube thoracostomy for acute trauma. Am J Surg. 1980;140:738–41.
85. Dickson RL, Gleisberg G, Aiken M, Crocker K, Patrick C, Nichols T, et al. Emergency medical services simple thoracostomy for traumatic cardiac arrest: Postimplementation experience in a ground-based suburban/rural emergency medical services agency. J Emerg Med. 2018;55:366–71. https://doi.org/10.1016/j.jemermed.2018.05.027.
86. Kasotakis G, Sideris A, Yang Y, de Moya M, Alam H, King DR, et al.; Inflammation and Host Response to Injury Investigators. Aggressive early crystalloid resuscitation adversely affects outcomes in adult blunt trauma patients: an analysis of the Glue Grant database. J Trauma Acute Care Surg. 2013;74(5):1215–21; discussion 1221–2. https://doi.org/10.1097/TA.0b013e3182826e13.
87. Morrison CA, Carrick MM, Norman MA, Scott BG, Welsh FJ, Tsai P, et al. Hypotensive resuscitation strategy reduces transfusion requirements and severe postoperative coagulopathy in trauma patients with hemorrhagic shock: preliminary results of a randomized controlled trial. J Trauma. 2011;70(3):652–63. https://doi.org/10.1097/TA.0b013e31820e77ea.
88. Duchesne JC, Heaney J, Guidry C, McSwain N Jr, Meade P, Cohen M, et al. Diluting the benefits of hemostatic resuscitation: a multi-institutional analysis. J Trauma Acute Care Surg. 2013;75(1):76–82. https://doi.org/10.1097/TA.0b013e3182987df3.
89. Story DA, Morimatsu H, Bellomo R. Hyperchloremic acidosis in the critically ill: one of the strong-ion acidoses? Anesth Analg. 2006;103(1):144–8.
90. Todd SR, Malinoski D, Muller PJ, Schreiber MA. Lactated Ringer's is superior to normal saline in the resuscitation of uncontrolled hemorrhagic shock. J Trauma. 2007;62(3):636–9.
91. Phillips CR, Vinecore K, Hagg DS, Sawai RS, Differding JA, Watters JM, et al. Resuscitation of haemorrhagic shock with normal saline vs. lactated Ringer's: effects on oxygenation, extravascular lung water and haemodynamics. Crit Care. 2009;13(2):R30. https://doi.org/10.1186/cc7736.
92. Wang Y, Guo W, Gao D, You G, Wang B, Chen G, et al. Effects of Plasma-lyte A, lactated Ringer's, and normal saline on acid-base status and intestine injury in the initial treatment of hemorrhagic shock. Am J Emerg Med. 2017;35(2):317–21. https://doi.org/10.1016/j.ajem.2016.10.007.
93. Neal MD, Hoffman MK, Cuschieri J, Minei JP, Maier RV, Harbrecht BG, et al. Crystalloid to packed red blood cell transfusion ratio in the massively transfused patient: when a little goes a long way. J Trauma Acute Care Surg. 2012;72(4):892–8. https://doi.org/10.1097/TA.0b013e31823d84a7.
94. Balogh Z, McKinley BA, Cocanour CS, Kozar RA, Valdivia A, Sailors RM, et al. Supranormal trauma resuscitation causes more cases of abdominal compartment syndrome. Arch Surg. 2003;138:637–43.
95. Kiraly LN, Differding JA, Enomoto TM, Sawai RS, Muller PJ, Diggs B, et al. Resuscitation with normal saline (NS) vs. lactated ringers (LR) modulates hypercoagulability and leads to increased blood loss in an uncontrolled hemorrhagic shock swine model. J Trauma. 2006;61(1):57–64.

96. Hahn RG, Lyons G. The half-life of infusion fluids: an educational review. Eur J Anaesthesiol. 2016;33(7):475–82. https://doi.org/10.1097/EJA.0000000000000436.
97. Pearce FJ, Lyons WS. Logistics of parenteral fluids in battlefield resuscitation. Mil Med. 1999;164(9):653–5.
98. Ley EJ, Clond MA, Srour MK, Barnajian M, Mirocha J, Margulies DR, et al. Emergency department crystalloid resuscitation of 1.5 L or more is associated with increased mortality in elderly and nonelderly trauma patients. J Trauma. 2011;70(2):398–400. https://doi.org/10.1097/TA.0b013e318208f99b.
99. Sobrino J, Shafi S. Timing and causes of death after injuries. Proc (Bayl Univ Med Cent). 2013;26:120–3.
100. Cap AP, Pidcoke HF, Spinella P, Strandenes G, Borgman MA, Schreiber M, et al. Damage control resuscitation. Mil Med. 2018;183(Suppl_2):36–43. https://doi.org/10.1093/milmed/usy112.
101. McGinity AC, Zhu CS, Greebon L, Xenakis E, Waltman E, Epley E, et al. Prehospital low-titer cold-stored whole blood: philosophy for ubiquitous utilization of O-positive product for emergency use in hemorrhage due to injury. J Trauma Acute Care Surg. 2018;84(6S Suppl 1):S115–9. https://doi.org/10.1097/TA.0000000000001905.
102. Bahr MP, Yazer MH, Triulzi DJ, Collins RA. Whole blood for the acutely haemorrhaging civilian trauma patient: a novel idea or rediscovery? Transfus Med. 2016;26(6):406–14. https://doi.org/10.1111/tme.12329. Epub 2016 Jun 29.
103. Nessen SC, Eastridge BJ, Cronk D, Craig RM, Berseus O, Ellison R, et al. Fresh whole blood use by forward surgical teams in Afghanistan is associated with improved survival compared to component therapy without platelets. Transfusion. 2013;53(Suppl. 1):107S–13S.
104. Zielinski MD, Jenkins DH, Hughes JD, Badjie KS, Stubbs JR. Back to the future: the renaissance of whole-blood transfusions for massively hemorrhaging patients. Surgery. 2014;155:883–6.
105. Spinella PC, Strandenes G, Rein EB, Seghatchian J, Hervig T. Symposium on fresh whole blood for severe hemorrhagic shock: from in-hospital to far forward resuscitations. Transfus Apher Sci. 2012;46:113–7.
106. Strandenes G, Skogrand H, Spinnela PC, Hervig T, Rein EB. Donor performance of combat readiness skills of special forces soldiers are maintained immediately after whole blood donation: a study to support the development of a prehospital fresh whole blood transfusion program. Transfusion. 2013;53:526–30.
107. Shlaifer A, Siman-Tov M, Radomislensky I, Peleg K, Shina A, Baruch EN, et al. Prehospital administration of freeze-dried plasma, is it the solution for trauma casualties? J Trauma Acute Care Surg. 2017;83(4):675–82. https://doi.org/10.1097/TA.0000000000001569.
108. Vu E. Data presented at special operations medicine scientific assembly, May 2015.
109. Shakur H, Roberts I, Bautista R, Caballero J, Coats T, Dewan Y, et al. Effects of tranexamic acid on death, vascular occlusive events, and blood transfusion in trauma patients with significant haemorrhage (CRASH-2): a randomised, placebo-controlled trial. Lancet. 2010;376(9734):23–32.
110. Gayet-Ageron A, Prieto-Merino D, Ker K, Shakur H, Ageron FX, Roberts I, Antifibrinolytic Trials Collaboration. Effect of treatment delay on the effectiveness and safety of antifibrinolytics in acute severe haemorrhage: a meta-analysis of individual patient-level data from 40,138 bleeding patients. Lancet. 2018;391(10116):125–32. https://doi.org/10.1016/S0140-6736(17)32455-8.
111. Morrison J, Dubose J, Rasmussen T, Midwinter M. Military application of tranexamic acid in trauma emergency resuscitation (MATTERs) study. Arch Surg. 2012;147(2):113–9.
112. Marsden M, Rossetto A, Duffield C, Woolley T, Buxton W, Steynberg S, et al. Prehospital tranexamic acid shortens the interval to administration by half in Major Trauma Networks: a service evaluation. Emerg Med J. 2019;36:395–400. https://doi.org/10.1136/emermed-2018-208118. Jun 19. pii: emermed-2018-208118.

113. El-Menyar A, Sathian B, Wahlen BM, Abdelrahman H, Peralta R, Al-Thani H, et al. Prehospital administration of tranexamic acid in trauma patients: A 1:1 matched comparative study from a level 1 trauma center. Am J Emerg Med. 2019. pii: S0735-6757(19)30293-1. [epub ahead of print].
114. Morrison JJ, Ross JD, Dubose JJ, Jansen JO, Midwinter MJ, Rasmussen TE. Association of cryoprecipitate and tranexamic acid with improved survival following wartime injury: findings from the MATTERs II Study. JAMA Surg. 2013;148(3):218–25.
115. CRASH-3 Trial Collaborators. Effects of tranexamic acid on death, disability, vascular occlusive events and other morbidities in patients with acute traumatic brain injury (CRASH-3): a randomised, placebo-controlled trial. Lancet. 2019;3394:1713–23. https://doi.org/10.1016/S0140-6736(19)32233-0.
116. CRASH-2 Collaborators, Intracranial Bleeding Study. Effect of tranexamic acid in traumatic brain injury: a nested randomised, placebo controlled trial (CRASH-2 Intracranial Bleeding Study). BMJ. 2011;343:d3795. https://doi.org/10.1136/bmj.d3795.
117. Sprigg N, Flaherty K, Appleton J, Al-Shahi Salman R, Bereczki D, Beridze M, et al. Tranexamic acid for hyperacute primary IntraCerebral Haemorrhage (TICH-2): an international randomised, placebo-controlled, phase 3 superiority trial. Lancet. 2018;391:2107–15.
118. Rowell S, et al. Use of tranexamic acid in patients with traumatic brain injury: results from the North American multi-center prehospital TXA for TBI trial. Proceeding of the American Academy of Neurosurgery, 4–10 May 2019, Philadelphia.
119. Morte D, Lammers D, Bingham J, Kuckelman J, Eckert M, Martin M. Tranexamic acid administration following head trauma in a combat setting: does tranexamic acid result in improved neurologic outcomes? J Trauma Acute Care Surg. 2019;87(1):125–9. https://doi.org/10.1097/TA.0000000000002269.
120. Lapostolle F, Sebbah JL, Couvreur J, Koch FX, Savary D, Tazarourte K, et al. Risk factors for onset of hypothermia in trauma victims: the HypoTraum study. Crit Care. 2012;16(4):R142.
121. Forristal C, Van Aarsen K, Columbus M, Wei J, Vogt K, Mal S. Predictors of hypothermia upon trauma center arrival in severe trauma patients transported to hospital via EMS. Prehosp Emerg Care. 2019;4:1–8. [epub ahead of print].
122. Strandenes G. Data presented at special operations medicine scientific assembly, May 2016.
123. Corso P, Finkelstein E, Miller T, Fiebelkorn I, Zaloshnja E. The incidence and economic burden of injuries in the United States. Inj Prev. 2015;21(6):434–40. https://doi.org/10.1136/ip.2005.010983rep.
124. Bell JM, Brelding M, Jenkins EL, Haarbauer-Krupa J. Report to congress: traumatic brain injury in the United States: epidemiology and rehabilitation. Atlanta: US Centers for Disease Control and Prevention; 2014. p. 18. Accessed 24 Nov 2019.
125. Spaite DW, Bobrow BJ, Kein SM, Barnhart B, Chikani V, Gaither JB, et al. Association of statewide implementation of the prehospital traumatic brain injury treatment guidelines with patient survival following traumatic brain injury. The Excellence in Prehospital Injury Care (EPIC) Study. JAMA Surg. 2019;154(7):e191152.
126. Wilson M, Hinds J, Grier G, Burns B, Carley S, Davies G. Impact brain apnea – a forgotten cause of cardiovascular collapse in trauma. Resuscitation. 2016;105:52–8.
127. Spaite D, Hu C, Bobrow B, Chikani V, Sherrill D, Barnhart B, et al. Mortality and prehospital blood pressure in patients with major traumatic brain injury implications for the hypotension threshold. JAMA Surg. 2017;152(4):360–8.
128. Feldman Z, Kanter M, Robertson CS, Contant CF, Hayes C, Sheinberg MA, et al. Effect of head elevation on intracranial pressure, cerebral perfusion pressure, and cerebral blood flow in head injured patients. J Neurosurg. 1992;76(2):207–11.
129. French L, McCrea M, Baggett M. The military acute concussion evaluation (MACE). J Spec Oper Med. 2008;1:68–77.
130. Stone M, Safadjou S, Farber B, Velazco N, Man J, Reddy SH, et al. Utility of the Military Acute Concussion Evaluation as a screening tool for mild traumatic brain injury in a civilian trauma population. J Trauma Acute Care Surg. 2015;79(1):147–51.

131. Wedmore IS, Kotwal RS, McManus JG, Pennardt A, Talbot TS, Fowler M, McGhee L. Safety and efficacy of oral transmucosal fentanyl citrate for prehospital pain control on the battlefield. J Trauma Acute Care Surg. 2012;73(6 Suppl 5):S490–5. https://doi.org/10.1097/TA.0b013e3182754674.
132. Moeller-Bertram T, Keltner J, Strigo IA. Pain and post traumatic stress disorder - review of clinical and experimental evidence. Neuropharmacology. 2012;62(2):586–97.
133. Polomano RC, Buckenmaier CC, Kwon KH, Hanlon AL, Rupprecht C, Goldberg C, et al. Effects of low-dose IV ketamine on peripheral and central pain from major limb injuries sustained in combat. Pain Med. 2013;14(7):1088–100.
134. Wenderoth BR, Kaneda ET, Amini A, Amini R, Patanwala AE. Morphine versus fentanyl for pain due to traumatic injury in the emergency department. J Trauma Nurs. 2013;20(1):10–5. https://doi.org/10.1097/JTN.0b013e31828660b5.
135. Hermens JM, Ebertz JM, Hanifin JM, Hirshman CA. Comparison of histamine release in human skin mast cells induced by morphine, fentanyl, and oxymorphone. Anesthesiology. 1985;62(2):124–9.
136. Tawfic QA. A review of the use of ketamine in pain management. J Opioid Manag. 2013;9(5):379–88.
137. Beaudoin FL, Lin C, Guan W, Merchant RC. Low-dose ketamine improves pain relief in patients receiving intravenous opioids for acute pain in the emergency department: results of a randomized, double-blind, clinical trial. Acad Emerg Med. 2014;21(11):1193–202.
138. Mahshidfar B, Rezai M, Abbasi S, Farsi D, Hafezimoghadam P, Mofidi M, et al. Intravenous acetaminophen vs. ketorolac in terms of pain management in prehospital emergency services: a randomized clinical trial. Adv J Emerg Med. 2019;3(4):e37. https://doi.org/10.22114/ajem.v0i0.130. eCollection 2019 Fall.
139. Butler FK, Kotwal RS, Buckenmaier CC, Edgar EP, O'Connor KC, Montgomery HR, et al. A triple-option analgesia plan for tactical combat casualty care: TCCC guidelines change 13-04. J Spec Oper Med. 2014;14(1):13–25.
140. Giannau C, Baldan M. War surgery: working with limited resources in armed conflict and other situations of violence, Volume 1. International Committee of the Red Cross. Geneva. 2013. p. 257.
141. Bowyer GW, Cooper GJ, Rice P. Small fragment wounds: biophysics and pathophysiology. J Trauma. 1996;40(Suppl):S159–64.
142. Mellor SG, Cooper GJ, Bowyer GW. Efficacy of delayed administration of benzylpenicillin in the control of infection in penetrating soft tissue injuries in war. J Trauma. 1996;40(3 Suppl):S128–34.
143. Giannau C, Baldan M, Molde A. War surgery: working with limited resources in armed conflict and other situations of violence, volume 2. International Committee of the Red Cross. Geneva. 2013. p. 78.
144. Pickett JR. Data presented at special operations medicine scientific assembly 2019.
145. Singh AK, Ditkofsky NG, York JD, Abujudeh HH, Avery LA, Brunner JF, et al. Blast injuries: from improvised explosive device blasts to the Boston Marathon bombing. Radiographics. 2016;36(1):295–307. https://doi.org/10.1148/rg.2016150114.
146. Cuske J. The lost art of splinting. How to properly immobilize extremities & manage pain. JEMS. 2008;33(7):50–64.; quiz 66. https://doi.org/10.1016/S0197-2510(08)70253-5.

The Explosive Mass Casualty Incident: Prehospital Incident Management and Triage

13

Richard B. Schwartz and Richard McNutt

Overview of Explosive Mass Casualty Incidents

Worldwide, the terrorist threat has increased dramatically since 2001 (Fig. 13.1). In 2016, the number of casualties from terrorist incidents was 59,435. Many of these international attacks utilized explosive devices and resulted in mass casualty incidents (MCIs). In the United States, annual explosion rates top 600/year and a majority are intentional bombings (Figs. 13.2 and 13.3) [1–11].

An MCI is an event that causes casualties in sufficient number or acuity to overwhelm the locally available medical and public health services and resources [12]. Large numbers of casualties alone can stress medical capabilities and resources. However, explosives are uniquely suited to cause MCIs due to their ability to affect large areas and numbers of people, produce severe and complicated injuries, cause massive structural damage, displace populations, and create environmental hazards (Table 13.1).

The characteristics of the bomb and explosion have a large impact on the resources needed for response and how to distribute them. A 2003 examination of 44 blast MCIs evaluated many of these differences [13]. Immediate mortality ranged from 0% to 68%, early (on-scene) mortality ranged from 0% to 4%, and late mortality ranged from 0% to 5%. ED utilization ranged from 26% to 100% of initial survivors.

Explosive MCIs also vary greatly in their epidemiological outcomes, time courses of resource needs, and overall use of resources. These vary in somewhat

R. B. Schwartz (✉)
Department of Emergency Medicine and Hospitalist Services, Augusta University Medical Center, Augusta, GA, USA
e-mail: rschwartz@augusta.edu

R. McNutt
Combined Army/Civilian Emergency Medicine Residency, Department of Emergency Medicine, Augusta University Medical Center, Augusta, GA, USA

D. W. Callaway, J. L. Burstein (eds.), *Operational and Medical Management of Explosive and Blast Incidents*, https://doi.org/10.1007/978-3-030-40655-4_13

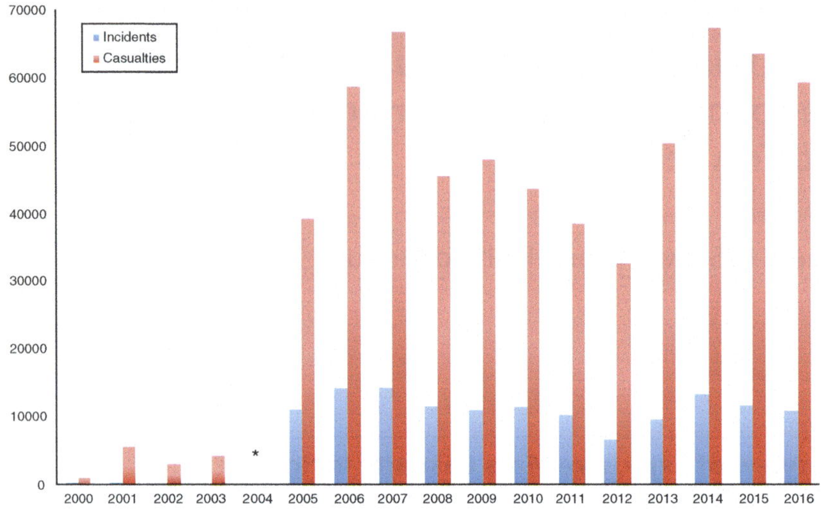

Fig. 13.1 Numbers of international terrorism incidents and casualties in 2000–2016 [1–9]. (*Data not available for 2004)

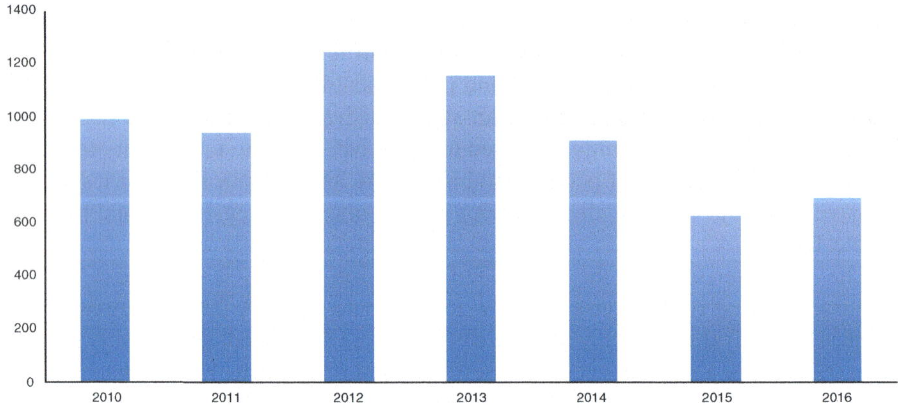

Fig. 13.2 Numbers of explosion incidents in the United States in 2010–2016 [10, 11]

predictable ways depending on the type of explosion, explosion setting, and blast sequelae [14]. This predictability can help emergency systems prepare for and react to explosive MCIs. The explosive incident characteristics useful for planning and predictive purpose include incident proximity to hospitals, explosive payload and mechanism of delivery, early warning and evacuation prior to detonation, open-air versus confined-space setting, and any structural collapse or fire. All of these characteristics have implications for MCI management, as well as anticipated impacts on number of patients, injury frequency, and injury severity. These effects are summarized in Table 13.2.

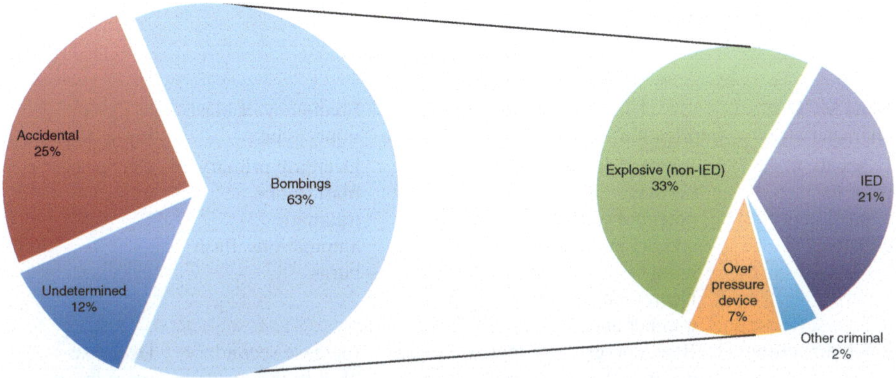
Accidental
25%
Bombings
63%
Undetermined
12%
Explosive (non-IED)
33%
IED
21%
Over
pressure
device
7%
Other criminal
2%

Fig. 13.3 United States explosions incidents types in 2016 [11]

Table 13.1 Relevant Explosive MCI Characteristics

High volume of casualties
Complex poly-trauma injuries may require specialized equipment and/or resources.
Structural damage resulting in casualty entrapment and prolonged extrications that overwhelm search, rescue, and evacuation capabilities
Contamination or environmental hazards may displace personnel from living or working areas
Ongoing security challenges and information management (i.e., social media) challenges

Table 13.2 Blast MCI characteristics and the implications and Anticipated impacts on hospitals

		Anticipated impacts		
Blast MCI characteristic	Implication	Numbers seeking emergency care	Frequency of blast injury type	Injury severity
Blast proximity to closest care center	1. Increased number of injured survivors will arrive at ED outside EMS 2. Decreased EMS transport time	Increased number at nearby hospitals	Increased primary blast injuries, traumatic amputations, and many minor injuries	Variable – more minor and more serious injuries
Vehicle-delivered explosive	1. Increase explosive magnitude 2. Structural collapse possible 3. Increase immediate deaths close to detonation point or inside collapse	Increase; may produce 100s to 1000s of injured survivors	Variable	Increased

(continued)

Table 13.2 (continued)

Blast MCI characteristic	Implication	Anticipated impacts		
		Numbers seeking emergency care	Frequency of blast injury type	Injury severity
Evacuation prior to explosion or collapse	1. Increase distance between potential victims and detonation point 2. Decreased number at risk	Decrease	Decrease primary blast injury, traumatic amputations, flash burns	Decrease
Open-air setting	1. Blast energy dissipated, but spread over greater area 2. Structural collapse unlikely 3. Decrease number of immediate deaths	Increase; may produce up to 200 injured survivors	Increase secondary blast injury	Decrease – more injuries minor
Confined space setting	1. Blast energy potentiated, but contained in lesser area 2. Increased number of immediate deaths inside space 3. Increased number of injured exposed to blast effects 4. Increased effects in smaller space (bus ≫ public room)	Decrease; usually produces <100 injured survivors	Increased primary blast injury, amputations, burns	Greatly increased
Structural collapse result	1. Increased explosive magnitude 2. Collateral damage outside structure possible 3. Increased number of immediate deaths inside collapse 4. Increased effects with taller building	1. Variable 2. Decreased number from inside structural collapse 3. Increased number from outside structural collapse 4. May produce 100s to 1000s of injured survivors	Increased inhalation injury, crush injury	Increased

Table 13.2 (continued)

Blast MCI characteristic	Implication	Anticipated impacts Numbers seeking emergency care	Frequency of blast injury type	Injury severity
Structural fire result	1. Increased number of victims inside structure exposed to smoke and fire 2. Increased effects with taller building 3. Increased evacuation time in high rise fire	Increased number from inside structure	1. Increase burns, inhalation injury 2. Increased inhalation injury in high rise fire	Variable

Modified from Halpern et al. [14], reproduced with permission
ED emergency department, *EMS* Emergency Management Services

Vehicle-delivered explosives often have a larger explosive magnitude and, if the vehicle is driven close to or into a structure, can cause collapse, thereby producing hundreds or even thousands of casualties to occupants and causing additional injury patterns. For example, explosives in a van were used to attack the World Trade Center in 1993. There were few deaths or injuries from the blast in an underground parking space, but it caused hundreds of casualties from smoke inhalation [15].

Explosions occurring in open-air setting compared to those in confined spaces, tend to decrease primary blast injury casualties because the blast energy is dissipated over a larger area. Victims close enough to sustain primary blast injury of the lungs or bowel tend to be killed outright by a combination of mechanisms, hence not becoming patients entering the medical system [14]. Although this tends to decrease the percentages of immediate deaths and overall injury severity, it tends to increase the percentage of initial survivors with secondary blast injuries requiring emergency medical system (EMS) intervention.

Explosions in confined spaces have their energy potentiated but concentrated in a smaller area [14]. This effect is enhanced by smaller structures or bombs placed in private or public transportation vehicles. This increases the chance of immediate deaths and increases the exposure to bomb additives [16]. Any increased number of immediate deaths acts to decrease the percentages of total victims seeking aid.

Structural collapse typically implies a larger explosion magnitude [14]. Collapse is likely to kill more people inside the structure as crush and inhalation injuries are compounded atop the injuries caused by the blast. For example, in the 1993 World Trade Center bombing, almost 88.8% of 546 casualties seeking hospital care were from smoke inhalation [17]. In addition, structural collapse often requires massive, specialized resources for rescue and result in high mortality, with delays in initial evaluation and stabilization. Should a fire result inside a building or vehicle, this will likely complicate extrication attempts, particularly in very tall buildings where vertical movement may be more difficult [14]. It may also require adjusting the prehospital treatment, because of ongoing risks to responders, combined burn-crush-blast injuries, and alterations in destination protocols.

It is important for the prehospital providers and on-scene Incident Command System (ICS) to be aware of these factors and impacts, as they can inform what resources they request, and how they request them. They can also help them understand higher-level decisions about where to route patients and why there are delays in resources. Regardless of the location, explosive MCIs present substantial risks to responders, such as ongoing terrorist threats, secondary explosions, unstable structures, and electrical and fire hazards. The response to such attacks requires a coordinated multi-jurisdictional approach, and this is best coordinated using the ICS. And all of these factors highlight the need for effective dynamic triage.

Incident Command in Explosive Mass Casualty Incidents

The initial chaos following a blast incident provides a difficult command, control, and logistics problem. How does one alert, marshal, and coordinate the assets necessary to effectively respond to a blast MCI? As noted in Chap. 6, emergency response organizations in the United States employ the National Incident Management System (NIMS) to structure emergency management activities related to preparedness, operational command, resource management, communication and information management, and maintenance [18]. Under NIMS, command and control of these activities is structured under the ICS to enable effective and efficient integration of facilities, equipment, personnel, procedures, and communications. Incidents of all types require the same broad functions in order to be managed successfully. The ICS breaks these functions out into the following areas: command, operations, planning, logistics, and finance/administration. The ICS seeks to accomplish these functions by leveraging its core principles of modular organization, integrated communications, manageable spans of control, transfer of command, and an incident action plan. Modular organization allows the ICS to be built, piece-by-piece, as assets and personnel arrive on scene. Integrated communications ensure that all elements of the response are in contact with each other. Manageable span of control ensures that no individual is directing more personnel than they are capable of personally overseeing. Transfer of command ensures appropriate, accurate, and timely handoff between commanders. An incident action plan ensures that there is a coherent framework for continued response to the incident.

Explosive MCIs are complex and highly dynamic with compressed response timelines that challenge the implementation of ICS. The keys to establishing an effective ICS after an explosive MCI is to start small, start early, and have a framework [12]. The ICS starts from the first step of the medical response as the initial responders designate an incident commander. As more personnel arrive on scene, the initial incident commander may transition command to a more capable person.

In the case of an explosive event, either law enforcement or fire department personnel will likely act as incident command (IC). Law enforcement is generally the IC if there is a persistent criminal threat with fire taking command once this threat is mitigated and the focus shifts to rescue. Command may change during the incident and the transfer of command must include a briefing, even if informal, including all essential information up until that point. Furthermore, all responding personnel must clearly understand when and to whom command has transitioned.

Manageable spans of control can be maintained as more personnel arrive by delegating responsibilities and organizing arriving personnel into well-defined teams with clear leadership, roles, and duties. Integrated communications must be maintained between arriving personnel, especially when a whole new organization (e.g., EMS) arrives. As more responders become available, these personnel can provide the planning, logistics, and finance functions (Fig. 13.4) that may not have been necessary during the initial response. The trend toward integrated warm-zone operations (e.g., Rescue Task Force), discussed in Chap. 15, is a model that facilitates improved communication during high-threat incidents such as the explosive MCI.

There is controversy as to the universality and effectiveness of the ICS in a dynamic MCI such as a terrorist bomb attack [19]. The ICS appears to be most effective under certain conditions. For instance, it may work best for events that are limited in duration, objectives, and scope. This would seem to make it well-suited for response to a blast incident. It also appears to work best when there is a shared vision for response among the participating organizations, there are strong working relationships among individual responders, and the individual responders are trained in, or familiar with, the ICS structure. This highlights the need to get organizational buy-in *before* an incident occurs, as well as the need to conduct integrated training exercises.

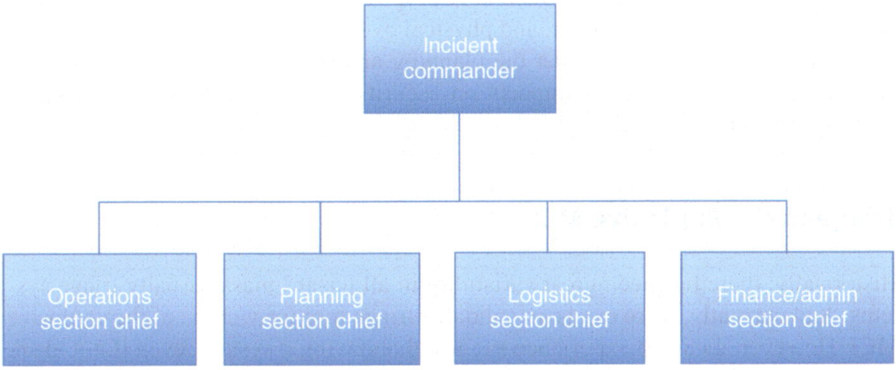

Fig. 13.4 Incident Command System structure [18]

Security Priorities in Explosive MCI Response

Security is paramount following an explosive MCI. Regardless of whether the explosion was intentional or accidental, secondary explosions, fires, structural collapse, and toxic inhalation can threaten first responders. In the case of intentional bombings, the possibility of additional security threats following the initial attack must be considered [10, 11, 20]. Secondary attacks on first responders—an initial attack may be a ruse to draw resources to the area in order to affect a larger attack—are an increasingly common tactic in terrorism. From the attacker's perspective, the concentration of emergency personnel provides a target-rich environment for a second explosive device or other follow-up attack. Thus, it is important for law enforcement and other security forces to be integrated into the ICS and the overall disaster response system. Security forces should maintain control of ingress and egress routes from the scene or scenes. They should also consider the area immediately surrounding them. These areas should be observed or cleared if suspicion is high enough. If an explosive device is suspected, bomb expert personnel, either law enforcement or military, need to be notified in order to deal with the threat. Figure 13.5 provides a rough guideline for the evacuation distances necessary depending on the type of threatening device [21]. Keep in mind that a clever terrorist might set a decoy to cause evacuation, with the real device set along the most likely evacuation routes and destinations, including hospitals.

As emergency responders, it is also important to note that nonprofessional bystanders at the scene will likely be the first responders to any blast incident [22]. The historical MCI focus on "crowd control" has largely evolved, acknowledging the important role active bystanders can play in reducing mortality. Lay public training courses that teach global sorting and provide a narrow range of LSI—generally open airway and hemorrhage control—can be important force multipliers. However, the extended presence of active bystanders on scene creates a host of security concerns including but not limited to threat of perpetrating secondary attack, increased victim load if follow-on incident, and physical overcrowding of response area. First responder agencies must consider the planning and response implications that this new reality brings including impacts on security, communication, and on-scene leadership roles.

Triage in the Explosive MCI

Historically, there has been great variability in all hazard mass casualty triage systems. And currently, there exists no validated triage tool for victims of the explosive MCI. However, data and experience suggest that having *a* system, even if not ideal, is more effective than a completely ad hoc response.

The Centers for Disease Control and Prevention (CDC) funded the development of standardized criteria known as the Model Uniform Core Criteria for Mass Casualty Triage (MUCC) [23–25]. The MUCC were integrated into the National Highway Traffic and Safety Administration (NHTSA) January 2017 guidance for

UNCLASSIFIED

Improvised Explosive Device (IED) Safe Standoff Distance Cheat Sheet

	Threat Description		Explosives Mass[1] (TNT equivalent)	Building Evacuation Distance[2]	Outdoor Evacuation Distance[3]
High Explosives (TNT Equivalent)	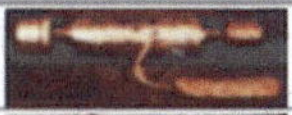	Pipe Bomb	5 lbs 2.3 kg	70 ft 21 m	850 ft 259 m
	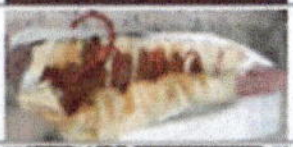	Suicide Belt	10 lbs 4.5 kg	90 ft 27 m	1,080 ft 330 m
	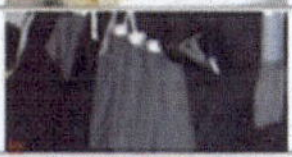	Suicide Vest	20 lbs 9 kg	110 ft 34 m	1,360 ft 415 m
	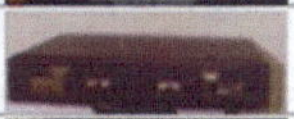	Briefcase/Suitcase Bomb	50 lbs 23 kg	150 ft 46 m	1,850 ft 564 m
	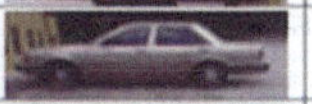	Compact Sedan	500 lbs 227 kg	320 ft 98 m	1,500 ft 457 m
	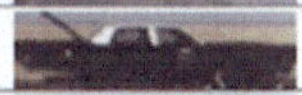	Sedan	1,000 lbs 454 kg	400 ft 122 m	1,750 ft 534 m
	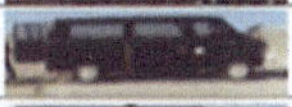	Passenger/Cargo Van	4,000 lbs 1,814 kg	640 ft 195 m	2,750 ft 838 m
	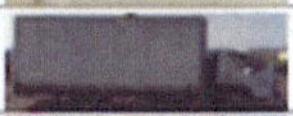	Small Moving Van/ Delivery Truck	10,000 lbs 4,536 kg	860 ft 263 m	3,750 ft 1,143 m
	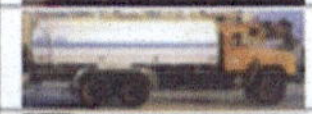	Moving Van/Water Truck	30,000 lbs 13,608 kg	1,240 ft 375 m	6,500 ft 1,982 m
		Semitrailer	60,000 lbs 27,216 kg	1,570 ft 475 m	7,000 ft 2,134 m
	Threat Description		**LPG Mass/Volume[1]**	**Fireball Diameter[4]**	**Safe Distance[5]**
Liquefied Petroleum Gas (LPG - Butane or Propane)	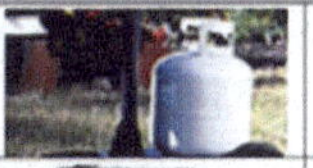	Small LPG Tank	20 lbs/5 gal 9 kg/19 l	40 ft 12 m	160 ft 48 m
	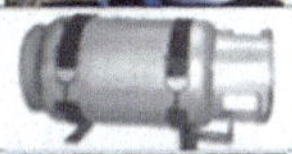	Large LPG Tank	100 lbs/25 gal 45 kg/95 l	69 ft 21 m	276 ft 84 m
	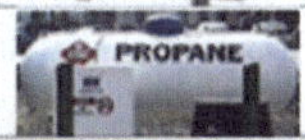	Commerical/Residential LPG Tank	2,000 lbs/500 gal 907 kg/1,893 l	184 ft 56 m	736 ft 224 m
	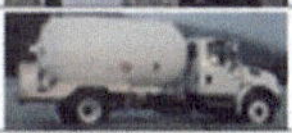	Small LPG Truck	8,000 lbs/2,000 gal 3,630 kg/7,570 l	292 ft 89 m	1,168 ft 356 m
	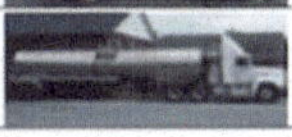	Semitanker LPG	40,000 lbs/10,000 gal 18,144 kg/37,850 l	499 ft 152 m	1,996 ft 608 m

[1]Based on the maximum amount of material that could reasonably fit into a container or vehicle. Variations possible.
[2]Governed by the abilty of an unreinforced building withstand severe damage or collapse.
[3]Governed by the greater of fragment throw distance or glass breakage/falling glass hazard distance. These distances can be reduced for personnel wearing basllistic protection. Note that the pipe bomb, suicide belt/vest, and briefcase/suitcase bomb are assumed to have a fragmentation characteristic that requires greater standoff distances than an equal amount of explosives in a vehicle.
[4]Assuming efficient mixing of the flammable gas with ambient air.
[5]Determined by U.S. firefighting practices wherein safe distances are approximately 4 times the flame height. Note that an LPG tank filled with high explosives would require a significantly greater standoff distance than if it were filled with LPG.

UNCLASSIFIED

Fig. 13.5 Improvised Explosive Device Safe Standoff Distance Cheat Sheet [21]

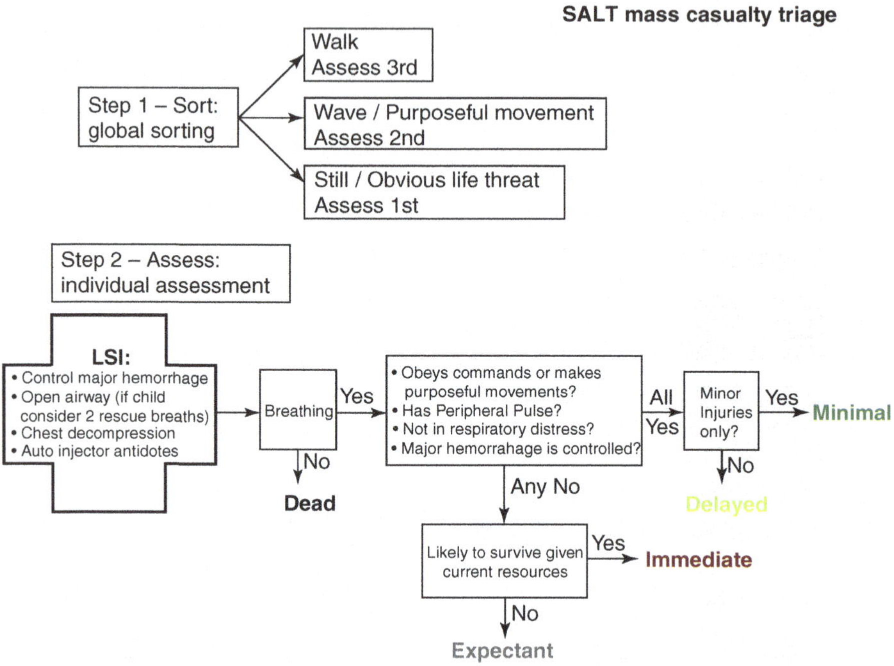

Fig. 13.6 SALT mass casualty triage [24]. LSI, lifesaving interventions

EMS education programs. SMART (not an acronym) and SALT (Sort, Assess, Lifesaving Interventions [LSI], Transport) triage are examples of MUCC-compliant triage systems. SALT triage (Fig. 13.6) is the most commonly used. It is a nonproprietary system that will be further described. Simple Triage and Rapid Treatment (START) is another commonly used triage system in the United States, but it is not MUCC-compliant and not in line with NHTSA guidance.

SALT triage and all MUCC-compliant systems utilize two steps: (1) global sorting of casualties and (2) LSI and individual victim assessment (see Fig. 13.6).

Global Sorting

All casualties are given clear, verbal commands augmented with hand signals regarding where to go and what to do in order to receive help. Those patients completely unable to respond to verbal commands are those most likely to require lifesaving interventions first. Thus, global sorting decreases the time it takes to get to those patients most in need of lifesaving interventions. Those casualties able to heed the instructions should be evaluated on scene and, if deemed low acuity, may be transported to designated facilities after scene clearance of more critical patients.

Individual Assessment

In SALT triage, there are no specific vital sign parameters to be memorized. Instead, the provider needs only to check for the presence of a peripheral pulse, the appearance of difficulty breathing and make a quick clinical assessment. This makes the triage scheme easier to remember, faster to apply, and usable for patients of all ages. All MUCC-compliant triage systems utilize the following triage categories: immediate (red), delayed (yellow), minimal (green), expectant (blue or gray), and dead (black). The categories can be remembered by using the mnemonic ID-MED and are consistent with US Military and North Atlantic Treaty Organization (NATO) triage categories.

The expectant category is resource-based and the use of this category changes depending on the magnitude of the event, the available resources, and the provider's level of training and comfort with using the category. The expectant category will only be needed if there are not enough resources available to meet demand. This allows providers to allocate scarce resources to potentially salvageable patients rather than applying resuscitation resources to those who are unlikely to survive. Labeling and identifying victims who are unlikely to survive as expectant is important to limit redundant triaging and so that resuscitation or comfort care can be provided when resources become available.

Casualties that are triaged as minimal may be transported to designated facilities after scene clearance of more critical patients. The consolidation of the minimal patients at the scene while more seriously injured patients are evacuated still requires resources. In an explosive incident, minor-appearing injuries with major life threats can be missed during the initial sorting. Medically, these victims will require a more thorough evaluation as soon as time permits. However, depending on the resources available, it may take several minutes or even hours before these patients can be given a more detailed evaluation. One mitigation strategy is to assign incoming personnel to the green zone as a re-triage officer. This person will operate in an environment with high patient-to-provider ratios and be responsible for re-triage, casualty accountability, and integrated operations with security personnel who will likely need to screen and interview all victims. Some patients who do not need urgent or emergent care can be reassured and sent home or to primary care follow-up, if adequately assessed at the scene.

The scene assessment needs to go beyond a triage assessment and must be provided by a practitioner who is familiar with injuries related to blasts. Patients with minor injuries should have no shortness of breath, abdominal pain, oropharyngeal petechia, and no penetrating wounds to the neck, thorax, abdomen, or over joints or major vascular structures.

All patients with concern for primary blast lung should be transported to a location with chest X-ray capabilities. Most patients with a concern for primary blast lung injury would be triaged as immediate or delayed depending on the severity of hypoxemia or respiratory distress. Symptoms and signs appear relatively early after exposure, and prolonged observation to rule out blast lung injury may not be necessary [26]. Other aspects of the patient should be assessed, such as presence of visible trauma, lung sounds, and abnormal vital signs (tachypnea or tachycardia) to determine if there is an underlying severe injury. Point-of-care ultrasonography (POCUS) can help discriminate between pneumothorax and potential primary blast lung injury in the field or in the hospital.

Providers should consider legality here, as they cannot legally prevent a patient from leaving the scene to seek aid wherever they choose. Thus, patients cannot be stopped from leaving the scene, only advised as to the best course of action. Similarly, due to the Emergency Medical Treatment and Active Labor Act (EMTALA), emergency departments cannot turn away patients who present seeking care, though they can be medically screened and assessed to not have a life-threatening condition and thereby made to wait while more-emergent patients are evaluated and treated.

Lifesaving Interventions

When employing a MUCC-compliant triage algorithm, providing lifesaving interventions is a formal process that is completed prior to assigning a triage category. Lifesaving interventions must be provided quickly and at any point in the SALT process. Lifesaving interventions include: controlling major hemorrhage, opening the airway, providing two rescue breaths for child casualties, decompression of any tension pneumothorax, and use of auto-injector antidotes, such as atropine and pralidoxime for a nerve-agent exposure. These interventions can be applied rapidly and may have a profound impact on survival. When the person performing triage is operating as part of a team, triage and LSI responsibilities can be split between responders.

Limitations of SALT Triage for Blast Victims

The global sorting process of MUCC-compliant triage utilizes verbal commands to sort the casualties. Tympanic membrane rupture has been reported between 9% and 45% of explosion casualties [27, 28]. Hearing injury from tympanic membrane injury and traumatic brain injury can complicate the sorting component of the SALT triage process. However, the remainder of the algorithm can be followed. It would be anticipated that fewer casualties would be able to follow verbal commands, yet a substantial number of them would still have purposeful movement and the algorithm could still be followed. Patients with only hearing changes would be triaged as minimal by SALT triage and would only need to have otoscopy by a medical provider eventually. While a high percentage of patients exposed to explosions will have TM injury, TM injuries are ***not*** predictive of other primary blast injury. Moreover, absence of TM injury ***does not*** rule out other primary blast injury [29].

Evacuation Priorities

MUCC-compliant triage was developed to establish treatment categories; however, it does not define the evacuation priority or process of moving patients from the scene to medical care. The US Military has established evacuation priority criteria (urgent, urgent surgical, priority, routine, and convenience) [30]. However, these are not easily applied to civilian EMS. As a general rule, the immediate patients should be evacuated first followed by delayed, expectant, and then minimal. *The likelihood of rapid decompensation can be used to prioritize patients in the same category*. For instance, if there were two patients with a penetrating torso injury, and one has altered mental status and respiratory distress and lacks a radial pulse, while the other has only respiratory distress, the former needs evacuation first. Clinical judgement will guide evacuation priority decisions on the scene.

In an explosive MCI, it may also be reasonable for minor patients to be evacuated along with, or in parallel to, higher-acuity patients. For instance, there may be room on an evacuation platform for a lower-acuity patient that is able to sit or stand and no higher-acuity patient able to occupy that space. There may also be unconventional evacuation platforms such as a school bus that can be considered for ambulatory patients.

An explosive MCI that occurs closer to a hospital often leads to more patients who self-transport and shorter EMS transport times [14]. The first patients may arrive within minutes, while the time delay to last patient arrival may be minutes or even days later [13]. It has been suggested that EMS tends to bring patients to the same hospital in order to decrease transport time and decrease turnaround time and because of lack of familiarity/access to routes to farther facilities [17]. The tendency in explosions close to hospitals is for the hospital to see more primary blast injuries as well as more major injuries like traumatic amputations, but also more minor injuries [17]. All these factors may overload that hospital and lead to inaccurate triage at that location. EMS should make efforts to distribute casualties rather than overloading the closest facility.

If the closest hospital becomes overloaded at the outset of an MCI response, one option to mitigate this is to have this hospital act as a casualty collection point (CCP). Patients can undergo further triage at the CCP hospital, and then as transportation resources are acquired, patients can be transferred to other facilities in order to maximize utilization of resources. These processes would correlate to the hospital-based "reevaluation phase" and "redistribution phase," respectively, which are discussed in Chap. 21—just that the main goal in this case would be to decompress the patient volume at the CCP facility instead of redistributing to obtain specialty services. Additionally, many casualties with relatively minor-appearing injuries may have self-evacuated to the nearest facility during the hospital-based "disordered arrival phase."

Critical patients have the potential to be under-triaged at hospitals following mass casualty incidents, particularly when highly visible, distracting injuries are concomitant with more serious, but less obvious, injuries [31]. Deceptively small entry wounds may hide serious internal injuries [32]. Therefore, care should be taken to not under-triage patients having secondary blast injuries with small wounds. Patients with traumatic amputation or injuries to four or more areas are likely to have associated intra-abdominal injury [33]. This also highlights the need for frequent reevaluation and re-triage throughout the continuum of care. If possible, the highest-acuity patients should be sent to the closest facility with appropriate capabilities, while lower-acuity patients are routed to farther away facilities.

Re-triage and Stabilization

Following initial triage and treatment and perhaps the first wave of evacuations, there are likely to be many patients still in need of transportation to medical facilities. These patients may need to wait a period of time for evacuation due to inadequate resources. Because of this, understanding the injury patterns produced by the different types of blast injuries, and their emergent interventions, can help ensure injuries are appropriately managed when prehospital care must be prolonged.

Patients should be reassessed as frequently as is feasible, and triage categories altered as their condition improves or worsens. As always, assessing and intervening on the ABCs (airway, breathing, and circulation) is of paramount importance. Using the typical tools of hospital-based triage—history, physical examination, and vital signs—may have significant rates of under- and over-triage. One study of non-MCI trauma patients suggested rates of over-triage of around 12% and under-triage of around 4% [34]. POCUS may be a useful adjunct in prehospital triage. Ultrasonographic imaging techniques can be taught in a short amount of time, units are portable, and images may be transmitted to receiving facilities or medical personnel and have been used in environments as diverse as space stations, medical transport, and combat support teams [35].

POCUS has been used in MCIs. For example, ultrasound was used as a primary screening tool in the 1988 Armenian earthquake, in which 530 ultrasound screening examinations were done with abdominal and retroperitoneal trauma being identified in 12.8% of the patients, with a 1% false-negative rate and no false positives [36]. In another earthquake MCI in Lushan China in 2013, START was compared to the Streamlined Focused Assessment with Sonography for Trauma (SFAST). When comparing the ability to predict the need for emergent surgery, START had an accuracy rate of 55.6%, sensitivity 51.9%, specificity 61.1%, positive predictive value (PPV) 66.7%, and negative predictive value (NPV) 45.8%; SFAST had an accuracy rate of 62.2%, sensitivity 59.3%, specificity 66.7%, PPV 72.7%, and NPV 52.2%. Although these are not impressive numbers for predicting the need for emergent surgery, they are better than a commonly used triage system. SFAST has not been compared to a MUCC-compliant triage system.

Prehospital POCUS was also studied in a prospective multicenter trial in Germany. They used the Prehospital Focused Abdominal Sonography for Trauma (PFAST) to evaluate 202 trauma patients for hemoperitoneum [37] and compared assessment by the emergency physician on-scene using physical examination and vital signs alone to PFAST assessment. The sensitivity was on par (93%) between the physician assessment and PFAST, but specificity of PFAST was 99%, compared to 52% for physician assessment. Accuracy of PFAST was 99%, compared to 57% for physician assessment. On-scene PFAST occurred a mean of 35 minutes earlier than FAST in the ED. Furthermore, prehospital management changed in 30% of the patients evaluated with PFAST, and PFAST results changed the choice of admitting hospital in 22% of patients. While not studied in an MCI, these findings suggest that prehospital POCUS may be useful for helping allocate scarce on-scene resources to the most seriously injured patients and to help with the evacuation priority. This is particularly true in the context of re-triage, as a patient with hemoperitoneum may not have a positive PFAST on initial examination, but may become positive as additional blood accumulates in the intraperitoneal space.

Conclusion

Explosions have a great potential to cause mass casualty incidents. A number of characteristics of a blast, including open air, enclosed space, building collapse, causing fire, vehicle delivered, hospital proximity, and prior evacuation, greatly affect the amount and type of casualties as well as the resource requirement for an effective prehospital response. Understanding how these factors are likely to affect casualty type and severity, as well as the necessary resources, can aid in the execution of an effective response. The triage process for MCIs should utilize a MUCC-compliant triage system for scene triage. There are a number of unique concerns related to explosive injuries that can complicate triage in the field setting. Preventing morbidity and mortality in MCIs is best accomplished using a well understood system of command and control (i.e., ICS), a practiced MUCC-compliant triage system (e.g., SALT), and a systems-based approach.

Pitfalls

- *Failure to correctly triage or re-triage a blast injury patient.* Lack of TM injury *should not* be taken as assurance that the patient has no serious, primary blast injury. Patients with primary blast injury to the lungs, or inhalation injury from fire/smoke, may rapidly progress from relative stability to emergent condition. Patient with small entry wounds may be hiding severe internal injuries.
- *Failure to establish ICS early and failure to grow the ICS as resources arrive.* Even with only a few responders on scene, it is important to start building an ICS so that command and control of the response is maintained. As additional resources arrive, they must be incorporated into the ICS so that overall command and control is maintained, thereby allowing appropriate allocation of resources to give the best chance of survival to the greatest number of patients.

- *Failure to allocate resources appropriately.* Given the complexity of blast MCI and the injuries it causes, triage, patient transport, and specialized response assets based on the mechanism of the blast can create major resource requirements that will cripple an unprepared system.

Pearls

- The possibility of additional accidental or intentional explosions is a paramount concern in any blast MCI, as there may be new or persistent threats after the initial casualties are produced.
- Due to limited resources available in an MCI assessment of evacuation, prioritization is essential. Evacuation categories may not line up exactly with triage categories and may be dependent on available evacuation platforms, as well as on-scene resources.
- Ultrasonography may be useful for initial triage, but particularly for retriage to help determine extended prehospital treatment and evacuation prioritization. It generally has higher sensitivity than physical examination and vital signs alone.
- Hearing, ear, and tympanic membrane findings are not reliable for field triage, neither to rule in nor rule out other serious injuries.
- A number of characteristics of a blast, including open air, enclosed space, building collapse, causing fire, vehicle delivered, hospital proximity, and prior evacuation, greatly affect the amount and type of casualties as well as the resource requirement for an effective response. Understanding how these factors are likely to affect casualty type and severity, as well as necessary resources, can aid in the execution of an effective response.

References

1. U.S. Department of State. Patterns of global terrorism 2003. Washington. http://www.state.gov/documents/organization/31912.pdf. Accessed 1 Apr 2018.
2. U.S. Department of State. Country reports on terrorism 2005. Washington. https://www.state.gov/j/ct/rls/crt/2005/. Accessed 1 Apr 2018.
3. U.S. Department of State. Country reports on terrorism 2010. Washington. https://www.state.gov/j/ct/rls/crt/2010/index.htm. Accessed 1 Apr 2018.
4. U.S. Department of State. Country reports on terrorism 2011. Washington. https://www.state.gov/j/ct/rls/crt/2011/index.htm. Accessed 1 Apr 2018.
5. U.S. Department of State. Country reports on terrorism 2012. Washington. https://www.state.gov/j/ct/rls/crt/2012/index.htm. Accessed 1 Apr 2018.
6. U.S. Department of State. Country reports on terrorism 2013. Washington. https://www.state.gov/j/ct/rls/crt/2013/index.htm. Accessed 1 Apr 2018.

7. U.S. Department of State. Country reports on terrorism 2014. Washington. https://www.state.gov/j/ct/rls/crt/2014/index.htm. Accessed 1 Apr 2018.
8. U.S. Department of State. Country reports on terrorism 2015. Washington. https://www.state.gov/j/ct/rls/crt/2015/index.htm. Accessed 1 Apr 2018.
9. U.S. Department of State. Country reports on terrorism 2016. Washington. [cited 2018 Apr 1]. Available from: https://www.state.gov/j/ct/rls/crt/2016/index.htm. Accessed 1 Apr 2018.
10. U.S. Bomb Data Center. Explosives incident report 2014. Washington. https://www.atf.gov/explosives/docs/report/2014-usbdc-explosive-incident-report/download. Accessed 2 Apr 2018.
11. U.S. Bomb Data Center. Explosives incident report 2016. Washington. https://www.atf.gov/explosives/docs/report/2016-explosives-incident-report/download. Accessed 2 Apr 2018.
12. Salome JP, Pons PT, McSwain NE, Butler FK, Chapeau W, Chapman G, et al., editors. Prehospital trauma life support. Military 8th ed. St. Louis: Jones and Bartlett Learning, 2014.
13. Arnold JL, Tsai M-C, Halpern P, Smithline H, Stok E, Ersoy G. Mass-casualty, terrorist bombings: epidemiological outcomes, resource utilization, and time course of emergency needs (part I). Prehops Disaster Med. 2003;18:220–34. https://doi.org/10.1017/S1049023X00001096.
14. Halpern P, Tsai M-CC, Arnold JL, Stok E, Ersoy G. Mass-casualty, terrorist bombings: implications for emergency department and hospital emergency response (part II). Prehosp Disaster Med. 2003;18:235–41. https://doi.org/10.1017/S1049023X00001102.
15. Quenemoen LE, Davis YM, Malilay J, Sinks T, Noji EK, Klitzman S. The World Trade Center bombing: injury prevention strategies for high-rise building fires. Disasters. 1996;20:125–32.
16. Leibovici D, Gofrit ON, Stein M, Shapira SC, Noga Y, Heruti RJ, et al. Blast injuries: bus versus open-air bombings—a comparative study of injuries in survivors of open-air versus confined-space explosions. J Trauma. 1996;41:1030–5.
17. Kapur G, Pillow M, Nemeth I. Prehospital care algorithm for blast injuries due to bombing incidents. Prehosp Disaster Med. 2010;25:595–60. https://doi.org/10.1017/S1049023X00008815.
18. Jensen J, Thompson S. The incident command system: a literature review. Disasters. 2016;40:158–82. https://doi.org/10.1111/disa.12135.
19. National incident management system training program. Washington, DC: Department of Homeland Security; 2011.
20. Kapur GB, Hutson HR, Davis MA, Rice PL. The United States twenty-year experience with bombing incidents: implications for terrorism preparedness and medical response. J Trauma. 2005;59:1436–44. https://doi.org/10.1097/01.ta.0000197853.49084.3c.
21. Department of the Army (U.S.). Improvised Explosive Device Safe Standoff Distance Cheat Sheet. Homeland Security Digital Library: https://www.hsdl.org/?view&did=440775. Accessed 1 Apr 2018.
22. King R, Larentzakis A, Ramly E. Tourniquet use at the Boston Marathon bombing: lost in translation. J Trauma Acute Care Surg. 2015;78:594–9. https://doi.org/10.1097/TA.0000000000000561.
23. Lerner E, Cone DC, Weinstein ES, Schwartz RB, Coule PL, Cronin M, et al. Mass casualty triage: an evaluation of the science and refinement of a national guideline. Disaster Med Public Health Prep. 2011;5:129–37. https://doi.org/10.1001/dmp.2011.39.
24. American College of Surgeons; Committee on Trauma. Model uniform core criteria for mass casualty triage. Disaster Med Public Health Prep. 2011;5:125–8. https://doi.org/10.1001/dmp.2011.41.
25. Federal Interagency Committee on Emergency Medical Services. National implementation of the model uniform core criteria for mass casualty incident triage: a report of the FICEMS. https://www.ems.gov/nemsac/dec2013/FICEMS-MUCC-Implementation-Plan.pdf. Accessed 8 July 2018.
26. Guzzi L, Argyros G. The management of blast injury. Eur J Emerg Med. 1996;3:252–5.
27. Almogy G, Lucia T, Richter E, Pizov R, Bdolah-Abram T, Mintz Y, Zamir G, et al. Can external signs of trauma guide management? Lessons learned from suicide bombing attacks in Israel. Arch Surg. 2005;140:390–3. https://doi.org/10.1001/archsurg.140.4.390.

28. Mellow SG, Cooper GJ. Analysis of 828 servicemen killed or injured by explosion in Northern Ireland 1970-1084: the hostile action casualty system. Br J Surg. 1989;75:1006–10. https://doi.org/10.1002/bjs.1800761006.
29. Mathews Z, Koyfman A. Blast injuries. J Emerg Med. 2015;49:573–87. https://doi.org/10.1016/j.jemermed.2015.03.013.
30. U.S. Army. Medical Evacuation. FM 4-02.2. Department of the Army. Washington, DC: Government Printing Office; 2007.
31. Arnold J, Halpern P, Tsai M-C, Smithline H. Mass casualty terrorist bombings: a comparison of outcomes by bombing type. Ann Emerg Med. 2004;43:263–73. https://doi.org/10.1016/S0196064403007236.
32. Hare S, Goddard I, Naraghi A, Dick A. The radiological management of bomb blast injury. Clin Radiol. 2007;62:1–9. https://doi.org/10.1016/j.crad.2006.09.013.
33. Almogy G, Mintz Y, Zamir G, Bdolah-Abram T, Elazary R, Dotan L, et al. Suicide bombing attacks: can external signs predict internal injuries? Ann Surg. 2006;243:541–6. https://doi.org/10.1097/01.sla.0000206418.53137.34.
34. Lehmann R, Brounts L, Lesperance K, Eckert M, Casey L, Beekley A, et al. A simplified set of trauma triage criteria to safely reduce overtriage: a prospective study. Arch Surg. 2009;144:853–8. https://doi.org/10.1001/archsurg.2009.153.
35. Wydo S, Seamon M, Melanson S, Thomas P, Bahner D, Stawicki S. Portable ultrasound in disaster triage: a focused review. Eur J Trauma Emerg Surg. 2016;42:151–9. https://doi.org/10.1007/s00068-015-0498-8.
36. Sarkisian AE, Khondkarian RA, Amirbekian NM, Bagdasarian NB, Khojayan RL, Oganesian YT. Sonographic screening of mass casualties for abdominal and renal injuries following the 1988 Armenian earthquake. J Trauma. 1991;31:247–50.
37. Walcher F, Weinlich M, Conrad G, Schweigkofler U, Breitkreutz R, Kirschning T, et al. Prehospital ultrasound imaging improves management of abdominal trauma. Br J Surg. 2006;93:238–42. https://doi.org/10.1002/bjs.5213.

Transporting Blast-Injured Patients 14

Hideaki L. Tanaka and Alex P. Keller IV

Introduction

Blast injuries are inherently difficult to address because of the various mechanisms involved in disrupting and damaging tissues. As described in other chapters, not all injuries will be readily visualized, so a high index of suspicion is paramount to appropriately consider ongoing care during transportation out of the field to a hospital or during transfer from one facility to another. This chapter will focus on the former. Although many principles will apply to both, especially if transporting by air, interfacility transfers are most often accomplished after casualties are somewhat stabilized and specialized teams are employed.

Transporting any patient increases risk. However, moving those with blast injuries can be especially precarious. Stable patients on the ground can easily become unstable in the air without any major change in patient pathophysiology due to changes in the environment associated with vehicular travel such as linear and angular accelerations and decelerations, noise, vibration, changes in humidity and temperature, and potential alterations in barometric pressure if altitude must be changed during ground or air transport. Hypoxia, pressure differentials, and expansion of closed gas-filled spaces are all challenges that need to be anticipated with ascent. Coupling this with the risk of dislodging lines and tubes during movement, transportation is by nature one of the most error-prone and perilous times. Unstable patients should not be moved, except in exigent circumstances where the risks are outweighed by the benefits of expeditiously delivering the patient to a higher level of care.

H. L. Tanaka (✉)
Military and Emergency Medicine, Uniformed Services University, Hurlburt Field, FL, USA

A. P. Keller IV
Military and Emergency Medicine, Uniformed Services University, United States Air Force, Athens, GA, USA

D. W. Callaway, J. L. Burstein (eds.), *Operational and Medical Management of Explosive and Blast Incidents*, https://doi.org/10.1007/978-3-030-40655-4_14

Transfer of patient care from one team to another is also a process that increases risk. If the transporting team is not the same as the one that provided the initial care, one handoff occurs before movement and effective communication of information must occur at this stage. Each time a handoff occurs, a new medical team takes ownership of a patient with whom they have not physically managed. Without a strong handoff, There is no history, no examination, no baseline, and no trends with which to compare other than the verbal report and written documentation provided. Independent evaluation of the patient from top to bottom is crucial each time a patient is received from another team. Receiving a detailed report of known injuries and documented treatments performed is also vital to successful patient transfer. Good verbal reports and written documentation enable longer-term trends to be noticed and occult pathophysiological problems to be identified.

Moving these types of patients requires careful thought and consideration to ensure a safe and efficient transport. The goal of this chapter is to identify the factors involved in the transportation of blast-injured patients. Identifying these individual factors will help in planning, which will be just as important as actually moving the patient.

Vehicular Movement

Whether moving a patient in a gurney through the halls of the hospital and into elevators, riding in an ambulance or commandeered vehicle, or flying in a helicopter, moving a patient takes coordination, ingenuity, and flexibility. All manners of transport are affected by space constraints, access issues, and suboptimal lighting. Noise and communication with transport team members and with patients will be hindered. Vibrations, especially in rhythm, can move lines, jostle sensitive tissues, and potentially dislodge clots.

Travel also may take a toll on the personnel providing care. If not prepositioned, a transport team is generated and needs to travel to pick up a patient. This may be the first transport of the day or the fifth. Team members may be fatigued, dehydrated, and fighting hunger which may more easily lead to mistakes [1, 2].

Ground Transport

Regardless of the primary transport modality, there will always be a component of movement on the ground. All hospital clinicians realize the inherent dangers of moving a patient from one floor to another, or from one hospital location to an imaging table and back. The same is true of ambulance transportation from the field to the hospital—airways become dislodged, lines become disconnected, and records lost. Even in the smoothest of civilian ambulances, noticeable jerks occur when driving over uneven terrain or bumps in roads. Although much of the movement is in two dimensions, there are numerous decelerations and accelerations with traffic, stoplights, and checkpoints—all of which can cause fluctuations in systemic blood pressure and intracranial pressure in supine patients.

Most urban ground transports are in the realm of minutes, as patients are taken to the closest hospital or regional trauma center. Depending on the area travelled, any unexpected issues can usually be addressed by stopping or diverting to the closest hospital for further stabilization and treatment. However, ground transport is often also slower than air travel and critical patients who need to travel longer distances are usually taken by air when weather allows.

Transportation in a rural setting is naturally different with limited resources and longer distances to care. Mutual assistance agreements and volunteer forces are crucial for this medical coverage, but the scopes of transporting provider practices are often variable. Roads may be unpaved and railroad crossings may be more frequently encountered. Coupled with longer transportation times, en route care is complicated with increased risk of deterioration of patient status while traveling [3], which will be further explained below.

Maritime Transport

Patient transportation may need to occur via water either to get to land or to get off a shore. Accidental explosions are not infrequent aboard powered watercraft. Handling fuel, volatile vapors in enclosed spaces, and potentially hazardous cargo all contribute. Boats and ships for various industries and commercial hauling rarely have robust medical resources during maritime operations. Even passenger cruise ships, which are generally prepared for austere medical care, cannot handle all problems.

Most maritime vessels are not built to transport injured patients. Further, all vessels are at risk of falling under rough water sufficient to cause untoward forces on patients and make patient care difficult. In regards to ship transport for long distances until a patient can be off-boarded to a boat or helicopter for ship-to-shore movement, a suitable location within the vessel for prolonged care may be needed. Most large vessels are designed to close off certain flooded sections to prevent capsizing. These chambers are secured via doors which are thick but narrow. Any movement of patients in ships should consider the effects movement may have on patients, especially as nonambulatory patients will need to be carried in narrow hallways, up or down steep stairwells, and through hatches. In terms of movement of a ship with rough seas, the lower and more central areas will be least affected; however, these can be more difficult areas to access and will require eventually moving the patient back up to a deck to off-board.

Seasickness, like airsickness, is a phenomenon that may affect both patient and medical providers. Medications to address motion sickness are thus important to treat patients, if side effects are inconsequential, but also to keep the transportation team involved in the treatment of those under their care. Two recommended medications are meclizine in oral tablet form or scopolamine. Although transdermal scopolamine via patch is readily available in the United States, a smaller yet just as effective intranasal dose is currently in the US Food and Drug Administration (FDA) fast-track approval process for use in the United States. Although ondansetron has been commonly used to treat motion sickness in the US military, used often by aeromedical evacuation crews to pretreat anticipated nausea and vomiting prior to aircraft flight, this medication is an antiemetic and is not designed to counter motion sickness. It will typically have less than desirable efficacy.

Air Transport

At some point, the speed of air travel outweighs the burden of establishing a helicopter landing zone or using a runway that may not be close to a treatment facility and will be beneficial for patients in getting care expeditiously. Typically, these are in rural settings or areas that are greater than an hour away by ground transport. This may also be impacted if roads are blocked, bridges are out, or traffic is snarled. Rotary-wing aircraft are prime modes of transport for medium-distance transport of one or two patients, due to their airspeeds of 120 knots or more, and need only an established helipad or improvised cleared helicopter landing zone. Airplane transport is ideal for extended distances, typically over 100 miles, as they can fly up to 500 knots, but need an established runway or possibly an expedient landing strip for more hardy aircraft.

Helicopter movement should be performed with the doors closed, although this may not always be feasible. Helicopters generally do not have pressurized cabins so attention should be paid to altitude during flight, mostly in regards to exposure. In the military, there is an old adage regarding the H-60 MEDEVAC helicopter: "If it is hot, cold, wet, dusty, or dark on the outside, it is hot, wet, cold, dusty, or dark on the inside." This serves as a reminder to flight medics to always package the patient appropriately to prevent hypothermia and other environmental insults. Patients transported by air, especially helicopters, should always be provided eye and ear protection. Rupture of the tympanic membrane from the overpressure of a blast is never a contraindication to hearing protection. In fact, disruption of the TM will result in more sound waves transmitting directly into the inner ear and, thus, may cause hearing damage that could be mitigated or prevented with simple foam earplugs.

Fixed-wing movement can take multiple forms as the variety of aircraft can range from small, single-engine propeller planes with a capacity for only one litter patient to enormous multi-engine jets that can carry over 100 patients. Some aircraft may also have medical oxygen systems built in to the airframe. Weight and space considerations generally are not as significant as they are for transportation in helicopters and small fixed-wing aircraft.

The type of aircraft may make a physiological difference to the patient during transportation. Most rotary-wing aircraft do not have the capability of controlling internal cabin pressure. Fixed-wing aircraft may have cabin pressurization systems, but smaller airplanes often may not. Furthermore, the types of pressurization in aircraft can vary between isobaric and constant differential. The typical setup in civilian aircraft is isobaric pressurization. It maintains a consistent cabin pressure that is set by the pilot, usually 6000–8000 feet above mean sea level (MSL) pressure. *Isobaric differential* is a pressurization scheme that keeps cabin pressure a specific percentage higher than the atmospheric pressure. Therefore, it will fluctuate throughout the flight as the aircraft changes altitudes. This scheme is most often encountered in military fighter jets to prevent explosive decompression when flying at very high altitudes, but is not typically used in aircraft that transport patients.

Altitude Effects on Oxygenation

The most crucial difference from maritime or most ground transportation compared to air movement is the pressure differential that is caused when flying at altitude. Taking anyone, especially a critically injured patient, from a lower altitude to this level of stress has physiologic consequences.

The common belief that there is less oxygen at altitude is actually oversimplified. The same percentage of oxygen exists at ground level and at any atmospheric altitude a rotary-wing or fixed-wing aircraft can fly. The difference is the partial pressure of oxygen at different altitudes. At higher altitudes, there is lower atmospheric pressure and thus less relative available oxygen for human consumption. This is conveyed by Dalton's law of reduced partial pressure of oxygen, which also hints that at certain elevated atmospheric levels, even with an F_IO_2 of 1.00, an intubated patient may not be receiving sufficient oxygen supplementation due to the low partial pressure of oxygen supplied. It is important to understand this concept as flying at higher altitudes will cause further difficulty with oxygenation, and similarly the inverse; if there are issues with maintaining oxygen saturations at altitude, decreasing the cabin altitude either via increased cabin pressure or by decreasing the flight altitude of the aircraft may improve patient oxygenation.

The end result of decreased oxygen is hypoxia. Hypoxia can lead to symptoms of headache, fatigue, decreased concentration, and decreased responsiveness. Hypoxia can be diagnosed by lower hemoglobin oxygen saturation levels on pulse oximetry (S_PO_2) and is normally treated by administering supplemental oxygen or otherwise increasing the F_IO_2. If increasing the amount of supplemental oxygen is impossible, positive end-expiratory pressure (PEEP) can be added with either noninvasive or invasive positive-pressure ventilation. Decreased S_PO_2 is typically secondary to hypopnea or apnea in a spontaneously breathing patient, but pneumothorax or progressive blast lung injury should be considered. Tension pneumothorax should be especially considered in the setting of unexpected hypotension. Intubated patients can be victim to inadvertent tube dislodgement inferiorly or superiorly, or frank endotracheal extubation from jostling during movement. Standard critical care ventilator concerns such as auto-PEEP and other causes of inadequate tissue oxygen delivery should also be considered.

Altitude Effects on Trapped Gases

Pneumothoraces are difficult to diagnose in any moving vehicle, but must be high on the list of considerations for blast-injured patients. A pneumothorax can easily develop as sequelae of blast exposure. Typically, by time of controlled transport, the diagnosis has been made. At the prehospital stage, decreased breath sounds on the associated side is noted along with loss of chest wall movement. However, an untreated pneumothorax at ground level can turn into a tension pneumothorax by the decreased relative ambient pressure in comparison to the stable pressure of an enclosed body cavity, causing gas expansion via Boyle's law. Thus, not declaring a pneumothorax to the transport team or failure to identify a pneumothorax before flight can be lethal, because they are notoriously difficult to detect in noisy vehicles. Critical hypotension or signs of shock may be attributed to internal hemorrhage, developing intrathoracic or intra-abdominal pathology with tension physiology not recognized, and circulatory collapse and arrest could ensue. All known pneumothoraces should be treated with a chest tube prior to flight. Point-of-care ultrasonography, if available, can be used to detect pneumothoraces prior to or during transportation [4, 5].

Probably more a consideration for transport team members and less critical patients, any type of Eustachian tube dysfunction may be amplified by ear block occurrences particularly on aircraft descent. It is typically easier to vent expanding air in the middle ear on ascent; but on descent, the squeeze on the middle ear of increasing external ambient air pressure can cause excruciating discomfort if not relieved via Valsalva maneuver. In these cases, oxymetazoline can work well to decongest any sinus tissue, but should only be used during the landing process, not just in order to fly. The worst outcome is usually a ruptured tympanic membrane, which normally heals well, though can sometimes be associated with permanent hearing loss. In blast-affected patients, tympanic membranes often already are ruptured by blast waves, and thus ear squeeze may be less of an issue.

Altitude Effects on Temperature and Humidity

Another concern of air travel is of hypothermia, which takes on importance as ambient temperature decreases with altitude. This decreased temperature will be an important consideration particularly in hemodynamically compromised patients or those with burns, which are certainly types of patients seen after explosions. Similarly, some helicopters fly with windows open and the air flowing in from rotor wash may cause circumstances ideal for evaporation and cooling. Although there are heating systems on aircraft and doors of rotary aircraft can be closed, combatting hypothermia will be an active concern to prevent the Lethal Triad from taking hold [6].

Some other considerations in a critically ill patient involve the decreased moisture in flying environments. The humidity at altitude can be as low as 4%, which will cause increased rates of dehydration via increased insensible losses. A burn patient who has lost the ability to retain moisture is a prime example of a blast-injured patient being affected by this phenomenon. In addition to preventing fluid loss by covering wounds appropriately, maintenance fluid rates will need to be increased. Coupled with the internal fluid shifts occurring in a low-pressure environment, homeostatic balance in an injured critical patient may easily be complicated. Intubated patients may experience thicker endotracheal secretions, which could lead to greater tendency for mucus plugs.

Altitude Effects on Venous Circulation

At altitude, the external ambient pressure, or lack thereof, can also affect venous return, as pooling of blood and fluid in dependent places will be magnified. The "coach class" syndrome referred to in the setting of commercial air travel is not only due to immobility in a cramped seat, but also due to increased propensity of stasis as the ground-level ambient pressure is removed and the venous vasculature is further relied upon to counter the effects of gravity.

Examining the Patient Prior to Movement

Examination of the blast-injured patient is done as with any other patient, but with special attention to the pulmonary system, musculoskeletal structures, abdominal hollow viscera, and central nervous system. The primary examination of addressing any airway issues, assessing adequacy of respirations, and then evaluating circulation is crucial. Exposing the patient for a secondary examination from top to bottom is a necessity, as findings can be subtle. In this manner, the approach should be similar to that for a ground medic who encounters a patient for the first time. A complete head-to-toe exam should be conducted to prevent missed injuries and establish baseline status prior to any movement.

A common mnemonic taught to Special Operations Forces is MARCH PAWS. This simple mnemonic has been shown to address all "battle injuries" and only missed a very small portion of non-battle injuries in a retrospective review of combat evacuations during Operation Enduring Freedom [7]. It gives a great framework to build upon and standardizes the primary and secondary examinations; the US military states that good use of the MARCH algorithm and practice of tactical combat casualty care is the basis for good prolonged field care, the latter of which some may consider akin to transport care. Below is the algorithm with some additions to more fully address the transport process:

M – Massive hemorrhage
A – Airway
R – Respiration
C – Circulation
H – Head injury, hypothermia/hyperthermia, and head-to-toe examination

P – Pain medication
A – Antibiotics
W – Wound dressings
S – Splinting, straps, spaghetti, and scribble

Massive hemorrhage should be addressed aggressively, although most of the focus during en route care shifts to ensuring tourniquets, pressure dressings, clamps, sutures, and staples are adequately preventing additional blood loss. All patients with massive hemorrhage or significant blood loss should receive 1 g of tranexamic acid (TXA), if it can be administered within 3 hours of sustaining the injury [8]. If 1 g TXA has already been given, a second dose should be given. The administration of TXA is increasingly a prehospital transport task.

Airway patency should be assured appropriately. This entails an assessment of breathing with confirmation of good ventilation via pulse oximetry. No significant intervention is required for a completely alert and oriented patient, unless respiratory distress or hypoxia is displayed. If lower oxygen saturations are seen, supplemental oxygen should be administered. However, new evidence has steadily been gathered suggesting harm of hyperoxia [9]. Although work has been focused on acute coronary syndrome treatment, there is evidence that patients may be harmed by too much supplemental oxygen via oxygen free radicals [9].

Patients with an altered mental status or concern of airway patency, inappropriately low or high respiratory rate, or concern for significant damage to lungs or tracheal-bronchial tree should receive further airway support based on provider experience and scope of practice. Secure airways are the first step in providing further ventilatory support in blast-injured lungs, although noninvasive positive-pressure devices may act as a bridge or act as definitive management [10]. In intubated or immediately postoperative patients being moved from one facility to another, fresh arterial blood gas values are important. Ventilator settings should be adjusted as needed. Respiratory rate should be controlled based on the specific clinical circumstances and desired effects.

Circulatory status should be frequently assessed during transport. Well-perfused distal extremities with good capillary refill is encouraging and should be trended over time. Maintenance fluids should be started if movement is anticipated to be an hour or more, but providers should also be wary of over-resuscitation. Any ongoing fluid administration should be monitored with serial pulmonary examinations, and appearance of any peripheral edema should be documented.

If a thermometer is available, core body temperature should be measured before transportation and en route if travel is prolonged. Core body temperature below 35 °C should be corrected prior to transportation, if possible, because it is only likely to be exacerbated, unless the internal warmth of the vehicle can be brought up to at least normal body temperature.

With blast injuries, intracranial injuries are very possible and may be hard to detect if mild. Initial mental status examination prior to transportation must be made, so that it can be trended through transportation and at arriving facility. Any evidence of deterioration should trigger immediate full neurological reexamination.

Any evidence of trans-tentorial herniation or impending herniation should instigate treatment to include hypertonic saline or mannitol administration. This treatment should not be given preventatively but only based on clinical findings and suspicion. Transport of any head-injured patients should generally occur in supine fashion with head elevated at 30 degrees and head first in fixed-wing aircraft due to the horizontal forces experienced at takeoff, although this may depend also on the length of the runway on landing and rapidity to full top after wheels touch the ground.

Pain assessment prior to transportation is important, because pain may be exacerbated by patient movement and affect hemodynamic stability. Furthermore, depending on patient-to-medical-attendant ratio, pain control may inadvertently become less of a priority while en route to higher levels of care. Pain documentation is also important for the receiving team as it can elucidate an otherwise subtle trend in patient status. The control of pain will be discussed later; however, traumatic experiences, such as being injured during a sudden and unexpected explosion, can be mitigated by dissociative medications such as ketamine, which has been suggested to lower rates of posttraumatic stress disorder (PTSD) in survivors [11].

Antibiotics are routinely administered to combat-wounded patients in the military setting. Prophylactic antibiotic administration in blast-injured patients is appropriate if any open, penetrating wounds are present. Ertapenem generally is a good antibiotic to administer due to good overall coverage for skin and soft tissue, as well as bowel flora. It may be administered either intravenously (IV) or intramuscularly (IM) and is typically dosed 1 g once every 24 hours.

Wound dressings should be applied to help protect exposed tissues, to prevent debris or contamination from further sullying open wounds, to provide comfort to the patient, and to indicate to providers later on in the chain of care to see where these wounds exist. Rotary-wing transportation particularly leads to flying dust and dirt which will adhere to any moist surface. Similarly, any engine-running on-load or offload particularly with propeller aircraft will present the same situation. If possible, all previously dressed wounds should be taken down and examined prior to patient movement. The exception would be fresh surgical dressings, which should be left to receiving surgeons to examine.

The original "S" in MARCH PAWS stood only for splinting, but can be extended to include "straps, spaghetti, and scribble." Splinting serves several purposes, as it helps to decrease pain and may prevent further aggravation of the injury due to movement of sharp bony ends. Cervical collars and padding of voids created by body shape in relation to a litter or cot can also be considered forms of splinting. Straps should be applied if a patient is packaged for transportation, but any injury that will be constantly monitored should be easily accessible. "Spaghetti" is a reminder to organize all lines, monitoring cables, and power cords that can be wrapped around the patient in hectic times or interfere with patient care or patient movement. Lines should be labeled and cables should be easily accessible or stowed prior to movement. Neatly kempt lines and tubes also set the stage for simple transportation and organized treatment, plus a professional handover at the receiving facility.

"Scribble" is a reminder to gather all documentation from the prior treatment team and complete all transportation documentation, so that the entire continuum of care can be followed throughout phases of patient management from the point of injury to definitive care and rehabilitation. Loss of this data may complicate or inhibit treatment and prevents future analysis for future quality improvement, identifying capability gaps leading to new medical developments, development of evidence-based best practice guidelines, and dissemination to the greater medical community. Moreover, with respect to compensation for occupational injuries and illnesses, it may affect benefits years or decades later if something was not documented appropriately.

In a multi-trauma patient, the eyes often do not receive immediate attention, and subtle injury can worsen with time. Any patient with significant eye discomfort, new pupil deformity or asymmetry, or any penetrating globe injury should have a rigid shield placed over the eye to protect it. A patch or any dressing that touches the eyelid or creates pressure on the globe should never be applied as an otherwise salvageable ruptured globe could be lost if additional force causes herniation of globe contents. Particular attention must be paid to communication with the patient who has both eyes covered to help keep them oriented and calm, since this induced blindness may cause significant anxiety.

The premise of en route care should always be to address conditions found prior to transport, with the knowledge that care during transportation will be limited and less than ideal. The multitasking needed to care for a critically injured patient is further complicated by added concerns of movement. If critical interventions are in any way anticipated, preparatory interventions should be made prior to transport. For example, although vasoactive medications can be used in peripheral lines in the short term, if they will be potentially used, a central IV line should be placed before movement. If a pneumothorax is noted, a chest tube should be placed even if considered clinically insignificant prior to transport. Additionally, if respiratory failure is anticipated in a self-breathing patient, the decision to intubate prior to flight should be strongly considered as the setting, space, and lighting in any transport platform will be less than ideal.

Before moving the patient, it is crucial to understand that further information will be unavailable during transport. The transport team should accept that once movement begins, further clinical data from the previous team will not be accessible unless a good handoff occurred. All questions regarding care should be anticipated and asked prior to departure. Similarly, any supplies that are unique or not carried by the transport team should be gathered prior to movement. In certain scenarios, patient movement may need to commence without appropriate handoff, but these situations exponentially heighten risk.

Transporting the Patient

Considering the manner of transport and optimizing the final mode of travel can be crucial in success of treatment. The vibrations of ground movement can often exacerbate fractures, especially unstable ones. Fat emboli can be dislodged from long-bone fractures and cause pulmonary emboli. Similarly, deep venous thromboses

(DVTs) can form from immobility and decreased diastolic pressure for venous return, which subsequently may be promulgated through the vasculature to the lungs. Air transport can further add complexity to the vibratory stimuli whether via rotary wing or fixed wing. Pressure differentials can also physiologically worsen disease or injury processes.

Packaging of the patient may certainly facilitate or complicate the task at hand. Pertinent not only to Emergency Medical Services (EMS) but to interfacility transfer as well, spine board immobilization for known or suspected fractures to minimize risk of further injury must be considered and weighed against the significant risk of skin pressure ischemia, especially with any patient who is sedated or paralyzed and unable to shift weight. Commonly, spinal patients can be safely transported on a padded cot or stretcher with cervical immobilization and precautions to logroll patients. The authors observed the British Critical Care Air Support Team routinely using a vacuum immobilizer to transport patients as it hugs the natural curves of the spine and molds to the patient. This tool is helpful as it provides support to a patient despite the stresses of movement and adds an increased level of safety via more evenly distributed weight that also minimizes mobility. However, it is another piece of equipment that must be maintained and carried. In all patients, particularly during longer transportation times, the possibility of pressure points causing further injury must be considered and actively addressed.

In all circumstances, the dangers of movement should be addressed proactively. Ear and eye protection should be considered for all. If the patient is conscious, an explanation of upcoming events should be communicated. A safety briefing, especially with regard to emergency egress of the vehicle, should be provided.

When straps are applied, hands and arms should be free in an awake and cooperative individual to allow for self-protection of the head or body if the litter or cot is accidentally dropped or rolled. Patients should also be properly secured to the litter or transport apparatus as well as to any vehicle or aircraft. Similarly, all monitoring equipment should be secured so that it does not become a projectile in the event of rough travel conditions and injure patients or providers, or become inoperable if damaged. "Spaghetti" should be neatly kept and out of the way, so excess loops are removed or hidden to avoid snagging on gear, personnel, vegetation, or vehicle parts during movement. If flying to altitude, cuffs on endotracheal tubes should be filled with saline rather than air to prevent balloon expansion and excessive pressure on the tracheal epithelium.

Appropriate equipment and supplies must be at hand to successfully transport (Table 14.1). Monitors, which have the capability to assess blood pressure, heart rate, oxygen saturation, end-tidal CO_2, and electrocardiographic (ECG) monitoring should be available. Suction and bag valve mask devices will be crucial for airway and respiratory management, including intubation kit and induction and maintenance medications. Ventilators should be chosen to provide the greatest capability for the smallest size. IV pumps can be temperamental due to air in the line and the physiologic expansion of gas at altitude, but do allow for precision administration of fluids. Otherwise, drips to gravity and push-dose meds can be given should this equipment be inoperable or unavailable.

Table 14.1 Equipment and supplies for en route care

Gear	Contents
Airway	Oxygen masks Bag valve mask Airway kit Suction Pulse oximetry
Ventilation	Ventilator Vent circuits Adaptors and regulators Blood gas analyzer
Trauma	Chest tubes Foley kits IV kits Central line kits Arterial line kits Surgical airway kit
Drugs	ACLS drugs General supportive medications Paralytics
Narcotics	Controlled substances including: Analgesics Sedatives
Support	Blood or blood products Fluids IV pumps Monitor/defibrillator Litters, straps, and restraints Blankets Infection control kit

The oxygen demands should be calculated per hour for each patient, and the supply should be commensurate with the need, but also exceed need in case of contingency. For example, if travelling by air for 4 hours with a patient taking 10 liters per minute of oxygen, 2400 liters of oxygen would be needed for the flight. However, time of shuttling from aircraft to pickup of patient and back, plus taxiing for takeoff and landing, and then final ground movement from aircraft to final destination should all be accounted for and factored into oxygen needs. This may necessitate another 90 minutes of care, which would equal an additional 900 liters, without including the reserve supply for emergencies. The US Aeromedical Evacuation teams typically add an additional two liters per minute to the baseline need while in flight, to address Dalton's law of decreased partial pressures [3]. This would indicate an extra 480 liters needed. For intubated patients, calculations should always be for 100% oxygen.

Most transportation vehicles do not generate their own oxygen and require cylinders or liquid oxygen. The source of oxygen is crucial to know and account for. One liter of liquid oxygen provides 804 liters of gaseous oxygen, whereas a D cylinder at 2200 PSI will provide for 352 liters of oxygen. Carrying multiple cylinders for transport is often not feasible for mobility or efficiency in movement.

Transport is often painful for patients, as injured extremities are inadvertently jostled and as shifts in body weight occur during exams and movement. Appropriate pain control should be provided to the patient at all times, but particularly prior to movement in anticipation of increased stimulation of pain receptors. The most turbulent times during aircraft transport is normally during takeoff and landing, thus providing pain medications immediately prior to these events may be beneficial. Proactive control is often more effective and requires lower overall amounts of analgesics than reactively administering pain medications.

Pain control can be accomplished in a myriad of fashions including ketamine, fentanyl, morphine, hydromorphone, acetaminophen, ibuprofen, naproxen, and other agents. Anxiolysis should also be considered as an adjunctive therapy especially in patients on ventilators for comfort. Research also suggests that early analgesia may reduce the potential for developing or worsening PTSD symptoms [11]. Advanced techniques such as a Bier block, hematoma block, or regional blocks should be considered by appropriately trained personnel for interfacility transfers or in a prolonged field care setting where resources may be limited or giving the patient narcotics may pose more operational/tactical risk. Neuromuscular blockade, only after pain has been addressed and sedation applied, could be used for short periods to increase compliance with ventilator treatment in a complicated patient.

The effect of all of analgesics and paralytics on blood pressure should be considered, especially in the complex blast patient at risk for hemodynamic compromise. Ensuring initial and ongoing resuscitation during transport is critical. It is important to remember that the nature of transport may create a resource-limited environment but damage control principles should be maintained. In general, vasopressors should only be used for euvolemic patients to maintain mean arterial pressure (MAP) at target levels or keep the patient's clinical status out of a shock state.

Head-injured patients, specifically those with intracranial hemorrhage, may require higher blood pressures. Cerebral perfusion pressure (CPP) is equal to MAP minus intracranial pressure (ICP). Head-injured patients with increased ICP will require higher MAP to maintain CPP. Most monitors will calculate MAP and display it in the same area as SBP and diastolic blood pressure (DBP). Providers should target a systolic blood pressure of greater than 100 mmHg and a goal for MAP in head injury of 65–70 mmHg [12].

Hypothermia represents a hazard to all trauma patients particularly during transport. Many potential sites of bleeding may be internal after blasts and easy to miss at any stage, though they tend to declare objective signs as time passes. Normal clotting is important to minimize blood loss as the Lethal Triad relationship is comprised of hypothermia, acidosis, and coagulopathy. Prevention of hypothermia is often overlooked during patient movement. Trauma blast and burn victims are at particular risk for hypothermia given the dermal damage, internal hypermetabolic states, and iatrogenic interventions such as casualty exposure for evaluation and fluid resuscitation. Providers should always strive for normothermia during initial resuscitations.

The danger of an unvented thoracic airspace in a critical patient should never be underestimated. A clinically significant pneumothorax measuring 2 cm of air around the rim of the hemithorax at ground level, or roughly a 30% pneumothorax [13], can expand 35% at cabin altitude of 8000 feet with all other parameters being equal. Considering that the greater pressure changes per foot of elevation are nearer sea level, lowering the cabin pressure can be a helpful intervention.

If a patient begins to decompensate, the patient should be exposed and a MARCH examination should be repeated. If on the ventilator, the patient should be detached and manually bagged while a full respiratory assessment is conducted. Fresh surgical wounds and any drains or suction devices should be exposed to ensure that no complications have arisen.

Point-of-care ultrasonography can be used to evaluate patients en route. However, any piece of equipment brought on vehicle, especially an aircraft, should be deemed safe via certification for use on mode of transport chosen. For example, considerations for medical gear include any interference it may cause to aircraft systems and vice versa with aircraft systems interfering with medical electronics. Altitude physiology affects humans, but may also affect equipment. It should not be assumed that all equipment brought on a transport mission will work outside of the hospital setting.

Importantly, all the documentation that will be performed during transport, especially in a mass casualty or active military operation, will be the only record of care for the patient. Everything should be documented as completely and concisely as possible so that the accepting team can easily scan the record for any pertinent information so that no patient care data is lost. Without complete and accurate records of care, quality improvement and lessons learned cannot be accomplished.

Living patients should not be transported with the dead. American Critical Care Air Transport and Aeromedical Evacuation teams have regulations preventing the cotransport of the living and dead [3]. Although some may attempt to maximize efficiency by cotransport, resistance should be given to this practice, as location of the dead may be useful to subsequent forensic investigations [14].

Handoff

The patient handoff should come from the primary medic who has been caring for the individual. A standard handoff in a MIST format (mechanism of injury, injuries sustained, symptoms and signs exhibited by the patient, and treatment provided) is a good foundation to build the discourse. This keeps the communication standard and brief. If elaboration is needed, this can easily be added to the relevant section. If transfer has gone as planned, lines will not be tangled and nothing unintentionally has been discontinued. This prevents time wasted untangling gear when passing off to the next level of care and prevents the need to reaccomplish procedures, thereby increasing patient safety. The team leader accepting handoff should be given all pertinent data and documentation, and the transferring team should be prepared to repeat the report of care in case senior personnel or consultants arrive.

Miscellaneous

Transportation safety is paramount. Secondary devices, suicide bombers, and IED imbedded are all possible discussions. Contamination from blasts can be a consideration, especially with dirty bombs, but those will likely have been considerations encountered prior to en route care teams accepting missions. One aspect of air transport that is a nonfactor is in regards to higher exposure to ionizing radiation at airline cruising altitude, and there is no evidence that this affects patients or medical teams during transport; normal ionizing radiation is a lifetime exposure risk.

Finally, hectic scenarios such as may occur after a blast event will undoubtedly complicate care. Events involving blasts in civilian scenarios are typically mass casualty events, with tens or hundreds of victims. Therefore, the concept of crew resource management (CRM) should be kept in mind. Typically found with aircrew in terms of risk management, the core of CRM involves situational awareness, crew coordination and integration, mission analysis including planning and debrief, task management, communication, and decision making as it involves risk management.

Some specific points to discuss with en route care involve the personnel involved. Although various trained individuals can be successful, those with prerequisite training include flight paramedics and critical care staff. Regardless of level of training, it is imperative that training and familiarization simulating patient movement occur before performing actual transport. Personnel involved must know the equipment and how to run it, as well as the actual mode of transportation and the intricacies involved with the airframe, vehicle, or watercraft. The physiological effects of travel should be introduced to team members prior to an actual mission.

There is inherent danger to transporting team members. Different from aircrew, convoy personnel, or shipmates, the medical team must be comfortable with the mode of transport and also care for the patient simultaneously. There have been documented instances of flight paramedics injured by impacts from rotor blades, ground medics being injured by doors or collisions with vehicles, and rescuers being struck by watercraft propeller blades. With that said, recent data indicate that air ambulances are the safest manner of flying in all rotary airframes [15]. Ideally, a trained transport team to include nonmedical crew will provide for the most reliable and safest manner of transport for the team and patient. For example, flying cargo and waiting on approach clearance and aircraft patterns is different from having priority medical clearance to approach direct to an airfield without loitering.

Motion sickness must also be considered and countermeasures should be identified. Even if the brightest and most capable medic is available to care for a patient, it is all for naught if the medic is incapacitated by the dynamic transport environment. Zofran is a standard medication that most medics will carry for treatment purposes, but meclizine or scopolamine should be considered for the treatment team. If this becomes an option for use, it should be tested on the ground while off-duty, to determine efficacy and side effect profile in each individual medic.

Conclusion

Moving blast-injured patients from one location to another to receive further advanced care is not an easy task. Blast phenomena lend to complicated wound patterns and injuries, with much of what is damaged not easily displayed to the naked eye. Those not aware of the effects of vehicular movement may not realize the importance of the physiological variations associated with transport—whether via ground, via water, or in the air.

Key Points

- Explosions often cause occult injuries, which can be exacerbated during transportation.
- If all blast injuries are not predicted or thoroughly evaluated prior to transport, patients may decompensate during travel.
- Multiple modes of transportation exist, and the best choice is dependent on scenario, stability of patients, time to higher or next-level care, and resources available at each end.
- Each mode of transportation has distinctive advantages, but also specific physiological stresses to individuals and medical conditions. Anticipating these stressors and subsequent effects on patients is a key to successful casualty movement.

Pitfalls

- Any transition of care is a particularly high-risk time. Medical errors can occur when crucial information is not effectively transmitted from one team to another.
- Transport by definition involves changes to a patient's physical location which can easily lead to pulled lines or tubes if safeguards are not made.
- Different modes of transport subject patients to various environmental changes which can lead to life-threatening physiological responses; be wary of air travel and changes with partial pressures of gas, which can lead to oxygenation issues, expansion of trapped gases, and exposure to cold temperatures and low humidity.

Pearls

- Using a checklist or pneumonic, such as MARCH-PAWS, can assist in providing optimal essential care before and during transportation.
- Conveying data in a MIST format verbally, in addition to transferring complete medical documentation, is helpful in quickly sharing information on injuries, assessments, treatments, and trends.
- Dedicated transportation teams trained in patient movement with practice and experience in casualty evacuation should lead to improved outcomes for morbidity and mortality, especially in blast-injured patients.
- Use of emerging technology, such as point-of-care laboratory and ultrasonography, may further enhance medical capabilities during transportation.

References

1. Armentrout JJ, Holland DA, O'Toole KJ, Ercoline WR. Fatigue and related human factors in the near crash of a large military aircraft. Aviat Space Environ Med. 2006;77(9):963–70.
2. Taylor-Phillips S, Stinton C. Fatigue in radiology: a fertile area for future research. Br J Radiol. 2019;14:20190043.
3. United States Air Force, School of Aerospace Medicine. Critical care air transport team notebook. San Antonio, TX: United States Air Force; 2009. 156 p.
4. Morrow D, Cupp J, Schrift D, Nathanson R, Soni NJ. Point-of-care ultrasound in established settings. South Med J. 2018;111(7):373–81.
5. Kozaci N, Avci M, Ararat E, Pinarbasili T, Ozkaya M, Etli I, et al. Comparison of ultrasonography and computed tomography in the determination of traumatic thoracic injuries. Am J Emerg Med. 2019;37(5):864–8.
6. Eastridge BJ, Costanzo G, Jenkins D, Spott MA, Wade C, Greydanus D, et al. Impact of joint theater trauma system initiatives on battlefield injury outcomes. Am J Surg. 2009;198(6):852–7.
7. Kosequat J, Rush SC, Simonsen I, Gallo I, Scott A, Swats K, et al. Efficacy of the mnemonic device "MARCH/PAWS" as a checklist for pararescuemen during tactical field care and tactical evacuation. J Spec Oper Med. 2017;17(4):80–4.
8. CRASH-2 collaborators, Roberts I, Shakur H, Afolabi A, Brohi K, Coats T, et al. The importance of early treatment with tranexamic acid in bleeding trauma patients: an exploratory analysis of the CRASH-2 randomised controlled trial. Lancet. 2011;377(9771):1096–101, 1101.e1–2.
9. Helmenhorst HJ, Schultz MJ, van der Voort PH, de Jonge E, van Westerloo DJ. Bench-to-bedside review: the effects of hyperoxia during critical illness. Crit Care. 2015;19:284.
10. Roberts S, Skinner D, Biccard B, Rodseth RN. The role of non-invasive ventilation in blunt chest trauma: systematic review and meta-analysis. Eur J Trauma Emerg Surg. 2014;40(5):553–9.
11. McGhee LL, Maani CV, Garza TH, Gaylord KM, Black IH. The correlation between ketamine and posttraumatic stress disorder in burned service members. J Trauma. 2008;64(2 Suppl):S195–8; Discussion S197–8.
12. McCafferty R, Neal C, Marshall S, Pamplin J, Bell R, Rivet D, et al. Joint Trauma System Clinical Practice Guideline (JTS CPG): neurosurgery and severe head injury (CPG ID:30). Current Publication. San Antonio, TX: Department of Defense Center of Excellence for Trauma (US), Joint Trauma System; 2017.
13. Sharma A, Jindal P. Principles of diagnosis and Management of Traumatic Pneumothorax. J Emerg Trauma Shock. 2008;1(1):34–41.
14. Ross D, Maggiore WA. Why are you transporting dead patients? J Emerg Med Serv [Internet]. 2007 [cited 2019 Jun 15]; [about 1 p]. Available from: https://www.jems.com/articles/2007/02/why-are-you-transporting-dead-1.html.
15. Wolfe F. Air ambulance leads US rankings of safest helicopter mission sets. Rotor Wing Int [Internet]. 2018 [cited 2019 Apr 15]; [about 1 p]. Available from: https://www.rotorandwing.com/2018/11/20/air -ambulance-leads-us-rankings-safest-helicopter-mission-sets/.

Risk-Related Zones of Prehospital Operations

15

E. Reed Smith Jr., Geoff Shapiro, Ofer Lichtman, and William Eisenhart

Introduction

Public safety medical responders often work in dynamic and unstable environments. Although efforts to mitigate threats are typically ongoing, the primacy of rescue for injured victims in the immediate aftermath of intentional and unintentional events often requires operations in areas with elevated, even imminent, risk. Medical rescue in post-blast areas is just one such example of operating in areas of high risk. Although the intentional use of explosives to injure and kill citizens is well known, unintentional or accidental explosions and subsequent post-blast operations are not uncommon in civilian emergencies. Events such as the chemical plant explosion in Crosby, Texas, on April 2, 2019 [1], and the 2013 ammonium nitrate explosion at the West Fertilizer Company storage and distribution facility in West Texas [2] that occurred while emergency services personnel were responding to a fire at the facility demonstrate not only the devastating power of these events, but also the difficult challenges and need for special considerations when operating in the post-blast environment.

E. R. Smith Jr. (✉)
Arlington County Fire and Police Department, Arlington, VA, USA

The George Washington University School of Medicine and Health Sciences, Washington, DC, USA

G. Shapiro
EMS and Operational Medical Training, Emergency Health Services Program, The George Washington University School of Medicine and Health Sciences, Washington, DC, USA

O. Lichtman
Rancho Cucamunga Fire Department, Rancho Cucamonga, CA, USA

W. Eisenhart
Yale University Physician Assistant Program, New Haven, CT, USA

D. W. Callaway, J. L. Burstein (eds.), *Operational and Medical Management of Explosive and Blast Incidents*, https://doi.org/10.1007/978-3-030-40655-4_15

Intentional use of explosives against military, government, public, and even medical facilities and personnel is well documented and has been employed by terrorists around the world for many years. Improvised explosive devices (IEDs) and vehicle-borne IEDs are considered by many terrorist groups to be cheap, easy to make, and extremely effective weapons. Explosive precursor materials are widely available, and the chemical recipes and mechanical plans for devices are easily accessed on the Internet and in print. Additionally, the mobility, flexibility, and ease of use of this weapon lend itself to stealthy and subtle deployment. For example, an explosive can be placed in a ubiquitous container such as a backpack that will not draw attention and then can either be set to detonate on a timer, can be command detonated in a suicide-homicide attack, or can be remotely command detonated once the individual who placed it is no longer in the area. This is the exact scenario and deployment of the two lethal explosive devices used in the 2013 Boston Marathon bombing. Explosives can also be placed and designed to be triggered by a victim months later, such as with a land mine. In essence, when used as an offensive weapon, explosive devices are limited only by the imagination of the designer and the one using it.

The "double bomb" is a common tactic used in intentional explosive mass casualty events to affect public safety responders. This term describes the tactic where a second explosive device is placed in a separate but geographically related area and then detonated on a delay with the purpose of creating additional casualties, especially among responders, disrupting the overall response, and creating chaos, confusion, and fear. Mistakenly thought by many to only occur in foreign countries, the double-bomb tactic was used on American soil by Eric Rudolph in his politically motivated bombing of the Atlanta Northside Family Planning Clinic in 1997 [3]. In this event, Rudolph detonated his first device inside the clinic, injuring six, and then detonated a second device on a delay in a nearby dumpster in an attempt to target first responders and evacuees from the clinic. Kip Kinkel, the 15-year-old assailant in the 1998 Thurston High School shooting in Springfield, Oregon, killed his parents the day before the shooting at the high school and booby-trapped his home with explosive devices intended to injure whomever found the bodies [4]. The double-bomb tactic has been used frequently to increase disruption and devastation in medical response worldwide. Internationally, from 1990 through 2014, at least 11 terrorist groups have detonated a device in one part of a city and then a second device at a nearby hospital to disrupt the medical response and injure those trying to save lives [3].

The risk of secondary devices is one of the many operational considerations that must be understood and mitigated during medical rescue operations. First responders must be aware of the tactics being used, the risks, and operational considerations and must be capable of conducting coordinated medical rescue operations for the wounded in the immediate aftermath of an explosive event and possibly even perform life safety and medical rescue operations in the vicinity of known but unexploded devices.

Traditionally, in the post-blast environment or when there is a potential explosive risk, the common public safety operational medical response has been to minimize risk to responders by taking a conservative approach: instead of initiating immediate coordinated rescue, a common standard operating procedure, at least on paper, is to "stage and wait" at a safe distance until the explosive risk is fully mitigated and the scene is totally secure. The idea of eliminating all risk to responders in active violence and in post-blast response is traditional fire and emergency medical services culture.

From day one of most fire and emergency medical services (EMS) training, students are taught that scene safety is paramount and that responder safety has the highest priority. However, in real-world incidents, many law enforcement, fire department, and EMS personnel, despite the risk and often without thought, have immediately reacted to an event, moving forward into uncleared, unsecured, and potentially dangerous areas to begin lifesaving rescue operations.

One well-known example of such spontaneous medical response into an area of high risk was the 2013 bombing near the finish line of the Boston Marathon. Despite a strongly traditional operational culture and a firm operational policy of "stage and wait" until the post-blast area was fully swept and cleared by the bomb unit, first responders from all public safety disciplines in Boston (police, fire/rescue, and EMS) instantly converged directly to the epicenters of the two blasts to provide immediate life rescue, treatment, and evacuation of the wounded [5]. In this and other cases, although suspicion for possible secondary devices or other threats existed, the subconscious urge to save lives as part of public safety first responder job identity and training became the operational driving force, and those professionals went to work despite the risk.

As the first responder community is looking to take on more of an "all-hazard model" approach, it may be time to look at a more modern "principles of risk" model for the future. In any incident the overall priorities should first be life safety, with incident stabilization second, and resource and property conservation third. Realizing that in the initial stages of the incident there is a short time frame to make the most impact on life safety, this would be when modern principles of risk should be deployed: (1) accept high risk to responder life to save a citizen life (conscious casualty), (2) accept mitigated risk to responder life to possibly save a citizen life (unconscious casualty), (3) accept no risk when there is no citizen life to save (obvious death), or (4) accept no risk when there are no casualties.

Given the operational truth that most public safety responders will not stage while there are citizens injured and in need of rescue, the only way to mitigate the increased risk to public safety is to give them a better understanding of that risk and provide the training, procedures, and operational knowledge for operations in these areas. This approach is similar to that employed by the US military. In the current War on Terror (WoT), many combat injuries incurred by US troops in Iraq and Afghanistan have been caused by the IED.

Early in the WoT, Explosive Ordnance Disposal (EOD) units were the only military personnel that were trained and empowered to mitigate and dispose of an IED. If an IED was discovered or detonated, all operations are halted until the immediate area had been swept and any unexploded ordinance had been prosecuted. However, as the number and frequency of IEDs requiring specialty EOD teams overwhelmed the limited availability of EOD personnel, the military countered by training frontline combat personnel to both identify explosive devices and to maneuver and operate in space around them despite the risk they represented. This training focused on teaching military line personnel to both identify key features of the device and initiate immediate action drills of extracting any casualties to areas of higher safety in order to minimize loss of life.

This chapter will discuss a similar operational approach for civilian systems and present the immediate action medical rescue tactics for public safety personnel responding to a post-blast scenario, or to a scenario in which there are casualties in need of rescue in locations near known but unexploded devices. The basis of the discussion will be considerations for operations and medical rescue in the different zones of prehospital operations and the application of the risk-benefit-ratio-based medical treatment paradigm of Tactical Emergency Casualty Care (TECC) for those injured.

Initial Actions on Scene of a Possible IED Incident

Upon initial response, the first arriving units must maintain a high index of suspicion and should recognize the pattern of widespread damage caused by an explosion. The reporting party that called 911, especially if that person is not directly involved, may not have known or may not have had direct situational awareness relevant to the true cause of the event and may wrongfully have reported only "smoke" or "fire" or "structural collapse" instead of correctly identifying the event as an explosion. As such, it is important for public safety response personnel to recognize scene details that could indicate an explosive device was detonated.

Explosives create destruction through distinct mechanisms: the rapid conversion of the explosive material (liquid or solid) to gas creates a destructive pressure wave and brisance; multiple projectiles from the device itself or from the surrounding environment are propelled outward at high velocity that create tearing and penetrating injuries; blast wind that can throw objects and people is created as the pressure wave moves through the air; and thermal injuries are caused from the heat of combustion of the explosive materials [6].

The pattern of destruction seen by first arriving personnel may provide clues to an explosive event. For example, an area with structural damage and widespread fragmented materials seemingly emanating from a charred epicenter should lead the first arriving units to initiate actions for response to an explosive event. Additionally, given the frequency of use of the double-bomb tactic, it is important for public safety response personnel to be trained in the key features of explosive devices and potential for additional accidental explosions to allow for recognition and identification. Any call type has the potential to involve explosives. For example, one of the two car bombs parked outside the Tiger Tiger London club in an attempted bombing in 2007 was not initially recognized as such; instead, it was ticketed for illegal parking and towed to an impound lot. It was not until much later that is was discovered to be a vehicle-borne IED [7].

Once recognized, either in a post-blast scene or with an unexploded live or suspicious device on scene, immediate notification of the situation and request for response should be made to the local EOD unit. The proximate blast area, or the potential blast and fragmentation area of an unexploded device, represents a direct and immediate threat to persons or providers and should be considered a hot zone (see Chap. 13 for information regarding estimated standoff distances). Direct threats in this area include, but are not limited to, fire, large fragmentation and unstable structural damage, and the potential for secondary devices or other additional explosions.

Recognizing the post-blast area and the apparent seat of the blast, responders should immediately position fire apparatus in a "V" with the front of each vehicle positioned towards the seat of the blast, creating a hasty area of refuge immediately behind the vehicles where, if additional explosions occurred, the blast overpressure wave and fireball would be channeled away and fragmentation would be absorbed by the structures of the vehicles. A safer area such as this can be considered a warm zone where risk exists, but it is not direct and immediate. Other potential warm zone areas could be established by using buildings and other terrain features to provide cover. For example, moving out of direct line of sight around the corner of a stable building will protect responders from ballistic and thermal trauma and minimize exposure to the shock wave. If using buildings for cover, be wary of corridor effects that create the potential for channeling of overpressure waves or overhanging features that could be damaged and fall.

Once a close warm zone area is created or identified, a hasty casualty collection point (CCP) should be quickly established in this area to receive patients as they are extracted by rescue personnel from the immediate blast area in the hot zone. An early operational priority should be to sweep this warm zone area for secondary explosive devices, although, even if swept, given the increased risk, time spent in this area should be minimized as much as possible (Fig. 15.1).

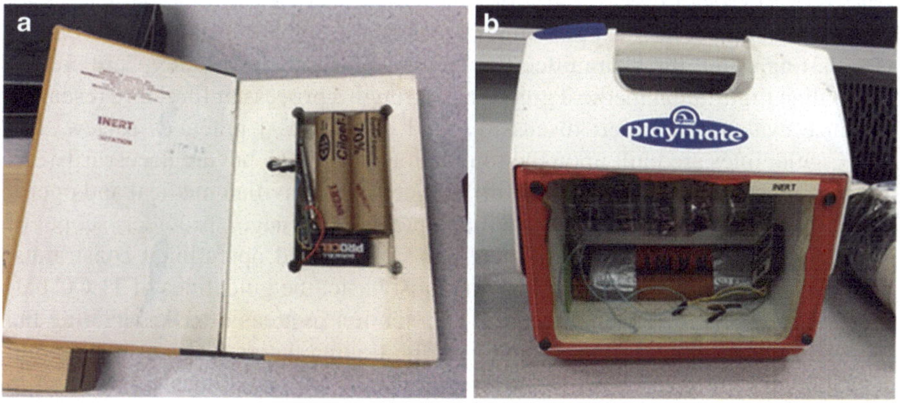

Fig. 15.1 (**a**, **b**) Examples of innovative improvised explosive devices

In cases where there is a known undetonated IED, any civilians and nonessential personnel in the area should be immediately moved outside the blast and fragmentation radius. Response personnel operating in the hot zone should be limited in number to only what is needed to effect rapid rescue of any casualties. Prior to initiating hot zone rescue operations, medical response personnel should determine "go/no go" criteria by using a checkdown method:

- *High threat, no victims:* no need for rescue so maintain cordon and safe standoff.
- *High threat, victims present:* determine rapid rescue method according to the priorities of life (civilian > public safety responder > perpetrator). Mitigate risk by utilizing the response concept of time-distance-shielding. Minimize the amount of time exposed to areas with high risk through coordinated rescue operations that involve rapid extrication. Additionally, rescue personnel functioning in this area should be wearing ballistic vests to provide some shielding. Utilize the same path of egress as entry to minimize additional disruption of the environment. Be aware of the surroundings and have an alternate egress route should it become necessary.
- *Low threat, victims present:* use safest ingress and egress means possible. Minimize environmental and evidence disturbance to extract victims.
- *Low threat, no victims:* maintain cordon and safe standoff distance.

Tactical Emergency Casualty Care: Medical Considerations in an IED Environment

Tactical Emergency Casualty Care (TECC) is a set of evidence-based and consensus best practice trauma care guidelines intended for civilian high-threat medical response [8]. The TECC guidelines are built upon the critical medical lessons learned by US and allied military forces over the past 18 years of conflict. Using the military combat medical guidelines of Tactical Combat Casualty Care (TCCC) as a starting point, the Committee for Tactical Emergency Casualty Care creates the civilian high-threat medical guidelines through a process of literature research, evidence evaluation, expert discussion, and civilian best practices review. The TECC guidelines are built upon the foundations of TCCC, but are necessarily different to meet the unique needs and differences of the civilian medical and operational environments, including civilian-specific language, provider scope of practice, population, civil liability, civilian mission and operational constraints, logistics, and resource acquisition. At its most basic, the guidelines of TECC balance the risk-benefit ratio for medical intervention in areas of risk, dictating the specific medical interventions to stabilize the trauma patient at or near the point of wounding and then effect rapid rescue. The TECC guidelines are applied in three different phases depending on the relationship between the provider and the actual or potential threat [9].

Risk-Related Zones of Prehospital Operations

Hot, warm, and cold zones are common terms used in civilian response communities. In addition to these, TECC guidelines use terms related to medical care appropriate in each zone, referred to as direct threat, indirect threat, and evacuation care. In scenarios involving risks from additional explosions (and other deliberate attacks discussed in Chap. 16), the most robust treatment and evacuation from the scene occurs from the cold zone/evacuation care area, although immediately lifesaving care may have to be performed in the hot zone/direct threat and warm zone/indirect threat locations (Fig. 15.2).

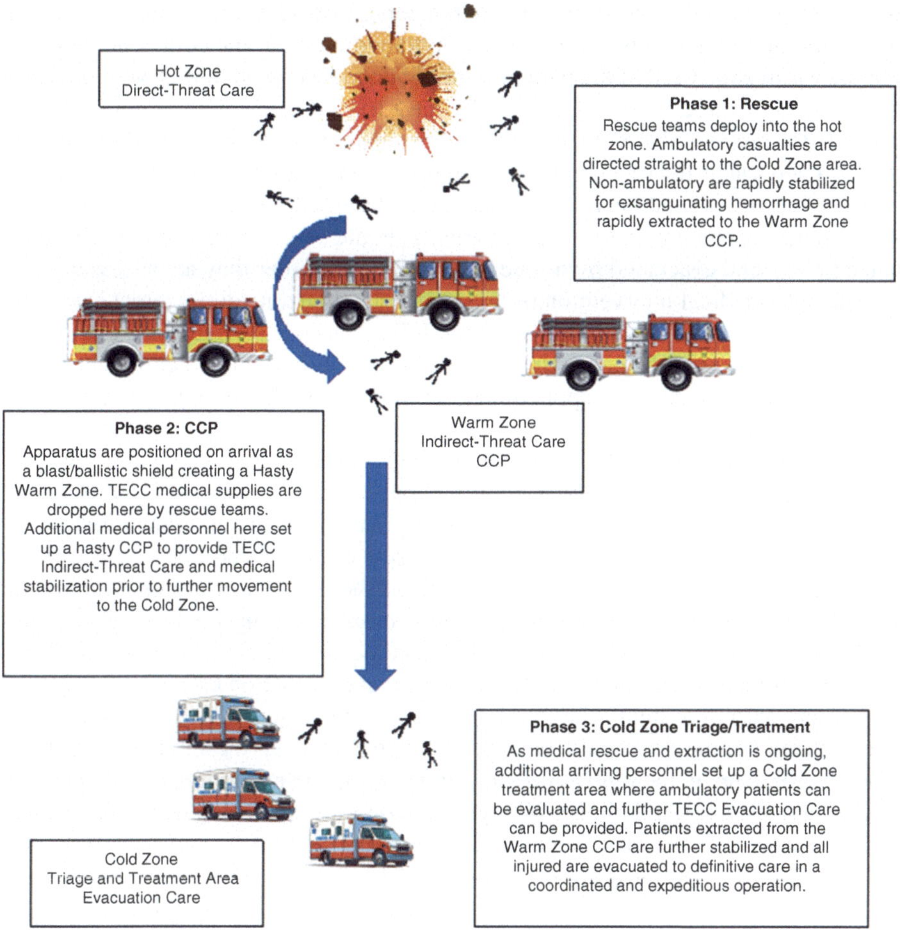

Fig. 15.2 Creating zones of care and casualty flow between risk-related zones

Hot Zone/Direct Threat

Any area of operations where there is a direct and immediate risk of injury to the provider and/or further injury to the patient should be considered a hot zone/direct threat area. As stated above, the estimated seat of the explosive in a post-blast area, or any area within the blast and fragmentation range of an unexploded device, represents the hot zone. Rescue personnel responding into this hot zone to effect victim rescue will have the primary role of direct threat care, point-of-wounding stabilization, and rapid extraction from the hot zone either to a CCP in the warm zone or, if appropriate, directly to the definitive care area in the cold zone.

The area of safety initially established using geography or apparatus positioning can be considered a warm zone and can be utilized as a close CCP if necessary. No formal triage should be performed in the hot zone. Instead, rescue personnel should direct ambulatory patients to quickly self-extract directly to the cold zone, bypassing the warm zone CCP. If the patient is ambulatory, has no obvious severe injuries, and can follow directions, they essentially have triaged themselves as not requiring immediate care and, therefore, do not need evaluation or treatment until they reach the assigned triage and treatment area in the cold zone. Patients with injuries incompatible with life should be visually marked as deceased but should not be moved. Any remaining nonambulatory viable patients should be assessed, stabilized as indicated below, and evacuated by rescue personnel in the order they are accessed.

The only medical intervention performed during hot zone/direct threat care is to stop immediately life-threatening bleeding. If there is no life-threatening compressible hemorrhage or if the hemorrhage is not immediately life threatening, no medical interventions need to be applied and the injured should be rapidly extracted to the warm zone CCP.

Direct pressure stops external bleeding. The rescuer should immediately apply—or have a bystander or even the patient, if capable, apply—pressure directly to the wound itself. For very large wounds or for amputations where applying direct pressure would be difficult or impossible, the rescuer can instead apply pressure by kneeling on the proximal inner arm to occlude the brachial artery or the femoral triangle to occlude the femoral artery. Once exsanguinating hemorrhage is controlled with direct pressure or proximal arterial occlusion, application of prefabricated tourniquets or compression devices will make extraction easier.

For any extremity injury that, in the opinion of the rescuer, is exsanguinating, a commercial tourniquet should be placed "high and over the clothes," meaning placed as high up on the limb as possible and overtop of any clothing—but not solid pocket items such as cell phones or keys—to stop life-threatening hemorrhage that, in the opinion of the rescuer, might lead to death during movement to the CCP. The decision to place a tourniquet versus a grab-and-go rapid extraction should be balanced with the amount of bleeding, the distance to safety, and the perceived risk of further injury to the rescuer and the patient. Spending time in the hot zone to apply a tourniquet is a consideration that must be balanced against the risk. If immediately indicated, the tourniquet should then be applied "high and tight," fully tightened and properly secured to prevent loosening. For commercial tourniquets, this process

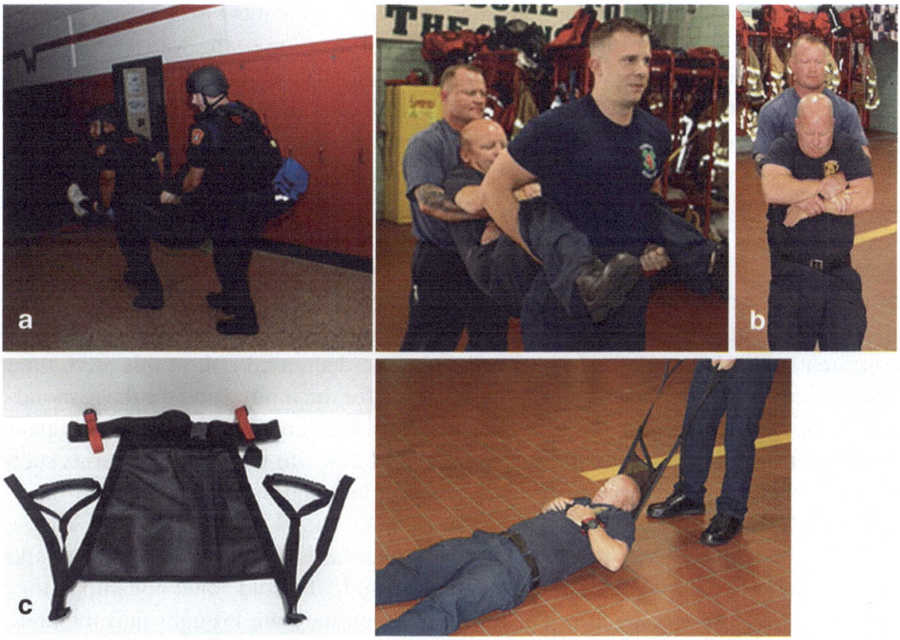

Fig. 15.3 Lifts, moves, and carries. (**a**) Fore-aft carry. (**b**) One-man elevated drag. (**c**) Rescue GrabStrap

should not take more than 60 seconds. If no tourniquet is available or the risk is too high to take the time to apply a tourniquet, direct pressure on the bleeding wound should be continued during extraction out of the hot zone.

All nonambulatory wounded persons should be extracted as rapidly as possible to the casualty collection point in the warm zone using an efficient technique such as the two-man fore-aft carry, the one-man elevated drag, or rescue equipment such as the GrabStrap™ (Fig. 15.3).

Warm Zone/Indirect Threat

Any area of operations where there is a potential, but not direct and immediate, threat of further injury to patients or providers should be considered as a warm zone. Examples include areas of safety intentionally created through apparatus positioning, as well as those identified in nearby areas with structural or geographical cover from shock waves and ballistic objects.

As stated above, a hasty CCP should rapidly be established in this warm zone. This CCP should be the initial destination for nonambulatory patients extracted from the hot zone and is where stabilizing medical care according to the indirect threat care principles of TECC will be applied. As such, in the initial phases of the response, as emergency responders arrive on scene and move forward to initiate rescue operations, TECC equipment and supplies from the Fire/EMS apparatus should be brought up to this CCP for medical stabilization in the warm zone. Fire/EMS medical personnel not involved in hot zone rescue and extraction operations should move into this CCP and be ready to accept care as patients are brought in by the rescue teams. A rapid transfer of care from the rescue team to medical personnel at the CCP allows the former to quickly return to the hot zone for continued rescue operations, while further medical stabilization is being provided in the warm zone by the latter.

This hasty CCP represents a pit stop during patient extraction, allowing for stabilization of immediately life-threatening injuries in a mitigated risk area close to the point of wounding prior to the continued movement to the cold zone/evacuation care treatment area or definitive care. Despite the decreased risk in this area, time spent here should be as minimal as possible, both for the injured and for the responders. By limiting care here to only immediately lifesaving stabilization, time spent here, and thus risk, is minimized. Management of non-life-threatening injuries such as fractures, non-hemorrhaging soft-tissue injuries, and small-to-moderate burns can be deferred until later.

No formal triage needs to be performed here either. Ambulatory patients should be directed to bypass this area and proceed straight to the cold zone; nonambulatory patients should be stabilized in the order in which they are brought into the area. Formal triage can occur in the next phase of care once the patients reach the cold zone where there is minimal threat to patients or providers.

The priority of care in this hasty CCP should follow the TECC indirect threat care guidelines. Although the MARCH^{2}E algorithm (Massive Hemorrhage, Airway, Respirations, Circulation and Resuscitation, Head Injury and Hypothermia Management, Everything Else) is described in the TECC guidelines, streamlining TECC even further to adapt to the austerity and meet the overarching goal of rapid movement of patients and personnel to safety is appropriate. By definition, any operational warm zone has inherent risk, but when compared to other scenarios, post-blast rescue or rescue operations when there is known unexploded ordinance falls on the higher end of the warm zone risk spectrum. For example, in response to the Boston bombing, each of the multitude of bags and backpacks left by those fleeing from the blast site had the potential to be secondary devices; as such, although there were no known tangible secondary explosive, the presence of many potential devices created a high-risk warm zone. In such operational cases when it is prudent to limit the amount of time spent in warm zone areas to the absolute minimum, TECC can be streamlined to address only the immediate life threat by limiting the medical treatment priorities to the mnemonic "SCAB-E": Situational Awareness, Circulation, Airway, Breathing, and Evacuate. Proceeded in a stepwise manner, this approach prioritizes care, not on the likelihood of injury, but on how rapidly lethal the injury can be. Bleeding control is prioritized, both because it is a likely injury in the blast scenario and because large vasculature injury can lead to irreversible hemorrhagic shock in minutes. Airway compromise and penetrating secondary blast injury to the torso are also likely in the severely wounded, and after hemorrhage control, compromised airways should be stabilized and any open or developing tension pneumothorax should be assessed for and treated prior to any further evacuation. At the responder's discretion, the full MARCH^{2}E care can then be performed during the evacuation care phase.

Situational awareness is listed first in the algorithm to remind the medical personnel operating in the warm zone CCP that they must "keep their head up," maintaining enhanced situational awareness in this area for additional, unrecognized threats. This includes not only secondary bombs, but structural damage from the blast that may lead to collapse. As a part of situational awareness, rapid egress routes from the warm zone CCP to other nearby safe havens should be identified.

Circulation in the algorithm means to assess for and treat any life-threatening extremity or junctional bleeding that was not addressed during direct threat care. Junctional hemorrhage is defined as bleeding from a non-torso wound that is too close to the hips or shoulders to place a proximal tourniquet.

The first medical priority during indirect threat care is to quickly assess for unrecognized or untreated exsanguinating hemorrhage and to reassess any tourniquet that was placed during direct threat care to ensure effective bleeding control after patient movement. If the tourniquet is effective, it should be left alone. If the tourniquet is found to be ineffective, it can be tightened further, or a second tourniquet can be placed immediately next to the first, ideally more proximal. The combination of two tourniquets adjacent to each other widens the area of circumferential pressure, increasing the compressive effect on the underlying vasculature. One other option for a fully tightened but still ineffective tourniquet is to leave it in place, but then fully expose the wound and apply a new deliberate tourniquet directly to the skin 2–3 inches proximal to the most proximal wound. If hemorrhage control is obtained with the deliberate distal tourniquet, the proximal ineffective tourniquet should be loosened but left in place.

If untreated life-threatening bleeding is identified, immediate direct pressure should be applied to the wound. The emphasis here is on treating exsanguinating hemorrhage only. Treatment for non-life-threatening bleeding may be deferred. With the exception of an amputation, which always needs a tourniquet regardless of bleeding, soft tissue wounds that are not bleeding heavily do not need to be addressed in this phase.

Hemorrhage control in this phase of care does not always have to be "tourniquet first"; the provider has three options for addressing hemorrhaging wounds: tourniquets, wound packing plus pressure bandage, and hemostatic gauze plus direct pressure. Each hemorrhage control intervention has strengths and weakness, and the decision on which method to employ should be based on the number and types of wounds versus the amount and type of hemorrhage-control supplies.

Tourniquets continue to be a rapid and effective hemorrhage control option in this phase and may be employed for any extremity wound with massive uncontrolled bleeding. Tourniquet application is the most effective method for controlling hemorrhage from an amputation; thus, all amputations, regardless of amount of bleeding, need a proximal tourniquet applied. In this phase of care, extremity wounds should be fully exposed and evaluated for extent, and the tourniquet applied in a deliberate manner directly to the skin in an appropriate location. If tourniquets are limited in supply, they may need to be prioritized for use on amputations, while other hemorrhage-control options are utilized for non-amputation-related extremity injuries.

Wound packing plus a circumferential pressure bandage is another effective hemorrhage control option in this phase. Prior to application of a pressure bandage, large and/or deep wounds should be fully packed with hemostatic or standard roller gauze, essentially creating a cotton plug to transmit the pressure applied at the surface deep into the wound onto the site of bleeding. If the wound is packed with plain gauze, direct pressure should be applied for 5–10 minutes. A concentric pressure bandage, either a manufactured pressure dressing/bandage or a plain elastic wrap, should then be applied over the packing to maintain direct pressure on the wound.

Hemostatic gauze packing plus direct pressure is the third option for hemorrhage control in this phase of care. Hemostatic gauze may be used on any bleeding wound, but should be prioritized for use on anatomically junctional wounds. These areas are traversed by large-caliber vasculature and anatomically are not amenable to tourniquet or pressure bandage. If a patient has a junctional wound such as to the femoral triangle or the carotid sheath, direct pressure should be immediately applied, followed by packing with hemostatic gauze and direct pressure for up to 3–5 minutes. Bandages should then be applied to keep the gauze packing in place.

One last consideration for hemorrhage control in this phase is the use of junctional tourniquets specifically for femoral junctional bleeding. If available, a junctional tourniquet such as the Junctional Emergency Tourniquet or the SAM Junctional Tourniquet should be applied for these life-threatening wounds. Additionally, there is a direct relationship between blast-induced traumatic lower limb amputation and open-book pelvic ring disruptions; thus, junctional tourniquets may have additional value of splinting the pelvis along with applying pressure into the femoral triangle.

Airway is the next step in the SCAB-E approach. The provider should assess for airway patency and provide basic airway maneuvers to attain and maintain an open airway. Allow the conscious and alert patient with facial injury to assume any position that best protects the airway, including sitting up and leaning forward. Concern for cervical injury and cervical immobilization should not dictate or compromise airway management. Even in the setting of an unstable cervical fracture, normal movements of the head may not injure the cervical spinal cord [10]. Additionally, in this phase of care, application of full spinal immobilization is too logistically cumbersome and manpower intense. Instead, employ spine injury-clearance protocols and, if indicated and available, facilitate spinal motion restriction by applying a semirigid cervical collar or an improvised blanket rolled into a horse collar.

Although advanced airway procedures may be performed by appropriately trained personnel operating within their scope of practice, endotracheal intubation requires more equipment, more time, and more personnel for post-intubation management. Deferring advanced airway procedures until the patient has been fully extracted to the cold zone should strongly be considered.

In place of advanced airway management, any occluded airway or any patient with altered mental status should have a nasopharyngeal airway (NPA) placed. This airway is easy to insert, useful regardless of gag reflex, and stable and has the added benefit of being transiently stimulating to patients with altered mental status. Concerns for intracranial placement of an NPA through a cribiform plate fracture in patients with facial trauma are largely unfounded and not reported in any meaningful incidence in the medical literature. Thus, there are almost no contraindications to their use in this scenario. Despite the low risk, however, proper training and proper technique during placement must be emphasized. For patients with severe facial injuries that are significantly compromising the airway, additional consideration can be given for appropriately trained and authorized personnel to secure an airway by surgical cricothyroidostomy.

Breathing assessment and management, during indirect threat care, is focused on assessing and improving respiratory mechanics. In blast injury, the risk to the respiratory system comes from both primary blast injury (i.e., blast lung) and from secondary penetrating injury to the chest wall. There is little that can be done in the hasty CCP for blast lung other than to recognize the symptom complex (see Chap. 12). Instead, the priority is to address penetrating chest injury that is compromising respiratory function by creating an open pneumothorax. Any penetrating wound to the torso above the level of the umbilicus, anterior or posterior, should be covered with a nonocclusive chest seal (one-way valve or channeled) that will prevent air from entering the chest cavity during inspiration yet allow any air inside the chest cavity to vent out, decreasing the risk of a tension pneumothorax [11].

Any patient with penetrating chest wounds, whether or not they were covered with chest seals, must be closely monitored for development of a tension pneumothorax. Symptoms may include increasing dyspnea or respiratory rate, gasping, increasing anxiety, or cyanosis.

Given the operational conditions, good respiratory assessment with palpation and auscultation will be challenging at best; thus, any patient with known or suspected thoracic injury (blast, blunt, or penetrating) who has respiratory distress, either initially or that develops during care, should have a needle thoracostomy performed by appropriately trained and authorized personnel. If there is no provider with the appropriate scope of practice immediately available to perform a needle decompression, the torso wound can be physically "burped" by uncovering the wound and massaging the tissue around the wound or gently pulling the wound edges apart to open the wound track back up, allowing intrapleural air to vent (Fig. 15.4).

Safe and effective locations for needle decompression include the second intercostal space at the midclavicular line, not medial to the nipple line and not directed towards the heart, and the fourth or fifth intercostal space at the anterior axillary line directed slightly posteriorly. At a minimum, needle/catheter devices should be 10–14 gauge to move enough air and 3¼ inches to reach the pleural space. Success is indicated by an improvement in the patient's symptoms. The needle should be removed and the catheter left in place, allowing it to vent the excessive intrathoracic pressure. If the first attempt is unsuccessful or only partially effective, or repeat decompression is necessary due to recurrence of tension physiology, another needle decompression should be performed on the same side at another location [12].

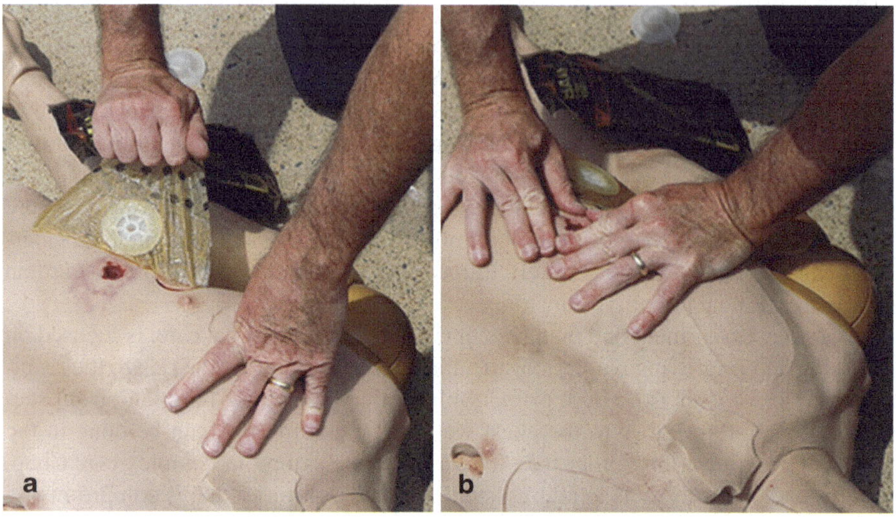

Fig. 15.4 (**a**, **b**) Manual "burp" of a chest wound for suspected tension pneumothorax

The final step in the SCAB-E indirect threat care management in the warm zone CCP is to reassess all interventions for continued effectiveness, perform a quick head-to-toe evaluation for any significant missed injuries that need stabilization, prevent hypothermia, and prepare the patient for further extraction to the cold zone. Any wounds discovered should be managed as above, and procedures to prevent heat loss should be instituted. Ideally, commercial hypothermia kits can be used, but improvised "burrito wraps" that consist of a vapor barrier, thermal barrier, and an inner reflective layer can be very effective [13]. At a minimum, a Mylar reflective blanket covered with a wool blanket can be utilized. The patient should then be allowed to assume a position of comfort or, if unconscious, placed in the lateral recumbent rescue position while awaiting evacuation to a triage and treatment area in the cold zone. No unconscious patient should ever be left by themselves in the supine position.

Limiting time in areas of higher risk is one of the risk mitigation strategies for patient and personnel protection. The overarching principle of high-threat rescue missions should be to deploy limited personnel into areas of high risk (hot zone), move the wounded to areas of mitigated risk (warm zone) for stabilization, and then further extricate to areas of relative safety (cold zone) for definitive care as expeditiously as possible. When sufficient personnel are available, patients should be extracted from warm zone CCP to cold zone triage and treatment area or directly to a waiting ambulance if one is available. Once all viable patients have been evacuated from the hot zone, stabilized in the warm zone CCP, and moved to the cold zone, medical operations in the hot and warm zones should be terminated.

Cold Zone/Evacuation Care

Initiating hot zone rescue operations, establishing a warm zone CCP, and providing personnel and resources to allow for indirect threat care stabilization of the wounded are the initial medical priorities on scene. However, identifying and establishing a cold zone treatment area is a close second. This should be established as early as practicable, clearly designated, and staffed with personnel and equipment to receive ambulatory casualties self-evacuating directly from the blast site and nonambulatory casualties who have been stabilized in and are being extracted from the warm zone CCP.

Ambulatory casualties directed out of the hot zone by the initial rescue teams will not have received any medical evaluation and, despite their ambulatory status, may have potentially life-threatening injuries. Young, healthy, well-conditioned people have the physiologic reserve to ambulate despite significant blast injuries by all mechanisms and, hence, should not be minimized or ignored, because they appear stable. Instead, any ambulatory person, especially any child carried into the cold zone, must be immediately evaluated for significant injuries.

When medical transport units are available, any severely injured patient that is brought into the cold zone area should be placed directly onto any available unit or immediate transport to receiving medical facility, in essence, bypassing the cold zone treatment area altogether. The immediate post-blast medical priority is to limit the time injured patients remain on scene.

When transport is available, TECC evacuation care can be performed during the transport by transporting medical crew. The tenet to follow is "get the red out," meaning prioritize evacuation of critical (red triage tag) patients. Ambulances should rarely stage on scene when there are patients that need transport, even if those patients do not have priority injuries. If transport resources are available, there is no need to hold "lower-priority" patients on scene in order to keep transport available for a more critical patient. Instead, deploy the available transport units as the patients are brought in from the hot zone or warm zone CCP following the mantra, "Ambulances should never wait on scene if patients are available, but patients may need to wait on scene until ambulances are available."

Controlled distribution of transported patients from the scene should be initiated as the first patients are leaving the scene. One important consideration in this distribution is that the minimally injured and worried well will predictably self-transport to the closet hospital. Thus, this hospital, regardless of trauma capability, will often be inundated with patients [14]. This pattern has been well documented after many of the recent intentional mass casualty events such as the shooting at the Route 91 festival in Las Vegas. The closest facility to the scene, Desert Springs Hospital, is a small community facility with a minimally staffed ED, and yet they received over 90 patients within the first hours of the event [15].

In the aftermath of any large-scale event, patients with lower triage designations should be transported to medical facilities farther away from the incident to decrease the medical surge at the closest medical facility. Additionally, operational consideration should be given to sending additional transport units directly to the closest hospital to enable secondary redistribution of patients after medical evaluation. Stable patients may be pushed to facilities farther out, allowing the closest facility to maintain capacity for the severely injured and unstable patients (see Chap. 21 for more information on this "redistribution phase").

Patient tracking procedures should be initiated in a coordinated fashion across the entirety of the medical system, including receiving facilities, to enable family reunification. Many "walking wounded" and even some severely wounded patients may be transported by other citizens directly to hospitals. As such, hospitals must assume responsibility along with Fire/EMS for patient tracking with information being fed into a coordinated system among all responder agencies for family notification and unification. Newer technology such as handheld barcode scanners and patient tracking via mobile facial recognition applications (www.FlingTrack.com) may help streamline this reunification process.

Once transport units are no longer immediately available, any patient brought into the cold zone treatment area from the CCP should be immediately reevaluated for efficacy of prior TECC interventions. Tourniquets and pressure bandages loosen while patients are carried or dragged, and some injuries may have been missed by providers under stress. As these patients are being reevaluated, they should be triaged according to local protocol for both priority of transportation and destination. There is no need to change principles of triage in the setting of field triage for blast injuries; however, additional considerations should be given for any patient with penetrating torso injury, even if they appear physiologically stable. Penetrating trauma to the torso should be considered as severe uncontrolled hemorrhage, and it should be assumed that the patient will go into uncompensated shock at any moment. These patients should have remote damage control procedures initiated in the cold zone treatment area and should be placed in the highest triage category even when physiologically stable.

The established cold zone should have additional personnel and the field medical resources that are standard for EMS systems. In this phase, these additional personnel and resources—including increased monitoring, diagnostic, and treatment modalities—should be devoted to increasing the level of care provided. Given the typically greater resources and personnel in the cold zone, the full evaluation and management guidelines of TECC evacuation care can be initiated, including interventions related to damage control resuscitation: permissive hypotension, limited administration of crystalloid fluids, hemostatic resuscitation, and hypothermia prevention. Pain control is emphasized as well.

The overarching medical priority for the cold zone triage and treatment area is to continue stabilizing any life-threatening wounds and to emphasize rapid evacuation to definitive treatment facilities with evacuation care en route. Efficient operations can lead to removal of all critical wounded from the scene in less than 30 minutes and all patients within an hour.

Conclusion

Operational medical response to explosive incidents, whether accidental or intentional, is a reality for public safety personnel. The post-blast environment represents unique operational considerations and challenges. Medical rescue in this environment should follow the priorities of life where first responders must put the lives of civilians first, but in a mitigated-risk operational approach. The post-blast environment and operations in the vicinity of unexploded ordinance environments carry risk for first responders, different but no less or no more dangerous than suppression activities, technical rescue, or other high-risk operations such as a Rescue Task Force [16].

As with all of these examples, the operational risk can be mitigated during the response by understanding the working environment, understanding the hazards, and mitigating risk through limiting time in areas of highest risk, creating warm zone areas with lower risk, rapidly stabilizing immediate life threats, and efficiently moving the wounded through the zones to definitive care. Once the wounded have been cleared, medical personnel should leave these zones of increased risk as well.

Key Points

- Recognize the key identifying features of the blast epicenter and post-blast environment.
- Recognize the potential for secondary explosions, any unexploded devices, good frontal and overhead protection, and the possibility of terrain or man-made structures to channel and magnify shock waves.
- Utilize vehicle positioning as a possible blast shield to create a hasty warm zone casualty collection point (CCP).
- Employ the phased medical care approach of Tactical Emergency Casualty Care to stabilize the immediate life threats and evacuate the patient in stages: hot zone to warm zone CCP to cold zone.

Pitfalls

- Delaying rescue operations for the wounded in a post-blast environment until the "all clear" signal is given following a formal explosive sweep by a specialized explosives ordinance handling team.
- Delaying medical care of immediately life-threatening injuries to extract the injured to an area of complete safety.
- Conducting medical rescue and treatment in the post-blast environment in the same manner conducted for non-high-threat environments.

Pearls

- Coordinate public safety operations to create areas of mitigated risk that allow for efficient patient access, rapid stabilizing medical care according to the Tactical Emergency Casualty Care Zones of Care, and prioritization of patient movement to definitive care while limiting time spent for personnel in high-risk areas.
- Immediately life-threatening injuries from explosives that can be stabilized in point-of-wounding care include hemorrhage, amputations, penetrating torso injury that compromises the mechanics of breathing and creates internal hemorrhage, airway compromise, trauma-induced coagulopathy, and hypothermia.
- Reassess the patient after each movement and at each phase of medical care to ensure all prior care remains effective and no important injuries are missed.
- Both the initial rescue operations and the back-end patient evacuation to definitive care at medical receiving facilities must be coordinated and communicated across all entities involved in the response.

References

1. Bagg J, Johnson A, Cumming J. Crosby, texas, chemical plant explodes twice, Arkema group says. Published online August 30, 2017. Accessed June 2019 at https://www.nbcnews.com/storyline/hurricane-harvey/harvey-danger-major-chemical-plant-near-houston-likely-explode-facility-n797581.
2. Taylor A. Texas's fertilizer plant explosion. Published online in the Atlantic, April 22, 2013. Accessed June 2019 at https://www.theatlantic.com/photo/2013/04/texass-fertilizer-plant-explosion/100501.
3. Mizell LR Jr, Smith ER Jr. Terrorism and the medical environment. Mizell: Bethesda, MD; 2016.
4. Friesen M. The Springfield school shooting: struggling with the Anguish. Published online in The Oregonian/OregonLive on May 23, 1998 and updated May 16, 2008. Accessed June 2019 at https://www.oregonlive.com/special/2008/05/the_springfield_school_shootin.html.
5. Gates JD, Arabian S, Biddinger P, Balnsfield J, Burke P, Chuhng S, et al. The initial response to the Boston Marathon bombing: lessons learned to prepare for the next disaster. Ann Surg. 2014;260(6):960–6. [PMID: 25386862].
6. Wightman JM, Gladish SL. Explosions and blast injuries. Ann Emerg Med. 2001;37(6):664–78. [PMID: 11385339].
7. Dodd V, Tran M, Oliver M, Laville S. Two car bombs found in London. Published online in The Guardian on June 29, 2007. Accessed June 2019 at www.theguardian.com/uk/2007/jun/29/terrorism.uksecurity.
8. Callaway D, Smith ER, Cain J, Shapiro G, Burnett W, McKay S, Mabry R. Tactical Emergency Casualty Care (TECC): guidelines for the provision of prehospital trauma care in high threat environments. J Spec Oper Med. 2011;11(3):104–22.
9. Callaway D, Smith ER, Cain J, Shapiro G, Burnett W, McKay S, Mabry R. The Committee for Tactical Emergency Casualty Care (C-TECC) evolution and application of TCCC guidelines to civilian high threat medicine. J Spec Oper Med. 2011;11(2).

10. Hauswald M. A re-conceptualisation of acute spinal care. Emerg Med J. 2013;30:720–3. https://doi.org/10.1136/emermed-2012-201847.
11. Limmer D, Limmer D, O'Keefe M, Dickinson E. Emergency care. 13th ed. (Legacy authors, Harvey D. Grant, Robert H. Murray, Jr., J. David Bergeron). Prentice Hall: Upper Saddle River, NJ; 2016.
12. Butler FK, Holcomb JB, Shackelford S. Management of suspected tension pneumothorax in tactical combat casualty care. J Spec Oper Med. 2018;18:19–35.
13. Auxier G. Wilderness medicine: your guide to treating illness or injury in the great outdoors. Contemp Pediatr. 2015;32(5):22–6.
14. Hogan DE, Waeckerle JF, Dire DJ, Lillibridge SR. Emergency department impact of the Oklahoma City terrorist bombing. Ann Emerg Med. 1999;34:160–7.
15. Harasim P, Munks J. Las Vegas-area hospital like 'War Zones' after strip massacre. Published online in the Las Vegas Review-Journal on October 2, 2017. Accessed June 2019 at https://www.review-journal.com/crime/shootings/las-vegas-area-hospitals-like-war-zones-after-strip-massacre/.
16. Smith E, Iselin B, Mckay W. Toward the sound of shooting: Arlington county, VA., rescue task force represents a new medical response model to active shooter incidents. JEMS. 2009;34(12):48–55.
17. Campbell J. International trauma life support for emergency care providers. 8th ed. Prentice Hall: Hoboken, NJ; 2016.

Tactical Emergency Medical Support

16

Rittik Chaudhuri, Ameen M. Jamali, and Nelson Tang

Introduction

Tactical Emergency Medical Support (TEMS) involves the multidimensional provision of medical care during and surrounding high-threat civilian law enforcement operations. TEMS providers, often embedded in special operations tactical teams, are tasked with providing potentially lifesaving care in high-risk and medically remote settings. The practice of TEMS has been influenced significantly by the extensive experience of military combat medics confronted with battlefield injuries. Current best practices in TEMS are driven by additional guidelines developed specifically to account for important differences between the military and civilian environments.

Tactical Emergency Medical Support

In the mid- to late 1960s, an emerging pattern of hostile mass-violence incidents across the United States led to the realization among law enforcement agencies that specialized elements were needed to effectively respond to crises beyond the routine capabilities of patrol officers [1]. The subsequent decades saw a proliferation of Special Weapons and Tactics (SWAT) and other "tactical" teams, which are now commonly deployed by police departments and law enforcement agencies throughout the United States. Today, the law enforcement tactical mission commonly includes responses to hostage or barricade incidents, high-risk warrant service, civil disturbances, dignitary and executive protection missions, maritime

R. Chaudhuri · A. M. Jamali · N. Tang (✉)
Center for Law Enforcement Medicine, Johns Hopkins Medical Institutions, Baltimore, MD, USA
e-mail: ntang@jhmi.edu

D. W. Callaway, J. L. Burstein (eds.), *Operational and Medical Management of Explosive and Blast Incidents*, https://doi.org/10.1007/978-3-030-40655-4_16

and dive operations, and explosive ordnance disposal. The potential for explosive devices and blast injuries to complicate many or all of these types of missions is increasingly recognized.

The emergence of TEMS followed closely the evolution of SWAT teams and has gained increasing recognition as an essential element of the modern law enforcement mission [2–5]. TEMS recognizes that law enforcement personnel engaged in special-operations-type missions are placed at high risk for traumatic injury often without the organized provision of dedicated or accessible medical care. Early functional parallels were drawn between these tactical officers and military combatants engaged in small-unit operations. Unlike their medic and corpsman counterparts embedded with teams of military operators, civilian Emergency Medical Services (EMS) providers historically lacked the training and skills to render lifesaving care to injured tactical officers in high-threat environments. Today, although singularly focused on medical effectiveness in operational settings, TEMS remains a heterogeneous entity rendered either by non-sworn medical providers with specialized training or law enforcement officers who maintain collateral skills as medics.

The goals of TEMS are broadly to facilitate the overall success and safety of high-risk law enforcement missions throughout all phases of tactical operations. Its primary objectives during a mission are injury prevention, resource allocation, and rapid initiation of emergency medical care. TEMS bolsters the on-scene command infrastructure by providing medical threat assessments, delivering immediate emergency medical care, and promoting the safety and health of law enforcement personnel. TEMS personnel further achieve their objectives by facilitating communications and interoperability between law enforcement, EMS, and the emergency health care system. During law enforcement operations, medical activities and casualty movements are coordinated between the command post, operational team leaders, and the medical support element. A fundamental tenet in TEMS is that law enforcement mission accomplishment will often supersede medical decision-making and the needs of individual casualties.

Integral to the advancement of TEMS has been the ongoing pursuit of medically effective practices specifically developed or adapted for the high-threat law enforcement environment. TEMS providers must be thoroughly prepared to manage both high-frequency/low-consequence and low-frequency/high-consequence medical and trauma scenarios [6, 7]. Best practices derived from emergency medicine and EMS remain the foundation for most clinical interventions performed in the course of tactical operations. Furthermore, TEMS has sustained longitudinal benefit from military medicine experiences and lessons learned in active theaters of combat.

Lessons from the Military

Prior to 1996, US military medics were trained according to the principles of Advanced Trauma Life Support (ATLS). Although the widespread implementation of ATLS had been credited with decreasing the mortality of trauma victims in the civilian in-hospital setting, many in the military medicine community recognized that it was poorly suited for their out-of-hospital mission sets. ATLS was developed by trauma surgeons establishing clinical standards for hospital-based care. It did not adequately address the needs of medics and corpsmen expected to balance mission-specific operational goals with the need to provide medical care for combat casualties. Military prehospital providers routinely had to provide that care under active enemy fire, with limited portable equipment, and in austere locations.

The US Special Operations Command (USSOCOM) recognized the shortcomings of using ATLS on the battlefield and in 1995 commissioned a study on how to improve survival from combat-related injuries. The following year, after extensive research on ballistic and blast wounding patterns from military weapons, which included medical records and autopsy data, a report entitled "Tactical Combat Casualty Care (TCCC) in Special Operations" was released [8]. This report, for the first time, described the integration of both tactics and medicine. The three major goals of TCCC are the delivery of lifesaving treatment to injured combatants, limiting the risk of additional injuries to casualties and providers, and mission success.

In order to achieve these goals, TCCC proposed dividing each mission into three phases based on threat levels and provided specific recommendations for the medical care appropriate during each phase. USSOCOM embraced TCCC and rapidly implemented its recommendations. Following positive feedback from the Special Operations community, the remainder of the US military adopted TCCC as well. Since its implementation, TCCC protocols have been credited with significantly reducing battlefield mortality [9, 10].

Adaptation to Civilian Casualty Care

In recent decades, high-capacity firearms and improvised explosive devices (IEDs) have been used with increasing frequency to target civilians [11]. In these incidents of intentional mass violence, law enforcement and medical responders are often forced to operate in an environment with significant similarities to a military combat zone. Confronted with the prospect of ongoing threats, including active shooter(s) or secondary explosive devices and patterns of injuries at least theoretically similar to those experienced by injured combatants, civilian public safety entities have been challenged with continually adapting their response capabilities. While TEMS had already broadly espoused medical approaches derived from its military counterparts, the need to establish more organized and standardized approaches to casualty care in the civilian high-threat setting became critical.

In the effort to develop civilian guidelines, important differences between the military and civilian settings must be recognized. Compared to their military counterparts, civilian prehospital responders are employed by a wider variety of agencies across multiple tiers of government and possess variable levels of training, scopes of practice, and prior experiences. Historically, medical care in high-threat environments is not intrinsic to the approaches of civilian prehospital care. Vulnerable populations in the civilian setting are diverse and not typically accounted for in the TCCC paradigm. These include pediatric, pregnant, and geriatric patients with variable baseline conditioning and physiologies. A myriad of physical settings for many acts of intentional mass violence exist in the civilian setting and can impact access to casualties and transport times to definitive medical care.

Tactical Emergency Casualty Care (TECC)

The Committee for Tactical Emergency Casualty Care (C-TECC) was founded in 2011 as a standing, independent, nonprofit organization comprised of operational and academic medical leaders with a unified mission to develop and maintain best practice guidelines for the provision of medical care during high-threat incidents. Translating key lessons learned from its military counterpart, the TECC guidelines promoted evidence-based management of casualties during tactical operations accounting for differences in civilian environments, resource allocations, patient populations, and responder scopes of practice. The C-TECC convenes formally twice annually to present scientific advances, emerging technology, and update TECC guidelines to further enhance the lifesaving mission. C-TECC membership includes leaders, subject matter experts, presenters and stakeholders from domestic and international law enforcement, EMS, fire/rescue, military, industry, and interested parties. TECC recommendations and guidelines are updated on a regular basis and available as open source resources [12, 13].

TECC protocols provide specific recommendations for medical care according to the threat level. In TECC nomenclature, the three phases of care are defined as follows [14]:

- *Direct Threat Care (DTC)*: This phase of care occurs at the scene of the injury, when the casualty and medical provider remain under some immediate threat (e.g., enemy weapons fire or civil disturbance, IEDs or accidental explosions, flooding or fire, etc.). The emphasis in DTC remains on mitigating the threat to prevent further casualties, moving the wounded to cover or an area of relative safety, and managing life-threatening extremity hemorrhage with tourniquets. The importance of various rescue and patient-movement techniques and rapid positional airway management is delineated in DTC. Medical care and operational requirements are the same for operators and all levels of TEMS providers during this phase of care.
- *Indirect Threat Care (ITC)*: This phase is initiated once the casualty is in a location of relative safety where there is less potential for responders being injured or casualties sustaining additional injuries. Assessment and treatment priorities in this phase focus on the preventable causes of death such as hemorrhage control, airway management, diagnosis and treatment of tension pneumothorax and hypovolemic shock, and prevention of hypothermia. Five different levels of providers are assigned TECC skill sets based on training and certification (Table 16.1).
- *Evacuation Care*: During this phase of care, efforts are initiated to move the casualty toward a definitive treatment facility. Most additional interventions

Table 16.1 C-TECC skill sets based on provider level

Provider level	Tourniquets[b]	Pressure bandage w/ packing	Hemostatic agents	Tourniquet de-escalation	Needle thoracentesis	Surgical airway	Nasopharyngeal airway	Bling airway insertion device
LEO[a]	X	X	X				X	
EMR or equivalent	X	X	X		X[c]		X	X
EMT	X	X	X	X	X[c]		X	X
Advanced EMT	X	X	X	X	X	X[c]	X	X
Paramedic	X	X	X	X	X	X	X	X

Courtesy of Committee for Tactical Emergency Casualty Care

[a]Law Enforcement Officer; may have CPR/basic first aid training

[b]Already included in National Registry of Emergency Medical Technicians (NREMT) Skill Sheets

[c]Only with proper training, specialized protocol and operational medical director approval

during this phase of care are similar to those performed during conventional EMS. Major emphasis is placed on reassessment of field interventions and continuation of damage control resuscitation (DCR).

Delays in the evacuation of injured patients may be caused by a number of factors, including the tactical situation, lack of appropriate transportation assets, and limitations imposed by inclement weather and adverse terrain. Tactical medical providers should be prepared to continue effective treatment in these situations, referred to as "prolonged field care." Although current TECC guidelines do not cover prolonged field care, recognizing the potential need to render care for extended durations in the field is important for TEMS providers. Planning for such contingencies and operational flexibility are critical to limiting morbidity and mortality when immediate evacuation is not possible.

Mechanisms of Blast Injuries

Explosions have the potential to cause a wide variety of physical injuries, which can range in severity from mild to life-threatening. It is important for TEMS providers to rapidly recognize these injuries, so that they may successfully triage and treat victims of a blast.

Blast injuries are often classified according to the mechanism of injury. The most common classification system divides injury mechanisms into four categories [15] and is discussed in detail in the introductory sections of this book. Briefly:

- *Primary blast injury* is caused by the pressure wave generated during an explosion. Immediately following combustion, air is rapidly compressed and forced outwards at high speed. The blast wave can move around barricades and is not mitigated by body armor.
- *Secondary blast injury* is caused by the acceleration of an object, which subsequently strikes an individual. The accelerated object can be from the bomb (shrapnel) or from the environment (debris or shattered glass). Most secondary blast injuries result in penetrating trauma. Body armor and armored vehicles offer some protection from secondary blast injury.
- *Tertiary blast injury* is caused by the acceleration of an individual, who subsequently strikes an object. In these cases, the force of the explosion lifts an individual off the ground and launches them through the air. Blunt trauma occurs much more frequently than penetrating trauma. However, as with secondary blast injuries, any organ system may be involved.
- *Quaternary blast injury* is caused by all other mechanisms not specifically described in the first three categories, including burns, inhalational injuries, chemical exposures, and crush injuries. These are increasingly relevant in response to multimodal attacks and urban operations.

Many blast casualties will suffer from a combination of the injury patterns described above, resulting in damage to multiple organs. TEMS providers should therefore understand how blasts affect the different organ systems, so that they can correctly assess and treat victims after an explosion.

TEMS Responses to Blast Incidents

A thorough understanding of the complex injuries that may result from explosions and blast incidents is key to effective recognition and clinical management in the prehospital phase of responses. (The injury patterns from blast are discussed extensively in Part I of this book.) Blast incidents are typically of such large scale and wide impact that TEMS resources are quickly overwhelmed, and these specialized teams end up playing a focused support role in the incident response.

Conventional EMS system-based providers will always significantly outnumber TEMS assets and ultimately provide the broad base of sustained responses to blast incidents, especially during the casualty transport phase. However, scene safety is a fundamental tenet of EMS care, with emphasis on provider safety the predominant consideration. In typical high-threat tactical incidents, this approach often limits early EMS provider access and initiation of emergency care of casualties within the law enforcement hot zone – the innermost perimeter of a tactical operation where the risk of ongoing harm is highest. By contrast, integrated TEMS providers with specialized training and ballistic protective equipment can initiate care in these environments thus bridging a critical gap between points of injury and conventional EMS resources.

TEMS by definition is intended to support exclusively tactical teams, a very small subset of overall law enforcement capacity. Operationally, TEMS providers typically deploy singly or in small numbers and are outfitted with finite, highly compact medical load outs designed to care for limited casualties resulting from isolated incidents. Consequently, the ability of TEMS providers to respond comprehensively to blast incidents resulting in mass casualties is limited. A key operational TEMS decision is when to transition from primary provider for the tactical team to a force multiplier, focused on leading teams of conventional EMS responders who do not routinely operate in high-threat environments.

The involvement of explosive devices in acts of intentional mass violence complicates the operational responses exponentially. Whether intended to cause injury or provide distraction, or both, the scope of actual threat in blast incidents is unknown during the initial phases of all responses. In some cases, whether explosions are intentional or accidental may not even be known. If the primary incident is an intentional explosion, the potential for delayed blasts that are set to inflict maximal damage to initial responders must be considered. The chaos that invariably follows an initial blast incident makes the detection or exclusion of a secondary explosive threat extremely difficult. If incidents involve shootings, stabbings, or vehicular trauma plus explosives, TEMS personnel are at particular risk for injury or death as secondary devices are most likely to harm those earliest responders in closest proximity.

Conclusion

Over the past 25 years, TEMS providers have become integral components of many law enforcement teams. These providers have specialized training and protective equipment that allows them to render lifesaving care in high-risk settings. They are uniquely positioned to initiate treatment of wounded patients immediately after the injury occurs, filling a critical gap in medical coverage between the point of injury and definitive medical care.

Injuries resulting from blast incidents are among the most complex that TEMS providers may encounter. Explosions have the potential to cause severe, complex injuries involving multiple organ systems. TEMS providers with a thorough understanding of the spectrum of blast injuries will be better prepared to support law enforcement personnel during high-risk operations and capable of effectively managing the injuries resulting from blast incidents.

Key Points

- TEMS providers are key subject matter experts related to blast injuries and can serve in both advisory roles and as force multipliers in MCI response.
- TEMS providers serve as critical liaisons during multiagency responses.
- TECC is the civilian standard of care for response to high-threat prehospital incidents including blast-related events.

Pitfalls

- Relying on TEMS teams to provide large-scale response to blast-related MCI
- Failing to create whole community high-threat response programs and instead relying solely on TEMS teams to responds to blast incidents

References

1. Tang N, Kelen GD. The role of tactical EMS in support of public safety and the public health response to a hostile mass casualty incident. Disaster Med Public Health Prep. 2007;1(1):S55–6.
2. Heiskell LE, Carmona RH. Tactical emergency medical services: an emerging subspecialty of emergency medicine. Ann Emerg Med. 1994;23:778–85.

3. McArdle DQ, Rasumoff D, Kolman J. Integration of emergency medical services and special weapons and tactics teams: the emergence of the tactically trained medic. Prehosp Disaster Med. 1992;7(3):285–8.
4. Jones JS, Reese K, Kenepp G, Krohmer J. Into the fray: integration of emergency medical services and special weapons and tactics (SWAT) teams. Prehosp Disaster Med. 1996;11(3):202–6.
5. Rinnert KJ, Hall WL. Tactical emergency medical support. Emerg Med Clin North Am. 2002;20:929–52.
6. Levy MJ, Smith R, Gerold KB, Alves DW, Tang N. Clinical encounters in tactical medicine: a mission-specific analysis of the Maryland State Police experience. J Spec Oper Med. 2014;14(2):98–104.
7. Tang N, Kubit J, Berrett OM, Levy MJ. A multiyear analysis of the clinical encounters of the ATF tactical medical program. J Spec Oper Med. 2014;14(3):102–6.
8. Butler FK, Hagmann J, Butler GE. Tactical combat casualty care in special operations. Mil Med. 1996;161(Suppl 3):1–16.
9. Kotwal RS, Montgomery HR, Kotwal BM, Howard RC, Butler FK, Mabry RL, et al. Eliminating preventable death on the battlefield. Arch Surg. 2011;146(12):1350–8.
10. Kotwal RS, Butler FK, Edgar EP, Shackelford SA, Bennet DR, Bailey JA. Saving lives on the battlefield: a joint trauma system review of pre-hospital trauma care in combined joint operating area – Afghanistan. J Spec Oper Med. 2013;13(1):77–85.
11. Goralnick E, Trimpont FV, Carli P. Preparing for the next terrorism attack: lessons from Paris, Brussels, and Boston. JAMA Surg. 2017;152(5):419–20.
12. Callaway DW, Smith ER, Cain J, Shapiro G, Burnett WT, McKay SD, et al. Tactical emergency casualty care (TECC): guidelines for the provision of prehospital trauma care in high threat environments. J Spec Oper Med. 2011;3:104–22.
13. Hartford B, Shapiro G, Marino M, Smith R, Tang N. Proceedings from the 2017 mid-year meeting of the committee for tactical emergency casualty care (C-TECC) and committee updates. J Spec Oper Med. 2018;18(1):160–1.
14. Guidelines. Committee for Tactical Emergency Casualty Care. http://c-tecc.org/guidelines. Accessed on 31 Aug 2018.
15. Burns GD, Wightman JM. Explosive events. In: Koenig KA, Schultz CH, editors. Koenig & Schultz's disaster medicine: comprehensive principles and practices. 2nd ed. Cambridge, UK: Cambridge University Press; 2016. p. 463–85.

Case Study: Primary Blast Injury in a Field Setting

17

Elon Glassberg, Avi Benov, and Avraham Yitzhak

On July 8, 2014, Israel launched Operation Protective Edge (OPE) in response to the kidnapping and murder of three Israeli teenagers and a massive rocket attack on the civilian population in southern Israel. The aim of the operation was to stop rocket fire from Gaza into Israel. The operation ended 50 days later, when a cease fire agreement was reached. The operation resulted in more than 700 casualties (including 74 fatalities) among the Israeli Defense Forces.

On July 30, 2014, a special forces team gained control of a tactically vital two-story building. While in the building, a previously planted large improvised explosive device (IED), positioned in the basement of the building, was detonated. All team members were injured, including a few that were positioned outside the building; one was buried under the rubble.

Four blast-injured soldiers were immediately designated for urgent evacuation with need of lifesaving intervention (LSI). Injuries included (1) penetrating abdominal trauma from blast fragments; (2) blunt head trauma with concussion; (3) penetrating ocular trauma and blunt chest trauma; and (4) buried under rubble with head, chest, and abdominal injuries. Injuries to the casualties designated for nonurgent

E. Glassberg (✉)
Israel Defense Forces Medical Corps, Ramat Gan, Israel

Department of Surgery, The Azrieli Faculty of Medicine, Bar-Ilan University, Safed, Israel

Uniformed Services University of the Health Sciences, Bethesda, MD, USA

A. Benov
Israel Defense Forces Medical Corps, Ramat Gan, Israel

Department of Surgery, The Azrieli Faculty of Medicine, Bar-Ilan University, Safed, Israel

A. Yitzhak
Israel Defense Forces, Department of Surgery, Soroka Medical Center, Beer Sheva, Negev, Israel

D. W. Callaway, J. L. Burstein (eds.), *Operational and Medical Management of Explosive and Blast Incidents*, https://doi.org/10.1007/978-3-030-40655-4_17

evacuation included tympanic membrane perforations and limb injuries with undisplaced fractures and soft-tissue abrasions.

In the aftermath of the explosion, the seriously injured team leader was replaced by one of the operators, who had been positioned on the roof of the building at the time of the explosion. He took command and directed the rescue efforts. Within minutes, the units' medical squad (consisting of a physician and three medics) arrived and started triaging and treating the casualties. The now-in-command 19-year-old sergeant seemed to be minimally affected by the blast. He was found to be fully conscious and "feeling well" with no overt external injuries. He was thus triaged for nonurgent evacuation, and he continued leading rescue efforts and directing the evacuation of the wounded and the dead.

However Ten minutes later, the sergeant reported some "dizziness" and difficulty breathing. His vital signs were found to be normal, except a heart rate of 106 beats per minute, which could have been expected for his level of emotional and physical activity. He was again triaged for nonurgent evacuation while efforts concentrated on the evacuation of the four seriously injured team members. The estimated time of arrival for the first evacuation helicopter was 20 minutes. At the evacuation point, the sergeant refused to be evacuated and allowed other team members to take priority in boarding the helicopter. Minutes later, the sergeant collapsed with pronounced dizziness, headache, cough, and hemoptysis. He was now tachypneic with respiratory rate of 30 breaths per minute, hemoglobin oxygen saturation of 88% on room air, blood pressure of 95/60 mmHg, and pulse rate of 75 beats per minute. His situation quickly deteriorated and, per Israeli Defense Forces Medical Corps protocol, advanced damage control resuscitation (DCR) was initiated at the point of injury and he was added to the list of urgent evacuations.

Out-of-hospital resuscitation included venous access, administration of reconstituted freeze-dried plasma (FDP) and ventilation. Within half an hour, the casualty was air-transported to a level-one trauma center, where he was diagnosed to be suffering from severe primary blast lung injury and hypovolemic shock. He was admitted to the intensive care unit, and a myriad of lifesaving interventions were initiated, including extracorporeal membrane oxygenation (ECMO), without success. The patient and two other team members were pronounced dead within 18 hours following their injuries.

In the after-action report, his teammates stressed the fact that the sergeant was on the roof of the building at the time of the explosion, wearing his body armor and helmet, and was functioning and feeling well immediately following the blast. The importance of the advanced care provided on the scene was also stressed by the surgeons at the trauma center, as it was their estimation that without it the patient would not have made it to the hospital alive.

Challenges

- *Operating in Hot and Warm Zones*: Poses Direct and indirect threats and to the responders (see Chaps. 11, 12, 13, and 14 for more information on scene safety). In this case, medical operations in a dense urban enviroment entailed specific challenges, that included booby-trapped buildings and three-dimensional threats (e.g., tall buildings with possible snipers, adversaries in the streets, and underground tunnels for hidden movements leading to surprise attacks). The potential for a "dirty bomb" to spread contamination with chemical, biological, or radiological (CBR) materials is always present.

- *Primary Blast Injuries (PBI)*: Primary blast injuries to internal structures present a specific challenge. Aside from tympanic membrane rupture with otorrhea, PBIs may not present with immediate symptoms or obvious signs of external trauma. The operator on the roof had been protected from secondary, tertiary, and quaternary blast injury but was still exposed to the high-explosive blast wave, which ultimately caused fatal blast lung injury. Clinical manifestations of blast intestinal injury may be even further delayed.
- *Providing Advanced Medical Care in the Field*: Bringing capabilities beyond those of the paramedic level to the prehospital environment *is extreemly challenging* a physician assistants, physicians, or surgical assets prestaged *before* an incident may not be able to employ their full capabilities under direct or indirect threat, wearing appropriate personal protective equipment, in the dark, exposed to temperature extremes or inclement weather. Rushing to extend medical care *after* an incident has occured, may also prove of limited contribution, especcialy when transportation to definitive care is significantly delayed (see Chap. 11).
- *Multiple Casualty Incident*: Medical support consisted of a single medical squad with a small number of prehospital providers confronted with multiple casualties, having to perform triage, provide care, conduct evacuation, and coordinate the rescue efforts. These are all extremely challenging, especially in high-threat environments and with relatively junior team members involved.
- *Rapid Evacuation*: Rapidly clearing casualties from the scene of an explosion is as critical, as it is difficult. Unless prestaged, transportation assets may take considerable time to arrive and to evacuate the casualties (see Chaps. 14 and 15 for more information on evacuation priorities). Ongoing threats may further delay evacuation by ground, water, or air vehicles.

Lessons Learned

- *Blast Wave Physics*: One does not need to be in a direct line of sight to the explosion to suffer primary blast injury! The casualty in this case was standing on the roof and was wearing his protective gear when the detonation occurred in the basement. Blast waves can wrap around objects and be magnified in small spaces. Awarness to this potential mechanism of injury should lead to a higher index of suspicion, where those impacted by the blast wave should be "over-triaged" initially or watched more closely after the exposure. That said, the importance of the protective gear should not be underestimated, as it helps prevent the much more common penetrating injuries (secondary balst injuries).
- *Advanced Life Support*: Responding with advanced provider allows for rapid application of advanced interventions that may be needed for lifesaving care (e.g., tube thoracostomies and blood products for resuscitation), all the while

acknowledging that operations in a Hot or Warm zone may be putting the care providers at significant risk.

- *Advanced Out-of-Hospital Damage Control Resuscitation*: When feasible and in anticipation of high-risk operations, teams capable of advanced DCR should be staged as close as possible to the potential points of injury is crucial for saving the lives of those seriously wounded. When feasible, rapid evacuation to a higher level of care in a more stable environment generally takes precedence, particularly if advanced en route care can be provided.
- *Timely Evacuation:* Effective casualty evacuation that balances care in the field, en route care capabilities, and time to definitive care poses a significant challenge and requires a well-coordinated effort.
- *Military-to-Civilian Translation*: Lessons learned in the military environment can be translated to civilian prehospital care. Although this case study concerned a military team, lessons could be easily applied to law enforcement teams (see Chap. 15), other specialized rescue teams, or even conventional EMS responders.

Case Study: 2013 Boston Marathon

18

Ricky C. Kue

Overview of the Incident

April 15, 2013, marked the 117th running of the Boston Marathon, an annual tradition occurring on the Patriot's Day holiday commemorating the Revolutionary War battles of Lexington and Concord. Runners began their journey from Hopkinton, Massachusetts, eastward into the City of Boston. At approximately 2:49 pm, everything changed. Two improvised explosive devices (IEDs) positioned less than 200 yards apart were detonated near the finish line on Boylston Street in a span of 13 seconds. The devices used were homemade bombs inside pressure cookers hidden in backpacks and placed among spectators.

Due to the size and nature of the Boston Marathon, the Boston Athletic Association (BAA) operated a medical support program using healthcare volunteers to staff the majority of medical tents near the finish line. Boston Emergency Medical Services (EMS) provided additional response support to the BAA along the race route, medical staffing within the tents, and ambulance transport to area hospitals. The intent of this robust medical support is to minimize unnecessary ambulance transports to hospitals and avoid emergency department (ED) overload by maximally managing runners in need of medical attention on site. The two finish line medical tents – Alpha and Bravo – had been operational since the start of the race.

Many volunteers and EMS personnel located near the finish line quickly recognized an intentional bombing incident once the explosions occurred. The medical response to the blasts was rapid and swift. First responders and BAA volunteers already on site had begun treatment and evacuation to ambulances already near the two sites. Casualty evacuation then shifted to the Alpha medical tent at the finish line. The Alpha tent quickly transitioned its operations from a medical aid station

---

R. C. Kue (✉)
Medical Corps, Vermont Army National Guard, Colchester, VT, USA

Boston University School of Medicine, Boston, MA, USA

D. W. Callaway, J. L. Burstein (eds.), *Operational and Medical Management of Explosive and Blast Incidents*, https://doi.org/10.1007/978-3-030-40655-4_18

to a casualty collection point (CCP). Inside the tent, casualties were quickly triaged and placed in treatment areas, with the most critical patients located closest to the ambulance loading zone. Care was limited to control of major external hemorrhage and other basic interventions in order to rapidly load patients onto waiting ambulances for transport to area trauma centers.

Overall, the prehospital medical response resulted in a total of 118 ambulance transports to a total of six area trauma centers. Approximately 30 critically injured patients were transported within 18 minutes, and all 80 critically injured patients were ultimately transported within 60 minutes of the first blast. The median time interval from scene departure to hospital arrival was 11 minutes. Based on available pooled data from all the Boston-area trauma centers, approximately 36% of the 127 patients evaluated arrived by means other than EMS. The majority of patients seen were spectators of the event (75%). Hospitals reported a total of 31 patients with signs of exsanguinating extremity wounds, with 84% (26/31) having had at least one or more tourniquets placed prior to ED arrival. A low rate of triage tag use as reported by receiving hospitals (0.8%) coupled with the relatively short median transport time was a result of the "scoop-and-run" approach by EMS in response to this incident.

Within 6 minutes of the initial blast, EMS was able to coordinate mutual-aid responses from other ambulance services within the area, increasing transportation capabilities from 16 ambulances detailed to the event to up to nearly 90 in all. Area hospitals received notification of the incident within 4 minutes of the initial blast and prepared for inbound patients. Dispatch Operations personnel were able to direct patient destinations for on-scene EMS personnel so that no one trauma center would be overwhelmed with patients coming from the scene. As a testament to the response by an entire trauma system, no single casualty transported by EMS to a hospital that afternoon died from their injuries.

The incident did not end in the metro-Boston area when the bombing scenes were cleared. A weeklong manhunt for the perpetrators ensued, ending in a large-scale search-and-apprehend operation 4 days later in Watertown, Massachusetts. In all, four fatalities occurred as a result of this incident, and numerous victims were left with permanent disabilities.

Challenges

- *Scene Safety*: Given that first responders and BAA volunteers were already on scene as part of the event, scene safety was an immediate concern after the blasts occurred. It was not feasible for responders and volunteers to "stage appropriately" until scene safety could be assured. Rather, responders and volunteers quickly began treatment and evacuation to nearby ambulances and the Alpha tent CCP.
- *Triage Tags*: Performing full triage in a large-scale mass casualty incident (MCI), including the use of triage tags that document prehospital care, is problematic because responders often do not have time to document care prior to loading for

evacuation from the scene. Additional time constraints were imposed in this incident given the safety concerns at both the blast sites and around the CCP. Limited triage prior to loading did occur based on injury patterns and severity; however, receiving hospitals should understand that documentation of triage categories and prehospital interventions may not be completed at the scene under some operational constraints and that hospital triage should be performed upon arrival, especially given the differences in available resources that could affect treatment decisions compared to the prehospital environment.

- *Tourniquet Availability*: Given the fluid and dynamic nature of the initial response at both blast sites, most first responders did not have readily available tourniquets or other bleeding-control kits on hand. Unlike the military, where tourniquet-containing individual first-aid kits (IFAKs) are issued and carried by troops at all times, most victims requiring initial control of extremity hemorrhage had improvised tourniquets placed by bystanders at the scene. A few prefabricated tourniquets were placed by EMS personnel.
- *Contamination Potential*: Communication of any concerns for chemical, biological, or radiological (CBR) hazards from scene to area hospitals did not occur as rapidly as the information did to Incident Commanders and the Unified Command Center. This left many hospitals unaware on whether the blast casualties required decontamination prior to transfer of care from EMS providers to ED staff.
- *Mental Health Services*: Coordination of mental health services through local, state, and federal resources became available within 2 days of the incident. In the aftermath, however, some first responders and volunteers voiced the need for mental health services sooner after the incident.

Lessons Learned

- *Incident Command System (ICS)*: ICS works well for MCIs when it is used as planned. Every year, the Boston Marathon is managed as a "preplanned" MCI, which allows for efficient management of the event. Having ICS roles already in place at the time of the bombing allowed for an instantaneous and seamless response.
- *Regional EMS Communications*: This network allowed for rapid response to the EMS mutual-aid request by area ambulance services, as well as notification to receiving hospitals. The Boston Area Ambulance Mutual Aid (BAMA) enabled direct communication between the City of Boston EMS Dispatch Center and participating EMS agencies to allow for immediate mutual-aid request and dispatch. The metro-Boston Central Medical Emergency Direction (CMED) Center within Boston EMS Dispatch Operations allowed for real-time communication with all regional hospitals, as well as direct communications with EMS field staff to evenly distribute patients to all facilities. This correlates to the Deliberate Arrival Phase discussed in Chap. 21.
- *Tactical Emergency Casualty Care (TECC)*: Integration of EMS warm-zone response methods gave first responders a patient-care approach that incorporated

the environmental threats faced during active-shooter and other hostile-action events. Active-shooter response training that occurred prior to the bombings, as well as the longstanding practice of prehospital tourniquet use under Boston EMS protocols, all contributed to the effective response by EMS that day.

- *Limited Field Medical Care*: With the rapid arrival of ambulances and crews to the CCP for transportation of casualties to hospitals, limiting medical care within the Alpha tent to lifesaving interventions such as hemorrhage control with tourniquets, basic airway maneuvers, bag-valve mask ventilation with airway adjuncts, and use of high-flow supplemental oxygen allowed for rapid loading and transport to available definitive care.
- *Bystander Utilization*: Bystander participation in casualty care on scene, despite their uncertain safety, demonstrated that MCI response policies and training should consider incorporating the general public as a "force multiplier" for first responders, as opposed to hysterical distractions used in exercises to provide "stress inoculation."

Dedication This chapter is dedicated to Captain Robert Y. "Sarge" Haley, Special Operations, Boston EMS, 1954–2017 (Fig. 18.1). As Captain of Special Operations for Boston EMS, Sarge is considered the architect for many of the successes described in this case study. Most of the successes did not occur by chance; rather, the response followed an MCI plan that had been rehearsed many times and developed over the years of his experience. Through his dedication and service to the Department and the community for which he served, Sarge has left a lasting legacy on the way in which EMS respond to disasters.

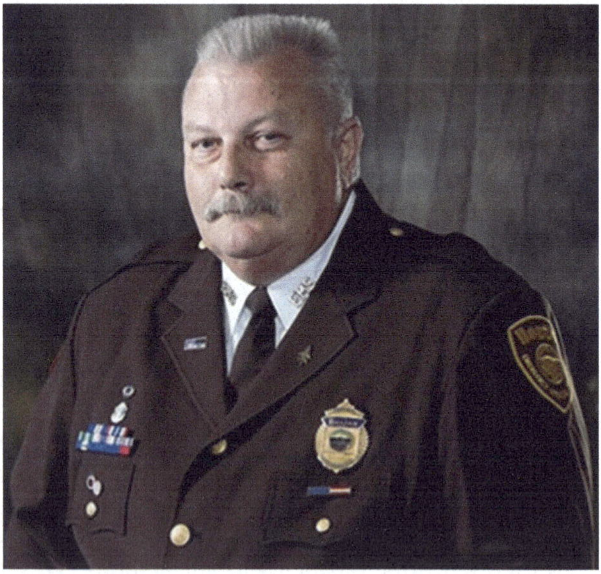

Fig. 18.1 Captain Robert Y. "Sarge" Haley

Part III

Emergency Department

Emergency Department Response to Explosive Incidents: Scope of the Problem and Operational Considerations

19

James P. Phillips and Drew Maurano

Introduction

This chapter provides a broad introduction to critical emergency department operations in response to an explosion-related mass casualty incident (MCI). Although malicious action as a cause is a common concern, not all explosive incidents are terrorism or intentional bombings. Storage facilities for petroleum products, fertilizer, and other chemicals and fireworks factories have exploded, resulting in tremendous loss of life in recent years [1–5]. The two deadliest events in recent US history were the 2013 West Fertilizer Company ammonium nitrate arson explosion that killed 15 and injured 160 [6] and the 2010 West Virginia coal mine dust explosion that killed 38 men [7]. Regardless of the intent surrounding the incident, all explosion-related MCIs have added layers of complexity tied to security, decontamination, information management, and complex polytrauma. Preparation is needed in all hospitals, not just those located in areas vulnerable to terrorism.

Scope of (Part of) the Problem

The Explosives Incident Report is an informational product prepared by the US Bomb Data Center, using incident data reported in the Bomb Arson Tracking System (BATS), that examines the total number of annual explosive-related incidents. It includes explosions and bombings, recoveries, suspicious packages, bomb threats, hoaxes, and explosives thefts or losses. In 2017, the most recent report, BATS captured a total of 687 explosions of which 335 were bombings. Both total explosive incidents and bombings decreased significantly since 2014. Total explosive

J. P. Phillips (✉) · D. Maurano
Department of Emergency Medicine, The George Washington University Hospital, Washington, DC, USA

D. W. Callaway, J. L. Burstein (eds.), *Operational and Medical Management of Explosive and Blast Incidents*, https://doi.org/10.1007/978-3-030-40655-4_19

incidents are down by 25%, and bombing incidents as a subset decreased by 48% over those 3 years [8]. Epidemiological statistics for accidental explosions are not included in this report.

The Disaster Surge Plan

The emergency department (ED) and hospital must have a plan to effectively manage explosive incidents. The US Department of Health and Human Services and the Centers for Medicare and Medicaid Services provide some general recommendations for effective healthcare facility disaster planning [9]. A hospital must develop a workable and relevant emergency operations plan (EOP). The structure recommended is an all-hazards approach that allows the ED to manage all disasters both internally and externally. Please refer to Chap. 24 in this textbook for detailed information on these topics.

The planning process should include a mechanism by which the EOP can be continually adapted in response to changing requirements and emerging threats. Changes in ED infrastructure, staffing models, trauma protocols, and supply availability may also force changes. Each hospital should develop and facilitate an emergency management committee composed of administrative, physician, nursing, and ancillary support department leaders. This committee should meet regularly to review significant hazards and modify the EOP as needed. Emergency plans should be exercised frequently to improve skill retention [10].

Command and Control

The ED frontline providers are generally responsible for recognizing a disaster/surge situation, communicating with hospital leadership, and coordinating other specialty engagement. Once the EOP is activated, major decision-making responsibility transfers from the ED attending to representatives of the hospital administration and emergency management committee. The Hospital Incident Command System (HICS) is a scalable administrative model designed to streamline this process [11]. The HICS is discussed in significant detail in Chap. 24 of this text.

Large explosive MCIs will likely require command and control functions to also incorporate local, federal, and private partners. Local health departments and healthcare coalitions can be integrated into all functions of the hospital management system to assist in resource acquisition, trauma and burn region-wide system activation, incident intelligence, and family reunification. For catastrophic events, the federal government can provide resources through mechanisms administrated by the Federal Emergency Management Agency and the Department of Health and Human Services.

Emergency Department Logistics

The resources available to an ED to provide care are critical to the management of mass casualties of any cause. Resources can be divided into four categories: staffing, services, space, and supplies. The planning phase for any MCI should include developing a system of activation, accountability, maintenance, and recovery within each category. This is vital to be able to sustain short-term and long-term operations, including care for patients who were not victims of the incident.

Each department should have a plan to expand their services. Support services such as laboratory, materiel management, and plant services must be ready to augment their capabilities to meet increased demand, operating room use, and equipment needs during a surge in patient volume. The medical services depend on the ability of the supporting services to parallel their expanding and changing needs.

Modification of existing hospital spaces during a surge event can expand the patient care footprint quickly. Large areas such as the cafeteria, atrium, and auditorium can be used alternatively as family reunification centers, personnel "triage" and staging sites, and care areas for minimally injured patients. Outpatient clinics, classrooms, and meeting spaces can be used as minor patient treatment areas, storage, or other uses. Each facility is unique, and the disaster plan should clearly delineate these sites for alternative use. The ED space, in particular, will need to be adapted to fit the needs of arriving patients and to maximize staff efficiency. Capacity can be created by converting non-critical care rooms into critical care capable spaces by adding needed monitoring equipment, procedure kits, ventilators, etc. Additional patient care spaces can be created by utilizing appropriate hallway beds and by converting single patient locations into multiple patient spaces. This can be done quickly but will also require additional critical care equipment, procedure materials, and other trauma/burn supplies. Doubling the critical patient load in an ED may tax the infrastructure. The logistical support for these types of changes must consider appropriate access to generator power, information technology services, food and water, and toilets for patients and staff.

Hospitals typically store 48–72 hours' worth of supplies to maintain normal operations. In a blast incident, those supplies may be quickly exhausted. The surge plan should detail means of obtaining additional supplies from distributors, the health department, and associated healthcare coalition partners. Supplies include, but are not limited to, medications, blood products, surgical materials, specialty items such as radiology contrast, lab-testing materials, and reagents. Sterile processing facility's staff and supplies should be immediately augmented for surgical equipment turnover. Members of the material management and sterile processing teams should be included in the operational branch of the HICS to ensure needs are being met.

Communications

Communication in a disaster is paramount to the success of most operations in the prehospital and hospital setting. The entire system of care requires effective communication, including but not limited to on-scene dispatch, hospital trauma notifications, staff recall, and real-time resource management. A PACE-based communication plan should be considered for each phase of operations to ensure redundancy of communication. PACE is a communication planning modality that stands for Primary, Alternative, Contingency, and Emergency:

- *Primary* – The primary or usual means of communicating during day-to-day operations.
- *Alternative* – The first "backup" system of communicating should the primary system fail.
- *Contingency* – Third-line communication system, the "backup to the backup."
- *Emergency* – The plan for when all prepared means of communication fail.

An example of the communication PACE plan in practice was during the May 22, 2011, EF-5 tornado that severely damaged St. John's Regional Medical Center in Joplin, Missouri. The damage destroyed portions of the hospital including its primary communication system. One hundred and eighty-three patients required vertical evacuation to safety without their primary system of communications, landline telephones. Cellular phone voice calling was expected to suffice as the alternative mode, but cellular voice calling was also unavailable. However, personal cellular phone text messaging and social media sites were available and were utilized as a contingency plan for communications, leading to a successful evacuation [12].

Communication with Prehospital EMS Providers

Except in rare circumstances, receiving hospitals will be notified to expect patients from the scene of an explosive incident prior to arrival. High-casualty events will require the local EMS dispatch center to coordinate with multiple hospitals quickly in an effort to distribute patients appropriately to prevent overwhelming any individual ED. The infrastructure for such communications and coordination differs by jurisdiction and city size. In small locales, there may be only a single EMS provider, hospital, and associated dispatch. In large cities, there are special communication centers in place to manage these tasks. During mass casualty situations, these centers play a key role in determining the appropriate location and timing for transport of triaged survivors to medical facilities. In the immediate aftermath of the Boston Marathon Bombing, the local Central Medical Emergency Direction Center (CMED) determined the number of patients each ED could accept and coordinated distribution of patients to each center. CMED centers play a role in assisting field medics with communications during an event by connecting them directly with medical control and receiving hospitals, managing radio channel usage, maintaining clear EMS communications procedures within a region, and providing interoperability with other public safety agencies [13]. Particularly during a multi-jurisdictional response, heavy or unreliable radio traffic may lead to confusion and operational mistakes. Most EMS systems employ redundant means of communications and multiple available frequencies of radio communication.

Communications Within the Hospital

Within the hospital environment, redundant means of communication are recommended even during normal working conditions. Barring power loss, telephones, pagers, and overhead announcements will serve as the primary means of communication between physicians, administrators, nurses, and departments during an MCI as well. In the event of power or phone losses, human "runners" can serve in lieu of telephones or pagers. Whatever the system, pre-incident planning and training are prerequisite to success.

Staffing Needs

A good disaster plan is not binary. It must be scalable and able to be tailored quantifiably to the number of injured patients expected. Hospitals should activate staff early in order to meet the projected demand. There must be a system of checking in, deployment, and accountability for staff members and volunteers. A majority of US hospitals operate at overcapacity on a daily basis. Limited staff availability could make it very hard to meet manpower needs during a mass casualty surge [14]. A system of rapid notification and recall of hospital staff is a mandatory plan component. Such systems include calling staff from a phone list, autodialing "robocalls," mass text messaging systems, and even television announcements.

Recall must include not only ED physicians and nurses but also trauma surgery, ICU, and anesthesia. Not to be forgotten is the need for inpatient medicine providers. While their utility may be quite limited in the care of arriving trauma victims, medicine staff should take immediate care of all boarding, recently admitted, and admission-pending patients. Nurses from critical care areas should be considered as options to support the ED. Instructions to recalled staff should provide clear, specific directions detailing exactly where to report so that they may be "triaged" to areas of need. Instructions should include known information on street closures, security measures, and potential threats. The logistics leadership should plan to provide food, water, and sleeping arrangements during the operational period. Technicians, medical students, EMS providers, and other qualified personnel can be utilized to transport patients within the hospital, as there may be a large increase in transport use, and also to monitor those patients being cared for in auxiliary locations.

Environmental services (EVS) staff deserve special mention. Without augmented housekeeping staff, ED and OR staff will be responsible for room cleaning and "turnover" which will cause significant delay and distraction from patient care. The

EVS leadership should be involved in disaster planning at least annually. Security staff will need to be augmented. In addition, they may have particular needs that they must address through contact with local law enforcement (such as extra armed staff).

Emergency Department Operations

Surge capacity in the healthcare sector can be defined as the maximum augmentation of resources available to care for the influx of an unexpectedly large number of patients [15]. Surge capacity is a critical function of a hospital's ability to manage mass casualties from a sudden event such as an explosion. Factors that determine surge capacity include availability of extra staff, supplies, and the number of empty licensed beds. The most critical means by which surge capacity can be increased is by discharging inpatients to home or other facilities when safe to do so. Reverse triage, a concept of discharging patients from the hospital early if they are considered low risk for any significant medical consequence that continued admission can prevent or treat, has been studied. If appropriately harnessed, it can be a major contributor to increasing surge capacity [16]. Depending on the size of the event, increasing patient capacity will require not only ED decompression but also the inpatient wards.

However, even if inpatients are identified who are appropriate candidates for immediate hospital discharge or transfer to unaffected inpatient facilities, completing these tasks is time-consuming, and inter-hospital transport ambulances may be limited. The nursing staff who routinely perform these tasks may be already involved in the disaster response elsewhere in the hospital and therefore may be unavailable. Temporizing options can be instituted in such a case. As patient rooms and physical space on medical wards become the priority need, patients awaiting discharge to home can be taken to a designated area elsewhere in the hospital. Such a "discharge waiting room" requires minimal staff and patient care supplies (wheelchairs, home oxygen, access to scheduled medications) while these stable patients await completion of their discharge paperwork. Additional inpatient capacity can be achieved by temporarily converting single patient rooms into multiple patient rooms. Noncritical patients in private rooms can be "doubled up" if space, electrical power access, and patient safety allow.

Decompressing the emergency department of patients is a critical immediate step when facing a large patient surge following an explosion. In an ideal situation, every patient would be accurately triaged in the ED, would receive relevant laboratory and radiological evaluation, and would be assessed by all necessary consultants. During a surge event, this may be impossible, and typical ED care may need to be abbreviated when it is safe to do so. In accordance with the Emergency Medical Treatment and Labor Act (EMTALA), all patients must undergo a medical screening evaluation (MSE) in the ED. Patients without an emergency medical condition identified during the MSE should be immediately discharged to home. Others will require admission to the hospital. For those patients, inpatient medicine teams must be prepared to accept patients into inpatient areas without delay, even if a full workup is incomplete by typical ED standards. Admitting internists, intensivists, and consultants should be prepared to complete patient workups and minor procedures on inpatient wards in a manner they are not accustomed to but are qualified to perform. Inpatient hallways should be used as overflow patient care areas to increase surge capacity. For this to work effectively, incorporation into drills and disaster planning is necessary. Because safety is the priority, the fire marshal should be involved in surge planning to help identify nontraditional patient care areas that can be safe and in accordance with local laws.

Patient Inflow

Patients will begin to arrive at nearby EDs via EMS and private vehicles. Depending on the location of the hospital and proximity of the incident, some may arrive by public transportation, ride-sharing services, taxi, or foot. Research has demonstrated a bimodal distribution of arrival, with less severely injured patients arriving to the ED by non-ambulance transportation prior to the more severely injured patients who required EMS transport [17]. ED mass casualty plans must include a plan to triage all arriving casualties, regardless of their prehospital triage designation. Those arriving by EMS are likely to have been sorted in the field by a standard triage method (i.e., SALT, START, JumpSTART). Reassessment is critical. Initial field triage may be inaccurate, or the patient's clinical condition may change after this initial assessment. A multiple-layer system of assessment and triage, although not validated, are likely to improve accuracy and reduce both over-triage and under-triage.

Following an explosive event, traffic may impair ingress and egress of transport vehicles and could affect patient outcomes. This is true at the scene of the event where patients are being loaded for transport to a hospital but equally importantly upon arrival to the receiving center. In areas where traffic is a preexisting concern, hospitals should include in their mass casualty plan strategies for traffic control around the hospital to allow continuous flow of transporting vehicles. Hospital security should have a plan to control movement of vehicles into and out of the ambulance bay to prevent a bottleneck. Additional unloading points at the hospital may be necessary and should be planned for in advance.

Security concerns include safety of the hospital itself. EDs have been targets of secondary attacks, and multiple recent violent attacks have led to lockdown of EDs for fear of such violence [18]. A manned defensive security perimeter that can be quickly implemented should be part of the disaster plan.

Patient Throughput

Triage

Efficient flow of patients through the ED is critical to accommodate a surge in complex victims of an explosive incident. Initial triage at the incident site may occur and be helpful in the setting of limited transport and large numbers of injured. However, recent mass casualty events in the United States demonstrate that on-scene triage systems are limited in their utility. Injured but ambulatory survivors are utilizing alternative modes of transport that bypass EMS to seek ED care (e.g., civilian vehicles, phone app-based ride-share vehicles) and may arrive before more critically injured patients [19, 20]. This bimodal arrival of patients will disrupt the ideal on-scene triage goal in which the sickest patients arrive to the ED first. Additionally, high rates of over-triage and under-triage using standard prehospital triage systems further reduce this desired orderly arrival. Therefore, it is imperative that mass casualty plans incorporate the designation of a triage officer, preferably an experienced physician, to perform secondary triage of patients arriving at the ED, re-sorting them to specific patient care areas and teams based upon their injury severity. Continuous reassessment of patients will detect both improvements and declines in their conditions and should be performed constantly during the surge.

Registration

The flow of patients through the ED can be delayed at multiple bottleneck points. One of these that can impede care significantly during an MCI is registration and provision of a hospital identification. During normal ED operations, traumatically injured patients are typically given temporary pseudonyms (e.g., Trauma Jack) and number in an effort to rapidly assign a hospital chart and facilitate the ordering and tracking of medications and imaging. During an MCI surge of trauma victims, this type of registration may lead to medical errors if the temporarily assigned identifications are confusing or too similar. It is likely that all EDs already have a naming convention for unidentified patients. However, those existing conventions may prove confusing or inadequate during simultaneous care of many unidentified patients. One of the receiving trauma centers during the Boston Marathon Bombing found in their after-action review that "critically ill patients were checked in with our unidentified patient naming convention; however, the names assigned with this convention were difficult to distinguish from one another on the ED electronic tracking board and in downstream clinical systems" [21]. This resulted in one near-miss event and prompted a revision of their naming system, taking into account the manner in which the names appeared on department computer screens, ID bracelets, etc. A system should be designed to reduce the possibility of such errors. This should include the creation of a preexisting disaster registration set – a large number of unique, temporary identifications that will allow for immediate patient tracking, medication administration, and accurate ordering and reporting of radiological studies.

Movement to Designated ED Care Area

Emergency department space is limited and creating patient care "zones" may be useful. Prior to recalling physicians and nurses for augmentation, staffing levels will be at their lowest. Casualties will require the most immediate level of care during that time. If possible, staff should be divided into care areas, and arriving patients assigned to those areas by the triage officer. Each individual should expect to manage multiple critical and lesser injured patients simultaneously during the stabilization phase while awaiting the arrival of additional staff.

As recalled ED providers arrive to help, "staff triage" should be performed by the lead emergency physician and the lead surgeon to assign them to appropriate zones and/or patients based upon their skill and experience. Medical students and volunteers can provide valuable help and should be used accordingly. Pathology staff are often overlooked in disaster planning, but their value is significant if fatalities are present. Deceased patients should be taken to the morgue as quickly as possible, and capacity may be quickly reached. Disaster plans should include contingencies for additional refrigerated space.

Trauma and resuscitation bays should be reserved for "red" (immediate care) patients that require intubation or immediate surgical evaluation. Grouping of "yellow" (delayed care) patients together in one zone will allow for efficient evaluation and continuous reevaluation. "Green" patients, or the so-called walking wounded and worried, should be rapidly assessed and isolated in large areas that can accommodate such a mass of low-acuity patients. Walking wounded patients post explosive incident may harbor occult life-threatening injuries, and clinicians should insure a regimented reassessment process is in place.

Clinical Care

The clinical aspects of care will vary depending upon many factors. Police and fire department reports, in addition to EMS triage on scene, will likely identify the type of explosion relatively early making it clear if the majority of survivors will present with injuries caused by primary blast injury from high-order explosives or with shrapnel, fragmentation, and burn injuries typically resulting from low-order explosive improvised devices. Primary blast lung injury can present in a delayed fashion, and the treatment is primarily medical. Trauma surgery teams will manage penetrating trauma, amputations, and soft tissue and CNS injuries operatively as needed. Extensive burns resulting from the blast and resulting fires may require stabilization and transfer if criteria for burn center admission are met.

Decontamination

Decontamination may be necessary after an explosion involving hazardous chemicals, chemical warfare agents, or biological weapons. The process typically involves disrobing and showering the patient using soap and water. If hazardous chemicals or agents are suspected, all patients and potentially exposed persons must be decontaminated prior to entry to the ED. The most common mass decontamination shower type is the "pop-up" style shower system designed to be rapidly set up outdoors. Inefficient processes may serve as an additional bottleneck to patient input and thus delay trauma care.

Criminal Evidence

Staff should be made aware that in the event that the explosive incident was an intentional attack, the clothing and belongings of patients should be considered evidence from a crime scene. Staff should follow law enforcement evidence preservation instructions. Additionally, the perpetrators of a bombing could be patients in the ED themselves and may require special security considerations. At Beth Israel Deaconess Medical Center, both brothers who perpetrated the Boston Marathon Bombings received care in the same emergency department just days after dozens of victims from their bombs were treated there. The surviving brother required surgery and a long hospital stay. There were significant security concerns associated with his residence in the same hospital where many of his victims still resided as patients requiring large-scale security staffing by local and federal agencies.

Radiology and Labs

The essence of a medical disaster is when patient needs exceed medical resources. In a mass casualty surge, radiological imaging and laboratory capabilities can become quickly overwhelmed. Following an explosive incident with large-scale shrapnel imaging, computed tomography (CT) imaging is the modality of choice to diagnose organ and CNS damage to determine the need for immediate surgical intervention. When CT availability is limited severely, it has been postulated that CT imaging should be reserved for CNS injury detection almost exclusively, relying upon thoracic and abdominal ultrasonography performed by experienced emergency specialists to detect internal injuries that warrant thoracic procedures or exploratory laparotomy/damage control surgery. A designated ultrasound team can perform serial exams on patients to reassess for newly detectable injury that may warrant intervention more quickly [22]. Bedside lab testing can be utilized if available for both quick results and to offload some of the burden from the hospital laboratory. The blood bank should be notified immediately when a traumatic mass casualty event has occurred, and the initial steps to procure additional blood products from other facilities should be explored.

Prioritization of Disposition

An additional layer of triage in the trauma bay may improve throughput. Following an explosive incident, a senior surgeon (ideally with knowledge of blast injury patterns) should serve as the leader in the "red zone" to determine timing and order of surgeries. This "OR gatekeeper" determines the ultimate need and order of emergent operative treatment and acts as the liaison between the ED and the OR [23]. Damage control resuscitation and surgery concepts, discussed elsewhere in this book, boosted surge capacity in the receiving hospitals following the 2005 London Transit bombings [24].

A senior intensivist may prioritize and direct traffic to intensive care units in the hospital. In 2016, an expert recommendation paper was published on critical care triage emphasizing key concepts including the following regarding ICU admissions during an MCI (Table 19.1) [25, 26].

Emergency Department Output

A mass casualty surge is not just an ED problem, it is a hospital and health system problem. Output includes admission to the hospital, transport to the OR, transport to the morgue, and discharge to home. The primary factors that will determine output from the ED include availability of hospital rooms and associated nursing coverage, manpower for the transport of patients to various locations within the hospital, and abbreviated registration. Just as the ED must be decompressed rapidly in anticipation of an immediate bolus of patients from the scene of an explosion, the entire hospital should be prepared to decompress inpatients, allowing for ongoing

Table 19.1 Key considerations regarding intensive care admission during a mass casualty incident [25, 26]

Triage criteria goals	Triage method choices	ICU decision-making
Objective Ethical Transparent Applied equitably Publicly disclosed	Who will likely benefit the most from the ICU care? "First come, first served" basis	Apply explicit inclusion and exclusion criteria to determine appropriateness for intensive care unit admission
Special considerations Consider transferring to alternative hospitals stable patients to maximize ICU space Transfer trauma patients to trauma centers if possible Transfer pediatric trauma patients to pediatric trauma centers if possible Transfer patients who meet appropriate criteria to burn centers if possible Pediatricians should be assigned to the triage area if children are among the victims		

admission output from the ED. As the response matures and the less critical yellow and green patients begin receiving care, output will transition from the OR/ICU/telemetry settings to the less acute care settings or to home. Stable patients requiring admission or specialty services should be considered for transfer to other hospitals remote from the response zone as local capacity is reached.

Media Relations

The media play a vital role in reporting information about an incident. The information disseminated to the public must be well coordinated, timely, and accurate in order to avoid confusion, anger, or the loss of public trust. During an incident, the hospital's public information officer (PIO) must work closely with other official information sources to provide "one message, many voices." This is an essential component of the HICS, which is discussed at length in a later chapter in this book. The hospital's PIO may use social media to disseminate information to the public [11]. During mass casualty and other high-profile medical events, hospital employees and visitors may choose to post information on social media sites. Employees should review their hospital social media policy to ensure compliance with confidentiality laws prior to posting potentially inflammatory statements or misinformation.

Patient Family Assistance

The HICS should designate a family reunification unit leader who will assist families in locating their loved one through the hospital's patient tracking program or the community's patient location system. Reunification of families with the deceased must also be a priority. For example, following a mass fatality event, the District of Columbia has a plan to establish a Family Assistance Center to collect antemortem information from family and friends of the missing and deceased in order to reunite them [27].

Conclusion

Explosions can result in large numbers of injured and dead. Drills and exercises practiced at the hospital level are necessary to prepare for surge events and must include all medical specialties. Normal hospital operations will be proportionally disrupted by the magnitude of the event. Disaster plans should be enacted to modify operations, recall necessary staff, and create additional surge capacity for the survivors. Special considerations include decontamination, security, involvement of specialists in disaster planning, media relations, and family assistance. Psychological care for the responding hospital staff should be provided free of cost.

Pitfalls

- Failure to conduct regular disaster drills and to familiarize new staff with disaster plans.
- Failure to coordinate disaster plans with local EMS agencies and their dispatching agents, the Department of Health, and the participating healthcare coalition.
- Failure to prepare inpatient medicine physicians for their role in the surge plan.
- Failure to have a nimble patient registration system for MCI surge.
- Failure to recognize the psychological stress experienced by staff members.

References

1. BBC News. Mexico fireworks blast: Dozens killed in Tultepec explosion. 2016. Available at: https://www.bbc.com/news/world-latin-america-38387239. Accessed 31 May 2018.
2. Beijing A. Tianjin explosion: China sets final death toll at 173, ending search for survivors. 2015. Available at: http://www.theguardian.com/world/2015/sep/12/tianjin-explosion-china-sets-final-death-toll-at-173-ending-search-for-survivors. Accessed 31 May 2018.
3. PTI. Sivakasi factory fire: 54 charred to death in the incident. 2012. Available at: https://timesofindia.indiatimes.com/city/chennai/Sivakasi-factory-fire-54-charred-to-death-in-the-incident/articleshow/16266391.cms. Accessed 31 May 2018.
4. Rajiv G. Kollam temple fire: death toll reaches 111, 40 badly wounded. 2016. Available at: https://timesofindia.indiatimes.com/city/thiruvananthapuram/Kollam-temple-fire-Death-toll-reaches-111-40-badly-wounded/articleshow/51795419.cms. Accessed 31 May 2018.
5. Hawley S. Fireworks factory explosion kills at least 47 outside Jakarta. 2017. Available at: http://www.abc.net.au/news/2017-10-26/indonesia-fireworks-factory-explosion-kills-dozens/9090478. Accessed 31 May 2018.
6. Reuters Staff. Ammonium nitrate stores exploded at Texas plant: state agency. 2013. Available at: https://www.reuters.com/article/us-usa-explosion-texas/ammonium-nitrate-was-cause-of-texas-explosion-state-agency-says-idUSBRE9460GP20130507. Accessed 31 May 2018.
7. MSHA. MSHA – News Release: US Labor Department's MSHA cites corporate culture as root cause of Upper Big Branch Mine disaster – Massey issued 369 citations and orders with $10.8 million in civil penalties. 2011. Available at: https://arlweb.msha.gov/MEDIA/PRESS/2011/NR111206.asp. Accessed 31 May 2018.
8. United States Bomb Data Center. Bomb Arson Tracking System. 2017 explosive incidents report. 2018. Available at: https://www.atf.gov/resource-center/docs/report/2017-explosives-incident-report-eir/download. Accessed 10 Mar 2019.
9. CMS. Survey and Certification Emergency Preparedness Initiative: SC emergency preparedness checklist revision. Department of Health and Human Services Centers for Medicare & Medicaid Services. 28 Feb 2014.
10. Kellermann AL, Peleg K. Lessons from Boston. N Engl J Med. 2013;368(21):1956–7.
11. California Emergency Medical Services Authority. Hospital Incident Command System guidebook. 5th ed. Sacramento: California Emergency Medical Services Authority; 2014.

12. Reynolds M. The Joplin tornado: the hospital story and lessons learned. Available at: http://docplayer.net/32123995-The-joplin-tornado-the-hospital-story-and-lessons-learned-marcia-reynolds-rn-bsn-msn-cphrm-mercy-health.html. Accessed 12 Mar 2019.
13. Massachusetts Department of Public Health. The Massachusetts emergency medical services communications plan. Boston: Massachusetts Department of Public Health Office of Emergency Services; 2013.
14. Kaji AH, Lewis RJ. Hospital disaster preparedness in Los Angeles County. Acad Emerg Med. 2006;13(11):1198–203.
15. Kelen GD, McCarthy ML. The science of surge. Acad Emerg Med. 2006;13(11):1089–94.
16. Kelen GD, McCarthy ML, Kraus CK, Ding R, Hsu EB, Li G, et al. Creation of surge capacity by early discharge of hospitalized patients at low risk for untoward events. Disaster Med Public Health Prep. 2009;3(2 Suppl):S10.
17. Mothershead JL. Local disaster response. In: Ciottone GR, editor. Ciottone's disaster medicine. 2nd ed. Philadelphia: Elsevier; 2016. p. 90–4.
18. Huffman A. The worst kind of emergency. Ann Emerg Med. 2016;68(5):A18.
19. Vales L. Iraq veteran took stranger's truck to transport Las Vegas shooting victims. 3 Oct 2017. Available at: https://www.cnn.com/2017/10/03/us/las-vegas-shooting-witness-taylor-winston-anderson-cooper-cnntv/index.html. Accessed 13 Jan 2019.
20. Frakt A. Uber, Lyft and the urgency of saving money on ambulances. 1 Oct 2018. Available at: https://www.nytimes.com/2018/10/01/upshot/uber-lyft-and-the-urgency-of-saving-money-on-ambulances.html. Accessed 13 Jan 2019.
21. Landman A, Teich JM, Pruitt P, Moore SE, Theriault J, Dorisca E, et al. The Boston marathon bombings mass casualty incident: one emergency department's information systems challenges and opportunities. Ann Emerg Med. 2015;66(1):51.
22. Shokoohi H, Pourmand A, Boniface K, Allen R, Petinaux B, Sarani B, et al. The utility of point-of-care ultrasound in targeted automobile ramming mass casualty (TARMAC) attacks. Am J Emerg Med. 2018;36(8):1467–71.
23. Gale SC, Donovan CM, Tinti M, Ahmed H, Gracias VH. Organization and operations management at the health care facility. Ann Emerg Med. 2016;69(1):S35.
24. Aylwin CJ, König TC, Brennan NW, Shirley PJ, Davies G, Walsh MS, et al. Reduction in critical mortality in urban mass casualty incidents: analysis of triage, surge, and resource use after the London bombings on July 7, 2005. Lancet. 2006;368(9554):2219–25.
25. Christian M, Joynt G, Hick J, Colvin J, Danis M, Sprung C. Chapter 7. Critical care triage. Intensive Care Med. 2010;36(S1):55–64.
26. American Burn Association. Guidelines for the operation of burn centers. J Burn Care Res. 2007;28(1):134–41.
27. Government of the District of Columbia. District of Columbia Family Assistance Center (FAC) Plan. 2016. Available at: https://files.asprtracie.hhs.gov/documents/13-family-assistance-center-plan-508.pdf. Accessed 9 Sept 2018.

Emergency Medicine: Combat Lessons Learned 20

Nicholas D. Drakos

Introduction

The practice of emergency medicine in the unique risk-context of the combat environment is at once the same but altogether different from the practice of civilian medicine [1–3]. The overarching challenge for medical providers serving in combat is optimally adapting their medical expertise to a dynamic, austere, and unfamiliar risk-context. Medical expertise is contextual [4, 5], and as we transition from the risk-context of civilian medicine to the risk-context of combat, we must transition and adapt our expertise, both task specific and operational [6]. Task-specific expertise entails the knowledge, experience, and critical decision-making that we apply to specific tasks within a medical problem-set, such as a blast injury. Operational expertise encompasses a broad understanding of a risk-context and a critical decision-making framework to understand and calculate trade-offs in that risk-context in order to optimally utilize available resources to resolve the problem-set and accomplish the goals of patient care.

Adapting expertise from the civilian risk-context to the combat risk-context requires emergency physicians to understand two critical concepts: *trauma as a problem-set* and *risk-context*. For critically injured patients, *trauma is a time-constrained problem-set* with three fundamental risk variables:

- Time: Physiologic dysfunction increases as time elapses without effective treatment. At some point in time, the patient will reach a terminal outcome – loss of life, limb, eyesight, fertility, or function.
- Diagnostic uncertainty: Emergency physicians require some threshold of diagnostic certainty to apply risk-optimal intervention and effectively treat the patient. Decreasing diagnostic uncertainty requires time, either in the form of

N. D. Drakos (✉)
Department of Emergency Medicine, Womack Army Medical Center, Fort Bragg, NC, USA

D. W. Callaway, J. L. Burstein (eds.), *Operational and Medical Management of Explosive and Blast Incidents*, https://doi.org/10.1007/978-3-030-40655-4_20

clinical assessment or the utilization of diagnostic modalities. Thus, the cost of diagnostic certainty is elapsed time and increased physiologic dysfunction.
- Intervention: All diagnostic and therapeutic interventions carry some risk of morbidity and mortality, either directly or through the risk of elapsed time required to implement them. Furthermore, as physiologic dysfunction increases, patients will generally require more therapeutic intervention, which means that the total applied risk of intervention generally increases with time [7].

The optimal intersection of these risk variables will yield the optimal resolution of the problem-set. Ultimately, the goal of emergency physicians treating critically injured patients is to apply the lowest effective interventional risk, with as much diagnostic certainty possible, in as little time as possible. However, the ability to accomplish this, and where the optimal intersection lies, is dependent upon *risk-context.*

Risk-context is defined by three domains: environment, system, and components. The environment is the product of political, social, economic, security, and infrastructure considerations. The environment has two critical implications with respect to trauma: it affects the nature and incidence of trauma, and it determines what systems can be supported and enabled to treat trauma. Trauma systems provide the operational framework within the environment for treating trauma. The components of trauma are the patients, medical providers, and medical supplies and equipment that define the trauma problem-set and coalesce within the system to resolve the trauma problem-set.

The civilian risk-context is a *complicated* predictability risk-context, while the combat risk-context is a *complex* adaptability risk-context. A complicated risk-context has multiple well-defined components with clear and often discernable relationships between them. The effect of these components on the trauma problem-set can generally be understood and anticipated. A *complex* risk-context has multiple components that are poorly defined and highly networked through ambiguous relationships. The effect of these components on the trauma problem-set cannot be easily understood or anticipated [8–10]. The combat environment has the potential to produce a high incidence of trauma that is unfamiliar to civilian emergency physicians by virtue of both its nature and scale, such as blast injuries and mass casualty incidents (MASCALs). Furthermore, the combat environment cannot support trauma systems with the same level of integration and predictability as US trauma systems. The relatively predictable environment in which US trauma systems are nested potentiates their ability to create systemic predictability and decreased risk through a focus on process at scale. The dynamic combat environment favors a trauma system based on a decentralized "Team of Teams" model [8]. This system potentiates the adaptability required in a dynamic environment. At the component-level within this system, emergency physicians and their medical teams ideally function as Mission Critical Teams (MCTs) to resolve the trauma problem-set, a type of Rapidly Emergent Complex Adaptive Problem Set (RECAPS) [6, 11].

Emergency physicians primarily develop and sustain their expertise in the civilian risk-context. They are critical components within robust and efficient systems who, as part of the trauma team, apply validated processes to optimally resolve the trauma problem-set. The expertise that emergency physicians develop is specific to this context, and the more "expert" the physicians become, the more their expertise manifests as habit patterns, a type of System I thinking, specific to the context where the expertise is developed [5, 12, 13]. In medicine, these habit patterns are termed scripts [14]. When emergency physicians transition from the civilian risk-context to the combat risk-context, they risk exposing their patients to the liability of negative habit pattern transfer; the risk that a habit pattern, applied out of context, will have an unintended or deleterious outcome [15]. Therefore, when emergency physicians are called to apply their expertise in the combat risk-context, they must recognize the contextual change, they must determine how the time-constrained trauma problem-set can be optimally resolved in the specific risk-context, and they must adapt.

Body

Blasts and explosions have been the most common mechanism of injury (MOI) for US combat casualties throughout the Global War on Terror (GWOT) and dating back to World War II [16, 17]. Conversely, explosive mechanisms of injury are not frequently encountered in the civilian medical setting [18]. Emergency physicians who have primarily developed and sustained their expertise in the civilian setting may not have developed certain task-specific expertise related to blast injuries.

Emergency physicians practicing in a combat theater must be experts in Tactical Combat Casualty Care (TCCC), Damage Control Resuscitation (DCR), and the Theater Tactical Evacuation (TACEVAC) system, which are the foundation of task-specific combat trauma expertise [2, 19, 20]. Aggressive but calculated use of these principles and resources in a well-integrated fashion throughout the GWOT has contributed to the lowest rates of US combat fatalities in modern history [21]. TCCC is the task-specific standard of care for "prehospital" combat medicine. TCCC recognizes three core objectives: (1) treat the casualty, (2) prevent additional casualties, and (3) complete the mission. It mitigates the primary causes of preventable death on the battlefield by focusing on the Massive Hemorrhage, Airway, Respiration, Circulation, and Hypothermia/Head Injury (MARCH) patient assessment and stabilization algorithm through three phases of care: (1) care under fire (CUF), (2) tactical field care (TFC), and (3) tactical evacuation (TACEVAC) [22, 23]. Emergency physicians should be capable of integrating the basic principles of TCCC by reading the TCCC guidelines, which are published and updated by the Joint Trauma System (JTS) Committee on Tactical Combat Casualty Care (CoTCCC) [24]. However, effective and efficient application of TCCC will require training under realistic conditions. DCR is a strategy for preventing or reversing the lethal triad of hypothermia, acidosis, and coagulopathy through the use of multiple treatment paradigms. It is typically employed once casualties have reached the care of a surgical-resuscitative asset. DCR focuses on early control of both compressible and noncompressible hemorrhage, hypotensive resuscitation with whole blood or fixed ratio blood product transfusion, and patient warming [25]. Tactical evacuation systems will be theater, location, and mission specific. Medical personnel must have open and frequent communication with medical operations personnel and combat leadership to maintain awareness of available evacuation platforms, medical resources on those platforms, evacuation times, and resources available at higher levels of care. These variables have the potential to change on a frequent basis due to multiple factors.

Explosive MOIs have the potential to produce significant polytrauma, and military emergency physicians must be familiar with the management of common injuries that result from the primary, secondary, tertiary, or quaternary effects of blast mechanisms [20, 26, 27]. It is important to understand both the acute management of these injuries and the management over hours to days in the event that emergency physicians face a prolonged field care (PFC) contingency. The Joint Trauma System (JTS) Clinical Practice Guidelines (CPGs) provide an excellent resource for DCR and PFC [28].

The military battlefield trauma system may be conceptualized as a trauma center that has been deconstructed and geographically distributed, with the emergency department trauma bay, operating rooms, and intensive care units connected by medical evacuation platforms. This system, outlined in military doctrine, is composed of four "Roles of Care" with increasing medical capabilities. Role IV describes large military medical centers such as those in the USA or Germany. Military emergency physicians serving in combat should expect to be deployed as part of a Role I, II, or III medical elements. Role I is the farthest forward and most austere, while Role III approximates the emergency department and trauma capabilities of a US Level I Trauma Center [3]. Increasingly, military emergency physicians are being deployed as part of non-doctrinal surgical-resuscitative teams composed of four to six medical providers and employed far forward in the battle space [6, 29]. Individual experiences, and the degree of adaptability required, will vary for emergency physicians depending where and how they are deployed.

The care of critically injured patients is a time-constrained problem-set that balances the risks of time elapsed without treatment, diagnostic uncertainty, and interventions [7]. Recognizing and understanding the limitations and trade-offs in this problem-set forms the basis of operational expertise in the combat setting. Time without effective treatment is equivalent to risk and will adversely affect the probability of morbidity and mortality. The lack of resources is cited as the limiting factor in the care of patients in the austere combat setting [2]. However, the overarching theater trauma system, with its increasing Roles of Care, provides all resources necessary for the diagnosis and treatment of complex trauma. The challenge is that patients are often separated from needed resources by time due to distance, logistics, weather, kinetic activity, and other factors such that, even where a robust tactical evacuation (TACEVAC) system exists, it may not be able to connect a patient with an optimal resource in the limited time afforded by their injuries. This dilemma becomes most acute when small medical elements are faced with mass casualty incidents (MASCALs), such as those often seen with improvised explosive device (IED) attacks [2]. Rather than focusing on an immediate lack of resources, emergency physicians must focus on the most efficient use of time in the care of critically injured patients in order to potentiate successful stabilization, evacuation, and definitive care. Operational parallels exist in the civilian sector as resources vary across prehospital systems, non-trauma centers, and trauma centers. This subtle shift in thinking drives more effective utilization of immediately available resources.

No clear standard of care exists to guide far forward surgical-resuscitative care [29]. This is, in part, because the dynamic nature of the risk-context makes a rigid standard elusive. US trauma systems represent a *complicated* predictability risk-context that exists to solve the time-constrained trauma problem-set for critically injured patients – patients are rapidly and reliably transported to resources capable of optimally efficient diagnosis and treatment. In the *complex* adaptability risk-context of the far forward combat environment, this is the ideal, but often not the case due to multiple factors. The result is that emergency physicians confront critical decisions that are different, more ambiguous, and more complex than in a civilian emergency department [9, 10]. Physical, environmental, and emotional adversity will compound the challenge of critical decision-making.

In response to blast multiple casualty incidents (MCIs), emergency physicians and medical teams will be forced to operate out of their comfort zone, requiring medical courage and a critical decision-making framework that is based on sound medical principles, tolerates uncertainty, and is clearly articulated and agreed upon by all team members [30]. The goal for emergency physicians and their teams is to function as MCTs capable of resolving Rapidly Emergent Complex Adaptive Problem Sets (RECAPS) across the combat risk-context spectrum to provide the best care possible under the prevailing circumstances at a given time and place [1, 6, 11]. Without certain immediate diagnostic capabilities, risk calculus may favor aggressive early intervention with a low level of diagnostic certainty. Emergency physicians must consider treating empirically to avoid deterioration and the lethal triad of hypothermia, acidosis, and coagulopathy [20]. Alternatively, when there is a high level of diagnostic certainty for imminently mortal pathology and the optimal interventional expertise is not immediately available, risk calculus may favor emergency physicians or other nonexperts performing certain life-saving interventions. For example, the JTS recognizes the potential need for, and past instances of, non-neurosurgeons performing emergency life-saving cranial procedures in the deployed setting and provides published guidance [31].

Developing and adapting operational expertise is a continuous process of recognizing changes in risk-context and potential contingencies; developing primary, alternate, contingency, and emergency (PACE) plans; rehearsing the plans; performing after action reviews (AARs) to improve the plans; and, ultimately, validating plans with high fidelity. It is critical to coordinate with nonmedical personnel on both medical and nonmedical tasks related to the efficient and effective care of patients. These include plans for communication, patient transload and transport, securing patient weapons and sensitive items, a "walking blood bank" (WBB) protocol for drawing fresh whole blood (FWB), work rest cycles for prolonged contingencies, and a MASCAL plan [32]. A plan for medical task sharing should be devised for medical and nonmedical personnel to optimize medical care in extremis [33]. This requires training, validation, documentation, and trust.

Translation to Civilian Setting

The *complicated* predictability risk-context of a US trauma system may be suddenly transformed to a *complex* adaptability risk-context in the event of a natural or man-made disaster, particularly large-scale intentional acts of violence such a bombing. This transformation occurs when one or more of the three risk-context domains – environment, system, components – experiences rapid and precipitous change. The 2013 IED attacks at the Boston Marathon, resulting in 281 casualties (127 of whom were transported to one of Boston's five adult Level I trauma centers or four pediatric trauma centers), offers a key example of a rapid transition from a complicated to complex risk-context [34].

This event transformed the environment, most immediately from a security standpoint, and injected an elevated level of uncertainty into what had been a predictable risk-context. Initially, in such events, it is unknown what exactly happened and whether the attacks are isolated and discrete or part of a broader and ongoing terrorist attack, possibly with the goal of targeting first responders and medical infrastructure. Within this uncertainty, the system and components must determine how to best allocate resources and effectively deliver care. Medical and emergency response systems and components adapted to the change in risk-context and performed exceptionally. This was largely a result of planning and preparation, which had the effect of prophylactically minimizing uncertainty. It was also the result of emergent adaptation.

The medical outcomes from the Boston Marathon Bombing benefited from the fact that the city had assumed an elevated emergency response posture for the marathon, which facilitated a favorable environment, placed key response systems on alert, and potentiated component response. Distinct actions were taken to structure the command climate through Incident Command System (ICS) use and control of the physical environment – roads were already closed to traffic, allowing for clear ingress and egress of EMS vehicles to and from the point of injury. Robust security and communications infrastructure were in place, accelerating scene safety and command and control at the incident site. Medical treatment capabilities were proximate to the time and location of injury with a staffed medical tent on scene that served as a casualty collection point for approximately 100 patients. One-hundred eighteen patients were evacuated directly to the hospital based on the severity of injury and concern regarding scene safety. The median transport time from the time of the explosions until patients reached the hospital was only 11 minutes. Patients were transported by multiple platforms including police vans [34, 35].

The use of prehospital tourniquets in the Boston Marathon Bombing response highlights both emergent adaptation and an area for significant improvement in response to civilian blast incidents. Among 29 patients with recognized extremity exsanguination, 27 had tourniquets applied at the point of injury. Ten were applied by EMS personnel, nine were applied by non-EMS personnel, and eight were applied by unknown individuals. None of these were commercial, purpose-designed tourniquets, and many only achieved control of venous bleeding without arterial hemorrhage control [36]. Tourniquets have been validated as a life-saving prehospital intervention for extremity hemorrhage on the battlefield in the GWOT [37]. The fact that tourniquets were utilized prehospital in Boston, and the fact that a significant percentage were placed by non-EMS personnel, demonstrates favorable component-level adaptation by EMS and bystanders alike. However, it also highlights the need for broader adaptation of, and training on, core combat trauma response tactics, techniques, and procedures.

Boston's Massachusetts General Hospital (MGH) rapidly initiated their disaster response plan, which had been rehearsed and implemented on previous occasions, such as blizzards. However, the initial challenges of responding to the incident were unprecedented in the history of the hospital. They received 39 patients in the immediate period after the bombing and made multiple emergent adaptations to potentiate an effective response. In the emergency department, dispositioned and low acuity patients were rapidly cleared to accommodate incoming casualties [35], the most severely injured patients went directly to the operating rooms without evaluation in the trauma bay, medical staff changed from using the electronic medical records (EMR) system to using paper charting as it became clear that the EMR was too time-consuming, and crystalloid and blood products were used judiciously to ensure both optimal resuscitation and resource utilization (David R. King, personal communication, 6 Mar 2019).

Driven by the time-constrained problem-set of multiple critically injured patients and a finite number of immediately available surgical resources, surgeons applied damage control surgery (DCS) techniques common on the battlefield. Surgical patients initially received the required level of surgical stabilization and nothing more. Surgeons later convened to review all of the surgical patients, catalogue the entirety of their injuries, and re-triage patients for follow-on interventions (David R. King, personal communication, 6 Mar 2019).

One of the challenges encountered at MGH in response to the bombing was that hospital staff, including attending surgeons, residents, and cafeteria employees, admirably insisted on staying at the hospital even as the initial chaos transitioned to a controlled response and less personnel were required. The hospital administration responded by bringing in cots and sleeping bags to facilitate a rested and optimally functioning staff (David R. King, personal communication, 6 Mar 2019). This mirrored a common challenge in the combat environment where military operations may last for days, and a deliberate work-rest cycle is critical to ensure the ability of medical providers to optimally function for prolonged periods.

Conclusion

It is important for emergency care providers to understand that the combat risk-context is markedly different from the civilian risk-context and that explosive-incident-related MCIs may require shifts in mindset. Teams must determine local best practices for effectively and efficiently solving the time-constrained blast injury problem-set including adaptations and trade-offs of civilian best practices. It is important to proactively integrate with all co-located medical and nonmedical assets to establish communication and participation in mission and contingency planning. And, the responders within and across health systems must plan, rehearse, perform AAR, and validate their response procedures to maintain currency. This cycle must be constantly repeated, particularly as risk-variables change (e.g., new mission sets, personnel changes, and asset availability).

Pitfalls

- Failure to understand and recognize the time-constrained problem-set that blast injuries represent, changes in risk-context, and associated contingencies
- An inability or unwillingness to adapt task-specific and operational medical expertise to changes in risk-context
- Failure to coordinate, plan, rehearse, perform AAR, and validate courses of action for multiple contingencies

Disclaimer The views expressed in this chapter are those of the author and do not reflect the official policy or position of the Department of the Army, the Department of Defense, or the US Government.

References

1. Giannou C, Baldan M. War surgery: working with limited resources in armed conflict and other situations of violence, vol. 1 [Internet]. Geneva: ICRC; 2010 [cited 2018 May 18]. Available from: https://www.icrc.org/eng/assets/files/other/icrc-002-0973.pdf.
2. Beekley AC, Bohman H, Schindler D. Modern warfare. In: Savitsky E, Eastridge B, editors. Combat casualty care: lessons learned from OEF and OIF. Fort Detrick: Borden Institute; 2012. p. 1–37.
3. Cubano MA, editor. Emergency war surgery. 4th ed. Fort Sam Houston: Borden Institute; 2013.
4. Pelaccia T, Tardiff J, Triby E, Ammirati C, Bertrand C, Dory V, et al. From context comes expertise: how do expert emergency physicians use their know-who to make decisions? Ann Emerg Med. 2016;67(6):747–51.
5. Croskerry P. Context is everything or how could I have been that stupid? Healthc Q [Internet]. 2009 [cited 2018 May 14];12:e171–6. Available from: http://www.longwoods.com/content/20945.
6. Drakos ND, Hardin RD, DuBose JJ, King DR, Johnson JC, Knipp BS, et al. In good conscience: developing and sustaining military combat trauma expertise. J Am Coll Surg. 2018;227(2):293–4.

7. Sarcevic A, Zhang Z, Kusunoki DS. Decision making tasks in time-critical medical settings. In: Proceedings of the 17th ACM international conference on supporting group work (Group '12). Oct 2012. p. 99–102.
8. McChrystal S, Collins T, Silverman D, Fussell C. Team of teams: new rules for engagement in a complex world. New York: Penguin Random House; 2015.
9. Kurtz CF, Snowden DJ. The new dynamics of strategy: sense-making in a complex and complicated world. IBM Syst J. 2003;42(3):462–83.
10. Snowden DJ, Boone ME. A leader's framework for decision making. Harv Bus Rev. 2007;85(11):68–76.
11. Cline P. Mission critical teams: towards a university assisted mission critical teams instructor cadre development program. Dissertation for Doctorate in Education, University of Pennsylvania Graduate School of Education. 2017.
12. Dowie J, Elstein A. Professional judgement: a reader in clinical decision making. New York: Cambridge University Press; 1988.
13. Wears RL, Schubert CC. Visualizing expertise in context. Ann Emerg Med. 2016;67: 752–4.
14. Charlin B, Boshuizen HP, Custers EJ, Feltovich PJ. Scripts and clinical reasoning. Med Educ. 2007;41:1178–84.
15. Merlin PW, Bendrick GA, Holland DA. Breaking the mishap chain: human factors lessons learned from aerospace accidents and incidents in research, flight test, and development. NASA Aeronautics Book Series. Washington, DC: US Government Printing Office; 2011.
16. Owens BD, Kragh JF, Wenke JC, Macaitis J, Wade CE, Holcomb JB. Combat wounds in operation Iraqi freedom and operation enduring freedom. J Trauma. 2008;64:295–9.
17. Belmont PJ, Schoenfeld AJ, Goodman G. Epidemiology of combat wounds in operation Iraqi freedom and operation enduring freedom: orthopaedic burden of disease. J Surg Orthop Adv. 2010;19(1):2–7.
18. Wilkerson RG, Lemon C. Blast injuries. Trauma Rep [Internet]. 2016 [cited 2018 May 14];17(3). Available from: https://www.ahcmedia.com/articles/137658-blast-injuries.
19. National Association of Emergency Medical Technicians [Internet]. TCCC-MP guidelines and curriculum, Clinton, MS. 31 Jan 2017 [cited 2018 May 14]; [multiple screens]. Available from: https://www.naemt.org/education/naemt-tccc/tccc-mp-guidelines-and-curriculum.
20. Nessen SC, Lounsbury DE, Hetz SP, editors. War surgery in Iraq and Afghanistan a series of cases, 2003–2007. Washington, DC: Borden Institute; 2008.
21. Eastridge BJ, Mabry RL, Seguin P, Cantrell J, Tops T, Uribe P, et al. Death on the battlefield (2001-2011): implications for the future of combat casualty care. J Trauma Acute Care Surg. 2012;73:S431–7.
22. USSOCOM Command Surgeon. Tactical trauma protocols. USSOCOM Office of the Command Surgeon Department of Emergency Medical Services and Public Health. 2013.
23. Gerhardt RT, Mabry RL, De Lorenzo RA, Butler FK. Fundamentals of combat casualty care. Modern warfare. In: Savitsky E, Eastridge B, editors. Combat casualty care: lessons learned from OEF and OIF. Fort Detrick: Borden Institute; 2012. p. 85–120.
24. Joint Trauma System Committee on Tactical Combat Casualty Care [Internet]. TCCC guidelines; 28 Aug 2017 [cited 2018 May 21]; [multiple screens]. Available from: http://jts.amedd.army.mil/index.cfm/committees/cotccc/guidelines.
25. Perkins JG, Beekley AC. Damage control resuscitation. In: Savitsky E, Eastridge B, editors. Combat casualty care: lessons learned from OEF and OIF. Fort Detrick: Borden Institute; 2012. p. 121–223.
26. Champion HR, Holcomb JB, Young LA. Injuries from explosions: physics, biophysics, pathology, and required research focus. J Trauma. 2009;66(5):1468–77.
27. Brevard SB, Champion H, Katz D. Weapons effects. In: Savitsky E, Eastridge B, editors. Combat casualty care: lessons learned from OEF and OIF. Fort Detrick: Borden Institute; 2012. p. 39–83.
28. Joint Trauma System [Internet]. Clinical practice guidelines; 3 May 2018 [cited 2018 May 14]; [multiple screens]. Available from: http://jts.amedd.army.mil/index.cfm/PI_CPGs/cpgs.

29. Edwards MJ, White CE, Remick KN, Edwards KD, Gross KR. Army general surgery's crisis of conscience. J Am Coll Surg. 2018;226(6):1190–4. https://doi.org/10.1016/j.jamcollsurg.2018.03.001. [epub ahead of print].
30. Rieke RD, Sillars MO, Peterson TR, editors. Argumentation and critical decision making. 6th ed. Boston: Allyn & Bacon; 2005.
31. Bell RS, McCafferty R, Shackelford S, Tomlin J, Dirks M, Neal C, et al. Emergency lifesaving cranial procedures by non-neurosurgeons in deployed setting. Joint Trauma System Clinical Practice Guidelines [Internet]. Apr 2018 [cited 2018 May 14]; CPG ID 68. Available from: http://jts.amedd.army.mil/assets/docs/cpgs/JTS_Clinical_Practice_Guidelines_(CPGs)/Emergency_Cranial_Procedures_by_Non-Neurosurgeons_Deployed_Setting_23_Apr_2018_ID68.pdf.
32. Joint Trauma System Clinical Practice Guidelines [Internet]. Fresh whole blood (FWB) transfusion. Oct 2012 [cited 2018 May 14]. Available from: http://jts.amedd.army.mil/assets/docs/cpgs/JTS_Clinical_Practice_Guidelines_(CPGs)/Fresh_Whole_Blood_Transfusion_24_Oct_2012_ID21.pdf.
33. Fakhri A, Aryankhesal A. The effect of mutual task sharing on the number of needed health workers at the Iranian health posts: does task sharing increase efficiency? Int J Health Policy Manag. 2015;4(8):511–6.
34. Gates JD, Arabian S, Biddinger P, Blansfield J, Burke P, Chung S, et al. The initial response to the Boston marathon bombing: lessons learned to prepare for the next disaster. Ann Surg. 2014;260(6):960–6.
35. Tomsho R. Determined response: MGH and the boston marathon bombing. Mass General Magazine [Internet]. 2014 [cited 2019 Mar 15]; [about 8 screens]. Available from: https://giving.massgeneral.org/boston-marathon-bombing-response/.
36. King DR, Larentzakis A, Ramly EP, The Boston Trauma Collaborative. Tourniquet us at the Boston marathon bombing: lost in translation. J Trauma Acute Care Surg. 2015;78:594–9.
37. Kragh JF, Littrel ML, Jones JA, Walters TJ, Baer DG, Wade CE, et al. Battle casualty survival with emergency tourniquet us to stop limb bleeding. J Emerg Med. 2011;41(6):590–7.

First Receivers: Managing Blast Injuries upon Hospital Arrival

21

John M. Wightman

Introduction

The first place a hospital is likely to receive persons injured during an explosive event is the emergency department (ED). Many of these victims will arrive under their own power, some will be driven to the hospital by nonmedical first responders or bystanders, and others will be transported via emergency medical services (EMS).

Casualties from the employment of military munitions are very rare in most civilian EDs, but the criminal use of improvised explosive devices (IEDs) is more common than many planners know. IEDs can be as small and simple as a pipe bomb or as large and complex as a tanker truck loaded with tons of ammonium nitrate mixed with fuel oil. The majority of these felonious acts are directed against only property, but collateral human injuries do occur. Terrorist IED attacks directed against people are also increasingly common [1]. Accidental and natural explosions occur throughout the world as well and create their own response complexities [2].

In explosive incidents, mechanisms and severities of injuries vary widely. The different types of blast trauma have been reviewed [2] and are covered in detail in Chap. 3. Using hospital admission rates as a gross surrogate marker of injury severity in victims who survive long enough to be admitted, pooled data from incidents involving 30 or more casualties suggest that terrorist bombings have high injury severities [3]. Arnold et al. noted admission rates of 13% for IEDs placed and detonated in open spaces and 19% for vehicle-borne improvised explosive devices (VBIEDs) but 58% for IEDs carried by an individual who committed suicide with detonation [3]. Aharonson et al. found that over a quarter of all initial survivors of

J. M. Wightman (✉)
Department of Military and Emergency Medicine, F. Edward Hébert School of Medicine, Uniformed Services University, Bethesda, MD, USA
e-mail: john.wightman@usuhs.edu

D. W. Callaway, J. L. Burstein (eds.), *Operational and Medical Management of Explosive and Blast Incidents*, https://doi.org/10.1007/978-3-030-40655-4_21

explosions perpetrated by suicidal bombers required management in an intensive care unit (ICU) compared to approximately 1 in every 15 patients with non-blast mechanisms of injury [4].

Situational Awareness

Clear communication between responders at the scene or scenes, the emergency operations center (EOC), and all facilities where casualties might be transported are essential. Understanding the location and characteristics of the incident and its impact on the surrounding population and infrastructure is the first step in preparing to receive casualties [5]. The epidemiology of injuries following terrorist bombings may be quite different depending on a number of factors. Many of these have been detailed in Chap. 13.

Detonation of IEDs in open spaces, especially when shrapnel has been intentionally added to the device, mostly causes secondary and tertiary blast injuries. Victims close enough to the epicenter of the explosion to sustain primary blast injury of internal organs are typically dead at the scene [6]. Bombings in enclosed spaces like commuter buses tend to leave a higher proportion of initial survivors with blast lung injury (BLI) and blast intestinal injury (BII), due to magnification of overpressure at surfaces in close proximity to victims [7, 8]. Building collapse leads to a high percentage of fatalities in the areas of structural failure [9, 10] and a higher proportion of crush injuries in those who survive [11]. After pooling data from 44 events causing 30 or more casualties, Arnold et al. observed that structural collapse and structural fire result in high initial death rates and relatively higher rates of hospital admissions [3].

Hospital proximity to incident site(s) may affect casualty flow, because not all victims will be transported by EMS. Following the April 19, 1995 detonation of a large VBIED outside the Murrah Federal Building in downtown Oklahoma City, Hogan et al. found that 80% (312/388) of victims were eventually treated and released from an ED. Some of the victims arrived at the nearest ED as early as 5 minutes after the explosion. These relatively less-injured patients were more likely to arrive at hospitals *before* the 19% of casualties injured seriously enough to require admission. Although only 33% of all victims arrived to the ED via ambulance, casualties transported by EMS were ten times more likely to be admitted (64% vs. 6%, respectively) [12]. Healthcare facilities relatively close to scenes of explosions should anticipate at least two waves of casualties: less serious first and then more serious [5]. The multiple coordinated IED attacks in London on July 7, 2005, are illustrative of patient flow challenges post-incident. The Royal London Hospital received 194 of the 775 total casualties. The maximum surge rate was 18 seriously injured patients per hour, and capacity was reached within the first 15 minutes [13].

A unified Incident Command System (ICS) or Central Medical Emergency Direction (CMED) can offer some control of patient flow if destination protocols are in place, coordinated with local health systems, and well-practiced [14]. The goal is to match available healthcare resources to medical and surgical needs. Although hospital capacity is a critical issue in destination protocols, clinical leaders must also understand that this is balanced with the duration for which an EMS asset will be off-line if transporting to more remote facilities.

A multiple-casualty incident (MCI) may be defined as one in which more casualties must be evaluated and managed than time allows to maintain the culturally customary standard of care, but any alterations or delays are unlikely to result in increased morbidity or mortality. A mass-casualty (MASCAL) incident may be defined as one during which the standard of care must be significantly altered for some patients in such a way as to decrease the likelihood of avoiding death or permanent disability in order to increase the likelihood of meaningful survival for a larger percentage of the affected population.

Two publications from Israel have described four phases of the out-of-hospital MASCAL response slightly differently [15, 16] and two phases of the in-hospital approach to surgical problems [15]. Blending these for the initial receivers at a fixed location providing emergency medical care, the following five phases are proposed:

1. *Disordered arrival phase*: casualties who have departed the scene under their own power or who have been transported by nonmedical first responders or bystanders arrive in the ED in a completely uncontrolled order. They may or may not have had any first aid rendered prior to arrival. Some may have life-threatening injuries, but most will have been ambulatory at some point in time, so the probability of an untoward outcome is diminished but not zero.
2. *Controlled arrival phase*: casualties who did not self-evacuate and arrive via EMS. These patients should be the most seriously injured of all victims en route to a given facility. Some out-of-hospital interventions should have been performed, and some information regarding patient injuries and physiological status should have been communicated prior to arrival.
3. *Deliberate arrival phase*: casualties are directed or transported to specific destinations to best match their needs with resources available at any given time. Facility destinations are usually controlled by a designated person or team under the ICS or CMED. Some casualties may be deliberately sent to facilities farther away, so as not to further burden hospitals close to the scene. After field medical-screening examinations, some victims may even be directed to urgent care centers or primary care offices the same day or next day.
4. *Reevaluation phase*: experienced emergency medicine or trauma providers reassess all remaining patients who received only field or preliminary triage. This occurs after disposition of critical patients or when surge staffing arrives. One recommended process is to conduct the reevaluation while bringing noncritical patients back through radiology to have any needed imaging studies performed prior to subsequent triage and treatment decisions [2]. This process acknowledges that radiological imaging is often the most saturated ancillary service in many MASCAL situations [3, 12].
5. *Redistribution phase*: patients are moved to where needed services can be most effectively and efficiently delivered. Once all victims have been evaluated

sufficiently to determine all resources needed emergently, patients can be redistributed to services or facilities where capability and capacity exist or will be soon augmented. This could involve *intra*-facility movement of patients (e.g., operating room (OR) for a surgical procedure that was not immediately necessary) or could involve *inter*-facility transfer when services are not available at the hospital where a patient might have been initially admitted.

Repeated assessments and re-triage should be accomplished during all phases.

Arrival Triage

Conventional ED triage protocols (e.g., Emergency Severity Index (ESI) [17], Canadian Triage and Acuity Scale (CTAS) [18]) may be too cumbersome to employ in a necessarily brief initial encounter without exact vital signs or other parameters used by the triage system. They may not effectively sort patients in situations with extraordinarily limited resources, because they assume a normal standard of emergency care.

During any MASCAL triage process, the principle of justly distributing limited resources for the greater good may supersede the right of individuals to make their own decisions regarding care—autonomy being a cornerstone of patient-provider relationships in other situations [19]. Patients and caregivers decide on their needs for emergency services [20], but the healthcare system must decide on what resources can or should be allocated to meet those needs.

Triage methodologies developed for out-of-hospital settings (e.g., Sort → Assess → Life-saving interventions → Treatment/Transport (SALT) [21]) may not be appropriate inside a hospital where resources not available in the field may be employed. The Simple Triage and Rapid Treatment (START) algorithm has gained wide popularity even in hospital disaster plans but was derived from bus crashes and then developed for field responses to earthquakes [22], so its applicability to initial triage at a healthcare facility for blast-injured trauma victims may be limited. No out-of-hospital or in-hospital MASCAL triage methodology has been retrospectively derived from real-world MASCAL situations, prospectively and consistently applied in a limited population, scientifically evaluated and modified as necessary, validated in a broader population or under different conditions, and then widely accepted for generalized employment. Until that rigorous assessment occurs [23, 24], no specific triage system can be recommended as the standard [25], especially not for one that might be better than another for blast-injured patients [2]. Hospitals and their EDs should choose a single triage system based on best available evidence, fully integrate it into their MCI planning, and train personnel to their internal standard.

Triage accuracy has operational implications. "Under-triage" (i.e., inadequate specificity) can result in potentially preventable morbidity or mortality in the acute phase. This can be mitigated through an MCI plan that integrates structured patient reassessments. Conversely, "over-triage" (i.e., excessive sensitivity) can result in over-expenditure of human and material resources on noncritical patients. The result is more rapid progression to operational saturation. Following the 2005 London bombings, over-triage was felt to be less when performed by trained responders [13]. Over-triage has been thought to have a direct relationship to overall event mortality rates [26], but scientific evidence of this is lacking. In essence, over-triage is only an issue *if* the receiving facility exceeds capacity to care for patients.

Incorrect triage decisions can affect outcomes [27] beyond the individual patient. Accordingly, triage should be thought of as a dynamic process, and a formal re-triage process must be in place to mitigate the initial sacrifice of detailed information for speed of decision-making. In a review of 19 MASCAL incidents from terrorist bombings, Ashkenazi et al. discovered that, out of 205 victim records examined, 11 to 18 (i.e., < 10%) may have been under-triaged (depending on the measure of injury severity) initially, but the true seriousness could later be detected with additional examinations [28].

Point-of-care ultrasonography (POCUS) may be a useful adjunct in evaluating critical patients. As a general screening examination for life threats of unknown cause under normal circumstances, the Rapid Ultrasound for Shock and Hypotension (RUSH) or extended RUSH protocols may be useful [29]. POCUS protocols with the largest body of evidence specifically for trauma patients in the ED are the focused abdominal sonography for trauma (FAST), the extended FAST (E-FAST), and the chest abdominal FAST (CA-FAST) protocols [30]. FAST has been suggested as a potential adjunct to the START triage system [31].

Sarkisian et al. reported the first use of POCUS in triage following a MASCAL event. The study examined abdominal imaging on 400 patients in a single facility during the first 72 hours after a magnitude 6.8 earthquake in Armenia in order to identify intra-abdominal organ injuries in need of operative intervention [32]. Blaivas as also noted use of the FAST protocol to prioritize simultaneous patients with penetrating cardiac injuries [33]. These reports are examples of interventions based on positive findings (i.e., actions based on the specificity or positive likelihood ratio (LR+) of the examination). Negative findings can also be useful decision criteria. For instance, the absence of anechoic fluid in the intraperitoneal and intrapleural cavities indicates that any cause of shock is unlikely due to life-threatening blood loss into these internal potential spaces.

Two detonations at the Boston Marathon on April 15, 2013 resulted in 281 casualties [34]. Emergency physicians at Brigham and Women's Hospital used POCUS to rule out or rule in intracavitary truncal hemorrhage in many patients during their ED assessments [35]. Although not used as a primary triage tool to direct casualties to specific locations in a facility, POCUS was used as an adjunct to triage patients for surgical services.

One POCUS protocol has been proposed for MASCAL situations, which goes by the acronym CAVEAT: chest, abdomen, vena cava, and extremities for acute triage [36, 37]. Imaging windows for the chest and abdomen are the most crucial and essentially constitute the examinations in the E-FAST protocol. Assessment of vena cava diameter and compressibility could be performed if time allows and the cause of any shock or hypotension is still in question.

POCUS has yet to be prospectively validated as an efficient and effective adjunct to any specific ED MASCAL triage system during an actual event. Over the courses of six combat deployments, this author has observed that decisions to perform needle thoracentesis for suspected tension pneumothoraces could be made clinically and did not require imaging of any kind. POCUS using the basic FAST protocol, while noting if anechoic fluid was present in the costophrenic angles, was more useful in allocating personnel resources to perform procedures (e.g., needle pericardiocentesis and tube thoracostomy) or expeditiously sending casualties to an OR than it was in assigning triage categories during MASCAL situations.

Some casualties will not be *in extremis* or present with multiple external injuries to cue the triage officer into the possibility of internal injuries due to the primary effects of the blast wave, and therefore, they may not be identified as being at risk for BLI or BII. One expert with experience in the Vietnam War suggested that "medical personnel should look for certain sentinel signs, such as a ruptured tympanic membrane, hypopharyngeal contusions, hemoptysis in the absence of external chest trauma, or subcutaneous emphysema" as potential associations with BLI [38].

During assessment of the airway, petechiae may be noted in the tissue of the hard or soft pallet or the posterior pharynx. This is a rare finding in the author's experience managing initial survivors [39], but based on experimental evidence [40], it may indicate trauma from a blast wave of sufficient magnitude to have also caused contusions of internal organs. This finding could be helpful if noted but likely has no predictive value if absent. Any blast event associated with hemoptysis or subcutaneous emphysema should prompt consideration of pulmonary trauma.

Rupture of one or both tympanic membranes does indicate exposure to a blast wave, but its presence does not predict the occurrence or progression of BLI [41], and it can be absent in persons exposed to significant blast loads due to a variety of factors such as head orientation and hearing protection. There is no need to perform otoscopy during the initial triage process. Clinical manifestations and pulse oximetry (S_PO_2) can be used to signal development of significant BLI.

Absolute S_PO_2 spot measurements and trends might be useful in predicting which patients are or are not likely to require mechanical ventilation in the first 24 hours after injury [2]. Otherwise, no absolute number or combination of vital signs have been identified to suggest occult primary BLI or BII. Non-POCUS imaging studies are unlikely to be rapidly available at the time of triage upon hospital arrival. No laboratory tests were found to be sensitive or specific in one animal study [42] and anything but basic laboratory testing is even less likely to be rapidly available at the point of care.

By whatever means triage for treatment is accomplished, the remainder of this chapter will base discussions on a typical five-category model for initial triage upon hospital arrival, because such systems are in common use and systems that use fewer groupings can be considered as modifications. The five categories most often used in MASCAL situations are named and coded by color: immediate/red, delayed/yellow, minimal/green, expectant/blue, and dead/black.

Standards of Care

Virtually every decision in MASCAL situations involves prioritization of two or more courses of action. When the standard of care must be significantly altered during a MASCAL situation, the concept of "minimum acceptable care" may be useful [2, 43]. If this model is to be truly accepted by the society being served, proposals should be debated within the community and its leaders, discussed among health departments at local and state levels, and socialized throughout each healthcare facility before an event occurs [44]. Ultimately, the success or failure of victim triage and treatment will be judged in multiple forums at multiple levels after the MASCAL circumstances have resolved. Any altered standard of care will also need to be applied to all other ED patients: those who may not have been affected by the casualty-generating explosion but who, nevertheless, still present to the ED requesting emergency services (i.e., the baseline volume).

Allocation of resources must be prioritized when there is not enough to go around for all patients. Even in facilities where major trauma is not part of routine practice, extra resources are typically dedicated to the seriously injured. When these resources are needed for multiple patients simultaneously, this standard may not be met. The time personnel and services can spend with each individual casualty must often be curtailed. History taking and physical examination should initially be focused on two things: (1) screening for life threats requiring emergent intervention and (2) gathering information necessary for clinical decision-making regarding additional studies or disposition from the ED.

The level of care may be increased from the "minimum" by sharing portable equipment between patients. POCUS may be a useful adjunct to relieve some of the burden for radiological services [35, 45]. Although no POCUS protocols specific for blast injuries exist at this time, standard applications for penetrating and blunt trauma would be appropriate, though the interpretation of findings and any action taken based on them may require alternative consideration.

One meta-analysis of POCUS for blunt trauma discovered relatively high specificity for detecting free fluid and organ lesions, but the negative likelihood ratio (LR-) for excluding abdominal injuries was only 0.23 [46]. The time to add organ-specific imaging would not likely be taken under MASCAL circumstances; however, the absence of free fluid would inform providers that the patient does not have more than 250–500 mL of blood in the peritoneal cavity at that time, so damage-control laparotomy might not be immediately necessary. Serial physical examinations coupled with POCUS may be helpful, keeping in mind that positive findings are generally more actionable. Negative findings often require additional testing at a later time yet may provide information that can reassure providers that any delay to more definitive decision-making is less likely to increase mortality or long-term morbidity. Prospective trials are needed to confirm this recommendation.

Immediate Threats to Life

Patients who are likely to have a poor outcome without rapid intervention are typically prioritized into an immediate/red or expectant/blue triage category. Patients in the immediate category receive immediate care. Patients in the expectant category do not. The only difference between the two is that sufficient resources are readily available to intervene for the potential benefit of immediate patients, but the resources necessary to reasonably improve outcomes for expectant patients are not available at the time any given triage decision is made.

The term "expectant" is often misunderstood when applied to casualties being triaged [2, 43]. Medical personnel should not "expect them to die." They should "expect to take care of them" when the required resources become available. If that cannot occur before they die, then that is an unfortunate reality of critical injuries when too many victims need to be managed in too short a time or when the seriousness of the injuries makes saving life impossible. Some patients in the blue category will be truly unsalvageable, but they still should not be placed in the black category until they are actually dead.

Massive Hemorrhage

Massive bleeding is always the first priority. Failure to control exsanguinating external hemorrhage is the primary cause of potentially survivable death in combat casualties. In a mixed population of 4596 deaths—73.7% due to explosions and 22.1% due to gunshot wounds—Eastridge et al. documented that 90.9% died from uncontrolled hemorrhage. Approximately one in every three of these had hemorrhage from the extremities where timely nonsurgical interventions could have made a difference [47].

Similarly refined data could not be found in the English-language literature concerning noncombat blast events. Any population-based conclusions must be inferred from other data. For instance, Mirza et al. examined deaths in Karachi over a 5-year period [48]. Not counting late deaths due to shock, they found that about two in every three bombing victims died of "shock from multiple injuries" separate from head, chest, and abdominal trauma—so this could be indirect evidence for exsanguinating extremity wounds.

Interventions for exsanguinating external hemorrhage are the same as those used in the field: direct pressure, tourniquets, and wound packing. Direct pressure should be employed first, while equipment or supplies are obtained and employed. Prefabricated tourniquets or pneumatic devices can be placed around extremities proximal to bleeding wounds or amputation remnants. Full exposure of patients may not have occurred when immediate intervention is necessary, so direct pressure and tourniquets are applied over clothing initially. Bony anatomical locations like joints and solid items in clothing pockets should be avoided when placing tourniquets. If the site(s) of massive hemorrhage cannot be determined at a glance, tourniquets are placed "high and tight" (i.e., as proximal on the extremity as possible) at an otherwise appropriate location.

Tourniquets should also be placed proximal to traumatic amputations, regardless of the degree of hemorrhage, because bleeding may resume as the casualty's physiological condition improves.

One group in Israel examined terror-related explosive events and discovered that the presence of vascular trauma was associated with poorer prognosis [49]. Nonetheless, a review of trauma solely in extremities, prehospital interventions for those injuries, and outcomes (e.g., deaths that might have been preventable with earlier hemorrhage control) has not yet been undertaken in Israel (Kobi Peleg, MD, MPH, personal communication). One Canadian study found a very low prevalence of tourniquets used in the field, but tourniquets placed in the ED may have improved survival [50]. In the United States, one retrospective study at a single institution comparing matched cases with penetrating extremity hemorrhage amenable to tourniquet application found that those who had tourniquet(s) applied in the field had a lower shock index on hospital arrival, required fewer blood products, and had fewer surgical procedures such as fasciotomy and amputation [51]. Another single-site US study came to similar conclusions and identified an increased risk of death: 4.5 times higher if hemorrhage control was delayed until hospital arrival [52].

Only one commercial purpose-built tourniquet was known to have been used on victims of the bombings at the Boston Marathon, despite 17 traumatic amputations of lower extremities in 15 victims and 12 others with major vascular injuries. Twenty-six other tourniquets were improvised and mostly ineffective on hospital arrival. Several casualties arrived at a hospital with active life-threatening extremity hemorrhage [53]. Whether or not two of the three on-scene deaths could have been prevented with rapid hemorrhage control in the field has been debated.

Junctional hemorrhage is represented by bleeding wounds too close to the hips or shoulders to place a proximal tourniquet. Direct pressure should be applied first. In the hospital setting, wounds can be packed with standard or "hemostatic" gauze followed by 2–3 more minutes of direct pressure [54]. The latter may be further categorized as procoagulants or muco-adhesive dressings, with many commercial products being equally efficacious if used in appropriate settings [55]. A relatively new device has been developed to inject multiple, small, rapidly expanding sponges into narrow channels that may be difficult to pack [56]. These approaches can also be used for neck wounds, which should be considered a junctional location as well.

For axillary and inguinal junctional wounds, a number of prefabricated devices have been marketed for exerting external pressure on femoral or axillary vessels and one for externally compressing the abdominal aorta. If efficacious in controlling bleeding, with or without wound packing, they have the advantage of freeing up a person who would otherwise have been applying direct pressure.

The continued effectiveness of tourniquets, other devices, and packing that may have been placed in an out-of-hospital setting to control external hemorrhage should be reassessed upon hospital arrival. Many of those placed after the Boston Marathon bombing were ineffective on hospital arrival (Ricky Kue, MD, MPH, personal communication). Vascular pressure can increase with prehospital resuscitation, and muscular relaxation can decrease the pressure being generated by a nonelastic tourniquet that is not retightened [57].

Although other methods are being researched, life-threatening internal hemorrhage can only be stopped through endovascular or surgical intervention at present. Resuscitative endovascular balloon occlusion of the aorta (REBOA) has been used with great success to temporarily arrest distal bleeding, thereby extending the time until damage-control surgery must be performed. REBOA has been effectively performed by both emergency physicians and surgeons in resource-constrained circumstances [58].

Emergency support of circulation, breathing, and airway should be addressed after life-threatening hemorrhage has been controlled. Damage-control resuscitation is covered in more detail in Chap. 22. The following paragraphs will briefly discuss some of the problems that are more likely to occur in blast-injured casualties than in victims of trauma by other mechanisms more commonly seen.

Tension Pneumothorax

Tension pneumothoraces are often identified when assessing respirations. The pathophysiology appears to be more complex than previously appreciated—and, in the setting of an ED resuscitation, possibly biphasic. Based on detailed measurements in a porcine model by Nelson et al., tidal volume in spontaneously breathing patients is likely to be progressively diminished by the increasing extrapulmonary intrathoracic pressure, which leads to advancing hypoxia and the potential for hypoxic cardiac arrest. Once a patient is exposed to positive-pressure ventilation (PPV), intrathoracic pressure may exceed central venous pressure and diastolic arterial pressure to cause a form of cardiogenic shock due to preload attenuation [59].

Tension pneumothoraces may be bilateral due to either penetrating trauma or internal rupture of lung tissue by a primary blast mechanism, so asymmetrical breath sounds may not be detectable [2]. Pizov et al. reported seven cases of bilateral tension pneumothoraces and two cases of unilateral tension pneumothorax out of 15 victims with BLI from IED detonations inside two commuter buses [60]. Although the prevalence of tension pneumothorax is reported in many event-based studies, no population-based epidemiological reports on the true incidence following explosive blast could be found.

Any set of the following conditions should prompt immediate performance of needle thoracostomy on the side of suspected tension pneumothorax: (1) shock and asymmetrical breath sounds, (2) penetrating trauma and progressive respiratory distress, or (3) traumatic cardiac arrest without obviously fatal wounds. Tension pneumothorax should also be considered with severe or progressive respiratory distress or low or rapidly decreasing hemoglobin oxygen saturation as measured by continuous S_pO_2.

If one needle thoracostomy fails to improve the patient's condition, another needle decompression should be performed on the same side at an alternate location. If that also does not provide relief, then one or two needle thoracostomies should be attempted on the opposite side [61]. Because they have been shown to be effective in the out-of-hospital setting [62], bilateral limited "finger" thoracotomies should be considered in moribund or arrested patients in the in-hospital

MASCAL setting. With the immediate life threat of tension physiology addressed, tube thoracostomies can be performed at the time of the thoracotomies or later as resources and time allow.

Blast Lung Injury

Pulmonary contusions are the primary manifestations of BLI, though disruption of lung tissue can also result in blood occluding airways and air leaks into the lung substance, pleural spaces, and pulmonary vascular system. Contusions of lung tissue may range from a few patchy areas beneath intercostal spaces to entire lungs, which inhibit gas exchange to various degrees [1, 63]. A BLI clinical prediction rule has been posted on MDCalc as "useful in guiding triage decisions in the setting of mass casualties" [64] but has not been prospectively validated and requires arterial blood-gas analysis, a known fraction of inspired oxygen, a plain radiograph of the chest, and determination of the presence or absence of any bronchopleural fistula(e)—none of which will be readily available during the initial triage process. On the other hand, the small retrospective case series of BLI patients [60] from which this putative scoring system was drawn did have some useful information regarding patients who are *unlikely* to require PPV [65], the cutoff for which can be roughly estimated as those not in shock who can maintain hemoglobin oxygen saturation of at least 75% breathing ambient air [2].

Contused lung tissue is less compliant than normal, so PPV has the potential to cause barotrauma to affected areas, which can increase the possibilities of tension pneumothoraces (see above) and arterial air embolism (AAE) (see below). Spontaneous negative-pressure ventilations are preferred whenever possible [65]. A trial of noninvasive PPV is a reasonable option in borderline cases [2]. A definitive airway and PPV will commit ICU resources to a patient.

Of 93 victims from two confined-space explosions seen at a single facility, Leibovici et al. found that 71 did not require mechanical ventilation, but of those diagnosed with BLI, 76% did require some period of PPV with intubation being accomplished in the field or within 2 hours of injury [8]. Primary BLI has been reported to be capable of progressing over the first 4 hours after the initial insult [66].

However, one study examining 647 survivors of 11 terrorist bombings in Israel found that none of the patients were diagnosed with BLI by physical examination or plain chest radiography within the first hour after injury subsequently developed BLI [41]. If not requiring intervention within the first hour after exposure to a blast wave, progression is much more likely to be slow and not life-threatening. A review of BLI short- and long-term outcomes has been conducted by Avidan et al. [63].

Massive Hemoptysis

Although rarely reported in the literature related to explosive events, another immediate threat to life is massive hemoptysis, when blood from torn lung tissue occludes the larger airways. The only interventions that are available are selective intubation of the lesser injured lung or performance of a thoracotomy to surgically stop pulmonary blood flow. With regard to the former in a resource-limited MASCAL situation, access to and expertise with specialized endotracheal tubes will be unlikely. An algorithm for blind intubation of one mainstem bronchus or the other has been proposed for use with conventional single-lumen tubes [1, 2].

Arterial Air Embolism

AAE can be a sequela of either primary or secondary blast trauma. Air can escape into pulmonary veins, flow to the heart, and be ejected into the systemic circulation. Embolic infarction may be clinically silent, but major syndromes related to cerebral/cerebellar, retinal, spinal, myocardial, mesenteric, renal, and other ischemic insults do occur.

If the side of the lung injury is known or strongly suspected by penetrating wounds, ED intervention includes lung isolation by selectively intubating the opposite mainstem bronchus [67]. The same algorithm for blind mainstem bronchial intubation used for massive hemoptysis could also be used for AAE or tension pneumothorax, so additional air does not enter the injured lung to transit into pulmonary veins or pleural spaces [1, 2]. Additional hospital-based treatments include operative lung exclusion and hyperbaric therapy [67].

Positioning the patient with the head at the level of the heart is important to lessen the likelihood of air embolism to the brain and eyes [38]. Another proposed but unproven method of decreasing the likelihood of cerebral or coronary AAE is to place the casualty in the recovery position turned 45° toward prone [65]. If the side of the injury is known, placing that side down will increase pulmonary venous pressure and increase the airway-to-vessel resistance. If the side of injury is not known or is bilateral, the left side down will place the coronary artery ostia at the lowest orientation relative to gravity.

The true prevalence of AAE after exposure to a blast wave is unknown. It is often not definitively diagnosed in living patients and is difficult to detect on autopsies even if specifically sought.

Other Serious Injuries

Casualties who do not require immediate intervention, but who have the potential to deteriorate or develop secondary problems over time, are typically assigned to a delayed/yellow category during the triage process. They must be monitored for changes in their conditions that might warrant more or less healthcare resources. Hospitals should consider where and how this monitoring occurs, taking into account current and expected patient inflow as well as status of inpatient resources (e.g., staffed OR suites, open hospital beds, professional and ancillary staffing).

Spinal Injury

In a retrospective study of 2667 victims of terror-related explosions, all had cervical collars placed at the scene, yet only nine had unstable cervical spine injuries, and only one of those had no identifiable neurological deficits on initial presentation [68]. On the other hand, the US military experience has revealed a large number of spinal injuries from IEDs and other explosives [69]. One army unit sustained 5.6 spinal injuries per 1000 combat-years [70], but these populations are not the same as most civilian blast-injured populations. Civilians close to IED detonations are often dead at the scene. During MASCAL situations with limited supplies, cervical collars may only be necessary for blast-injured casualties with neurological deficits on examination.

Ocular Injury

No definitive evidence for primary blast ocular injury exists outside the laboratory [71]. Nonetheless, penetrating and nonpenetrating wounds have been reported to occur in 10–15% of victims from explosive events [72]. In the 2013 Boston incident, 13.4% of casualties transported to trauma centers had eye injuries in addition to multiple other injuries [73]. A thorough examination with magnification is required [74, 75]. POCUS may be a useful bedside adjunct once life-threatening injuries have been considered and managed [76]. Definitive imaging of the globes may involve either or both ultrasonography and computed tomography (CT) as complementary tests [77].

Blast Intestinal Injury

BII is, in general, relatively uncommon following intentional bombings, but it carries a high risk for morbidity and mortality [78, 79]. It deserves special mention, because symptoms can be subtle [65] and delayed bowel perforation can occur up to a week or more after initial injury [80, 81]. The most common symptom is tenesmus, and the most common sign is hematochezia, but neither of these have been reported to be particularly sensitive or specific [2]. Pain may be diffuse, localized, or referred to the shoulders, back, or testicles [38]. CT may be useful if images demonstrate abnormalities [82, 83], but it is less sensitive for detecting bowel injury without gas-releasing perforation than it is for other injuries [84, 85]. POCUS is also relatively insensitive for bowel injury in the absence of hemoperitoneum [86]. When applying negative likelihood ratios from existing trauma literature, the pretest probability of bowel injury is likely higher following exposure to a blast wave than it is for blunt trauma, and this should be kept in mind when interpreting physical examinations and imaging results for clinical decision-making.

Orthopedic Injury

Imaging services are often the most taxed during MASCAL events. Radiology was the most heavily employed support service following the VBIED explosion in Oklahoma City [12]. In addition to standard POCUS for immediately life-threatening injuries, one protocol has suggested using this bedside imaging modality to examine for pulmonary contusions as well [30]. POCUS may also be useful in lieu of radiography to detect foreign bodies [87, 88] and underlying fractures, particularly around the midshafts of long bones [89, 90]. Extremity examinations are part of the proposed CAVEAT protocol to augment MASCAL triage when time allows for these additional views [36].

Burn Injury

Thermal trauma resulting in burns is another important mechanism of injury, either directly due to the explosion (i.e., quaternary blast injury) or due to ignition of clothing, vehicles, buildings, or surrounding vegetation [91]. The number of burned casualties will vary greatly by the type of explosion. Industrial accidents are notorious for producing large fireballs and ongoing chemical fires. Terrorists can also construct intentionally incendiary devices [92, 93]. No studies could be identified that have addressed any differences in airway, ventilation, or circulatory management of thermal injuries in the presence of concomitant blast trauma with or without BLI.

Miscellaneous Injuries

Patients who are unlikely to have any significant sequelae from their injuries are typically assigned to a minimal/green triage category. This does not mean that they will not need significant resources at another time. Some of these injuries include superficial wounds, simple closed fractures, mild traumatic brain injury (TBI), and emotional distress. Until proven otherwise, the "worried well" should also be placed in the green/minimal triage category pending an appropriate evaluation.

Mild Traumatic Brain Injury

TBI may occur without external evidence of blunt or penetrating trauma. Mild TBI is sometimes more difficult to uncover than moderate or severe TBI, especially in the absence of any known period of abnormal consciousness or mental functioning. Structured screening algorithms can be useful for this purpose [94]. The Defense and Veterans Brain Injury Center (DVBIC) offers a number of free tools for acute screening, such as the Military Acute Concussion Evaluation (MACE) [95], and for follow-up for persistent symptoms. In general, the prognosis after mild TBI is good, but cases must first be detected, and professional evaluation might be indicated [96].

Wound Contamination

Tetanus immunization standards are appropriate for all open wounds. The possibility of embedded bacterial, fungal, and viral pathogens must also be considered. Biological agents can be intentionally added to make a dirty bomb, debris from the environment can contaminate wounds, and human blood and tissue from other victims can penetrate the skin when propelled by the energy of a high-explosive detonation. Issues surrounding prophylaxis against blood-borne pathogens have been reviewed [97].

Admission and Transfer

No prospective trials have evaluated any particular admission criteria or algorithm for blast-injured casualties. All retrospective studies have reported admission rates based on clinical judgment. With the exception of BII, most blast injuries can be detected during the reevaluation phase of management. CT imaging can be the linchpin of decision-making regarding disposition.

Transfers to other hospitals should be based on matching available resources in the facility where the patient is and other facilities where the patient could be sent. Trauma care has been shown to be better at trauma centers, but many routinely operate at near-maximum capacity [98]. Following detonation of a high-yield explosive in the region a trauma center serves, it may be overwhelmed with victims during the disordered and perhaps controlled arrival phases. Sending patients who do not need the unique services of a trauma center occurs even when a MASCAL incident has not occurred [99]. Centers with specialty capabilities (e.g., burn care and hyperbaric therapy) may also be potential destinations for patients in facilities without these services. Discussions must occur between sending and receiving facilities to determine where needed resources can be delivered in a time frame that will make a difference in outcome without placing the patient at unacceptable risk during transport.

The disposition of blast victims with penetrating trauma should fundamentally be no different than for those sustaining non-blast trauma [2]. Because fragments of explosive devices, any shrapnel added to IEDs, and debris picked up from the environment may be propelled at very high initial velocities yet cause only tiny puncture wounds, every wound has the potential to cause internal damage. When not associated with abnormal physiological parameters or other immediate concerns suggested by trajectory, wounds should be further assessed during the reevaluation phase after imaging resources become more available.

Even after negative CT imaging, patients with any abdominal complaint such as pain or discomfort, nausea or vomiting, tenesmus, or hematochezia should be observed for development of primary BII over the next 2–3 days.

With regard to the potential for primary BLI, pulse oximetry and plain chest radiography should be sufficient to exclude any problems that might require intervention or an additional period of observation for asymptomatic patients being clinically considered for discharge. Patients with lingering chest pain not ascribed to specific surface wounds, unresolved dyspnea, wheezing on auscultation, prolonged expiratory phase on forced exhalation, or any imagining abnormalities should be observed for at least several hours to watch for progression or resolution. If space and personnel resources are needed for other victims during a MASCAL situation, admission or transfer may be appropriate.

Discharge

Numerous descriptions of individual explosive events [1] and articles pooling data from multiple incidents [100–103] have shown that the majority of initial survivors are able to be discharged from the ED without admission to the hospital. More recent incidents have had different results, likely as a result of different response types.

Over 2000 people were injured by multiple simultaneous IED detonations in Madrid on March 11, 2004. Almost all casualties transported to hospitals were taken to only two trauma centers. Just over half of the initial survivors were managed in EDs, and 47% of those were discharged the same day. However, in this event, many were initially managed in rapidly deployed field hospitals as part of the emergency disaster response or in primary care clinics throughout the city [104]. Therefore, the overall rate of initial survivors not admitted was 73%, despite the closed spaces in which these bombings occurred.

Following the 2005 bombings at four separate London locations, 722 casualties were distributed to six hospitals. One trauma center reported receiving 27 seriously injured casualties, but did not report admission rates on the other 167 "walking wounded" [13]. In Boston, 281 victims of two explosions in close proximity were distributed to 26 area hospitals in 2013. Of the 127 casualties seen at trauma centers, 52 (41%) were not admitted [34].

Community standards for discharge instructions related to specific injuries should be applicable. Standards of care in this regard would not require adjustment in most MASCAL situations; because, unless space is critically needed for the care of other patients during the arrival phases, the time at which discharge decisions are made will usually be during the reevaluation phase after the last anticipated victim has arrived and been assessed.

Patients ultimately diagnosed with mild TBI by history or neurocognitive screening tests (e.g., MACE) can be discharged under community standards applicable to concussions sustained by blunt mechanisms, preferably into a setting with another responsible individual who is familiar with the patient's baseline neuropsychological functioning, and can be observed for subtle changes in level of consciousness, mood or behavior, and symptoms such as headache and difficulty concentrating. In a study of war veterans with mild TBI caused by blast, blunt, and combined injuries, there were no substantial differences in post-concussive symptoms based on mechanism [105]. The DVBIC has posted recommendations, clinical tools, and fact sheets for progressive return to activities [106].

Acute, subacute, and chronic mental health issues in blast-injured casualties have become more well-known and well-studied since the events of 9/11 and the subsequent Global War on Terrorism [107, 108]. Post-traumatic stress reactions and post-traumatic stress disorder (PTSD) occur with some frequency [109]. Patients being discharged from the ED should be made aware of these possibilities and instructed to seek care for any concerns. If these patients return to the ED at a later time with complaints of new or persistent symptoms, they should be thoroughly evaluated with full knowledge that psychological PTSD and physical TBI symptoms and signs often overlap [96, 110]. The DVBIC offers free information, clinical tools, and fact sheets for clinicians and patients [111].

Tympanic membrane rupture is not a problem requiring immediate care. Full otoscopic evaluation in the ED is recommended when time allows, but discharge with a 72-hour referral to an otorhinolaryngologist for a detailed examination and possible middle ear irrigation would be appropriate when space and time are at a premium during a MASCAL scenario.

No matter what injuries a patient has sustained, discharge must include a safe plan and comprehensive written instructions. If discharged earlier than desired during a MASCAL situation, scheduled return to the ED or other medical setting for delayed reevaluation may be appropriate.

Conclusion

Victims of explosions are uncommon in civilian EDs, but when encountered, polytrauma from multiple mechanisms may rapidly strain even the most robust healthcare system. Some patients may have unique injuries with which some healthcare personnel may not be familiar. Multiple casualties may present simultaneously or in rapid succession. All this may complicate triage and treatment decisions upon hospital arrival and throughout courses of care in EDs. Knowledge, planning, and rehearsals are the keys to mitigating potentially preventable morbidity and mortality.

Key Points

- Explosions may cause isolated or polytraumatic injuries by multiple mechanisms, one of which is primary blast injury caused by translation of atmospheric wave energy into the body.
- Exsanguinating hemorrhage must be controlled immediately.
- Tension pneumothoraces may manifest quickly, occur bilaterally, and cause cardiac arrest by both hypoxic respiratory and obstructive vascular mechanisms. Decompression of the chest by needle thoracentesis or simple finger thoracotomy on the affected side(s) can be immediately lifesaving.

- Mass-casualty situations may necessitate difficult triage decisions and alterations of normal standards of care.
- When resources are limited at the time they are needed at any given location, only three options remain: (1) bring required resources to the patient, (2) move the patient to where needed resources are available, or (3) defer allocating potentially beneficial resources until a later time.

Pitfalls

- Not being aware of injuries that may initially be clinically occult could lead to delayed diagnosis as symptoms manifest or lead to erroneous interpretation of symptoms. Important examples include traumatic brain injury, arterial air embolism, blast lung injury, and blast intestinal injury.
- Unnecessary or excessive positive-pressure ventilation or intravascular fluid administration can exacerbate blast-induced brain or lung injury.
- Sight-threatening eye injuries and limb-threatening compartment syndromes can be missed in victims with other critical injuries or casualties who cannot communicate or participate in an examination of vision.

Disclaimer The opinions and assertions herein are the private views of the author and are not to be construed as official or as reflecting the views of the Uniformed Services University, Department of the US Air Force, US Department of Defense, or the US government.

References

1. Wightman JM, Kharod CU. Explosive events. In: Koenig KA, Schultz CH, editors. Koenig & Schultz's disaster medicine: comprehensive principles and practices. 1st ed. Cambridge: Cambridge University Press; 2010. p. 393–422.
2. Burns GD, Wightman JM. Explosive events. In: Koenig KA, Schultz CH, editors. Koenig & Schultz's disaster medicine: comprehensive principles and practices. 2nd ed. Cambridge: Cambridge University Press; 2016. p. 463–85.
3. Arnold JL, Ming-Che T, Halpern P, Smithline H, Stok E, Ersoy G. Mass-casualty, terrorist bombings: epidemiological outcomes, resource utilization, and time course of emergency needs (part I). Prehosp Disaster Med. 2003;18:220–34.
4. Aharonson-Daniel L, Klein Y, Peleg K. Suicide bombers form a new injury profile. Ann Surg. 2006;244:1018–23. https://doi.org/10.1097/01.sla.0000225355.06362.0f.
5. Halpern P, Ming-Che T, Arnold JL, Stok E, Ersoy G. Mass-casualty, terrorist bombings: epidemiological outcomes, resource utilization, and time course of emergency needs (part II). Prehosp Disaster Med. 2003;18:235–41.
6. Wightman JM, Wayne BA. Explosives. In: Roy MJ, editor. Physician's guide to terrorist attack. Totowa: Humana; 2004. p. 363–77.
7. Katz E, Ofek B, Adler J, Abramowitz HB, Graus MM. Primary blast injury after a bomb explosion in a civilian bus. Ann Surg. 1989;209:484–8.

8. Leibovici D, Gofrit ON, Stein M, Shapira SC, Noga Y, Heruti RJ, et al. Blast injuries: bus versus open-air bombings—a comparative study of injuries in survivors of open-air versus confined-space explosions. J Trauma. 1996;41:1030–5.
9. Mallonee S, Shariat S, Stennies G, Waxweiler R, Hogan D, Jordan F. Physical injuries and fatalities resulting from the Oklahoma City bombing. JAMA. 1996;276:382–7.
10. Kalebi AY, Olumbe AK. Forensic findings from the Nairobi U.S. Embassy terrorist bombing. East Afr Med J. 2006;83:380–8.
11. Glenshaw MT, Vernick JS, Li G, Sorock GS, Brown S, Mallonee S. Factors associated with injury severity in Oklahoma City bombing survivors. J Trauma. 2009;66:508–5. https://doi.org/10.1097/TA.0b013e31815d9b72.
12. Hogan DE, Waeckerle JF, Dire DJ, Lillibridge SR. Emergency department impact of the Oklahoma City terrorist bombing. Ann Emerg Med. 1999;34:160–7.
13. Aylwin CJ, König TC, Brennan NW, Shirley PJ, Davies G, Walsh MS, et al. Reduction in critical mortality in urban mass casualty incidents: analysis of triage, surge, and resource use after the London bombings on July 7, 2005. Lancet. 2006;368:2219–25.
14. Department of Homeland Security. National response framework. 4th ed. Washington: Department of Homeland Security; 2019. https://www.fema.gov/media-library/assets/documents/117791. Accessed 27 Feb 2020.
15. Stein M, Hirschberg A. Medical consequences of terrorism: the conventional weapon threat. Surg Clin North Am. 1999;79:1537–52.
16. Einav S, Feigenberg Z, Weissman C, Zaichik D, Caspi G, Kotler D, et al. Evacuation priorities in mass casualty terror-related events: implications for contingency planning. Ann Surg. 2007;239:304–10.
17. Gilboy N, Tanabe T, Travers D, Rosenau AM. Emergency severity index (ESI): a triage tool for emergency department care, version 4. Implementation handbook, 2012 edition. Rockville: Agency for Healthcare Research and Quality; 2011.
18. Canadian Association of Emergency Physicians. The Canadian triage and acuity scale: combined adult/paediatric educational program, version 2.5b. Participant's manual, 2012 edition. Ottawa: CTAS National Working Group; 2012.
19. Moskop JC, Iverson KI. Triage in medicine, part II: underlying values and principles. Ann Emerg Med. 2007;49:282–7. https://doi.org/10.1016/j.annemergmed.2006.07.012.
20. ACEP Board of Directors. Definition of an emergency service. Irving: American College of Emergency Physicians; 2015. https://www.acep.org/patient-care/policy-statements/definition-of-an-emergency-service/#sm.0001p08bjv1s0dvuqbo152rnmt6dr. Accessed 27 Feb 2020.
21. Lerner BE, Schwartz RB, Coule PL, Weinstein ES, Cone DC, Hunt RC, et al. Mass casualty triage: an evaluation of the data and development of a proposed national guideline. Disaster Med Public Health Prep. 2008;2(Suppl 1):S25–34. https://doi.org/10.1097/DMP.0b013e318182194e.
22. Benson M, Koenig KL, Schultz CH. Disaster triage: START, then SAVE—a new method of dynamic triage for victims of catastrophic earthquake. Prehosp Disaster Med. 1996;11:117–4.
23. Laupacis A, Sekar N, Stiell IG. Clinical prediction rules: a review of suggested modifications of methodological standards. JAMA. 1997;277:488–94.
24. McGinn TG, Guyatt GH, Wyer PC, Naylor CD, Stiell IG, Richardson WS. Users' guides to the medical literature, XXII: how to use an article about clinical decision rules. JAMA. 2000;284:79–84.
25. Jenkins JL, McCarthy ML, Sauer LM, Green GB, Stuart S, Thomas TL, et al. Mass-casualty triage: time for an evidence-based approach. Prehosp Disaster Med. 2008;23:3–8.
26. Frykberg ER. Medical management of disaster and mass casualties from terrorist bombings: how can we cope? J Trauma. 2002;53:201–12.
27. Kennedy K, Aghababian RV, Gans L, Lewis CP. Triage: techniques and applications in decision making. Ann Emerg Med. 1996;28:136–44.
28. Ashkenazi I, Turégano-Fuentes F, Einav S, Kessel B, Alfici R, Olsha O. Pitfalls to avoid in the medical management of mass casualty incidents following terrorist bombings: the hospital perspective. Eur J Trauma Emerg Surg. 2014;40:445–50. https://doi.org/10.1007/s00068-014-0403-x.

29. Seif D, Perera P, Mailhot T, Riley D, Mandavia D. Bedside ultrasound in resuscitation and the rapid ultrasound in shock protocol. Crit Care Res Pract. 2012;2012:503254. https://doi.org/10.1155/2012/503254.
30. Zanobetti M, Coppa A, Nazerian P, Grifoni S, Scorpiniti M, Innocenti F, et al. Sonography for trauma during the primary survey in the emergency department: the CA-FAST protocol. Eur J Trauma Emerg Surg. 2015; https://doi.org/10.1007/s00068-015-0620-y.
31. Sztajnkrycer MD, Baez AA, Luke A. FAST ultrasound as an adjunct to triage using the START mass casualty triage system: a preliminary descriptive system. Prehosp Emerg Care. 2006;10:96–102. https://doi.org/10.1080/10903120500373058.
32. Sarkisian AE, Khondkarian RA, Amirbekian NM, Bagdasarian NB, Khojayan RL, Oganesian YT. Sonographic screening of mass casualties for abdominal and renal injuries following the 1988 Armenian earthquake. J Trauma. 1991;31:247–50.
33. Blaivas M. Triage in the trauma bay with the focused abdominal sonography for trauma (FAST) examination. J Emerg Med. 2001;21:41–4.
34. Gates JD, Arabian S, Biddinger P, Blansfield J, Burke P, Chung S, et al. The initial response to the Boston Marathon bombing: lessons learned to prepare for the next disaster. Ann Surg. 2014;260:960–6. https://doi.org/10.1097/SLA.0000000000000914.
35. Kimberly HH, Stone MB. Clinician-performed ultrasonography during the Boston Marathon bombing mass casualty incident. Ann Emerg Med. 2013;62:199–200.
36. Stawicki SP, Howard JM, Pryor JP, Bahner DP, Whitmill ML, Dean AJ. Portable ultrasonography in mass casualty incidents: the CAVEAT examination. World J Orthop. 2010;1:10–9. https://doi.org/10.5312/wjo.v1.i1.10.
37. Wydo SM, Seamon MJ, Melanson SW, Thomas P, Bahner DP, Stawicki SP. Portable ultrasound in disaster triage: a focused review. Eur J Trauma Emerg Surg. 2016;42:151–9. https://doi.org/10.1007/s00068-015-0498-8.
38. Phillips YY, Zajtchuk JT. The management of primary blast injury. In: Bellamy RF, Zajtchuk R, editors. Conventional warfare: ballistic, blast, and burn injuries. Ft Sam Houston: Borden Institute; 1991. p. 295–336.
39. Wightman JM. Pathophysiology of primary blast injury. Ann Emerg Med. 2017;70:104–5.
40. Rössle R. Pathology of blast effects. In: German aviation medicine: World War II. Washington: Office of the Surgeon General of the United States Air Force; 1950. p. 1260–73.
41. Leibovici D, Gofrit ON, Shapira SC. Eardrum perforation in explosion survivors: is it a marker of pulmonary blast injury? Ann Emerg Med. 1999;34:168–72.
42. Harmon JW, Sampson JA, Graeber GM, Phillips Y, Richmond D. Readily available serum chemical markers fail to aid in diagnosis of blast injury. J Trauma. 1988;28(1 suppl):S153–9.
43. DeMers G, Wightman J. Mass-casualty preparedness and response. In: O'Connor FG, Schoomaker EB, Smith DC, editors. Fundamentals of military medicine. Ft. Sam Houston: Borden Institute; 2019. p. 503–29.
44. Health Systems Research Inc. Altered standards of care in mass casualty events. Rockville: Agency for Healthcare Research and Quality; 2005.
45. Berger FH, Körner M, Berstein MP, Sodickson AD, Beenen LF, McLaughlin PD, et al. Emergency imaging after a mass casualty incident: role of the radiology department during training for and activation of a disaster management plan. Br J Radiol. 2016;89(1061):20150984. https://doi.org/10.1259/bjr.20150984.
46. Stengel D, Bauwens K, Sehouli J, Porzsolt F, Rademacher G, Mutze S, et al. Systematic review and meta-analysis of emergency ultrasonography for blunt trauma. Br J Surg. 2001;88:901–12. https://doi.org/10.1046/j.0007-1323.2001.01777.x.
47. Eastridge BJ, Mabry RL, Seguin P, Cantrell J, Tops T, Uribe P, et al. Death on the battlefield (2001–2011): implications for the future of combat casualty care. J Trauma Acute Care Surg. 2012;73(6 suppl 5):S431–7. https://doi.org/10.1097/TA.0b013e3182755dcc.
48. Mirza FH, Parhyar HA, Tirmizi SZA. Rising threat of terrorist bomb blasts in Karachi: a 5-year study. J Forensic Legal Med. 2013;20:747–51. https://doi.org/10.1016/j.jflm.2013.04.014.
49. Heldenberg E, Givon A, Simon D, Bass A, Almogy G, Kobi Peleg K. Civilian casualties of terror-related explosions: the impact of vascular trauma on treatment and prognosis. J Trauma Acute Care Surg. 2016;81:435–40. https://doi.org/10.1097/TA.0000000000001123.

50. Passos E, Dingley B, Smith A, Engels PT, Ball CG, Faidi S, et al. Tourniquet use for peripheral vascular injuries in the civilian setting. Injury. 2014;45:473–7. https://doi.org/10.1016/j.injury.2013.11.031.
51. Smith AA, Ochoa JE, Wong S, Beatty S, Elder J, Guidry C, et al. Prehospital tourniquet use in penetrating extremity trauma: decreased blood transfusions and limb complications. J Trauma Acute Care Surg. 2019;86:43–51. https://doi.org/10.1097/TA.0000000000002095.
52. Scerbo MH, Holcomb JB, Taub E, Gates K, Love JD, Wade CE, et al. The trauma center is too late: major limb trauma without a pre-hospital tourniquet has increased death from hemorrhagic shock. J Trauma Acute Care Surg. 2017;83:1165–72. https://doi.org/10.1097/TA.0000000000001666.
53. King DR, Larentzakis A, Ramly EP. Tourniquet use at the Boston Marathon bombing: lost in translation. J Trauma Acute Care Surg. 2015;78:594–9. https://doi.org/10.1097/TA.0000000000000561.
54. Bennett BL, Littlejohn LF, Kheirabadi BS, Butler FK, Kotwal RS, Dubick MA, et al. Management of external hemorrhage in tactical combat casualty care: chitosan-based hemostatic gauze dressings. J Spec Oper Med. 2013;13:12–29.
55. Bennett B, Littlejohn L. Review of new topical hemostatic dressings for combat casualty care. Mil Med. 2014;179:497–514. https://doi.org/10.7205/MILMED-D-13-00199.
56. RevMedX™. XSTAT®. https://www.revmedx.com/xstat/. Accessed 27 Feb 2020.
57. Wall PL, Duevel DC, Hassan MBWelander JD, Sahr SM, Buising CM. Tourniquets and occlusion: the pressure of design. Mil Med. 2013;178:578–87.
58. Manley JD, Mitchell BJ, DuBose JJ, Rasmussen TE. A modern case series of resuscitative endovascular balloon occlusion of the aorta (REBOA) in an out-of-hospital, combat casualty care setting. J Spec Oper Med. 2017;17:1–8.
59. Nelson D, Porta C, Satterly S, Blair K, Johnson E, Inaba K, et al. Physiology and cardiovascular effect of severe tension pneumothorax in a porcine model. J Surg Res. 2013;184:450–7. https://doi.org/10.1016/j.jss.2013.05.057.
60. Pizov R, Oppenheim-Eden A, Matot I, Weiss YG, Eidelman LA, Rivkind AI, et al. Blast lung injury from an explosion on a civilian bus. Chest. 1999;115:165–72.
61. Butler FK, Holcomb JB, Shackelford S, Montgomery HR, Anderson S, Cain JS, et al. Management of suspected tension pneumothorax in tactical combat casualty care. J Spec Oper Med. 2018;18:19–35.
62. High K, Brywczynski J, Guillamondegui O. Safety and efficacy of thoracostomy in the air medical environment. Air Med J. 2016;35:227–30. https://doi.org/10.1016/j.amj.2016.04.002.
63. Avidan V, Hersch M, Armon Y, Spira R, Aharoni D, Reissman P, et al. Blast lung injury: clinical manifestations, treatment, and outcome. Am J Surg. 2005;190:927–31. https://doi.org/10.1016/j.amsurg.2005.08.022.
64. Kim J, Polk T. Blast lung injury severity score. MDCalc. https://www.mdcalc.com/blast-lung-injury-severity-score#evidence. Accessed 27 Feb 2020.
65. Wightman JM, Gladish SL. Explosions and blast injuries. Ann Emerg Med. 2001;37:664–78. https://doi.org/10.1067/mem.2001.114906.
66. Caseby NG, Porter MF. Blast injuries to the lungs: clinical presentation, management and course. Injury. 1976;8:1–12.
67. Ho AM, Ling E. Systemic air embolism after lung trauma. Anesthesiology. 1999;90:564–75.
68. Klein Y, Arieli I, Sagiv S, Peleg K, Ben-Galim P. Cervical spine injuries in civilian victims of explosions: should cervical collars be used? J Trauma Acute Care Surg. 2016;80:985–8. https://doi.org/10.1097/TA.0000000000001040.
69. Blair JA, Possley DR, Petfield JL, Schoenfeld AJ, Lehman RA, Hsu JR. Military penetrating spine injuries compared with blunt. Spine J. 2012;12:762–8. https://doi.org/10.1016/j.spinee.2011.10.009.
70. Schoenfeld AJ, Goodman GP, Belmont PJ. Characterization of combat-related spinal injuries sustained by a US Army Brigade Combat Team during Operation Iraqi Freedom. Spine J. 2012;12:771–6. https://doi.org/10.1016/j.spinee.2010.05.004.
71. Abbotts R, Harrison SE, Cooper GL. Primary blast injuries to the eye: a review of the evidence. J R Army Med Corps. 2007;153:119–23.

72. Centers for Disease Control and Prevention. Explosions and blast injuries: a primer for clinicians. https://www.cdc.gov/masstrauma/preparedness/primer.pdf. Accessed 27 Feb 2020.
73. Yonekawa Y, Hacker HD, Lehman RE, Beal CJ, Veldman PB, Vyas NM, et al. Ocular blast injuries in mass-casualty incidents: the marathon bombing in Boston, Massachusetts, and the fertilizer plant explosion in West, Texas. Ophthalmology. 2014;121:1670–6. https://doi.org/10.1016/j.ophtha.2014.04.004.
74. Harlan JB, Pieramici DJ. Evaluation of patients with ocular trauma. Ophthalmol Clin N Am. 2002;15:153–61.
75. Weichel ED, Coyler MH. Combat ocular trauma and systemic injury. Curr Opin Ophthalmol. 2008;19:519–25. https://doi.org/10.1097/ICU.0b013e3283140e98.
76. Ritchie JV, Horne ST, Perry J, Gay D. Ultrasound triage of ocular blast injury in the military emergency department. Mil Med. 2012;177:174–8.
77. Wightman JM, Hurley LD. Emergency department management of eye injuries. Crit Decis Emerg Med. 1998;12(7):1–11.
78. Owers C, Morgan JL, Garner JP. Abdominal trauma in primary blast injury. Br J Surg. 2011;98:168–79. https://doi.org/10.1002/bjs.7268.
79. Turégano-Fuentes F, Pérez-Diaz D, Sanz-Sánchez M, Alfici R, Ashkenazi I. Abdominal blast injuries: different patterns, severity, management, and prognosis according to the main mechanism of injury. Eur J Trauma Emerg Surg. 2014;40:451–60. https://doi.org/10.1007/s00068-014-0397-4.
80. Paran H, Neufeld D, Schwartz I, Kidron D, Susmallian S, Mayo A, et al. Perforation of the terminal ileum induced by blast injury: delayed diagnosis or delayed perforation? J Trauma. 1996;40:472–5.
81. Cripps NPJ, Cooper GJ. Risk of late perforation in intestinal contusions caused by explosive blast. Br J Surg. 1997;84:1298–303.
82. Hare S, Goddard I, Ward P, Naraghi A, Dick A. The radiological management of bomb blast injury. Clin Radiol. 2007;62:1–9. https://doi.org/10.1016/j.crad.2006.09.013.
83. Zissin R, Osadchy A, Gayer A. Abdominal CT findings in small bowel perforation. Br J Radiol. 2009;82:162–71. https://doi.org/10.1259/bjr/78772574.
84. Brody JM, Leighton DB, Murphy BL, Abbott GF, Vaccaro JP, Jagminas L, et al. CT of blunt trauma bowel and mesenteric injury: typical findings and pitfalls in diagnosis. Radiographics. 2000;20:1525–36. https://doi.org/10.1148/radiographics.20.6.g00nv021525.
85. Butela ST, Federle MP, Chang PJ, Thaete FL, Peterson MS, Dorvault CJ, et al. Performance of CT in detection of bowel injury. AJR. 2001;176:129–35. https://doi.org/10.2214/ajr.176.1.1760129.
86. Chiu WC. Abdominal injuries without hemoperitoneum: a potential limitation of focused abdominal sonography for trauma (FAST). J Trauma. 1997;42:617–23.
87. Horton LK, Jacobson JA, Powell A, Fessell DP, Hayes CW. Sonography and radiography of soft-tissue foreign bodies. AJR. 2001;176:1155–9. https://doi.org/10.2214/ajr.176.5.1761155.
88. Davis J, Czerniski B, Au A, Adhikari S, Farrell I, Fields MJ. Diagnostic accuracy of ultrasonography in retained soft tissue foreign bodies: a systematic review and meta-analysis. Acad Emerg Med. 2015;22:777–87. https://doi.org/10.1111/acem.12714.
89. Dulchavsky SA, Henry SE, Moed BR, Diebel LN, Marshburn T, Hamilton DR, et al. Advanced ultrasonic diagnosis of extremity trauma: the FASTER examination. J Trauma. 2002;53:28–32.
90. Brooks AJ, Price V, Simms M, Ward N, Hand CJ. Handheld ultrasound diagnosis of extremity fractures. J R Army Med Corps. 2004;150:78–80.
91. Chukwu-Lobelu R, Appukuttan A, Edwards DS, Patel HDL. Burn injuries from the London suicide bombings: a new classification of blast-related thermal injuries. Ann Burns Fire Disasters. 2017;30:256–60.
92. Gomez Morell PA, Naif FE, Palao Domenech R, Sospedra Carol E, Bañuelos Roda JA. Burns caused by the terrorist bombing of the department store Hipercor in Barcelona. Part 1. Burns. 1990;16:423–5.
93. Jimenez-Hernandez FH, Lliro Blasco E, Leiva Oliva R, Caicedo JC, Bañuelos Roda JA. Burns caused by the terrorist bombing of the department store Hipercor in Barcelona. Part 2. Burns. 1990;16:426–31.

94. Rosenfeld JV, McFarlane AC, Bragge P, Armondo RA, Grimes JB, Ling GS. Blast-related traumatic brain injury. Lancet Neurol. 2013;12:882–93. https://doi.org/10.1016/S1474-4422(13)70161-3.
95. Defense and Veterans Brain Injury Center. Military Acute Concussion Evaluation 2 (MACE 2). https://dvbic.dcoe.mil/material/military-acute-concussion-evaluation-2-mace-2. Accessed 27 Feb 2020.
96. Swanson TM, Isaacson BM, Cybroski CM, French LM, Tsao JW, Pasquina PF. Traumatic brain injury incidence, clinical overview, and policies in the US Military Health System since 2000. Public Health Rep. 2017;132:251–9. https://doi.org/10.1177/0033354916687748.
97. Edwards DS, Barnett-Vanes A, Narayan N, Patel HD. Prophylaxis for blood-borne diseases during the London 7/7 mass casualty terrorist bombing: a review and the role of bioethics. J R Army Med Corps. 2016;162:330–4. https://doi.org/10.1136/jramc-2015-000546.
98. MacKenzie EJ, Rivara FP, Jurkovich GJ, Nathens AB, Frey KP, Egleston BL, et al. A national evaluation of the effect of trauma-center care on mortality. N Engl J Med. 2006;354:366–78. https://doi.org/10.1056/NEJMsa052049.
99. Ciesla DJ, Sava JA, Street JH, Jordan MH. Secondary overtriage: a consequence of an immature trauma system. J Am Coll Surg. 2006;206:131–7. https://doi.org/10.1016/j.jamcollsurg.2007.06.285.
100. Hadden WA, Rutherford WH, Merrett JD. The injuries of terrorist bombings: a study of 1532 consecutive patients. Br J Surg. 1978;65:525–31.
101. Pyper PC, Graham WJH. Analysis of terrorist injuries treated at Craigavon Area Hospital, Northern Ireland, 1972–1980. Injury. 1983;14:332–8.
102. Adler J, Golan E, Golan J, Yitzhaki M, Ben-Hur N. Terrorist bombing experience during 1975–79: casualties admitted to the Shaare Zedek Medical Center. Isr J Med Sci. 1983;19:189–93.
103. Rodoplu U, Arnold JL, Tokyay R, Ersoy G, Cetiner S, Yücel T. Mass-casualty terrorist combings in Istanbul, Turkey, November 2003: report of the events and the prehospital emergency response. Prehosp Disaster Med. 2004;19:133–45.
104. Turégano-Fuentes F, Pérez-Díaz D, Sanz-Sánchez M, Ortiz Alonso J. Overall assessment of the response to terrorist bombings in trains: Madrid, 11 March 2004. Eur J Trauma Emerg Surg. 2008;34:433–41. https://doi.org/10.1007/s00068-008-8805-2.
105. Lippa SM, Pastorek NJ, Benge JF, Thornto GM. Postconcussive symptoms after blast and nonblast-related mild traumatic brain injuries in Afghanistan and Iraq war veterans. J Int Neuropsychol Soc. 2010;16:856–66. https://doi.org/10.1017/S1355617710000743.
106. Defense and Veterans Brain Injury Center. Progressive return to activity following acute concussion/mild TBI clinical suite. https://dvbic.dcoe.mil/material/progressive-return-activity-following-acute-concussionmild-tbi-clinical-suite. Accessed 27 Feb 2020.
107. Tanielian T, Jaycox LH, editors. Invisible wounds of war: psychological and cognitive injuries, their consequences, and services to assist recovery. Santa Monica: RAND Corporation; 2008.
108. Lowell A, Suarez-Jimenez B, Helpman L, Zhu X, Durosky A, Hilburn A, et al. 9/11-related PTSD among highly exposed populations: a systematic review 15 years after the attack. Psychol Med. 2018;48:537–53. https://doi.org/10.1017/S0033291717002033.
109. US Department of Veterans Affairs National Center for PTSD. How common is PTSD? https://www.ptsd.va.gov/PTSD/understand/common/index.asp. Accessed 27 Feb 2020.
110. Bryant R. Post-traumatic stress disorder vs traumatic brain injury. Dialogues Clin Neurosci. 2011;13:251–62.
111. Defense and Veterans Brain Injury Center. http://dvbic.dcoe.mil/resources. Accessed 27 Feb 2020.

The Role of Blood Products in Damage Control Resuscitation in Explosion-Related Trauma

22

Jansen N. Seheult and Mark H. Yazer

Introduction

Damage control resuscitation (DCR) of the massively bleeding trauma patient comprises early intervention with blood products to replete intravascular volume, restore tissue oxygenation, and correct coagulopathy until surgical hemostasis can be achieved. Blood product resuscitation in the emergency department (ED), and also in the prehospital setting, must be coordinated, prompt, multifaceted, and evidence-based and should incorporate the appropriate use of laboratory tests and adjunct therapies, which facilitate DCR and damage control surgery. Hemostatic resuscitation should also address the management of the acute and delayed complications of massive transfusion including electrolyte imbalances, interstitial edema, acidosis, and hypothermia.

Uncontrolled or refractory hemorrhage accounts for up to 40% of trauma-related mortality among injured civilian patients admitted to trauma centers, and up to 5% of general civilian trauma patients require a massive transfusion [1, 2]. Mass casualty events (MCE) associated with blast injuries, such as civilian bombings, can place an even greater strain on a hospital's, or even a region's, blood product inventory due to the number of casualties involved, the unpredictability of the events, and the distribution and severity of injuries [3].

J. N. Seheult
Department of Pathology, University of Pittsburgh Medical Center, Pittsburgh, PA, USA

M. H. Yazer (✉)
University of Pittsburgh, Pittsburgh, PA, USA
e-mail: myazer@itxm.org

D. W. Callaway, J. L. Burstein (eds.), *Operational and Medical Management of Explosive and Blast Incidents*, https://doi.org/10.1007/978-3-030-40655-4_22

Historical Review of Blood Product Resuscitation in Blast Injury

To treat the injuries that patients sustained during the London, England, bombings of 2005, hospitals ordered a total of 978 units of red blood cells (RBC), 36 doses of platelets (PLT), 141 units of plasma, and 300 doses of cryoprecipitate from the National Blood Service in the United Kingdom [4]. However, less than half (440) of the RBC units ordered by hospitals were ultimately transfused to a total of 25 critically ill patients. Most of the units were transfused within the patients' first 36 hours of admission: 336 of the RBC units, along with 106 units of plasma, 235 units of cryoprecipitate, and 29 PLT doses. Those casualties who had sustained traumatic amputations required the greatest number of blood products.

During the Boston marathon bombing in 2013, 281 people were injured and cared for at 26 hospitals. Of the 75 patients admitted for further management at trauma centers, close to 12% required immediate transfusion of RBCs in the ED [5]. Data from two of the Boston hospitals showed that 168 uncrossmatched group O RBC units were issued to 58 injured patients. There were two massive transfusion protocol (MTP) activations at those two hospitals, and thirteen patients were transfused with 48 RBC and 35 plasma units within 24 hours of admission [6].

The Israeli experience with blood product transfusion at a single level 1 trauma center following 17 civilian bombing attacks from 2000 to 2005 found that close to 40% of blast-injured patients required blood products [7]. The 53 transfused patients received a total of 524 RBC units, 42 whole blood (WB) units, and 449 plasma units. Close to half of all of the RBC units transfused to these 53 patients were given within the first 2 hours of admission. While only a quarter of these patients (14/53) required a massive transfusion, those that did require a massive transfusion used more than 75% of all of the RBC units transfused during the study period (399 RBC units), and these 14 patients were transfused with a mean of 28.5 (range: 10–59) RBC units.

The military experience with 26 MCEs from 2003 to 2004 during Operation Iraqi Freedom is similar (average number of RBC units transfused per patient: 1.4 ± 0.8), with 22% of all evacuated casualties from an MCE requiring transfusion and 4.2% requiring a massive transfusion [8]. There were more massive transfusions administered to patients injured by discrete explosion-related events compared with patients injured from firefights (9.6% vs. 4.0%, respectively, $p < 0.05$). It is also clear that blast injury to certain organ systems, such as the lungs, confers an even higher blood product requirement during their resuscitation. Of the 11.2% of patients admitted to a NATO Role 3 hospital in Afghanistan from January 2008 to March 2013 with a primary blast lung injury, the majority received a massive transfusion (average of 33.4 ± 38.3 RBC units per patient over 24 hours) [9].

Coagulopathy of Trauma

Traditional models that ascribe the etiology of coagulation defects in an injured patient to the trauma itself and to the effects of the ensuing resuscitation effort, such as hemodilution, hypothermia, acidosis, and coagulation factor depletion, do not fully explain the clinically observed defects. More recently, a newly recognized coagulopathic process occurring within the first few hours of injury in up to 24% of trauma patients and resulting from dysregulation of multiple procoagulant, anticoagulant and fibrinolytic pathways, and the so-called early trauma-induced coagulopathy (ETIC), has been described [10, 11]. There have been two main mechanisms proposed to explain the pathogenesis of ETIC: (1) activation of protein C by thrombin-thrombomodulin complexes resulting in degradation of plasminogen activator inhibitor 1 (PAI-1) [12, 13], an important inhibitor of fibrinolysis, and (2) overwhelming release of tissue plasminogen activator (tPA) from the vascular endothelium (Fig. 22.1) [14].

Modern resuscitation of traumatically injured patients involves minimizing hypothermia and acidosis and reversing the ETIC. Due to the deleterious consequences of administering large quantities of isotonic crystalloid or colloid solutions, including but not limited to clot disruption, dilutional coagulopathy, and pro-inflammatory

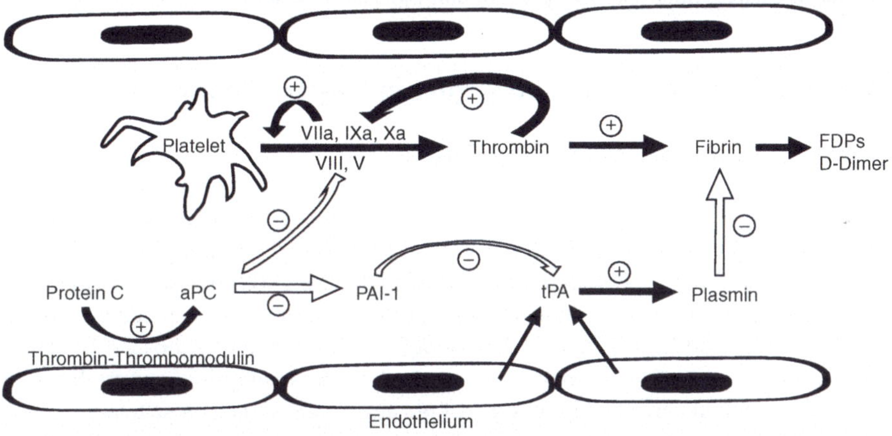

Fig. 22.1 Mechanisms of early trauma-induced coagulopathy. Protein C is activated by thrombin-thrombomodulin complexes. Activated protein C inactivates factors V and VIII and plasminogen activator inhibitor-1 (PAI-1). Damage to the endothelium stimulates release of tissue-type plasminogen activator (tPA). Inactivation of PAI-1 and release of tPA both contribute to the hyperfibrinolysis observed in the early trauma period. aPC activated protein C, FDPs fibrin degradation products

effects of these fluids on the endothelial glycocalyx [15–18], there has been a paradigm shift toward the early use of blood products and the limitation of crystalloid and colloid fluids, which are physiologically inert insofar as they do not have oxygen-carrying capacity or supply coagulation factors [19].

Massive Transfusion Protocol

Massive transfusion protocols (MTPs) facilitate the rapid delivery of blood products to a bleeding patient via a formal institutional response procedure. MTP activation usually occurs at the first point of contact with the injured trauma patient in the ED [20], although there is a survival benefit to providing blood products even before the patient arrives in the ED [21, 22]. Development of an MTP is an institutional affair and requires a multidisciplinary approach involving physicians, nurses, and laboratory staff. Factors such as staffing levels and competency; communication pathways; facilities for laboratory monitoring, including at the point of care; and logistics of specimen and blood product transportation and proper storage in order to minimize waste should be considered in implementing an MTP. Retrospective data suggest improved survival after implementation of an MTP [23–25], likely resulting from enhanced communication between the clinical staff and the transfusion service and/or optimization of blood product availability and transportation leading to earlier transfusion of plasma and platelet products.

Blood Product Transfusion Strategies in Massive Hemorrhage

Fixed-Ratio Component Therapy (FRCT)

A fixed-ratio component transfusion (FRCT) strategy aims to recapitulate the contents of whole blood using blood components, which is especially important in the early stages of DCR. Proposed in the 1980s and 1990s in the military setting, FRCT gained popularity in the civilian trauma setting in the late 2000s based on mathematical models and retrospective studies that purported to show a survival benefit among those who received higher ratios of plasma:RBCs compared to those with lower ratios [26, 27]. In 2007, Borgman et al. reported a significantly lower mortality rate among those who received a higher ratio of plasma to RBCs (i.e., close to a 1:1 ratio) compared to those who received a lower plasma:RBC ratio in a retrospective study of 246 military patients receiving massive transfusion at an Army Combat Support Hospital. However, survivor bias (i.e., patients who lived longer because they were less severely injured received more plasma) likely had a major impact on this result [28]. A series of retrospective civilian trauma studies that followed failed to clarify the benefits of FRCT due to important confounding factors that were present in these studies that limit their generalizability and the strength of their conclusions [29, 30].

The prospective, observational, multicenter, major trauma transfusion (PROMMTT) study, which was a prospective study conducted at ten level 1 trauma centers in the United States, examined the relationship of in-hospital mortality to early transfusion of plasma and/or platelets and to plasma:RBC and platelet:RBC ratios during the first 6 hours of resuscitation [31]. In this study, a low plasma:RBC transfusion ratio (<1:2) was associated with increased mortality only in the first 24 hours after admission, while the subsequent risk of death at 30 days was not related to the plasma:RBC or platelet:RBC ratio. The Pragmatic Randomized Optimal Platelet and Plasma Ratios (PROPPR) trial, which followed and which remains the largest randomized controlled trial to date on FRCT in trauma, found no differences in the primary outcomes of 24-hour and 30-day all-cause mortality in the 680 traumatically injured patients who were randomized to receive plasma, platelets, and red blood cells in a 1:1:1 ratio versus a 1:1:2 ratio [32]. However, the investigators did note that several secondary outcome analyses favored the 1:1:1 ratio group, including reduced exsanguination as the primary cause of death within 24 hours of admission and achieving anatomical hemostasis. The major limitation of the PROPPR trial was the absence of an intervention arm where the patients' resuscitations were guided by something other than FRCT, such as goal-directed resuscitation based on conventional laboratory testing or viscoelastic tests (VETs). Therefore, while there appears to be no significant difference in survival using a 1:1:1 ratio versus a 1:1:2 ratio in DCR, the question of the most effective technique for resuscitating bleeding trauma patients remains elusive.

Goal-Directed Component Therapy (GDCT)

Goal-directed component therapy (GDCT) aims to replace the specific hemostatic factors that the patient is missing, thus minimizing over- and under-transfusion, wastage, and the incidence of transfusion-related complications. In this regard, GDCT represents a lean, more individualized approach to DCR compared to FRCT. In GDCT, laboratory tests of hemostasis and oxygen-carrying capacity form the basis for decisions regarding blood product use. The utility of GDCT in guiding the dynamic resuscitation of a trauma patient was, in the past, limited by the typically long turnaround time of traditional laboratory testing such as the complete blood count (CBC), prothrombin time (PT), activated partial thromboplastin time (aPTT), and fibrinogen assays. However, more recently, the use of global tests of coagulation, mainly VETs such as thromboelastography (TEG) and rotational thromboelastometry (ROTEM), has made this approach more practical and feasible allowing earlier detection of coagulopathy and more accurate prediction of transfusion requirements compared with conventional coagulation assays (CCAs) [33, 34]. VETs, when offered at the point of care, can provide actionable results pertaining to the activity of coagulation factors (including fibrinogen) and platelet count and function within 30 minutes and can also provide information about hyper- and hypo-fibrinolysis within 60 minutes [35]. Thus, information derived from the tracings can be used to guide real-time blood component therapy. Additional benefits of VETs are that they are performed using whole blood, thus accounting for the patient's red cell contribution to the fibrin clot [36], and that they can be performed at the patient's core temperature, accounting for the potential effect of hypothermia on coagulation factor activity (although the importance of temperature-adjusted VET is still debatable) [37].

The following optimal thresholds have been suggested for TEG-guided massive transfusion resuscitation: plasma transfusion for a TEG-activated clotting time (TEG-ACT) > 128 seconds, cryoprecipitate transfusion for an α-angle <65°, platelet transfusion for a maximal amplitude (MA) < 55, and antifibrinolytic agents for an LY30 > 5%, although these recommendations should be considered in the context of the patient's clinical situation [38]. Studies comparing GDCT to FRCT have shown promising results [39, 40]. A pragmatic, randomized clinical trial (RCT), which included 111 patients admitted to a level 1 trauma center, demonstrated a survival benefit of TEG-directed MTP compared to CCA-guided MTP (80.4% vs. 63.6%, $p = 0.049$) [40].

The benefits and limitations of FRCT and GDCT have been extensively debated [41]. In the explosion-related MCE, the volume of high-acuity patients may place logistical and operational challenges on broad use of VETs. Based on the available evidence and practical experience, utilizing an FRCT strategy in the early stages of DCR when laboratory results are not immediately available appears to be a reasonable approach, as it emphasizes plasma replacement for the significant minority of trauma patients who are coagulopathic upon presentation in the ED. As soon as the results of VETs and/or CCAs are available, however, there should be a transition to GDCT for the remainder of the resuscitation.

Operational Aspects of an MTP

An institutional MTP should contain clear guidance on the following: the criteria for MTP activation, including who is authorized to initiate it; a validated mechanism for notification of the transfusion service/blood bank and general laboratory; an algorithm outlining the CCAs, VETs, and other tests, such as blood gases and ionized calcium levels, their frequency, and details about specimen types and transportation to the laboratory; blood product preparation and delivery guidelines including predetermined MTP package contents; and other patient care needs such as blood warmers and nursing care (Fig. 22.2).

What Constitutes a Massive Transfusion and When Should an MTP Be Initiated?

Massive transfusion has traditionally been defined as the transfusion of 10 or more RBC units within 24 hours [42, 43]; however, more recent pragmatic definitions include (1) transfusion of four or more RBC units within 1 hour with anticipation of continued need for blood product support [44] and (2) replacement of 50% of the total blood volume within 4 hours [45]. Predicting which hemorrhaging trauma patient is likely to require a massive transfusion can be difficult during the early stages of resuscitation. Trauma team clinical judgment appears to be the most frequently used trigger for MTP activation, followed by hypotension and administration of uncrossmatched blood products [46].

Two commonly used composite scoring systems, which have proven to be accurate in the prediction of which civilian trauma patients will require a massive transfusion, are presented in Table 22.1 [47, 48]. While these scores have been validated

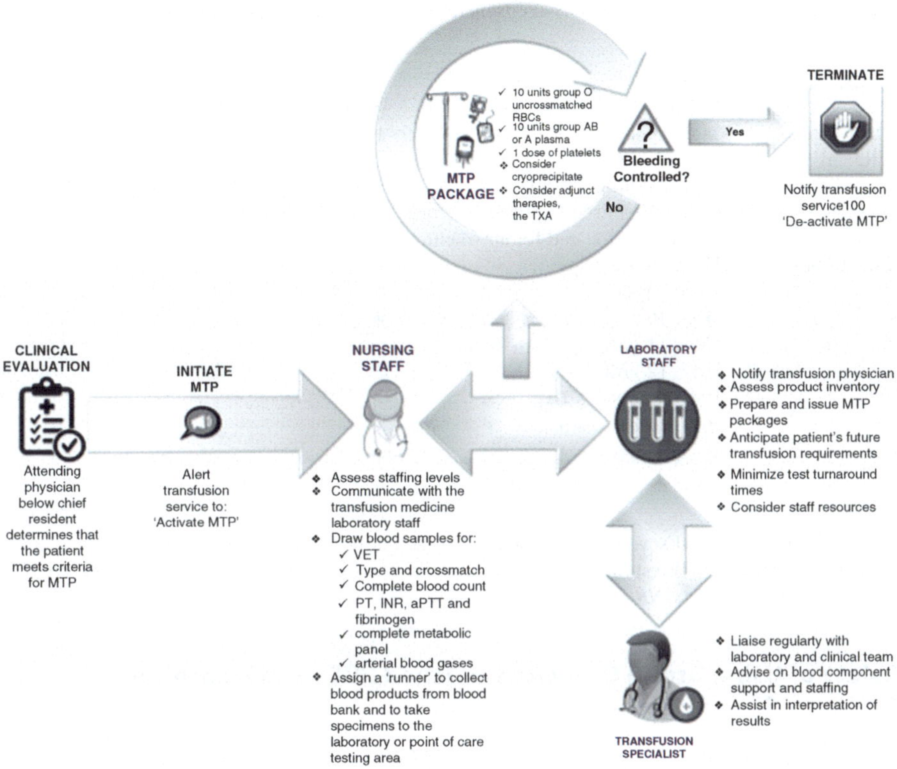

Fig. 22.2 Sample massive transfusion protocol (MTP) algorithm. Note that the contents of the MTP package can vary by institution. PT prothrombin time, aPTT activated partial thromboplastin time, INR international normalized ratio, TXA tranexamic acid, VET viscoelastic tests

extensively in general civilian trauma populations, their accuracy in the civilian and military blast injury settings remains to be verified. In fact, one study of 137 civilian blast injury patients identified between January 1993 and November 2012 in the TraumaRegister DGU of the German Trauma Society (TR-DGU) reported that the Trauma Associated Severe Hemorrhage (TASH) score underestimated the probability for transfusion of more than 10 units of packed red blood cells (5.0% estimated vs. 12.5% actual) [49].

MTP Packages

During an MTP activation, blood components are issued from the transfusion service/blood bank in rounds until the MTP is deactivated. MTP packages issued in this fashion contain RBCs and plasma (in coolers) and platelets (at room temperature) in a close to 1:1:1 ratio. The number and type of blood products in each MTP round should be based on the needs of the individual institution. Additionally, trauma centers usually store uncrossmatched group O RBCs in an easily accessible location in the trauma bay, with or without thawed plasma.

Table 22.1 Prediction tools for massive transfusion in the civilian post-trauma and liver transplantation settings [43, 44, 46]

	TASH Score		ABC Score	
	Criteria	Score	Criteria	Score
Demographic	Male gender	1		
Clinical	HR > 120 b/min	2	SBP < 90 mm Hg	1
	Free abdominal fluid	3	HR > 120 b/min	1
	Clinically unstable pelvic fracture	6	Penetrating mechanism	1
	Open or dislocated femur fracture	3	Positive FAST	1
Laboratory	Hb < 7 g/dl	8		
	Hb < 9 g/dl	6		
	Hb < 10 g/dl	4		
	Hb < 11 g/dl	3		
	Hb < 12 g/dl	2		
	Base excess < −10	4		
	Base excess < −6	3		
	Base excess < −2	1		
Maximum score		*29*		*4*
Threshold		*≥18*		*≥2*

TASH trauma-associated severe hemorrhage, *Hb* hemoglobin, *HR* heart rate, *ABC* assessment of blood consumption, *SBP* systolic blood pressure, *FAST* focused abdominal sonography for trauma, *MT* massive transfusion, *INR* international normalized ratio

Safety of Using Group O Uncrossmatched RBCs and Transition to Group-Specific Blood Components

Uncrossmatched group O RBCs can be issued quickly from the transfusion service or, if available, can be obtained from the trauma bay refrigerator for transfusion to a recipient of unknown ABO group. Group O RBCs are used since they will be compatible with the recipient's preformed anti-A and/or anti-B isohemagglutinins. The risk of a hemolytic transfusion reaction with uncrossmatched group O RBCs, even in patients with active alloantibodies against minor (i.e., non-A/ on-B) red cell antigens, is very low [50–52]. No acute hemolytic transfusion reactions were identified in one study of 581 uncrossmatched group O RBCs transfused to 161 patients [53]. In another study, only one out of 262 patients who received uncrossmatched group O RBCs had a hemolytic transfusion reaction, and the etiology of hemolysis was not firmly linked to the receipt of the incompatible RBC units [54]. Based on these safety data, lifesaving uncrossmatched RBCs should not be withheld from the resuscitation of a hemodynamically unstable trauma patient while awaiting group-specific products and the results of the antibody detection test.

Samples for ABO blood group determination, antibody detection, and RBC crossmatch should ideally be collected prior to transfusion of uncrossmatched RBCs, or as early in the resuscitation as possible, and should be sent to the blood bank as soon as possible. A check-ABO sample, required at many institutions in the United States, serves to confirm the ABO group in patients without a historic ABO group on file at the blood bank, thereby helping to prevent ABO mismatched transfusions by detecting wrong blood in tube (WBIT) miscollections [55]. Once the patient's samples have been received in the transfusion service, ABO-group-specific blood products can usually be provided by the blood bank within 15 minutes, and crossmatched RBCs can be provided within an hour, as long as an unexpected antibody to minor red cell antigens is not identified. Such unexpected antibodies are detected in ~5% of transfused patients [56], require further investigation to identify the nature of the antibody, and then find compatible RBC units; this process usually takes several hours to complete. After the testing is completed and if no unexpected antibodies are identified, crossmatched RBCs can be issued within minutes of ordering if an electronic crossmatch system is in place in the hospital's transfusion service.

The transition to ABO-group-specific blood products is especially important in the case of plasma products, since it helps conserve the often-limited AB plasma inventory (AB donors comprise only 4% of all donors in Caucasian cohorts), which can be rapidly depleted in an MCE setting. Trauma centers can supplement the limited AB plasma inventory by using group A plasma (see the Section "Thawed Plasma and Low-Titer Group A Plasma").

Platelets are generally transfused without regard to donor and recipient ABO groups in adult patients in the United States due to chronic shortages of this product. Given that there have been very few reports of hemolysis among recipients of incompatible plasma, group-specific platelets are not usually required in most adult settings [57, 58].

Use of Rh(D)-Positive Products in Rh(D)-Negative or Rh(D) status Unknown Patients

Rh(D)-negative group O uncrossmatched RBCs are generally reserved for transfusion to females of childbearing potential due to the risk of Rh(D) alloimmunization (~21% for RBCs [59–61] and 1.4% for platelets [62]) and the potential for the resulting anti-D to cause severe hemolytic disease of the fetus and newborn (HDFN) [63]. The criteria for using Rh(D)-positive RBCs in Rh(D)-negative patients and in patients whose Rh(D) group is unknown should be clearly defined in the institution's standard operating procedures. The transfusion service may choose to switch massively bleeding Rh(D)-negative or Rh(D) status unknown men, and women who are no longer of childbearing potential, to Rh(D)-positive products after their gender and age are confirmed, in an attempt to conserve the Rh(D)-negative RBC inventory. However, it is important to remember that a potentially lifesaving transfusion with Rh(D)-positive RBCs or platelets should *not* be withheld from a female of childbearing potential if she is Rh(D)-negative, or if her Rh(D) group is unknown, and Rh(D)-negative RBCs or platelets are not available.

Thawed Plasma and Low-Titer Group A Plasma

Plasma is the preferred fluid for the replenishment of coagulation factors and the treatment of ETIC in order to avoid dilutional coagulopathy in the massive transfusion setting [64]. Both fresh frozen plasma (FFP), which is plasma frozen within 8 hours of collection, and plasma frozen within 24 hours of collection (PF24) can be stored in the liquid state for a maximum of 24 hours in the refrigerator after thawing [65]. Thawed plasma, on the other hand, can be stored for up to 5 days after thawing and is a practical solution for trauma centers, especially those with an institutional response plan for MCEs, since these units can be thawed ahead of time and stored in the trauma bay refrigerator. The longer storage period also reduces wastage and constraints on the blood bank's inventory.

As mentioned earlier, the transition to ABO-group-specific plasma is important for preserving the limited AB plasma inventory. As a result, there has been renewed interest in the use of group A plasma in DCR of bleeding trauma patients, with 97% of 61 surveyed level 1 trauma centers in the United States reporting that they maintained group A thawed plasma. Of those surveyed, 88% stated that group A plasma was immediately available for use in a resuscitation, and 69% reported use for trauma patients of unknown ABO group [66]. Of the centers that use group A plasma for massively bleeding patients, 62% do not limit the amount of group A plasma that can be administered to a recipient of unknown ABO group, and 79% do not titer the anti-B level in the group A plasma. The safety of group A plasma transfusion to recipients of unknown ABO group can be inferred from the very low rate of hemolytic transfusion reactions following the transfusion of ABO-mismatched platelet units, which contain the same amount of plasma as a plasma unit [65, 67]. Also the results of the retrospective Safety of The use of group A plasma in Trauma (STAT) study demonstrated no increase in in-hospital or early (<24 hours after admission) mortality or hospital length of stay between group A versus B and AB trauma patients who were resuscitated with at least one unit of group A plasma [68].

Cold-Stored Low-Titer Group O Whole Blood

The use of cold-stored, low-titer group O whole blood (LTOWB) for the management of civilian trauma patients is now expanding because of its many advantages compared to conventional component therapy. These advantages include a smaller volume of anticoagulants, preservatives, and additive solutions in the whole blood that leads to less dilution of hemostatic factors and platelets, reduced fluid redistribution to the interstitial fluid compartment, fewer donor exposures, and the simplification of the logistics of DCR as all the components of whole blood can be administered in one bag instead of up to four [69–71]. Platelets stored in the cold (1–6 °C) demonstrate improved function compared with room temperature-stored platelets in in vitro studies, and agitation of the whole blood is not required to preserve platelet function [72–76]. The decision on what constitutes a "low-titer" LTOWB unit remains at the discretion of each institution and should be selected based on the institution's tolerance of risk from hemolysis among non-group O recipients versus the extent of donor deferrals (i.e., a very low-titer threshold will result in a very low risk of hemolysis but a high rate of donor deferrals) [77]. At the authors' center, a critical titer threshold of <50 for both anti-A and anti-B is used to mitigate the risk of immediate hemolysis, but titers of <256 have also been successfully utilized [78].

Transfusion of up to four units of LTOWB has been demonstrated to be safe in civilian trauma patients with no demonstrable clinical or biochemical evidence of hemolysis observed in a retrospective study of 102 non-group O recipients compared to 70 group O recipients [79, 80]. Clinical outcomes, such as mortality and length of stay, among a propensity-matched cohort of 135 recipients of up to four units of LTOWB compared to 135 recipients of conventional components were also similar, with perhaps a faster resolution of an elevated admission lactate concentration among the LTOWB recipients [81]. Based on the initial safety profile and outcome data, at least 15 centers in the United States are now using LTOWB in the initial resuscitation of trauma patients [78, 80, 82, 83]. LTOWB could also prove to be the ideal prehospital resuscitation fluid since it provides plasma and functional platelets early in the resuscitation and since it can be stored and transported in the same way as RBC units, which are already used in the prehospital setting at certain institutions. A study comparing the outcomes of trauma patients who will be randomized to receive LTOWB versus RBC units alone in the prehospital setting commenced in the autumn of 2018 and is expected to be completed in late 2021 (Pragmatic Prehospital Group O Whole Blood Early Resuscitation Trial, PPOWER, NCT03477006).

Adjunct Therapies in Massive Transfusion

Primary hyperfibrinolysis has been reported in 34% of trauma patients requiring massive transfusion [84, 85]. Tranexamic acid (TXA) and epsilon-aminocaproic acid are lysine analogues, which inhibit fibrinolysis by reversibly antagonizing the lysine-binding site on plasminogen and plasmin [86]. The Clinical Randomization of an Antifibrinolytic in Significant Hemorrhage 2 (CRASH-2) trial demonstrated that the administration of TXA to bleeding trauma patients within the first 3 hours of injury reduced the risk of death due to bleeding without an increase in vascular occlusive events [87]. VETs may be useful in differentiating those patients with primary hyperfibrinolysis who are most likely to benefit from antifibrinolytic agents from those with physiologic fibrinolysis or fibrinolysis shutdown who may not require these agents [88, 89].

Given the limited retrospective efficacy data [90] and the absence of a prospective randomized controlled trial, the decision to use prothrombin complex concentrate (PCC) in DCR should be assessed on a case-by-case basis. There is no definitive data on the safety and efficacy of desmopressin, a synthetic analogue of the antidiuretic hormone vasopressin, in the treatment of trauma-related hemorrhage, and the use of activated recombinant factor VIIa (rFVIIa) is no longer recommended as an adjunct therapy in DCR [91, 92].

Disaster Preparedness in the Civilian Blood Bank

Disaster preparedness vis-à-vis blood product use has been extensively reported from the military experience [8, 93]. Much of the civilian literature describing how civilian hospitals and their transfusion services and blood banks have prepared for such an event derives from the experiences gained from terrorist attacks with a large number of ensuing casualties [6, 7, 94–99]. An in silico analysis of the effect of various-sized MCEs performed using military and civilian transfusion requirements revealed that many of the hospitals that would have received injured patients would have had their stocks of group O (universal donor) RBCs exhausted in a median of 10 hours or fewer depending on the number of casualties [98]. It is thus imperative that civilian hospitals have an emergency plan in place for how their blood banks will supply products to injured patients during an MCE and rapidly restock their inventories. Some critical aspects to consider include the reserves of products located at the receiving facility, their major blood suppliers, and other regional hospitals. Having a disaster plan agreed upon by the hospitals that are most likely to receive injured patients and those that would not likely receive patients but would use their inventory of products to resupply those that do before the MCE occurs is essential for the seamless activation of the disaster plan.

Beyond the physical proximity of these resources, the delivery mechanism of the blood products to the treating hospitals must also be considered; streets might become impassable due to evacuations or crime scene investigation limiting the ability to move blood products by car or van, public transit might be halted, and "no fly" zones might be imposed limiting helicopter movement. The same conditions that might limit the movement of blood products between hospitals and the blood centers might also prevent donors from attending blood donation drives to resupply the blood center. In addition, unlike canned food goods, RBCs have a short shelf life such that they cannot be stockpiled in a liquid form indefinitely. While RBCs can be frozen, thawing them is usually a manual process that can take several hours, and thawing the large number of RBCs that might be required in an MCE is impractically slow. Therefore, relying on a blood center's inventory of frozen RBCs for the initial resuscitation of the first wave of casualties is not likely to be a practical solution when liquid RBCs are urgently needed. Thus, not only should the disaster plan detail the willingness to provide blood products, but also rehearsals of how the products would be transported under various conditions that might occur during an MCE should regularly take place.

Conclusion

The evidence indicates that the early intervention with blood products in severely injured trauma patients saves lives. Supplying blood products prehospital is the ideal way to begin the resuscitation, and the rapid and appropriate activation of the hospital's MTP when the patient arrives at the ED helps to ensure that the clinical team has the blood products that are necessary to continue the resuscitation. The ideal formula for resuscitating massively bleeding trauma patients is currently unknown, but starting with an FRCT strategy in the early stages of DCR followed by a transition to GDCT when the results of VETs and/or CCAs become available would seem reasonable. Uncrossmatched group O RBCs can be issued quickly from the transfusion service or, if available, can be obtained from the trauma bay refrigerator. The use of group A plasma in DCR can help to preserve the blood bank's often-limited AB plasma inventory. LTOWB use in DCR is expanding because of its many advantages compared to conventional component therapy. The use of TXA in DCR is well-established, but the evidence is not as strong for other adjunct therapies. A rehearsed disaster plan, which includes consideration of blood product reserves, blood supply agreements, and logistics of blood product transportation during an MCE, is of critical importance.

Pitfalls

- Not having an institutional MTP or uncertainty about how to activate it
- Failure to administer blood products early in the resuscitation to patients who require it
- Not having a rehearsed disaster plan in place before it is required

References

1. Sauaia A, Moore FA, Moore EE, Moser KS, Brennan R, Read RA, et al. Epidemiology of trauma deaths: a reassessment. J Trauma. 1995;38:185–93.
2. Como JJ, Dutton RP, Scalea TM, Edelman BB, Hess JR. Blood transfusion rates in the care of acute trauma. Transfusion. 2004;44:809–13.
3. DePalma RG, Burris DG, Champion HR, Hodgson MJ. Blast injuries. N Engl J Med. 2005;352:1335–42.
4. Glasgow SM, Allard S, Doughty H, Spreadborough P, Watkins E. Blood and bombs: the demand and use of blood following the London Bombings of 7 July 2005--a retrospective review. Transfus Med. 2012;22:244–50.
5. Gates JD, Arabian S, Biddinger P, Blansfield J, Burke P, Chung S, et al. The initial response to the Boston marathon bombing: lessons learned to prepare for the next disaster. Ann Surg. 2014;260:960–6.
6. Quillen K, Luckey CJ. Blood and bombs: blood use after the Boston Marathon bombing of April 15, 2013. Transfusion. 2014;54:1202–3.
7. Bala M, Kaufman T, Keidar A, Zelig O, Zamir G, Mudhi-Orenshat S, et al. Defining the need for blood and blood products transfusion following suicide bombing attacks on a civilian population: a level I single-centre experience. Injury. 2014;45:50–5.
8. Beekley AC, Martin MJ, Spinella PC, Telian SP, Holcomb JB. Predicting resource needs for multiple and mass casualty events in combat: lessons learned from combat support hospital experience in Operation Iraqi Freedom. J Trauma. 2009;66:S129–37.
9. Aboudara M, Mahoney PF, Hicks B, Cuadrado D. Primary blast lung injury at a NATO Role 3 hospital. J R Army Med Corps. 2014;160:161–6.
10. MacLeod JB, Winkler AM, McCoy CC, Hillyer CD, Shaz BH. Early trauma induced coagulopathy (ETIC): prevalence across the injury spectrum. Injury. 2014;45:910–5.
11. Brohi K, Singh J, Heron M, Coats T. Acute traumatic coagulopathy. J Trauma. 2003;54:1127–30.
12. Dobson GP, Letson HL, Sharma R, Sheppard FR, Cap AP. Mechanisms of early trauma-induced coagulopathy: the clot thickens or not? J Trauma Acute Care Surg. 2015;79:301–9.
13. Brohi K, Cohen MJ, Ganter MT, Matthay MA, Mackersie RC, Pittet JF. Acute traumatic coagulopathy: initiated by hypoperfusion: modulated through the protein C pathway? Ann Surg. 2007;245:812–8.
14. Chapman MP, Moore EE, Moore HB, Gonzalez E, Gamboni F, Chandler JG, et al. Overwhelming tPA release, not PAI-1 degradation, is responsible for hyperfibrinolysis in severely injured trauma patients. J Trauma Acute Care Surg. 2016;80:16–23; discussion –5.

15. Holcomb JB, Jenkins D, Rhee P, Johannigman J, Mahoney P, Mehta S, et al. Damage control resuscitation: directly addressing the early coagulopathy of trauma. J Trauma. 2007;62:307–10.
16. Neal MD, Hoffman MK, Cuschieri J, Minei JP, Maier RV, Harbrecht BG, et al. Crystalloid to packed red blood cell transfusion ratio in the massively transfused patient: when a little goes a long way. J Trauma Acute Care Surg. 2012;72:892–8.
17. Duchesne JC, Heaney J, Guidry C, McSwain N Jr, Meade P, Cohen M, et al. Diluting the benefits of hemostatic resuscitation: a multi-institutional analysis. J Trauma Acute Care Surg. 2013;75:76–82.
18. Blumberg N, Cholette JM, Pietropaoli AP, Phipps R, Spinelli SL, Eaton MP, et al. 0.9% NaCl (normal saline) – perhaps not so normal after all? Transfus Apher Sci. 2018;57:127–31.
19. Myburgh JA, Mythen MG. Resuscitation fluids. N Engl J Med. 2013;369:2462–3.
20. Dunbar NM, Olson NJ, Szczepiorkowski ZM, Martin ED, Tysarcyk RM, Triulzi DJ, et al. Blood component transfusion and wastage rates in the setting of massive transfusion in three regional trauma centers. Transfusion. 2017;57:45–52.
21. Sperry JL, Guyette FX, Brown JB, Yazer MH, Triulzi DJ, Early-Young BJ, et al. Prehospital plasma during air medical transport in trauma patients at risk for hemorrhagic shock. N Engl J Med. 2018;379:315–26.
22. Shackelford SA, Del Junco DJ, Powell-Dunford N, Mazuchowski EL, Howard JT, Kotwal RS, et al. Association of prehospital blood product transfusion during medical evacuation of combat casualties in Afghanistan with acute and 30-day survival. JAMA. 2017;318:1581–91.
23. Riskin DJ, Tsai TC, Riskin L, Hernandez-Boussard T, Purtill M, Maggio PM, et al. Massive transfusion protocols: the role of aggressive resuscitation versus product ratio in mortality reduction. J Am Coll Surg. 2009;209:198–205.
24. Cotton BA, Au BK, Nunez TC, Gunter OL, Robertson AM, Young PP. Predefined massive transfusion protocols are associated with a reduction in organ failure and postinjury complications. J Trauma. 2009;66:41–8; discussion 8–9.
25. Zaydfudim V, Dutton WD, Feurer ID, Au BK, Pinson CW, Cotton BA. Exsanguination protocol improves survival after major hepatic trauma. Injury. 2010;41:30–4.
26. Hirshberg A, Dugas M, Banez EI, Scott BG, Wall MJ Jr, Mattox KL. Minimizing dilutional coagulopathy in exsanguinating hemorrhage: a computer simulation. J Trauma. 2003;54:454–63.
27. Ho AM, Dion PW, Cheng CA, Karmakar MK, Cheng G, Peng Z, et al. A mathematical model for fresh frozen plasma transfusion strategies during major trauma resuscitation with ongoing hemorrhage. Can J Surg. 2005;48:470–8.
28. Borgman MA, Spinella PC, Perkins JG, Grathwohl KW, Repine T, Beekley AC, et al. The ratio of blood products transfused affects mortality in patients receiving massive transfusions at a combat support hospital. J Trauma. 2007;63:805–13.
29. Duchesne JC, Hunt JP, Wahl G, Marr AB, Wang YZ, Weintraub SE, et al. Review of current blood transfusions strategies in a mature level I trauma center: were we wrong for the last 60 years? J Trauma. 2008;65:272–6; discussion 6–8.
30. Snyder CW, Weinberg JA, McGwin G Jr, Melton SM, George RL, Reiff DA, et al. The relationship of blood product ratio to mortality: survival benefit or survival bias? J Trauma. 2009;66:358–62; discussion 62–4.
31. Holcomb JB, del Junco DJ, Fox EE, Wade CE, Cohen MJ, Schreiber MA, et al. The prospective, observational, multicenter, major trauma transfusion (PROMMTT) study: comparative effectiveness of a time-varying treatment with competing risks. JAMA Surg. 2013;148:127–36.
32. Holcomb JB, Tilley BC, Baraniuk S, Fox EE, Wade CE, Podbielski JM, et al. Transfusion of plasma, platelets, and red blood cells in a 1:1:1 vs a 1:1:2 ratio and mortality in patients with severe trauma: the PROPPR randomized clinical trial. JAMA. 2015;313:471–82.
33. Jeger V, Zimmermann H, Exadaktylos AK. Can RapidTEG accelerate the search for coagulopathies in the patient with multiple injuries? J Trauma. 2009;66:1253–7.
34. Plotkin AJ, Wade CE, Jenkins DH, Smith KA, Noe JC, Park MS, et al. A reduction in clot formation rate and strength assessed by thrombelastography is indicative of transfusion requirements in patients with penetrating injuries. J Trauma. 2008;64:S64–8.

35. Hanke AA, Horstmann H, Wilhelmi M. Point-of-care monitoring for the management of trauma-induced bleeding. Curr Opin Anaesthesiol. 2017;30:250–6.
36. Ogawa S, Szlam F, Bolliger D, Nishimura T, Chen EP, Tanaka KA. The impact of hematocrit on fibrin clot formation assessed by rotational thromboelastometry. Anesth Analg. 2012;115:16–21.
37. Cundrle I Jr, Sramek V, Pavlik M, Suk P, Radouskova I, Zvonicek V. Temperature corrected thromboelastography in hypothermia: is it necessary? Eur J Anaesthesiol. 2013;30:85–9.
38. Einersen PM, Moore EE, Chapman MP, Moore HB, Gonzalez E, Silliman CC, et al. Rapid thrombelastography thresholds for goal-directed resuscitation of patients at risk for massive transfusion. J Trauma Acute Care Surg. 2017;82:114–9.
39. Johansson PI, Sorensen AM, Larsen CF, Windeløv NA, Stensballe J, Perner A, et al. Low hemorrhage-related mortality in trauma patients in a level I trauma center employing transfusion packages and early thromboelastography-directed hemostatic resuscitation with plasma and platelets. Transfusion. 2013;53:3088–99.
40. Gonzalez E, Moore EE, Moore HB, Chapman MP, Chin TL, Ghasabyan A, et al. Goal-directed hemostatic resuscitation of trauma-induced coagulopathy: a pragmatic randomized clinical trial comparing a viscoelastic assay to conventional coagulation assays. Ann Surg. 2016;263:1051–9.
41. Howley IW, Haut ER, Jacobs L, Morrison JJ, Scalea TM. Is thromboelastography (TEG)-based resuscitation better than empirical 1:1 transfusion? Trauma Surg Acute Care Open. 2018 Jan 8;3(1):e000140.
42. Raymer JM, Flynn LM, Martin RF. Massive transfusion of blood in the surgical patient. Surg Clin North Am. 2012;92:221–34. vii
43. Sharpe JP, Weinberg JA, Magnotti LJ, Croce MA, Fabian TC. Toward a better definition of massive transfusion: focus on the interval of hemorrhage control. J Trauma Acute Care Surg. 2012;73:1553–7.
44. Moren AM, Hamptom D, Diggs B, Kiraly L, Fox EE, Holcomb JB, et al. Recursive partitioning identifies greater than 4 U of packed red blood cells per hour as an improved massive transfusion definition. J Trauma Acute Care Surg. 2015;79:920–4.
45. Mitra B, Cameron PA, Gruen RL, Mori A, Fitzgerald M, Street A. The definition of massive transfusion in trauma: a critical variable in examining evidence for resuscitation. Eur J Emerg Med. 2011;18:137–42.
46. Camazine MN, Hemmila MR, Leonard JC, Jacobs RA, Horst JA, Kozar RA, et al. Massive transfusion policies at trauma centers participating in the American College of Surgeons Trauma Quality Improvement Program. J Trauma Acute Care Surg. 2015;78:S48–53.
47. Yucel N, Lefering R, Maegele M, Vorweg M, Tjardes T, Ruchholtz S, et al. Trauma Associated Severe Hemorrhage (TASH)-Score: probability of mass transfusion as surrogate for life threatening hemorrhage after multiple trauma. J Trauma. 2006;60:1228–36; discussion 36–7.
48. Cotton BA, Dossett LA, Haut ER, Shafi S, Nunez TC, Au BK, et al. Multicenter validation of a simplified score to predict massive transfusion in trauma. J Trauma. 2010;69(Suppl 1): S33–9.
49. Kulla M, Maier J, Bieler D, et al. Civilian blast injuries: an underestimated problem?: results of a retrospective analysis of the TraumaRegister DGU(R). Unfallchirurg. 2016;119: 843–53.
50. Boisen ML, Collins RA, Yazer MH, Waters JH. Pretransfusion testing and transfusion of uncrossmatched erythrocytes. Anesthesiology. 2015;122:191–5.
51. Yazer MH, Waters JH, Spinella PC, Cap CA, Fahie CRL Sr, Gourdine E, et al. Use of uncrossmatched erythrocytes in emergency bleeding situations. Anesthesiology. 2018;128:650–6.
52. Radkay L, Triulzi DJ, Yazer MH. Low risk of hemolysis after transfusion of uncrossmatched red blood cells. Immunohematology. 2012;28:39–44.
53. Dutton RP, Shih D, Edelman BB, Hess J, Scalea TM. Safety of uncrossmatched type-O red cells for resuscitation from hemorrhagic shock. J Trauma. 2005;59:1445–9.
54. Goodell PP, Uhl L, Mohammed M, Powers AA. Risk of hemolytic transfusion reactions following emergency-release RBC transfusion. Am J Clin Pathol. 2010;134:202–6.

55. Goodnough LT, Viele M, Fontaine MJ, Jurado C, Stone N, Quach P, et al. Implementation of a two-specimen requirement for verification of ABO/Rh for blood transfusion. Transfusion. 2009;49:1321–8.
56. Saverimuttu J, Greenfield T, Rotenko I, Crozier J, Jalaludin B, Harvey M. Implications for urgent transfusion of uncrossmatched blood in the emergency department: the prevalence of clinically significant red cell antibodies within different patient groups. Emerg Med (Fremantle). 2003;15:239–43.
57. Cid J, Harm SK, Yazer MH. Platelet transfusion – the art and science of compromise. Transfus Med Hemother. 2013;40:160–71.
58. Josephson CD, Castillejo MI, Grima K, Hillyer CD. ABO-mismatched platelet transfusions: strategies to mitigate patient exposure to naturally occurring hemolytic antibodies. Transfus Apher Sci. 2010;42:83–8.
59. Yazer MH, Triulzi DJ. Detection of anti-D in D- recipients transfused with D+ red blood cells. Transfusion. 2007;47:2197–201.
60. Gonzalez-Porras JR, Graciani IF, Perez-Simon JA, Martin-Sanchez J, Encinas C, Conde MP, et al. Prospective evaluation of a transfusion policy of D+ red blood cells into D- patients. Transfusion. 2008;48:1318–24.
61. Frohn C, Dumbgen L, Brand JM, Görg S, Luhm J, Kirchner H. Probability of anti-D development in D- patients receiving D+ RBCs. Transfusion. 2003;43:893–8.
62. Cid J, Lozano M, Ziman A, West KA, O'Brien KL, Murphy MF, et al. Low frequency of anti-D alloimmunization following D+ platelet transfusion: the anti-D alloimmunization after D-incompatible platelet transfusions (ADAPT) study. Br J Haematol. 2015;168:598–603.
63. Koelewijn JM, de Haas M, Vrijkotte TG, Bonsel GJ, van der Schoot CE. One single dose of 200 microg of antenatal RhIG halves the risk of anti-D immunization and hemolytic disease of the fetus and newborn in the next pregnancy. Transfusion. 2008;48:1721–9.
64. Agaronov M, DiBattista A, Christenson E, Miller-Murphy R, Strauss D, Shaz BH. Perception of low-titer group A plasma and potential barriers to using this product: a blood center's experience serving community and academic hospitals. Transfus Apher Sci. 2016;55:141–5.
65. Roback JD, Caldwell S, Carson J, Davenport R, Drew MJ, Eder A, et al. Evidence-based practice guidelines for plasma transfusion. Transfusion. 2010;50:1227–39.
66. Dunbar NM, Yazer MH, Biomedical Excellence for Safer Transfusion C. A possible new paradigm? A survey-based assessment of the use of thawed group A plasma for trauma resuscitation in the United States. Transfusion. 2016;56:125–9.
67. Fung MK, Grossman BJ, Hillyer CD, et al. Technical manual. 18th ed. Bethesda: American Association of Blood Banks (AABB); 2014.
68. Dunbar NM, Yazer MH. Biomedical Excellence for Safer Transfusion (BEST) Collaborative and the STAT Study Investigators. Safety of the use of group A plasma in trauma – The STAT Study. Transfusion. 2017 Aug;57(8):1879–84.
69. Yazer MH, Cap AP, Spinella PC, Alarcon L, Triulzi DJ. How do I implement a whole blood program for massively bleeding patients? Transfusion. 2018;58:622–8.
70. Spinella PC, Pidcoke HF, Strandenes G, Hervig T, Fisher A, Jenkins D, et al. Whole blood for hemostatic resuscitation of major bleeding. Transfusion. 2016;56(Suppl 2):S190–202.
71. Seheult JN, Stram MN, Sperry J, Spinella PC, Triulzi DJ, Yazer MH. In silico model of the dilutional effects of conventional component therapy versus whole blood in the management of massively bleeding adult trauma patients. Transfusion. 2019;59:146–58.
72. Pidcoke HF, McFaul SJ, Ramasubramanian AK, Parida BK, Mora AG, Fedyk CG, et al. Primary hemostatic capacity of whole blood: a comprehensive analysis of pathogen reduction and refrigeration effects over time. Transfusion. 2013;53(Suppl 1):137S–49S.
73. Jobes D, Wolfe Y, O'Neill D, Calder J, Jones L, Sesok-Pizzini D, et al. Toward a definition of "fresh" whole blood: an in vitro characterization of coagulation properties in refrigerated whole blood for transfusion. Transfusion. 2011;51:43–51.
74. Reddoch KM, Pidcoke HF, Montgomery RK, Fedyk CG, Aden JK, Ramasubramanian AK, et al. Hemostatic function of apheresis platelets stored at 4 degrees C and 22 degrees C. Shock. 2014;41(Suppl 1):54–61.

75. Nair PM, Pidcoke HF, Cap AP, Ramasubramanian AK. Effect of cold storage on shear-induced platelet aggregation and clot strength. J Trauma Acute Care Surg. 2014;77:S88–93.
76. Yazer MH, Glackin EM, Triulzi DJ, Alarcon LH, Murdock A, Sperry J. The effect of stationary versus rocked storage of whole blood on red blood cell damage and platelet function. Transfusion. 2016;56:596–604.
77. Yazer MH, Seheult J. Who's afraid of incompatible plasma? A balanced approach to the safe transfusion of blood products containing ABO-incompatible plasma. Transfusion. 2018;58:532–8.
78. Yazer MH, Spinella PC. The use of low titer group O whole blood for the resuscitation of civilian trauma patients in 2018. Transfusion. 2018;58:2744–6.
79. Seheult JN, Triulzi DJ, Alarcon LH, Sperry JL, Murdock A, Yazer MH. Measurement of haemolysis markers following transfusion of uncrossmatched, low-titre, group O+ whole blood in civilian trauma patients: initial experience at a level 1 trauma centre. Transfus Med. 2017;27:30–5.
80. Seheult JN, Bahr M, Anto V, Alarcon LH, Corcos A, Sperry JL, et al. Safety profile of uncrossmatched, cold-stored, low-titer, group O+ whole blood in civilian trauma patients. Transfusion. 2018 Oct;58(10):2280–8.
81. Seheult JN, Anto V, Alarcon LH, Sperry JL, Triulzi DJ, Yazer MH. Clinical outcomes among low-titer group O whole blood recipients compared to recipients of conventional components in civilian trauma resuscitation. Transfusion. 2018 Aug;58(8):1838–45.
82. Pivalizza EG, Stephens CT, Sridhar S, Gumbert SD, Rossmann S, Bertholf MF, et al. Whole blood for resuscitation in adult civilian trauma in 2017: a narrative review. Anesth Analg. 2018 Jul;127(1):157–62.
83. McGinity AC, Zhu CS, Greebon L, Xenakis E, Waltman E, Epley E, et al. Prehospital low-titer cold-stored whole blood: philosophy for ubiquitous utilization of O-positive product for emergency use in hemorrhage due to injury. J Trauma Acute Care Surg. 2018;84:S115–s9.
84. Farrell NM, Wing HA, Burke PA, Huiras P. Addition of tranexamic acid to a traumatic injury massive transfusion protocol. Am J Health Syst Pharm. 2015;72:1059–64.
85. Kashuk JL, Moore EE, Sawyer M, Wohlauer M, Pezold M, Barnett C, et al. Primary fibrinolysis is integral in the pathogenesis of the acute coagulopathy of trauma. Ann Surg. 2010;252:434–42; discussion 43–4.
86. McCormack PL. Tranexamic acid: a review of its use in the treatment of hyperfibrinolysis. Drugs. 2012;72:585–617.
87. Roberts I, Shakur H, Coats T, Hunt B, Balogun E, Barnetson L, et al. The CRASH-2 trial: a randomised controlled trial and economic evaluation of the effects of tranexamic acid on death, vascular occlusive events and transfusion requirement in bleeding trauma patients. Health Technol Assess. 2013;17:1–79.
88. Roberts I. Fibrinolytic shutdown: fascinating theory but randomized controlled trial data are needed. Transfusion. 2016;56(Suppl 2):S115–8.
89. Moore EE, Moore HB, Gonzalez E, Sauaia A, Banerjee A, Silliman CC. Rationale for the selective administration of tranexamic acid to inhibit fibrinolysis in the severely injured patient. Transfusion. 2016;56(Suppl 2):S110–4.
90. Joseph B, Aziz H, Pandit V, Hays D, Kulvatunyou N, Yousuf Z, et al. Prothrombin complex concentrate versus fresh-frozen plasma for reversal of coagulopathy of trauma: is there a difference? World J Surg. 2014;38:1875–81.
91. Dutton RP, Parr M, Tortella BJ, Champion HR, Bernard GR, Boffard K, et al. Recombinant activated factor VII safety in trauma patients: results from the CONTROL trial. J Trauma. 2011;71:12–9.
92. Lin Y, Moltzan CJ, Anderson DR, ; National Advisory Committee on Blood and Blood Products. The evidence for the use of recombinant factor VIIa in massive bleeding: revision of the transfusion policy framework. Transfus Med 2012;22: 383–394.
93. Propper BW, Rasmussen TE, Davidson SB, Vandenberg SL, Clouse WD, Burkhardt GE, et al. Surgical response to multiple casualty incidents following single explosive events. Ann Surg. 2009;250:311–5.

94. Soffer D, Klausner J, Bar-Zohar D, Szold O, Schulman CI, Halpern P, et al. Usage of blood products in multiple-casualty incidents: the experience of a level I trauma center in Israel. Arch Surg. 2008;143:983–9; discussion 9.
95. Dann EJ, Bonstein L, Arbov L, Kornberg A, Rahimi-Levene N. Blood bank protocols for large-scale civilian casualty events: experience from terrorist bombing in Israel. Transfus Med. 2007;17:135–9.
96. Bloch YH, Schwartz D, Pinkert M, Blumenfeld A, Avinoam S, Hevion G, et al. Distribution of casualties in a mass-casualty incident with three local hospitals in the periphery of a densely populated area: lessons learned from the medical management of a terrorist attack. Prehosp Disaster Med. 2007;22:186–92.
97. Ramsey G. Blood component transfusions in mass casualty events. Vox Sang. 2017;112:648–59.
98. Glasgow S, Vasilakis C, Perkins Z, Brundage S, Tai N, Brohi K. Managing the surge in demand for blood following mass casualty events: Early automatic restocking may preserve red cell supply. J Trauma Acute Care Surg. 2016;81:50–7.
99. Doughty H, Glasgow S, Kristoffersen E. Mass casualty events: blood transfusion emergency preparedness across the continuum of care. Transfusion. 2016;56(Suppl 2):S208–16.

Pediatric Considerations

23

Guyon J. Hill and Katherine Remick

Introduction

Children are at risk of sustaining life-threatening injuries from acts of terrorism, industrial accidents, or the recreational use of explosives such as fireworks or pyrotechnics. In areas of conflict, children may be exposed to unexploded ordinance, land mines, or improvised explosive devices (IEDs). Pediatric patients are especially susceptible to blast injuries due to the same kinetic energy being transmitted over a relatively smaller mass in addition to key differences in anatomy and physiology. These factors also increase the risk for multisystem injuries. In areas of conflict and civilian settings, children will not have the benefits of protective attire such as body armor, ballistic eyewear, helmets, or other equipment available to military personnel. In any setting, healthcare providers with minimal pediatric experience may be called on to care for children with life-threatening injuries as a result of explosives.

Historically, there is little available evidence describing the scope of pediatric blast injuries. However, recent terrorist incidents and military conflicts have greatly enhanced our knowledge in this area [1–4]. Blast injuries can cause both blunt and

G. J. Hill (✉)
Department of Emergency Medicine, C. R. Darnall Army Medical Center, Fort Hood, TX, USA

Department of Pediatrics, Dell Children's Medical Center, Austin, TX, USA

K. Remick
San Marcos Hays County EMS System, San Marcos, TX, USA

National EMS for Children Innovation and Improvement Center, Houston, TX, USA

Austin-Travis County EMS System, Austin, TX, USA

Dell Medical School at the University of Texas at Austin, Austin, TX, USA

Dell Medical School, Austin, TX, USA

Department of Pediatrics, Dell Children's Medical Center, Austin, TX, USA

D. W. Callaway, J. L. Burstein (eds.), *Operational and Medical Management of Explosive and Blast Incidents*, https://doi.org/10.1007/978-3-030-40655-4_23

penetrating trauma as well as thermal burns. All of these can be life-threatening and have special implications in the pediatric age range. Blast injuries in children are further compounded by unique patterns of injury and distinct differences in anatomy and physiology. A number of other key factors that may increase or complicate the severity of injuries include:

1. The child's proximity to the blast
2. The type and composition of the explosive
3. Location of the child when the blast occurred (i.e., an enclosed space, next to a barrier, or submerged)
4. Presence of projectiles in the device
5. Potential for radiological or biological contamination

In an emergency situation, the varied developmental stages and behavioral characteristics of children can make the care of these children even more challenging. During terrorist events or disasters, children may choose to hide in their immediate vicinity, which may increase their risk of entrapment and delay discovery. They may also be less able to discern suitable escape routes [5]. Providers should expect children to be at higher risk of disorientation due to the trauma, separation from family and caregivers, and developmental regression. Given these factors, children may be more prone to developing post-traumatic stress disorder in the aftermath of a disaster. Thus, the pediatric blast-injured patient creates a rare challenge, especially for providers unaccustomed to caring for severely injured children.

Overview of Blast Injuries in Children

Blast injuries are commonly classified as primary to quaternary [6]. Primary blast injuries (PBIs) are a significant cause of mortality and are generally caused by high-order explosives, and injuries result from the overpressure of the blast wave. PBIs primarily affect organs that are either air-filled or contain an air-fluid interface such as tympanic membranes, blood vessels, the gastrointestinal tract, or the lungs. The classification of secondary blast injury is used to describe penetrating injuries caused by shrapnel or other flying debris. This classification usually causes the greatest number of injuries. Tertiary blast injury refers to injuries caused by acceleration and deceleration forces as individuals being propelled by the blast wind into other objects. These injuries can affect any organ and are unique to high-energy explosions. Children and those in close proximity to the blast are disproportionately affected due to the transfer of energy and their smaller size, respectively. Tertiary blast injuries can account for a considerable proportion of pediatric injuries and can cause injuries such as skull fractures, intracranial hemorrhage, long bone fractures, and traumatic amputations [1]. The classification of quaternary blast injury includes burns (thermal or chemical), inhalational injuries from toxic fumes, crush injuries, and the exacerbation of chronic illnesses such as asthma. These injuries contribute to delayed mortality. An additional classification that may sometimes be used is quinary. This designation refers to a hyperinflammatory state that cannot be explained by other categories of blast injury. It may also be used to refer to illnesses, diseases, or injuries caused by contamination of the explosive device with chemical, biological, or radiological substances (i.e., "dirty bombs") [7, 8]. Not included in this classification system are the psychological trauma and residual effects such as post-traumatic stress disorder (PTSD) that can result from these situations.

When approaching pediatric patients with blast injuries, it is important to consider key differences in anatomy and physiology. These variances can cause challenges during resuscitation especially if providers are inexperienced in caring for critically injured pediatric trauma patients. As hypoxia is the most common cause of cardiac arrest in children, optimal airway management is critical to the survival of pediatric patients injured by explosives. Several anatomic differences make airway management more difficult in children and make pediatric patients more prone to complications. Because resistance to flow is proportional to the radius to the fourth power (Poiseuille's law) and the pediatric airway is narrower, the same degree of swelling in children can cause significant airway obstruction. This also predisposes them to bronchospasm. Children have relatively shorter tracheas making it more likely to inadvertently perform a right mainstem intubation. Children also have proportionally larger heads making it more difficult to align the airway and cervical spine; padding beneath the upper back may be needed to achieve a neutral position. In addition to the difficulty in maintaining pediatric airway skills, optimal pediatric airway management requires having different-sized devices for different-sized children. Last, due to challenges in anatomic assessment, there are age limitations on surgical cricothyrotomy.

Children respond to hemodynamic losses primarily by increasing heart rate rather than altering cardiac contractility. Thus, in general, children are able to maintain normal blood pressure despite up to a 25% or greater loss of blood volume [9]. As hypotension is a late finding, other signs such as tachycardia or tachypnea, altered mental status, delayed capillary refill, or mottled skin may be more reliable indicators of a child in shock. Due to differences in metabolism and absorption, all medication doses and resuscitation fluid volumes in children are weight-based. Providers need to ensure the correct dose of medication is given. The simple misplacement of a decimal point can result in administration of 10–100 times the intended dose. Due to their high ability to compensate, children who are initially alert and at baseline should still warrant further evaluation for the presence of any of the following: abnormal behavior such as excessive sleepiness or irritability, seizure activity, persistent vomiting, loss of consciousness, or evidence of a cerebrospinal fluid (CSF) leak [9].

Common Blast Injury Patterns in Children

Severe head trauma is the most frequent cause of death for children involved in blast events [1, 2]. Traumatic brain injuries (TBIs) from primary blast injury can include hemorrhage, edema, concussions, diffuse axonal injury (DAI), or infarction due to gas emboli as is seen in blast lung [1]. It can be difficult to assess TBI in children, particularly in the preverbal child. Age-based neurologic assessments exist for children of all ages, and emergency departments (ED) would benefit from maintaining ready access to such tools. In addition, TBI can occur in the absence of loss of consciousness. Validated algorithms for the assessment of such children should be considered [10].

Pulmonary contusions are the most common traumatic thoracic injury in children and the most frequent fatal form of primary blast injury (PBI) among initial survivors [11–13]. However, pulmonary injuries from the primary blast may vary and include lung contusion, blast lung, alveolar rupture, air embolism, and acute respiratory distress syndrome (ARDS) [6]. Pulmonary PBI commonly results in symptoms of cough, chest pain, dyspnea, or hemoptysis. Clinical findings may consist of tachypnea, hypoxia, respiratory distress, cyanosis, decreased or adventitious breath sounds, crepitus, subcutaneous emphysema, or pneumomediastinum. The majority of patients will have other associated thoracic injuries such as pleural effusions, pneumothoraces, hemothoraces, and fractures as well as extrathoracic injuries. Unlike adults, pulmonary contusions in children can occur without rib fractures as the more compliant and elastic chest wall allows kinetic energy to be transmitted to intrathoracic structures [14]. When rib fractures are present, they portend significant force and are correlated with the presence of other injuries.

While most children will have at least mild degrees of respiratory distress, tachypnea, or hypoxemia, providers should suspect a pulmonary contusion in any child exposed to a significant blast, even in the absence of physical exam findings or signs of chest wall injury. One study of pediatric pulmonary contusions noted that more than half lacked abnormal findings on physical exam [15]. Yet, it is important that providers recognize the potential risks imposed by the presence of pulmonary contusions. Pneumonia is the most common complication and can develop in 20–50% of patients [16, 17]. ARDS is an infrequent complication of pulmonary contusions in children but carries an exceedingly high mortality rate. While ARDS can result from shock related to other bodily injuries, it can also result from direct lung injury [18, 19]. Regardless, the long-term outcomes for children with pulmonary contusions are generally excellent and are associated with much lower rates of long-term respiratory sequelae than adults [20, 21].

The term "blast lung" has traditionally been used to describe pulmonary barotrauma causing severe pulmonary contusions and other findings following a blast injury. It typically presents early in the clinical course and, in addition to pulmonary contusions, can include hemothorax, pneumothorax, pneumomediastinum, pulmonary edema, and other injuries. Chest radiographs and CT may demonstrate diffuse bilateral infiltrates in a "butterfly" pattern within the first few hours, and findings can be progressive until 24–48 hours [22]. Positive-pressure ventilation may be required for severe cases of blast lung. Patients with blast lung can also experience stroke-like symptoms, blindness, or death from an air embolism in the brain or spinal cord. The risks for air embolism are increased for those on positive-pressure ventilation. Treatment is generally supportive and includes 100% oxygen. Hyperbaric oxygen has been shown to be effective in patients with neurologic symptoms [23]. Air emboli can also enter the coronary circulation which can present as a cardiac arrhythmia or myocardial infarction. Pulmonary injury cannot be excluded in patients with intact tympanic membranes (TMs) in the absence of pulmonary symptoms; indeed, recent studies have shown that isolated pulmonary blast injury can occur in patients without TM rupture [24, 25].

Abdominal injuries due to blasts are more likely in children than in adults. In addition to the same force being applied to a smaller area, there are also several notable anatomic differences that make this more likely. Children have thinner and less muscular abdominal walls and more pliable and smaller ribs conferring less protection. Children also have proportionally larger abdominal organs making the liver and spleen the most likely to be injured by either penetrating or blunt trauma. Air- and fluid-filled structures in the abdomen and pelvis are especially susceptible to PBI. Possible injuries include retroperitoneal hematomas, subcapsular hematomas, lacerations of solid organs, mesenteric ischemia, and scrotal or testicular rupture. Of note, intestinal PBI is more common when the victim is submerged. While performing focused abdominal sonography for trauma (FAST) ultrasound may have some utility in the detection of fluid collections or solid organ injuries, it cannot rule out bowel or mesenteric injuries. Recent studies have concluded that FAST is not as sensitive in the pediatric population as it is in adults and may miss intra-abdominal injuries requiring intervention [26, 27]. Computed tomography (CT) imaging is required to identify such injuries in otherwise stable patients if there is a high index of suspicion and in unstable patients requiring early surgical intervention. Occult abdominal blast injuries may go undetected until complications develop.

The most common PBI injury that occurs involves the tympanic membrane (TM), as it is extremely vulnerable to the effects of the blast [28]. Injuries may include tympanic membrane rupture, ossicle fracture or dislocation, or isolated hemotympanum. Inner ear injuries may also occur and can cause hearing loss, vertigo, and tinnitus [29, 30]. As many as half of tympanic membrane perforations caused by barotrauma will need to be surgically repaired [29, 30]. While historically used as a marker to predict other injuries, there is no data to support TM rupture as a surrogate for primary blast injury in pediatrics.

Cervical spine injury should be considered in any child with head or neck injury. Due to a proportionally larger head and weaker neck musculature, children are more susceptible to cervical spine injury in the C1–C3 area [9]. Pediatric patients with neurologic findings on presentation or with resolution of transient symptoms may have significant injuries to the spinal cord and/or spinal column in the absence of abnormalities noted on radiographs or CT. Termed spinal cord injury without radiographic abnormality (SCIWORA), the majority of cases occur in the cervical region in children less than 8 years of age. Most children will have demonstrable injuries on MRI [9, 31]. In addition to complaining of neck or back pain, the affected child may present with neurologic deficits such as paralysis, weakness, loss of pain or sensation, or paresthesia. They may also present with apnea, bradycardia, and hypotension if in spinal shock.

Primary blast injury can result in numerous other injuries in children including transient complete or partial paralysis, eye injuries such as globe rupture and hyphema, and facial fractures [32, 33]. Even in the absence of obvious external trauma, PBI may cause cardiovascular shock likely due to a vagally mediated mechanism. Patients will typically present with bradycardia, hypotension, and hypoxemia and will not show evidence of compensatory vasoconstriction [32]. Last, traumatic amputations can occur as a result of the high-pressure blast wave (PBI) passing through long bones. In addition to primary blast injuries, children can suffer considerable injury from secondary and tertiary blast effects. Blunt trauma to the chest may cause cardiac contusions or arrhythmias. Traumatic asphyxiation is an entity unique to children and results from the compression of the chest or abdomen combined with inspiration against a closed glottis. The diagnosis is usually made by physical findings and may include petechiae on the upper chest and face, conjunctival hemorrhages, or facial edema and cyanosis. Treatment is generally supportive and consistent with the resuscitation of other pediatric traumatic injuries.

Treatment Considerations for Children with Blast Injuries

While many principles of prehospital care and emergency medical treatment remain constant when treating children, we will highlight key differences or areas that require special attention or emphasis. Steps taken in the prehospital setting can have a dramatic impact on lowering the morbidity and mortality of pediatric patients exposed to blasts. Serial examinations will increase the chances of detecting an injury as the traumatized child may be difficult to examine initially. When possible, minimizing the separation from parents and other family members will decrease distress and make children easier to treat and transport. In the prehospital setting, the immediate priority after a blast of any kind is scene safety. As there is a continuum of emergency care, it is critical that all medical teams (out-of-hospital and in-hospital) work collaboratively. Optimal care provided at the scene and en route will help ensure pediatric blast-injured patients arrive alive at treatment facilities. While mass casualty incidents (MCI) and triage are addressed elsewhere, triage strategies such as JumpSTART, Smart, SALT, or Sacco can be used to effectively triage children [34].

Traumatic amputations are common, and extremity hemorrhage should be addressed immediately at the scene with a tourniquet or manual compression. Tourniquets should be reassessed every time the patient is moved to ensure they are effective and have not been dislodged. Commercially available, purposed-designed tourniquets will work on most children. For those where the arm circumference is too small for it to be effective, a roll of gauze can be placed between the arm, and the tourniquet or direct pressure can be applied if necessary. A review of pediatric war casualties ages 4–17 years old failed to note any pediatric-specific issues and found the same survival rate as in adults [35]. Providers should pay particular attention to any signs of respiratory distress such as tachypnea or retractions as well as signs of chest wall injury. Providers should also inspect the child's chest for symmetric rise and fall (especially if they are altered) and auscultate for bilateral breath sounds when feasible. In children, tension pneumothoraces can develop quickly because the thoracic cavity is smaller and mediastinal structures are more mobile.

This diagnosis should be considered in any child that is hypoxic and hypotensive. Either missing or not managing this complication can be especially dangerous if the patient is transported via a helicopter or partially pressurized military aircraft. Pulse oximetry should be monitored in all patients if possible, and consider supplemental oxygen with a goal of 94–99% during transport and in the ED for those thought to be close to the explosion or those in enclosed areas. The decision to intubate a child in the prehospital setting must be carefully undertaken. Field intubation of the child is very resource intensive, requires the necessary equipment for the size of the child and provider experienced in pediatric airway management, and may diminish the ability to care for multiple other casualties depending on the situation and number and severity of injured patients. There is also some evidence that rapid sequence intubation in the field may not confer a benefit over bag-valve-mask [36, 37]. Care must be taken when spinal motion restriction is applied to place children in an anatomic position. Cervical collars and spinal motion restriction should not be applied automatically solely due to the age of the child [38]. Children have an especially large body surface area for their mass and can lose heat by radiation, convection, and evaporation. It is imperative to keep children warm throughout the continuum of care as this population is especially at risk for hypothermia and becoming more acidotic and coagulopathic during transport and in the ED [3].

In the emergency department (ED), there is no change to the primary, secondary, or tertiary surveys. Any patient with pulmonary symptoms or suspected inhalational injury or thoracic trauma should receive supplemental oxygen, and high-flow oxygen may be beneficial if available. Maintain a low threshold for placing intraosseous access if there is difficulty obtaining intravenous access. Special attention should be paid during the survey to explore areas that may hide small penetrating injuries such as the axilla, groin, and buttocks. Also inspect carefully for penetrating eye injuries, corneal injuries, or other ocular complications. If decontamination is necessary, it should be done in the presence of the parents when possible, and very close attention should be paid to mitigating hypothermia.

Hemorrhagic shock is the leading preventable cause of death after blast injuries. An initial bolus of 20–30 mL/kg of normal saline or Ringer's lactate can be given to children at risk of shock. Transfusion of blood products should be initiated if resuscitation volume exceeds 60 mL/kg, and consider earlier utilization in the case of hemorrhagic shock or anticipated massive transfusion. Massive transfusion in a pediatric patient is generally defined as when half or more of their circulating blood volume or greater than 40 mL/kg is expected to be replaced in 24 hours [5, 39]. The principles of damage control resuscitation that apply to adults can be applied to children. The ratio of blood products transfused to patients that have suffered combat-related trauma has been proven to reduce mortality with the 1:1 plasma to red blood cell (RBC) units being optimal during massive transfusion [5, 40]. The use of blood warmers will help prevent hypothermia and exacerbation of the acute coagulopathy of trauma. Also consider the use of tranexamic acid (TXA) in injuries less than 3 hours old. Early administration has been associated with a decrease in mortality and blood product utilization in severely injured adults [41]. Numerous pediatric surgery studies have shown TXA is associated with decreased blood loss and a decreased need for blood product transfusion [42]. A wartime review of pediatric trauma patients that received TXA showed that it was independently associated with decreased mortality despite the patients having greater injury severity, hypotension, acidosis, and coagulopathy. Patients receiving TXA also had no increase in thromboembolic complications, had decreased ventilator dependence, and improved neurologic status upon discharge [43].

Laboratory studies to consider ordering in the emergency department (ED) include urinalysis, complete blood count, and blood chemistries. Prothrombin time (PT), partial thromboplastin time (PTT), international normalized ratio (INR), and fibrinogen should be ordered in any patient with ongoing or suspected hemorrhage. Providers should also consider carboxyhemoglobin, especially in the case of an explosion in an enclosed space or if it was accompanied by a fire. Children can also develop cyanide toxicity if they were exposed to burning plastics. Creatine kinase may be beneficial to exclude rhabdomyolysis in suspected crush injuries, compartment syndromes, severe burns, or cases of delayed extrication. Providers should consider a screening EKG when there is concern for a cardiac contusion and cardiac biomarkers in the setting of EKG abnormalities suggestive of ischemia.

Chest radiographs should be obtained in all children that are significantly injured, with any pulmonary symptoms, with any physical exam findings consistent with thoracic trauma, or where pulmonary contusion is otherwise suspected. While the radiographs may initially appear normal in children with clinical findings consistent with pulmonary contusions, repeat studies are not needed if the child remains stable. As pulmonary contusions can evolve over hours, observation and repeat studies may be warranted for patients with a significant mechanism. Progression of the findings later in the clinical course may indicate complications of blast lung such as pneumonia or ARDS. The consolidations seen are generally in the areas of impact and are nonanatomic. Computed tomography (CT) of the chest solely for this purpose is generally not needed as, despite the increased sensitivity, it is unlikely to change management in the stable patient with normal oxygen saturation [44, 45]. CT scans may be helpful in the evaluation of other associated thoracic injuries. Intubation may be required but is rarely necessary for isolated pulmonary contusion. For those that require mechanical ventilation, they will benefit from positive end expiratory pressure (PEEP) [46]. Care is primarily supportive, and placement of the child with the injured portion of the lung in a dependent position may improve perfusion to the uninjured lung [47]. Pain relief can potentially be augmented by the utilization of intercostal nerve blocks. Other imaging studies to consider include radiographs of the cervical spine, pelvis, or extremities based on the significance of the mechanism or the physical examination. CT of the head, chest, and/or abdomen/pelvis may be indicated to identify other associated injuries. Providers should consider admitting any pediatric blast victim with continued abdominal pain even without an obvious source as injuries such as intestinal hematomas may be difficult to detect and can take 12–36 hours to present. MRI should be obtained when available in cases of SCIWORA in children with neurologic deficits (present or resolved) and no abnormalities noted on plain spine radiographs or CT to identify other injuries.

Fluid administration should be judicious in patients with pulmonary contusions or blast lung without the presence of shock to avoid causing edema in the contused lung tissue. Patients presenting with hypotension and bradycardia thought to be due to cardiovascular PBI may benefit from atropine or a vasopressor [33]. Providers need to initiate antibiotics in children with worsening respiratory status and fever as they may be developing pneumonia as a complication of their pulmonary contusions. These findings may be difficult to distinguish on radiographic studies. Providers may also consider prophylactic antibiotics for open wounds and consider systemic antifungals if there is potential for biological material in the wounds. Providers should consider delayed closure for contaminated wounds. Postexposure prophylaxis may be advised especially in the case of a suicide bomber. Crush or burn injuries should be treated per standard protocols, and shrapnel wounds are treated as low-velocity gunshot wounds. Ensuring appropriate pain treatment if a child has sustained serious injuries is necessary. Tetanus immunization should be updated in all patients with penetrating trauma if greater than 5 years from their last update. The last dose in the five-dose series is typically given at 4–6 years of age and another update given at 11–12 years of age. Tetanus immune globulin should also be given for those that are unimmunized or incompletely immunized. Pediatric patients should be transferred to a specialty center that is properly prepared to care of severely injured pediatric trauma patients as soon as feasible.

Impact of Blast Injuries in the Pediatric Population

The recent conflicts in Iraq and Afghanistan have allowed us to better understand the impact of blast injuries on pediatric patients. Blast injuries, particularly those caused by improvised explosive devices, have been the predominant mechanism of injury for pediatric patients admitted to US and coalition medical facilities [2–4, 48]. Evidence suggests that pediatric patients suffering blast injuries have increased injury severity and mortality when compared with either local adults or service members [2, 48, 49]. These effects are more pronounced in younger patients, and patterns of injury vary with age. One study concluded that pediatric patients less than 8 years of age who were predominantly injured by a blast mechanism had increased injury severity scores and higher in-patient mortality (18% vs. 4%) when compared with older children and adults [49]. Another study showed increased in-patient mortality in those less than 6 years of age when compared with older children and adults [50]. Additionally, children less than 8 years of age have more severe head and neck injuries and less severe extremity injuries when compared with those older than 8 years or adults. Amputation rates tend to increase with age [2, 51, 52].

Pediatric blast injury patients are more resource intensive than adult patients. The majority of pediatric blast patients are admitted to intensive care units, and hospitalization durations are almost twice that of adult patients at the same facilities [3, 48–50]. The rate of transfusion for children injured by explosives was higher than for those injured by any other mechanism. Estimates of blood transfusion rates have ranged from 15% to 42% [2, 3]. Reported overall mortality rates have ranged from 7% to 18.5% with head injury being the most common fatal injury [2, 52].

Conclusion

Children are at increased risk of sustaining life-threatening blast injuries. Compared to adults, pediatric patients are more likely to have head and neck injuries, burns, and more severe physiologic derangement. Additionally, children are more resource intensive than adult blast victims and carry higher mortality rates. Hypotension is a late finding for children in shock; providers should not wait until blood pressure drops to intervene. It is important to pay attention to other signs such as tachycardia, tachypnea, and mental status as potential indicators of shock. Most critical is that prehospital- and hospital-based emergency care providers possess and maintain proficiency with pediatric-specific equipment, supplies, and treatment guidelines. Institutions and healthcare administrators play a crucial role in ensuring a high level of day-to day pediatric readiness, so children with severe traumatic injuries receive optimal care [53]. Despite significant gaps, pediatric-specific needs should be incorporated into each hospital's mass casualty plan and drills [54].

Pitfalls

- Hypotension is a late finding for children in shock, and providers should not wait until this point to intervene. Pay particular attention to tachycardia, tachypnea, mental status, delayed capillary refill, or mottled skin as other potential signs of a child in shock.
- Children experience higher injury severity, more head and neck injuries, and less extremity injuries when compared with adults. Pediatric blast-injured patients are also more resource intensive than adult patients.
- It is important for prehospital- and hospital-based providers and institutions to possess and maintain day-to-day proficiency with pediatric-specific needs, so they are optimally able to care for children in the setting of disasters, including blast events. Length-based resuscitation tapes can assist providers in determining essential drug doses and resuscitation volumes for fluids and blood products.

References

1. Quintana D, Jordan F, Tuggle D, Mantor P, Tunell W. The spectrum of pediatric injuries after a bomb blast. J Pediatr Surg. 1997;32(2):307–11.
2. Edwards M, Lustik M, Eichelberger M, Elster E, Azarow K, Coppola C. Blast injury in children. J Trauma Acute Care Surg. 2012;73(5):1278–83.
3. Schauer S, Hill G, Naylor J, April M, Borgman M, Bebarta V. Emergency department resuscitation of pediatric trauma patients in Iraq and Afghanistan. Am J Emerg Med [Internet]. 2018 [cited 24 July 2018]. Available from: https://doi.org/10.1016/j.ajem.2018.01.
4. Schauer S, April M, Hill G, Naylor J, Borgman M, De Lorenzo R. Prehospital interventions performed on pediatric trauma patients in Iraq and Afghanistan. Prehosp Emerg Care [Internet]. 2018 [cited 24 July 2018]. Available from: https://doi.org/10.1080/10903127.2018.1439130.

5. Fuenfer M, Creamer K, Borden Institute W. Pediatric surgery and medicine for hostile environments. Washington, DC: United States Department of Defense; 2017.
6. Explosions and blast injuries a primer for clinicians [Internet]. Cdc.gov. 2018 [cited 9 July 2018]. Available from: https://www.cdc.gov/masstrauma/preparedness/primer.pdf.
7. Greer N, Sayer N, Kramer M, Koeller E., Velasquez T. Prevalence and epidemiology of combat blast injuries from the Military Cohort 2001-2014 [Internet]. Washington, DC: Department of Veterans Affairs (US); 2016 Feb. Executive summary. Available from: https://www.ncbi.nlm.nih.gov/books/NBK447480/.
8. Kluger Y, Nimrod A, Biderman P, Mayo A, Sorkin P. The quinary pattern of blast injury. Am J Disaster Med. 2007;2(1):21–5.
9. Blast injuries fact sheet for professionals [Internet]. Emergency preparedness - preparing hospitals for disasters. CDC; 2009 [cited 2018Jul11]. Available from: http://www.calhospitalprepare.org/sites/main/files/file-attachments/blast_fact_sheet_professionals-a.pdf.
10. Kupperman N, Holmes JF, Dayan PS, et al. Identification of children at very low risk for clinically-important brain injuries after trauma: a prospective cohort study. Lancet. 2009;374(9696):1160–70.
11. Cooper A, Barlow B, DiScala C, String D. Mortality and truncal injury: the pediatric perspective. J Pediatr Surg. 1994;29(1):33–8.
12. Peclet M, Newman K, Eichelberger M, Gotschall C, Garcia V, Bowman L. Thoracic trauma in children: an indicator of increased mortality. J Pediatr Surg. 1990;25(9):961–6.
13. Holmes J, Sokolove P, Brant W, Kuppermann N. A clinical decision rule for identifying children with thoracic injuries after blunt torso trauma. Ann Emerg Med. 2002;39(5):492–9.
14. Allen G. Pulmonary contusion: are children different? J Am Coll Surg. 1997;185(3):229–33.
15. Bonadio W, Hellmich T. Post-traumatic pulmonary contusion in children. Ann Emerg Med. 1989;18(10):1050–2.
16. Bliss D, Silen M. Pediatric thoracic trauma. Crit Care Med. 2002;30(Supplement):S409–15.
17. Clark G, Schecter W, Trunkey D. Variable affecting outcome in blunt chest trauma. J Trauma. 1986;26(7):671.
18. Allen G, Cox C. Pulmonary contusion in children: diagnosis and management. South Med J. 1998;91(12):1099–106.
19. Davis S, Furman D, Costarino A. Adult respiratory distress syndrome in children: associated disease, clinical course, and predictors of death. J Pediatr. 1993;123(1):35–45.
20. Haxhija E, Nores H, Schober P, Hollwarth M. Lung contusion-lacerations after blunt thoracic trauma in children. Pediatr Surg Int. 2004;20(6):412.
21. Kishikawa M, Yoshioka T, Shimazu T, Sugimoto H, Yoshioka T, Sugimoto T. Pulmonary contusion causes long-term respiratory dysfunction with decreased functional residual capacity. J Trauma. 1991;31(9):1203–10.
22. Barnard E, Johnston A. Blast lung | NEJM [Internet]. N Engl J Med. 2013 [cited 2018Jul17]. Available from: https://www.nejm.org/doi/full/10.1056/NEJMicm1203842.
23. Dunbar BM, Fox R, Watson B, Akrill P. Successful late treatment of venous air embolism with hyperbaric oxygen. Postgrad Med J. 1990;66:469–70.
24. Leibovici D, Gofrit O, Shapira S. Eardrum perforation in explosion survivors: is it a marker of pulmonary blast injury? Ann Emerg Med. 1999;34(2):168–72.
25. Harrison C, Bebarta V, Grant G. Tympanic membrane perforation after combat blast exposure in Iraq: a poor biomarker of primary blast injury. J Trauma. 2009;67(1):210–1.
26. Calder B, Vogel A, Zhang J, Mauldin P, Huang E, Savoie K, et al. Focused assessment with sonography for trauma in children after blunt abdominal trauma. J Trauma Acute Care Surg. 2017;83(2):218–24.
27. Holmes J, Kelley K, Wootton-Gorges S, Utter G, Abramson L, Rose J, et al. Effect of abdominal ultrasound on clinical care, outcomes, and resource use among children with Blunt Torso Trauma. JAMA. 2017;317(22):2290.
28. Kumar M. Blast injuries. Med J Armed Forces India. 2011;66(4):309–11.
29. Tungsinmunkong S, Chongkolwatana C, Piyawongvisal W, Atipas S, Namchareonchaisuk S. Blast injury of the ears: the experience from Yala Hospital, Southern Thailand. J Med Assoc Thail. 2007;90(12):2662.

30. Ritenour A, Wickley A, Ritenour J, Kriete B, Blackbourne L, Holcomb J, et al. Tympanic membrane perforation and hearing loss from blast overpressure in operation enduring freedom and operation Iraqi freedom wounded. J Trauma. 2008;64(Supplement):S174–8.
31. Leonard J, Jaffe D, Kuppermann N, Olsen C, Leonard J. Cervical spine injury patterns in children. Pediatrics. 2014;133(5):e1179–88.
32. Desaga H. Blast Injuries. In: German aviation medicine, World War II, vol. 2. Washington, DC: U.S. Government Printing Office; 1950.
33. Irwin R, Lerner M, Bealer J, Mantor P, Brackett D, Tuggle D. Shock after blast wave injury is caused by a vagally mediated reflex. J Trauma. 1999;47(1):105–10.
34. Lyle K, Thompson T, Graham J. Pediatric mass casualty: triage and planning for the prehospital provider. Clin Pediatr Emerg Med. 2009;10(3):173–85.
35. Kragh J, Cooper A, Aden J, Dubick M, Baer D, Wade C, et al. Survey of trauma registry data on tourniquet use in pediatric war casualties. Pediatr Emerg Care. 2012;28(12):1361–5.
36. Gausche M, Lewis R, Stratton S, Haynes B, Gunter C, Goodrich S, et al. Effect of out-of-hospital pediatric endotracheal intubation on survival and neurological outcome: a controlled clinical trial. JAMA. 2000;283(6):783–90.
37. Schauer S, Naylor J, Hill G, Arana A, Roper J, April M. Association of prehospital intubation with decreased survival among pediatric trauma patients in Iraq and Afghanistan. Am J Emerg Med. 2018;36(4):657–9.
38. Fischer P, Perina D, Delbridge T, Fallat ME, Salomone JP, Dodd J, et al. Spinal motion restriction in the trauma patient – a joint position statement. Prehosp Emerg Care. 2018;22(6):659–61.
39. Neff L, Cannon J, Morrison J, Edwards M, Spinella P, Borgman M. Clearly defining pediatric massive transfusion. J Trauma Acute Care Surg. 2015;78(1):22–9.
40. Borgman M, Spinella P, Perkins J, Grathwohl K, Repine T, Beekley A, et al. The ratio of blood products transfused affects mortality in patients receiving massive transfusions at a Combat Support Hospital. J Trauma. 2007;63(4):805–13.
41. CRASH-2 trial collaborators, Shakur H, Roberts I, Bautista R, Caballero J, Coats T, et al. Effects of tranexamic acid on death, vascular occlusive events, and blood transfusion in trauma patients with significant haemorrhage (CRASH-2): a randomised, placebo-controlled trial. Lancet. 2010;376(9734):23–32.
42. Urban D, Dehaeck R, Lorenzetti D, Guilfoyle J, Poon M, Steele M, et al. Safety and efficacy of tranexamic acid in bleeding paediatric trauma patients: a systematic review protocol. BMJ Open. 2016;6(9):e012947.
43. Eckert M, Wertin T, Tyner S, Nelson D, Izenberg S, Martin M. Tranexamic acid administration to pediatric trauma patients in a combat setting. J Trauma Acute Care Surg. 2014;77(6):852–8.
44. Kwon A, Sorrells DL Jr, Kurkchubasche AG, Cassese JA, Tracy TF Jr, Luks FI. Isolated computed tomography diagnosis of pulmonary contusion does not correlate with increased morbidity. J Pediatr Surg. 2006;41:78.
45. Rodriguez RM, Friedman B, Langdorf MI, Baumann BM, Nishijima DK, Hendey GW, et al. Pulmonary contusion in the pan-scan era. Injury. 2016;47:1031.
46. Hamrick MC, Duhn RD, Carney DE, Boswell WC, Ochsner MG. Pulmonary contusion in the pediatric population. Am Surg. 2010;76:721.
47. Ruddy RM. Trauma and the paediatric lung. Paediatr Respir Rev. 2005;6:61.
48. Borgman M, Matos R, Blackbourne L, Spinella P. Ten years of military pediatric care in Afghanistan and Iraq. J Trauma Acute Care Surg. 2012;73:S509–13.
49. Matos R, Holcomb J, Callahan C, Spinella P. Increased mortality rates of young children with traumatic injuries at a US Army Combat Support hospital in Baghdad, Iraq, 2004. Pediatrics. 2008;122(5):e959–66.
50. Spinella P, Borgman M, Azarow K. Pediatric trauma in an austere combat environment. Crit Care Med. 2008;36(Suppl):S293–6.

51. Schauer S, April M, Naylor J, Hill G, Arana A, Oh J, et al. The pediatric blast injury: out-of-hospital and emergency department resuscitation and resource utilization in Iraq and Afghanistan. Ann Emerg Med. 2017;70(4):S89.
52. Thompson D, Crooks R, Clasper J, Lupu A, Stapley S, Cloke D. The pattern of paediatric blast injury in Afghanistan. J R Army Med Corps. 2017; JRAMC-2017-000795.
53. Joint policy statement—guidelines for care of children in the emergency department. Pediatrics. 2009;124(4):1233–43.
54. Gausche-Hill M, Ely M, Schmuhl P, Telford R, Remick KE, Edgerton EA, et al. A national assessment of pediatric readiness of emergency departments. JAMA Pediatr. 2015;169(6):527–34.

Organization, Operations, Management, and Their Role in Surge Capacity and Mass Casualty Incidents

24

Meg S. Femino, Sage Guerke Weikel, and Ritu R. Sarin

Introduction

Mass casualty incidents (MCI) are defined differently among hospitals; a hospital may simply define an MCI when normal hospital operations and resources are exceeded. The parameters that will matter most in responding are the number of patients involved, their injury acuity, and current hospital capacity. Changes in any of these can overwhelm a hospital's ability to care for these patients during regular operations. In blast injuries, patients usually present with little or no notice and can rapidly deplete multiple critical resources, become a logistical challenge due to surge, and impede the ability to provide adequate care. The best approach in organization and operations management is to employ the Hospital Incident Command System (HICS) to utilize and leverage the whole hospital system to optimize care and resource utilization. In this chapter, special attention will be placed on emergency department (ED) operations.

M. S. Femino (✉)
Emergency Management, Department of Health Care Quality, Beth Israel Deaconess Medical Center, Boston, MA, USA
e-mail: mfemino@bidmc.harvard.edu

S. G. Weikel
Emergency Management, Department of Healthcare Quality, Beth Israel Deaconess Medical Center, Roxbury, MA, USA

R. R. Sarin
Department of Emergency Medicine, Beth Israel Deaconess Medical Center, Boston, MA, USA

D. W. Callaway, J. L. Burstein (eds.), *Operational and Medical Management of Explosive and Blast Incidents*, https://doi.org/10.1007/978-3-030-40655-4_24

Assumptions

The following are assumed based on an analysis of real-world events and after-action reporting:

- Patients will self-present to the emergency department (ED) without prior emergency medical service (EMS) triage or other lifesaving interventions [1].
- The sickest will arrive later than the less acute via EMS [2].
- Less acute patients may present to hospitals far away from the blast site and out of harm's way [3].
- Family and victims may be separated.
- Some victims from a blast will require specialty care—pediatric, burn, trauma, surgical subspecialties, and obstetrics [4].
- Patients may have significant internal injuries that may be delayed or overlooked [5].
- The majority of patients will not be critically injured [2].
- Criminal intent should be considered unless otherwise notified.

Challenges of Blast Incidents and MCI

The major challenge all hospitals face when dealing with a disaster of any nature is an outstripping of critical resources, the lack of which could prove to be a major threat to patient care or to the institution itself. When addressing resource utilization, and the need for surge capacity in the planning and response, these are often broken down into categories of space, staff, and supplies [6]. In the case of blast-related MCIs, there is strong historical data from prior events on what these limited resources tend to be [7, 8] (Table 24.1).

While the vast majority of blast-related MCIs occur outside of hospitals, the new trend in asymmetric terrorist attacks can lead to concerns that hospitals and healthcare providers will be secondary targets [9]. This brings up the primary consideration of the need for increased security services around these types of intentional events. These services are necessary to minimize access points to the facility, manage patient and staff needs inside the hospital, redirect spontaneous volunteers, and perform screenings of arriving emergency medical services (EMS) vehicles, patients, staff, and visitors for secondary devices [10].

With the arrival of patients comes the added uncertainty as to whether there will be additional attacks or if a perpetrator is among the wounded. Responder safety is paramount, and adding security at the ED is necessary, at least initially. In addition, there is a possible hazardous materials threat when an explosion occurs. Depending on the size and scale of a hazmat event, there may need to be a decontamination operation that protects hospital workers from exposure. A hospital-based hazmat team can further deplete already scarce resources in the forms of staffing, operating space, and medical supplies such as stretchers and/or backboards, triage equipment, etc.

Table 24.1 Critical resources for hospitals after blast events

Space	ED observation unit (for minimum of 6 hours of monitoring noncritical patients) Intensive care units Step-down units Monitored space for an operating room holding area Operating rooms Alternate space for low-acuity (green) patients Monitored postoperative recovery areas Burn bed capacity Space for psychological counseling or intervention Families seeking information on potential victims Space to coordinate spontaneous volunteers and extra staff
Supplies	Blood products Ventilators Sterile OR kits Orthopedic surgical supplies Intravenous fluids Thoracostomy tubes Prophylactic antibiotics Tetanus vaccine Radiation decontaminants and antidotes Personal protective equipment
Staff (medical)	Trauma surgeons Vascular surgeons Orthopedic surgeons Neurosurgeons Plastic surgeons Anesthesiologists and experienced airway management providers Surgical and medical intensivists Emergency medicine physicians Experienced triage officers Psychiatrists Nurses—ED, OR, PACU, critical care Operating room technicians Social workers
Staff (nonmedical)	Security Lab technicians Radiology technicians Pharmacists Facilities staff Transporters Environmental service Registration staff Emergency managers Public information officers

Staffing needs to provide medical care in relation to blast injuries will include trauma surgeons, vascular surgeons, orthopedic surgeons, neurosurgeons, plastic surgeons, anesthesiologists, surgical and medical intensivists, emergency medicine physicians and experienced triage officers, nursing staff, psychiatrists, social workers, perioperative staff, and a high-functioning incident management team [9]. The specific needs for these medical providers will be expanded on in later chapters.

Clinical support staff needed in all times of crisis such as lab technicians, radiology technicians, pharmacists, facilities staff, registration staff, transport, environmental services, safety officers, and emergency managers will be a must in these scenarios as well [9].

During blast events, critical spaces that will be limited in almost all hospitals are ED spaces to allow for minimum monitoring of many noncritical-presenting patients, intensive care units for critical airway monitoring for patients with or at high risk of developing acute respiratory distress syndrome (ARDS), operating rooms and monitored postoperative recovery areas, and burn bed capacity [9, 11–14]. Additionally, space will need to be found for families seeking information on potential victims and patients and staff requiring psychological counseling or intervention and space to coordinate spontaneous volunteers and extra staff. As in most disaster scenarios involving a surge of patients, alternate care site identification for special patient populations will be key to provide decompression of the ED.

When planning for supplies that may become limited, critical items include blood products, ventilators, orthopedic surgical supplies, sterile OR kits, intravenous (IV) fluids, thoracostomy tubes, prophylactic antibiotics, tetanus vaccines, and, in the event of a radiation dispersal device (RDD), appropriate decontaminants and personal protective equipment (PPE) [7–9].

Focus on System Approach and HICS

Emergent events often do not fit "business as usual" management for hospital operations. Due to patient care demands that may arise from the incident, multiple internal operations and business processes may also be affected by a greater-than-normal demand on specific critical services such as surging patient beds, increased staffing needs, and supply allocation, and due to the critical nature of blast wounds, day-to-day processes may not work fast enough to save lives such as electronic charting. Since disasters can impact several areas simultaneously and different activities are necessary to manage each affected area, routine business management processes may be inadequate.

Most hospitals across the nation have developed Emergency Operations Plans (EOPs) that address the coordinated response to extraordinary emergencies such as mass casualty incidents, fires, hazardous spills, loss of utilities, explosions, security threats, and civil disorder, all of which can occur during a blast event. The objective of the plan is to use resources in an effective manner should interruption or greater-than-normal demand of a critical service occur. The use of a hospital EOP and Hospital Incident Command System (HICS) brings order and coordination to the additional demands created by these complex situations.

The purpose of the all-hazard EOP is to set the parameters for implementation of the plan and outline functional areas that are always the same regardless of the emergency such as communication, alert and notification, and resource management, as well as outline the duties and responsibilities of critical departments, HICS roles, and the Emergency Operations Center. The EOP has an all-hazards approach, and event-specific plans are layered in as annexes to the main plan [15].

An EOP is not a substitute for thinking; instead, it provides organizational structure for dealing with emergencies. An EOP is not a "cookbook" for dealing with specific situations that may certainly arise in the course of an emergency. It does not and is not intended to substitute for analyzing what needs to be done and undertaking appropriate actions in situations that will arise and which must be acted upon quickly by those responding.

Incident Command System (ICS) was introduced by the National Forest Service in the 1980s but not widely adapted for US hospitals until post September 11. In 2003, the Homeland Security Presidential Directive-5 (HSPD-5) became law, introducing the National Incident Management System (NIMS) [15]. NIMS provides a template for government, private sector, and nongovernment organizations to work together during incidents and emergencies. HICS provides a flexible framework, organizational structure, and chain of command for response activities in the hospital. It is utilized for planned and unplanned facility or patient-driven events and can be used across the emergency management cycle regardless of hospital size, location, patient acuity, patient volume, or hazard type. The HICS toolbox is comprehensive and has outlined roles and responsibilities, incident response guides, building in accountability, and resource management [15].

Blast events are considered to be a low-frequency, high-impact event in most areas of the United States. Outside of war zones, they produce military-style injuries in civilian populations, and patients are treated at civilian hospitals [14]. Low-frequency, high-impact events are extraordinarily complex to manage due to lack of planning, lack of critical or sufficient resources, lack of surge capacity across the nation, and lack of clinical treatment expertise. That said, well-practiced incident management and clinical teams can quickly make critical adjustments to operational strategies to respond as effectively as possible. The hospital incident management team and EOP should be activated immediately upon notification of an event-generating blast-type injuries. It should be assumed that the response to such an event will be widespread across the hospital, and community integration will be significant. It is imperative to quickly get a situational awareness picture, including where the event was (open vs. closed space) [4], how many patients were affected, how significant of injuries are on scene, and proximity of event to your hospital, so you can begin to establish a common operating picture.

The hospital should prepare for a mass casualty with surgical trauma due to the mechanism of injury. Many strategies should be implemented simultaneously as detailed below.

Hospital Operations

Activation of the EOP, HICS, and the Command Center

Once the ED has been alerted of a mass casualty incident involving a blast, the notification should be escalated immediately to activate the hospital incident management systems and processes. There should be a command center, or post-activation and functional roles should be delegated. This activation may recall critical staff and will get the incident management team in place for a hospital-wide response. Examples of HICS positions to be activated are shown in Fig. 24.1.

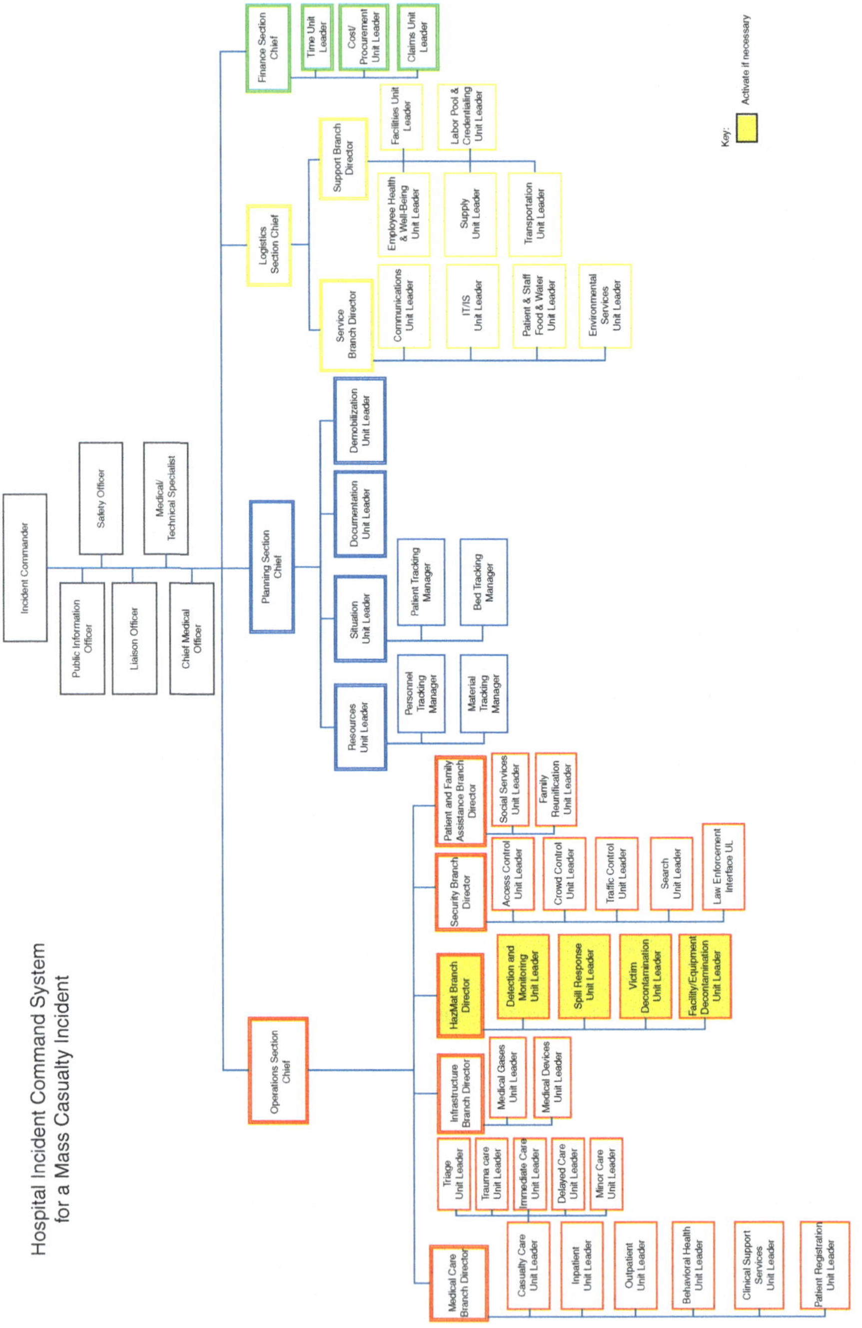

Fig. 24.1 Examples of HICS positions to be activated

The Purge-to-Surge

Regardless of an ED's protocol for MCI triage, some acutely injured patients will need to be fast-tracked to certain service areas such as the operating room or intensive care unit (ICU). It is necessary to implement MCI patient management at the time of notification. After receiving word that an explosion with casualties has occurred, a receiving hospital must act fast, because at any given moment, it is expected that a hospital is operating at a 64%+ occupancy with either a full operating room schedule or limited OR staff due to a holiday or weekend [16]. Many hospitals often operate at a much higher capacity with admitted patients boarding in the emergency department a common occurrence. Clearing critical space in anticipation of a significant rise in patient volume is known as "purge-to-surge." A large portion of inpatients can indeed be "purged" (discharged) or otherwise placed in the hospital within a 24- to 72-hour time period in the event of an MCI [17]. It is believed that 50+% of bed space can be made available within the first 24–48 hours [17, 18]. Specific, critical areas that need to be purged of less acute patients include the emergency department, the operating rooms, the intensive care units, and the radiology suite (if portable radiology equipment is unavailable), as these are the units most likely to be backed up during an MCI [19].

Patient surge has the potential to happen quickly. The emergency department must have a well-thought-out and practiced plan to rapidly decant the ED. This involves immediately sending all admissions with bed assignments to the floors. Staff from accepting floors should deploy to the ED to pick up the patient and receive a handoff to avoid delays in waiting for transport or clinicians to receive report. It also allows the ED to determine and identify acuity zones for incoming patients based on available information. The ED acuity zoning should be identified and staffed with the most appropriate ED and triage personnel. The most experienced ED providers should staff the high-acuity zone and triage zones. Lower-acuity patients can wait in the ED lobby after being triaged. They may be moved once the ED has transferred the higher-acuity patients to appropriate treatment areas. Typically, less injured patients will present to the ED from the scene before the more critically injured who require EMS transport. ED staff must be aware of this "second wave phenomena" and take care not to fill up all ED beds with lower-acuity patients at the expense of incoming more critically injured victims [2].

Nontraditional Alternate Care Sites

During a patient surge, it may be necessary to treat patients in nontraditional areas. Plans often assign low-acuity patients to lobbies or ambulatory clinics. Other space-utilization strategies include moving patient triage outside the hospital and using the OR patient waiting area or postanesthesia care unit (PACU) as a critical care unit or preoperative holding unit. Additional space considerations include a family waiting and reunification area, location for media staging, labor pool, and, if the event was intentional, an area for law enforcement to interview hospital staff.

Security Considerations

A primary goal is to keep the hospital staff and facilities safe from security threats and/or hazardous exposures. The hospital may need to consider restricting access, limiting or restricting visitors, and searching and screening patients, staff, ambulances, and private vehicles before they approach the building if there is a potential of criminal intent. There will need to be a law enforcement liaison for law enforcement partners arriving to assist or investigate [10].

Communication

In the event of a large-scale mass casualty blast incident, coverage of the event will most likely be broadcasted on TV and in the media. It is imperative that a public information officer be activated to manage the media messaging, briefings, and requests. Hospitals should also be communicating with their employees on the situation, if they need to come in, what they need to bring (badges, clothes), and what they should prepare for. External partners, patients, and visitors will also need to be notified and updated on current hospital situation and changes to any hospital operations.

Staffing

In a highly visible event, hospitals should prepare to set up a labor pool as staff will see this unfolding on TV and self-present to the hospital. While many are well-meaning and want to help, they may not have the skill sets needed. A labor pool will divert staff from frontline areas and organize staff by critical skill sets and can be ready to deploy the appropriate employee to the appropriate area of need. A buddy system should be considered for those employees working in an unfamiliar unit, providing them with just-in-time training and an evaluation of performance. If external staff is being utilized, there should also be an emergency credentialing and a badging process in place within the labor pool.

Emergency Department Operations

The Three-Minute Huddle

At the time of event notification, the resource nurse and ED attending should gather the entire unit team and lay out the plan for response, delegate tasks and positions (Table 24.2), and identify any alternate care plans such as treating low-acuity patients in the lobby, moving triage outside, having more than one triage area, and sending ED patients awaiting surgery to ICU or alternate spaces. Identify immediate assistance you may need from the hospital's resources, types of medical staff, staff from the inpatient units, extra housekeeping to turn over rooms, transport to bring patients upstairs and move stretchers and wheelchairs, security to control

Table 24.2 Emergency department incident management roles for a mass casualty incident

Role	Filled by	Critical tasks
Medical care branch director	ED attending and/or trauma attending	With CCUL, brief staff, delegate roles, and establish treatment protocols Determine medical care needs and physician staffing needs in all areas of the ED In tandem with trauma attending, prioritize care and resources for patients—OR, vents, etc. Establish two-way radio communication with the casualty care unit leader Communicate regularly with the casualty care unit leader to align expectations and situational status Communicate to command center medical staff support and resource needs known Brief command center periodically of current ED situation and project future patient care conditions and resource needs Alert command center of any changes in standards of care
Casualty care unit leader	ED charge nurse	Develop an incident action plan with the medical care director Delegate ED roles with the current staffing Regularly brief treatment area leaders with medical care director and establish two-way radio communication Determine safety and security needs in all treatment areas and communicate to the safety/security officer Assess problems and treatment needs and customize the staffing and supplies in each area Work with command center in communicating alternate care sites needed Receive, coordinate, and forward requests for personnel and supplies to the labor pool unit leader, medical care director, and material supply unit leader Communicate regularly situation, projected resource, and staffing needs to command center
Triage unit leader	Senior ED nurse	Establish triage area or areas Establish based on projected numbers and acuity number of triage staff needed Assess problem and triage-treatment needs relative to specific incident Identify staging areas for patients—red, yellow, green, and black Request stretchers, wheelchairs, and transport personnel to triage areas Request resource needs from the casualty care unit leader (CCUL) Communicate regularly situation, projected resource, and staffing needs to CCUL
Trauma care unit leader	Senior ED nurse	Establish patient treatment priorities with the ED attending Identify a senior surgeon to stay out of the OR to be a liaison with the senior ED attending Continually monitor and reassess all MCI patients for changes in status and new evolving needs Communicate surgical service lines needed to the chief medical officer Monitor OR availability and communicate projected needs to the command center and OR leads Communicate regularly situation, projected resource, and staffing needs to CCUL

(continued)

Table 24.2 (continued)

Role	Filled by	Critical tasks
Immediate care unit leader	ED nurse	Assess situation/area for supply and staffing needs. Request staff and supplies from the labor pool and supply unit leaders. Request medical staff support through CCUL Obtain an adequate number of patient transportation resources from the transportation unit leader to ensure the movement of patients in and out of the area Communicate regularly situation, projected resource, and staffing needs to CCUL
Delayed care unit leader	ED nurse	Assess situation/area for supply and staffing needs. Request staff and supplies from the labor pool and supply unit leaders. Request medical staff support through CCUL Ensure the rapid disposition and flow of treated patients from the delayed treatment area Communicate regularly situation, projected resource, and staffing needs to CCUL
Minor care unit leader	ED nurse	Establish minor care treatment area. This may be best in an alternate area to create more ED room for the more acute. Assess situation/area for supply and staffing need. Request staff and supplies from the labor pool and materials supply unit leaders. Request medical staff support through CCUL Obtain an adequate number of patient transportation resources from the transportation unit leader to ensure the movement of patients in and out of the area Ensure a rapid, appropriate disposition of patients treated within minor treatment area Communicate regularly situation, projected resource, and staffing needs to CCUL

access, and social work to reconcile families and patients. Discuss how and who is prioritizing patients for surgery, as this may be a rate limiter to getting care and therefore impact survival.

Set Up a Call Center

The nature of blast injuries may make it hard to identify victims, and the ED may become overrun with calls from families and friends looking for loved ones. It is crucial to set up a call center rapidly to divert these calls from the main ED desk. Social work staff is a good choice to manage the call center because they can coordinate with other hospitals and emergency operations centers to assist in finding loved ones and reunite families.

Patient Tracking

Due to the mechanism of injury, many critical patients may present immediately and will need immediate care to manage lifesaving interventions. These patients cannot wait to be registered and may present with no identification. Patient tracking may take an extended time, and it will be necessary to track patients across a region/state as patients will present or be sent to multiple hospitals from the scene [20]. Hospitals should have a process in place to begin patient care immediately without a name or identification. Hospitals will often employ "dummy" charts with a live medical record attached to be able to order labs, diagnostic radiology, pharmaceuticals, and blood products and avoid delays that can cost lives.

Logistics

Depending on acuity and volume of patients received, it may be necessary to identify a person to manage all the logistics. This person can be the point person for equipment, OR, blood bank, and other resource needs of these patients. They should track and close all requests and physically be within hearing distance in the areas set up for critical patients. This process funnels all requests through one person, and this person communicate the needs to the command center and tracks if the request has been filled or still pending. Ideally, this person has a clinical background, and he or she may be able to determine alternate equipment and supplies if the hospital is running out of a product (e.g., alternative OR kits, ventilator options, etc.).

Triage

Considerations on altering the triage process may be crucial in these types of events in order to manage the surge of critical patients. Not only should triage be staffed up, in primary triage, it may be sorted by only triage color, mental status, and the presence of a pulse. The best person conducting triage is not extra staff who are being utilized in the ED but instead the person most seasoned at conducting triage and performing rapid patient assessment. In some hospital systems in the US, this may be primarily nursing or a combined team of nurses and physicians, while in other countries, this may be a physician only. At the time of specific MCI events, it may be a combined team that includes surgeons [21–23]. Triage interventions should be damage control only. Triage should work like a pit stop, just to stratify critical, emergent, and low-acuity patients (red, yellow, green). Staff should clearly understand that triage is a dynamic process; in a blast scenario, patient conditions can change rapidly, and this must be managed through continual triage.

Lower-Acuity Patients (Green)

These patients can be triaged and wait in a lobby area or diverted to an ambulatory area of the hospital to wait or receive treatment. As injuries may not be readily apparent, these patients should be monitored closely and periodically re-triaged for any changes in acuity [24].

Critical Patients (Red)

High-acuity patients should be stabilized, be prioritized for OR, and/or utilize the postanesthesia care unit (PACU) to hold OR patients as they wait for OR time.

The PACU can be used pre and post OR as a critical care holding area, as the staff has the critical care skill set and equipment to safely care for this level of patient.

Family Reunification Waiting Area

In a mass casualty, families will be concerned and/or searching for loved ones almost immediately, and it may take a prolonged period of time to locate all the victims. These families pose unique challenges to the hospital and should be provided an area to gather as they wait for word on their loved ones. Staffing this area with social workers, pastoral care staff, and clergy to reunify family, provide psychological first aid, help with identifying victims without identification, and locate separated family members at other locations is key [25].

Staffing

In the immediacy, critical care and PACU nurses all have good skill sets to come help in the ED until extra ED staff are able to arrive. Floor nurses can manage the routine patient care in the ED and can assist the ED nurse in the non-acute areas. The hospital should have a plan on how they deploy non-ED nurses to the ED during a mass casualty. Policies often have the floor nurses come down to the ED to pick up admissions and get a quick report to help clear the ED. Rely on ED leadership to call in extra ED medical and nursing staff. In-house anesthesia, critical care intensivists, and hospitalists can assist the ED and trauma teams for a period of time. As the command center opens, the Chief Medical Officer should be getting the medical staff needed to assist with these patients.

Documentation

Documentation practices during blast events are often limited and inconsistent. It is essential to track any care that has been performed so that the next care providers are aware and to help with the later financial and medical needs of these patients in the months and years following the event. Often, patients have minimal information that may be written on their bodies with markers as they are rapidly sent from the ER to the OR. Planning should include streamlined documentation processes, including downtime paper charting and predesignated charts for unidentified criticals. This has proved to be faster than trying to continue with the EMR.

What Is Currently Best Practice?

Current best practices in hospital operations and management after blast events run the spectrum from executing coordinated command and control at the hospital level to continuous drilling to executing dynamic triage.

HICS

Utilization of the HICS approach is fairly standard in hospitals in the US and allows for the most organized approach to managing the chaos inherent in these types of events [15].

Drilling

A hospital plan is only useful if staff are familiar with how to execute it. Continuous drilling of various sections of the plan, patient surge, utilizing a call-out list, and heightened security measures allow for improvements and comfort with the plan at the time of a true crisis. Staff will often develop a "muscle memory" for what they need to do when the plan is enacted. This is critical in these low-frequency, high-impact events. This was cited as one of the reasons for such a successful medical response after the Boston Marathon bombings in 2013 [26].

As with any low-frequency, high-impact event, training and maintaining competency of staff is arduous. Most staff members are already overburdened with training on procedures they utilize daily, never mind an event that rarely occurs. That said, these high-impact events are on the rise nationally, and hospitals must be prepared to handle MCIs across the spectrum [27]. Staff may experience a "fog of war," or uncertainty in situational awareness, immediately following notification of an event. In order for staff to minimize confusion and empower action once an event occurs, they must have a plan to refer to and have developed muscle memory so they know the strategies that need to be immediately implemented to respond effectively [22]. This can be accomplished by drilling and exercises. Large, full-scale scoping exercises take significant resources, time, and funding to accomplish. Hospitals need to hold these types of exercises to walk staff through the entire plan and to also practice practical coordination with internal and external partners. Exercises help to identify and fix noted gaps in plans.

Large-scale exercises are not always necessary and may even be impractical for what is being drilled. If drilling an entire plan is too cumbersome, it may be prudent to divide your plan into pieces and drill each piece individually. An example of this technique is to routinely activate specific parts of the plan, such as expediting identified patients to floors during an ED high census due to a need for ED decompression. While this does not test the patient surge plan, per se, it does practice one of its integral processes. Another example is to ask floors to send staff members to the ED during a small-scale MCI to practice the buddy system, which helps non-ED staff members get used to deploying to the ED for a short period of time.

It is also effective to bring your incident management team together to manage smaller events, as this builds their capacity in working with each other in Hospital Incident Command System roles [28]. The more practiced all staff are, the more critical thinking skills they will have developed, which will allow for greater flexibility in management of the event based on its specific nuances [28, 29].

The more muscle-memory staff has, the faster the response will come together. If the plan is rarely practiced, undeveloped, and/or not properly vetted through the organization, it will be reflected in the outcome [22].

Comprehensive MCI ED Plan

A critical aspect of a successful response is to have a well-developed, well-thought-out, and well-exercised plan that is available to staff [27]. The plan should not only address all the ED strategies but should cast the net over the entire hospital for a coordinated response. A major gap is that many hospitals only rely on the ED for an MCI response, when in reality the response requires the whole hospital community. The more automated the hospital response is, the quicker that effective strategies affecting patient outcomes will be implemented. Having a plan in place that outlines the responding department's immediate roles and responsibilities, knowing what resources will come to the ED initially, and having other departments prepare for a surge is key to a good outcome.

Resource Management

The types of injuries associated with explosions typically tend to be resource-intensive and require specialized needs [5]. This poses a problem to hospitals that only have a finite number of resources. It is also problematic in that the type of blast can change what resources a hospital might utilize. More severe blasts tend to produce patients that require more surgeries, have a higher-frequency of ICU visits, and remain in the hospital longer [4]. Once capacity and capabilities are known, the team should begin immediate prioritization for the resources that will become scarce. This process should be coordinated between ED senior attending, trauma or surgical senior attending, and nursing leadership. The group should agree on goals. Once Incident Command is up and running, they need to be looped into the prioritization scheme and work on further capacity if needed.

Small Zones

While treating an MCI, the combination of patient volume and acuity can quickly overwhelm providers. By creating small zones of one to three beds where a smaller team of physicians and nurses provides care while the patients are moved in as space becomes available helps allow the medical team to focus on the care of the patients at hand while overall patient flow and management are being overseen by more senior staff. Many accounts after recent MCIs indicate similar techniques have been used with positive effects [30, 31].

Dynamic Triage

Medical staff need to understand that MCI and blast victims can often appear well in the initial stages of an event and decompensate within the first 6 hours.

Dynamic and continuous triage that adjusts for changes in resources and potential acute changes in patients' needs is critical in these types of events [9, 31].

Expanding Ventilator Capacity

After these types of events, there will likely be increased numbers of patients who require ventilator support. While there is federal capacity to send resources to states with increased need [32], there is a high likelihood of a critical ventilator shortage in the first 6 hours after an event. As a temporizing measure until more resources are acquired, it is possible to pair patients of similar size while increasing the tidal volume and using Y-tubing [33, 34].

Zero Preventable Deaths

The work of the National Academies and the Hartford consensus has shifted the focus of providing care in the civilian world based on lessons learned in the battlefield. One of the easier techniques to implement is the early use of tourniquets for major hemorrhage control [35, 36]. While these will be applied prehospital, maintaining them in the ED will allow for more unstable patients to have OR access sooner while still allowing for these patients with critical extremity injuries to still receive care in a timely fashion.

Conclusion

While hospitals and EDs cannot be prepared for every potential disaster or threat, the use of HICS and a strong EOP with an all-hazards approach gives systems the best chance for a successful response in the case of a blast-related event. Frequent drilling of various sections of the plan in all hospital spaces allows for the most comfort in transition of care at the time of an event and will likely help optimize patient outcomes.

Pitfalls

- The hospital incident management team is not familiar with their roles, responsibilities, and their interconnectedness.
- Lack of hospital wide practice for mass casualty situations and processes
- Lack of clinical discipline affecting resource utilization: reverting to day-to-day decisions, inability to tolerate practicing "greatest good for the greatest number," and practicing general trauma care as opposed to care optimized for blast victims

References

1. Reilly M, Markenson D. Hospital referral patterns: how emergency medical care is accessed in a disaster. Disaster Med Public Health Prep. 2010;4(3):226–31. Available from https://doi.org/10.1001/dmp.2010.30.
2. Hammond J. Mass casualty incidents: planning implications for trauma care. Scand J Surg. 2005;94:267–71.
3. Gates JD, Arabian S, Biddinger P, Blansfield J, Burke P, Chung S, Yaffe MB. The initial response to the Boston Marathon bombing: lessons learned to prepare for the next disaster. Ann Surg. 2014;260(6):960–6. Available from https://doi.org/10.1097/SLA.0000000000000914.
4. Rozenfeld M, Givon A, Shenhar G, Renert L, Peleg K. A new paradigm of injuries from terrorist explosions as a function of explosion setting type. Ann Surg. 2015. Available from: https://doi.org/10.1097/SLA.0000000000001338.
5. DeWitte M, Tracy E. Challenges of blast injuries. Adv Emerg Nurs J. 2005;27(3):176–9.
6. Kearns RD, Cairns BA, Cairns CB. Surge capacity and capability. A review of the history and where the science is today regarding surge capacity during a mass casualty disaster. Front Public Health. 2014;2(2):29.
7. Severance HW. Mass-casualty victim "surge" management. Preparing for bombings and blast-related injuries with possibility of hazardous materials exposure. N C Med J. 2002;63(5):242–6.
8. Propper BW, Rasmussen TE, Davidson SB, Vandenberg SL, Clouse WD, Burkhardt GE, et al. Surgical response to multiple casualty incidents following single explosive events. Ann Surg. 2009;250(2):311–5.
9. Ciottone GR, Biddinger PD, Darling RG, Fares S, Keim ME, Molloy MS, et al. Ciottone's disaster medicine. Philadelphia: Elsevier Health Sciences; 2015.
10. De Cauwer H, Somville F, Sabbe M, Mortelmans LJ. Hospitals: soft target for terrorism? Prehosp Disaster Med. 2017;32(1):94–100.
11. Frykberg ER. Medical management of disasters and mass casualties from terrorist bombings: how can we cope? J Trauma. 2002;53(2):201–12.
12. Li G-Q, Hou S-K, Yu X, Meng X-T, Liu L-L, Yan P-B, et al. A descriptive analysis of injury triage, surge of medical demand, and resource use in an university hospital after 8.12 Tianjin Port explosion, China. Chin J Traumatol. 2015;18(6):314–9.
13. Kuo L-W, Yen C-I, Fu C-Y, Pan C-H, Hsu C-P, Hsiao Y-C, et al. The role of preliminary hospitals in the management of a mass burn casualty disaster. Burns. 2018;44(4):800–6.
14. Peleg K, Jaffe DH. Israel Trauma Group. Are injuries from terror and war similar? A comparison study of civilians and soldiers. Ann Surg. 2010;252(2):363–9.
15. Hospital Incident Command System. Guidebook. 5th ed: California Emergency Medical Services Authority; 2014. p. 1–170.
16. Ellison A, Cohen J. 230 hospital benchmarks. Becker's Hospital Review. 2017; Available from: https://www.beckershospitalreview.com/lists/230-hospital-benchmarks-2017.html. Accessed 26 Aug 2018.
17. Davis DP, Poste JC, Hicks T, Polk D, Rymer TE, Jacoby I. Hospital bed surge capacity in the event of a mass-casualty incident. Prehosp Disaster Med. 2005;20(3):169–76. Available from: https://doi.org/10.1017/S1049023X00002405.
18. Kelen GD, McCarthy ML, Kraus CK, Ding R, Hsu EB, Li G, et al. Creation of surge capacity by early discharge of hospitalized patients at low risk for untoward events. Disaster Med Public Health Prep. 2009. Available from https://doi.org/10.1097/DMP.0b013e3181a5e7cd.
19. Campion EM, Juillard C, Knudson MM, Dicker R, Cohen MJ, Mackersie R, et al. Reconsidering the resources needed for multiple casualty events: lessons learned from the crash of Asiana airlines flight 214. JAMA Surg. 2016;13:1–6. Available from: https://doi.org/10.1001/jamasurg.2015.5107.

20. Landman A, Teich JM, Pruitt P, Moore SE, Theriault J, Dorisca E, et al. The Boston Marathon Bombings Mass casualty incident: one emergency department's information systems challenges and opportunities. Ann Emerg Med. 2015;66(1):51–9.
21. Navarro AP, Hardy E, Oakley B, Mohamed E, Welch NT, Parsons SL. The front-line general surgery consultant as a new model of emergency care. Ann R Coll Surg Engl. 2017;99(7):550–4.
22. Carles M, Levraut J, Gonzalez JF, Valli F, Bornard L. 16 authors, a full list of authors is available in the appendix. Mass casualty events and health organisation: terrorist attack in Nice. Lancet. 2016;388(10058):2349–50.
23. Gates JD, Arabian S, Biddinger P, Blansfield J, Burke P, Chung S, et al. The initial response to the Boston marathon bombing: lessons learned to prepare for the next disaster. Ann Surg. 2014;260(6):960–6.
24. Kleber C, Cwojdzinski D, Strehl M, Poloczek S, Haas NP. Results of in-hospital triage in 17 mass casualty trainings: underestimation of life-threatening injuries and need for re-triage. Am J Disaster Med. 2013;8:5–11.
25. Pandya A, Katz CL, Smith R, Ng AT, Tafoya M, Holmes A, et al. Services provided by volunteer psychiatrists after 9/11 at the New York City family assistance center. September 12-November 20, 2001. J Psychiatr Pract. 2010;16:193–9.
26. Gawande A. "Why Boston's Hospitals were ready." The New Yorker 2013. Why Boston's Hospitals were ready. https://www.newyorker.com/news/news-desk/why-bostons-hospitals-were-ready. Accessed 22 July 2018.
27. Moore K. Stop the bleeding: the Hartford consensus. J Emerg Nurs. 2017;43(5):482–3.
28. Shooshtari S, Tofighi S, Abbasi S. Benefits, barriers, and limitations on the use of Hospital Incident Command System. J Res Med Sci. 2017;22(1):36.
29. Hsu E, Jenckes M, Catlett C, Robison K, Feuerstein C, Cosgrove S, et al. Effectiveness of hospital staff mass-casualty incident training methods: a systematic literature review. Prehosp Disaster Med. 2004:191–9.
30. Orlando Health Disaster Response Project. https://www.orlandohealth.com/campaigns/g6iv8jkzop719. Accessed 22 July 2018.
31. Menes K, Tintinalli J, Plaster L. How one Las Vegas ED saved hundreds of lives after the worst mass shooting in U.S. History. EP Monthly. November 3, 2017. http://epmonthly.com/article/not-heroes-wear-capes-one-las-vegas-ed-saved-hundreds-lives-worst-mass-shooting-u-s-history/. Accessed 22 July 2018.
32. Ajao A, Nystrom SV, Koonin LM, Patel A, Howell DR, Baccam P, et al. Assessing the capacity of the US Health Care System to use additional mechanical ventilators during a large-scale public health emergency. Disaster Med Public Health Prep. 2015;9(6):634–41.
33. Neyman G, Irvin CB. A single ventilator for multiple simulated patients to meet disaster surge. Acad Emerg Med. 2006;13(11):1246–9.
34. Hick JL, Rubinson L, O'Laughlin DT, Farmer JC. Clinical review: allocating ventilators during large-scale disasters--problems, planning, and process. Crit Care. 2007;11(3):217.
35. National Academies of Sciences, Engineering, and Medicine. A National Trauma Care System: integrating military and civilian trauma systems to achieve zero preventable deaths after injury. Washington, DC: The National Academies Press; 2016.
36. Jacobs LM. Joint Committee to create a National Policy to enhance survivability from Intentional Mass Casualty shooting events. The Hartford consensus IV: a call for increased National Resilience. Conn Med. 2016;80(4):239–44.

25 Case Study: Emergency Department Response to the Boston Marathon Bombing

Czarina E. Sánchez and León D. Sánchez

Introduction

The Boston Marathon, the world's oldest annual marathon, brings over 20,000 runners and 500,000 spectators to this highly competitive race. On April 15, 2013, a few hours after the start of the race, two improvised explosive devices (IEDs) detonated near the finish line killing 3 people and injuring 279 [1]. The first explosion occurred at 2:49 pm on Boylston Street approximately 100 ft before the finish line. Seconds later, a second IED exploded along the same street. The IEDs were fabricated with pressure cookers and low-grade explosives and were placed where spectators watch runners cross the finish line. The bombs contained nails and metal shards which led to secondary blast injuries from the projectiles. The medical response primarily involved Boston's five level 1 adult trauma centers, but 26 hospitals in the surrounding area received patients, with a total of 118 ambulance transports from the scene.

Main Challenges

The emergency response to this incident presented challenges from the initial assessment at the scene to the area-wide coordination and hospital care. Given the spectator volume of the marathon, Boston had prepared for a mass casualty incident

C. E. Sánchez
Emergency Department, Brooke Army Medical Center, Fort Sam Houston, TX, USA

L. D. Sánchez (✉)
Harvard Medical School, Boston, MA, USA

Department of Emergency Medicine, Beth Israel Deaconess Medical Center, Boston, MA, USA
e-mail: lsanche1@bidmc.harvard.edu

D. W. Callaway, J. L. Burstein (eds.), *Operational and Medical Management of Explosive and Blast Incidents*, https://doi.org/10.1007/978-3-030-40655-4_25

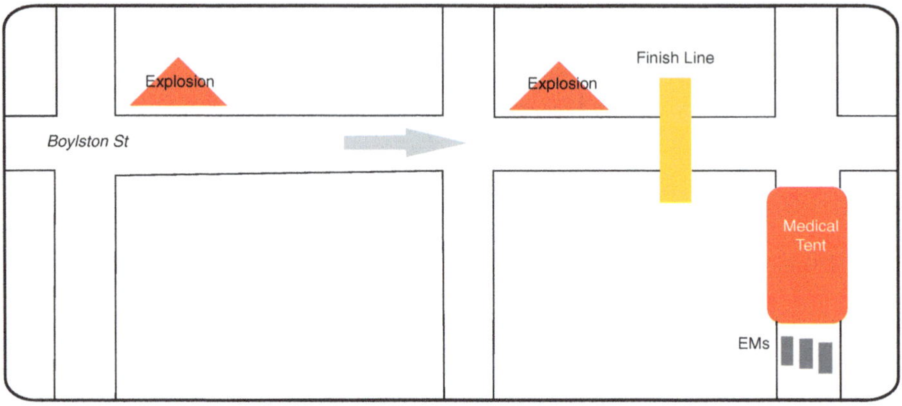

Fig. 25.1 Boston Marathon bombing scene diagram

(MCI) with a citywide incident management system. Hospitals added additional staffing and planned for the anticipated patient volume surge. On scene, a large medical tent was staged a short distance after the finish line to treat ill runners. Emergency medical services (EMS) were also stationed nearby to provide hospital transport [2] (Fig. 25.1). The initial challenge, as in any mass casualty incident, was the need for rapid triage. A significant advantage in this case was the number of medical staff already available at the finish line. Wheelchairs and volunteers waiting to help runners completing the marathon were instead used to transport victims to the medical tent. At the tent, patients were quickly evaluated by a triage team and directed to care areas for minor, moderate, and severe injuries. Maintaining standard field triage categories helped simplify this complex task. Victims with minor injuries were given first aid. Those with more significant injuries were stabilized and severe trauma patients moved for immediate transport by EMS to the surrounding trauma facilities. The first patient was transported from the scene 8 minutes after the explosion, and 100% of patients were transported within 1 hour [3]. The construction of the IEDs led to mostly lower body injuries from the explosions. Rapid hemorrhage control with tourniquets during triage was important, and Boston police officers are now equipped with purpose-designed tourniquets [4].

Another common challenge in MCIs is appropriate area-wide communication. The preestablished emergency operations center (EOC) helped distribute information and guide incident response decisions. Boston utilized WebEOC, a computer server, to help manage the flow of information during an incident [5]. WebEOC users can post information and communicate with all other users and provide real-time updates. The Internet connectivity of the system allows the EOC to operate outside one single physical location. Because of the high volume of calls, cellular phones were not reliable and communication was limited to the police radio system [4]. Integration with citywide partners was crucial to the well-developed response. While the possibilities for harm are endless, preparing for likely situations will provide a structure to respond in time of need. Predefined roles and responsibilities between the various state, local, and private agencies allowed for the successful effort in an event that could have otherwise overwhelmed the city [2].

One of the main challenges at the hospital level is the acute surge in patients. This difficulty was ameliorated by the excellent EMS response and balanced transfer of patients to the various hospitals. Also, the medical tent at the finish line provided surge capacity by holding a significant number of low-acuity victims. This action minimized the traditional initial emergency department surge of low-acuity patients post MCI and allowed facilities to focus resources on the more critical patients. Though the transport of patients from the scene was very rapid, hospitals were notified via the disaster radio within 5 minutes of the blasts. This early radio and EOC communication allowed hospitals to prepare for the MCI.

The following example highlights the response timeline for one of Boston's level 1 trauma centers, Beth Israel Deaconess Medical Center, where 24 patients from the bombings were treated. The disaster radio alert prompted the activation of the hospital's emergency operations plan. The patients in the emergency department (ED) were quickly assessed and either discharged or admitted to open beds for the incoming patients from the site. This occurred promptly as the hospital already had a system in place to facilitate movement out of the ED. Also based on prior planning, a HAZMAT tent was prepared for decontamination and incoming patients were scanned with a Geiger counter as it was unknown whether the explosions had chemical or radiological components. Security was established in cooperation with local police force within 30 minutes. Entrances were manned and everyone cleared prior to entering the hospital. A lobby was set up as a family center to provide a gathering space for people searching for loved ones.

Proper patient identification and tracking was a challenge. Part of the ED's standard operating procedures is a chart system which allows patient registration without full patient information. Preformatted "EU critical" charts allow the use of regular ordering and tracking system at times of large patient influx. This process streamlined registration and allowed order placement without delay. However, this system is not fail-proof, as multiple patients have the same "last name" increasing the chances of medication and charting errors. The triage at the hospital was coordinated by an ED attending who designated patient flow to different rooms. The bombings occurred at change of shift which provided immediate doubling of physician coverage in the ED. Physician teams were assigned to specific rooms, and patients were brought to them to allow the team to focus on one patient at a time rather than dealing with the whole event. This separated direct patient care from the management of resources, allowing caregivers to concentrate on individual patients in a way as close to their daily routine as possible. In a similar fashion, a surgery attending determined whether patients were going directly to the operating room or the ICU for later intervention. As an indicator of injury severity, 16 of the 24 patients required amputations (Fig. 25.2).

The pattern of injuries from the bombings led to the impromptu development of the Mass Casualty Service (MCS). This interdepartmental service was organized to

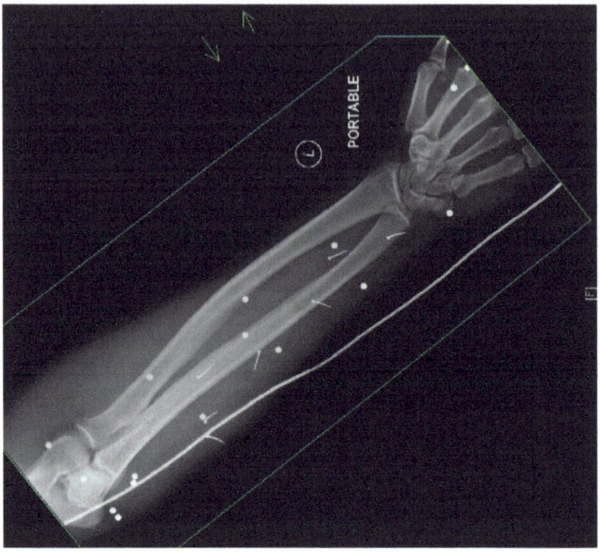

Fig. 25.2 Upper extremity x-ray with lodged nails and BBs

allow the central coordination of staged procedures across different services such as trauma, orthopedics, and plastics. For outpatient care, the MCS clinic provided one location for the multidisciplinary care of patients, including wound care and social work. While the rapid medical response was crucial to the positive outcomes, the long-term impact of a tragic event such as this should be considered to provide care beyond the critical first few hours. Providing psychological support, such as debriefing and providing a structure for discussion or counseling, is also important to help prevent negative psychological effects in both patients and staff.

Lessons Learned

- Have a plan. Preestablished MCI plans enabled the successful emergency response.
- Train on a recurrent basis to develop interagency coordination and provide the structure for real-word events.
- Anticipate the need for crowd control. Coordination with law enforcement and staff is crucial to control what can easily become a very chaotic space.
- Recognize long-term impact of event and need for multidisciplinary interaction.
- MCI response is like a marathon. It requires significant preparation, practice, and dedication.

References

1. Gates J, Arabian S, Biddinger P, Blansfield J, Burke P, Chung S, et al. The initial response to the Boston Marathon Bombing. Ann Surg. 2014;260(6):960–6. https://www.ncbi.nlm.nih.gov/pmc/articles/PMC5531449/.
2. Boston Marathon Bombings: the positive effect of planning and preparation on response [Internet]. Fema.gov. 2013 [cited 16 May 2018]. Available from: https://emilms.fema.gov/IS0235c/assets/BostonMarathonBombingsPositiveEffectsOfPreparedness.pdf.
3. 2013 Boston Bombings response & recovery [Internet]. Delvalle.bphc.org. 2018 [cited 16 May 2018]. Available from: https://delvalle.bphc.org/mod/page/view.php?id=610.
4. Stelter L. Boston Commish: 3 lessons learned from marathon bombing [Internet]. PoliceOne. 2013 [cited 16 May 2018]. Available from: https://www.policeone.com/chiefs-sheriffs/articles/6547563-Boston-Commish-3-/.
5. Cahill J. WebEOC fusion for disasters and everyday use [Internet]. Domestic Preparedness. 2008 [cited 16 May 2018]. Available from: https://www.domesticpreparedness.com/healthcare/webeoc-fusion-for-disasters-and-everyday-use/.

Case Study: Management of Blast Incidents in Israel

26

Avraham I. Rivkind

Case Report

The Sbarro Pizzeria suicide bombing took place on August 9, 2001 in a two-story building located on a busy crossing in downtown Jerusalem, Israel. The terror attack occurred at 2pm, when the restaurant was filled with customers and pedestrian traffic was at its peak. Fifteen civilians (and the bomber) were immediately killed including seven children and a pregnant woman. The blast injured 130 civilians. The bomber was wearing an improvised explosive device (IED) containing 8–10 kg of military-grade explosive material accompanied by a large amount of shrapnel such as nails, nuts, bolts, ball bearings, and rat poison; the shrapnel intensified the effects of penetrating trauma (Fig. 26.1). Following the attack, victims suffering from a combination of blast, penetrating injuries, and burns were brought to local hospitals.

There are four emergency departments (ED) in Jerusalem, and severely injured victims are preferentially evacuated to the only level 1 trauma center in the city, Hadassah University Hospital (HUH). In the event of a mass casualty incident (MCI), emergency medical services (EMS) crews are instructed to send severely injured casualties particularly to HUH over the nearest hospital despite in this instance it being located furthest of the four hospitals from the Sbarro Pizzeria (9.5 km, 6 mi). Due to HUHs broad range of experience with MCIs, blast injury, and triage, we have much experience in recognizing and treating complex injuries. Among the injured in this attack, a 14-year-old girl sustained multiple penetrating shrapnel wounds to her chest and lower limbs resulting in diffuse and severe soft tissue and bone damage (see Fig. 26.1). Massive blood loss required a total amount of 120 units of blood, FFP, and platelets to be transfused before an order was given to administer an injection of NovoSeven,

A. I. Rivkind (✉)
Department of General Surgery and Trauma, Hadassah Medical Center, Jerusalem, Israel
e-mail: AviR@hadassah.org.il

D. W. Callaway, J. L. Burstein (eds.), *Operational and Medical Management of Explosive and Blast Incidents*, https://doi.org/10.1007/978-3-030-40655-4_26

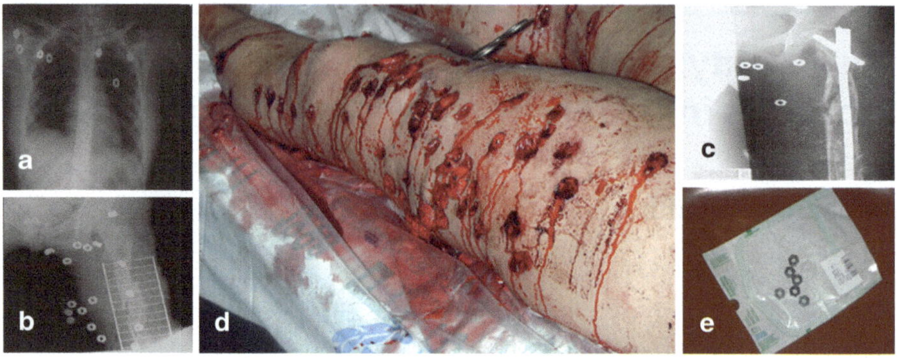

Fig. 26.1 A 14-year-old girl who was standing in proximity to the suicide bomber. She sustained multiple penetrating wounds to her chest and lower limbs (**a**, **b**, **d**). Comminuted femoral fracture and extensive soft tissue damage (**c**). Thigh showing multiple shrapnel entrance wounds (**d**). Some of the shrapnel removed from the patient (**e**)

a recombinant-activated factor VIIa. Activated VIIa was typically used to treat bleeding patients with hemophilia, and although it was not approved for a trauma situation, we have encouraged its use in exsanguinating trauma patients as an adjunct to medical and surgical hemostasis.

The availability of professional personnel, operating rooms, and ICU beds dictates the capacity of a medical center to handle an MCI. Approximately one-third of admissions to the ED within an hour of an MCI will be hospitalized as ED casualties usually correlate to the number of critically wounded [1]. This allows a general timeline for the management of hospital resources, and in-hospital teams can prepare accordingly for expected injuries. We have incorporated a multidisciplinary centrally coordinated and graded approach to handle our need to realign resources. As soon as the initial EMS report of an MCI is received, all available personnel are recruited in order of seniority and irrespective of call schedules by telephone landlines via a structured list, not via pagers or cellular phones which have been reported to crash due to overload at these times.

The ED is evacuated to provide physical space for incoming casualties by transferring existing patients to different floors, and incoming patients are admitted to the children's hospital located on the ground floor adjacent to the ED, which has oxygen and air that can be brought down from the ceiling (Fig. 26.2). The wide corridor opposite the ED leading to the outpatient clinics is additionally used to accommodate patients, essentially utilizing any available space outside the ED. Recovery rooms are evacuated to make room for temporary ICU beds while the ICU itself is alerted to relocate any patients they are able to other departments. All non-emergent studies, outpatient clinics, and scheduled operating room procedures are halted or rescheduled so all available personnel and resources can be redirected to the treatment of casualties. Elective computed tomography (CT) scans and, if necessary, magnetic resonance imaging (MRI) scans are also cancelled, thereby freeing up the radiography suites until the situation is stable.

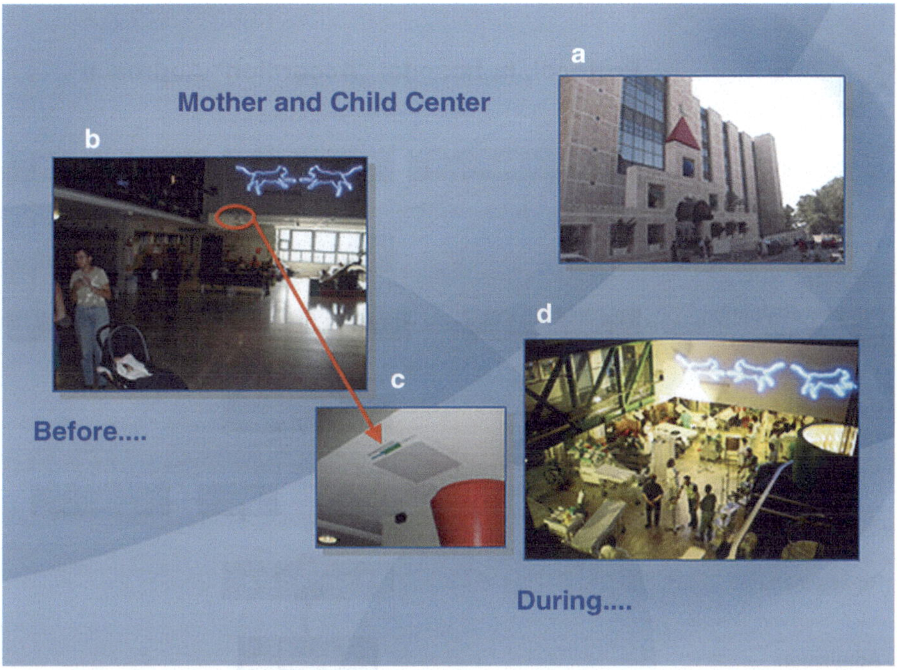

Fig. 26.2 Incoming casualties are admitted to the Mother and Child Center, which is reconfigured into a temporary ED. External building pictured upper right (**a**). Oxygen and air can be brought down from the ceiling when needed (**b**, **c**). During a mass casualty incident (**d**)

The ED Setup

The ED at HUH is divided into a designated trauma room with the capacity to simultaneously treat ten severely injured patients and a general admitting area that admits moderate to lightly injured victims. During a MCI, the latter are directed to an observation area after initial evaluation and examined once chaos subsides [2]. On arrival at the ED, surgical personnel are organized into predetermined teams of general surgeons, or subspecialty teams such as orthopedics, plastic surgery, and neurosurgery, and allotted to prearranged areas. The general surgeons lead the teams, initially examining each patient and determining the need for further examination by the subspecialty teams. Each team is led by an attending physician and includes two surgical residents and one or two anesthesiologists.

Surgeon-in-Charge: The Accordion Approach

We introduced a specialized, intensified approach to trauma care based on the guidelines for trauma management (Fig. 26.3). This includes hands-on close senior supervision beginning with prehospital triage and hospital preparedness and continuing

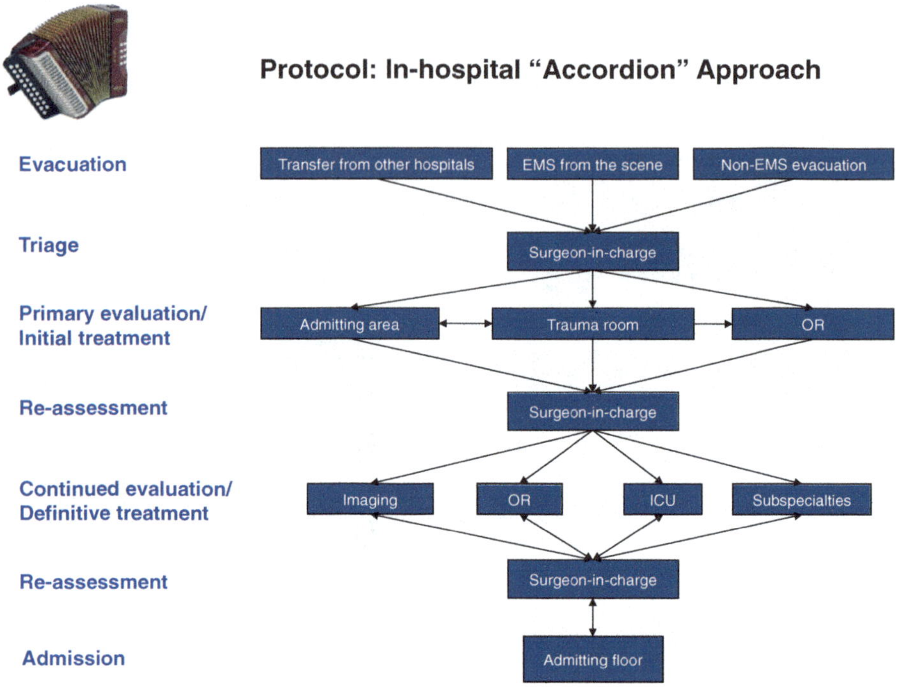

Fig. 26.3 The "accordion" approach. A definite chain of command is established via a centrally coordinated effort centered on the surgeon-in-charge. EMS, emergency medical services; OR, operating room; ICU, intensive care unit

with transportation, arrival, all surgical procedures, and hospital treatment through the discharge of the patient and completion of rehabilitation [3]. To ensure such senior supervision, the most experienced trauma surgeon available is designated as the surgeon-in-charge (SIC). The SIC receives each patient at the ambulance-unloading point and examines them outside the ED, triaging them into either the trauma room or the admitting area according to the presence of immediate life- or limb-threatening injuries and the degree of respiratory compromise. Attention is given to the moderately injured, whose injuries may be most immediately life-threatening. Initially, care should be withheld only from victims with severe and obvious brain injuries [4].

The SIC does not participate in surgical procedures in the first phases of triage and evaluation but rather determines operating room priority and accompanies the most severely injured victims into the trauma room. He orally communicates his findings to the treating teams and returns to receive the next incoming EMS crew and continue triage. The SIC is responsible for determining preferences for utilization of limited resources such as OR availability, ICU admissions, and CT and angiographic studies. Bedside sonograms as well as plain radiographs are performed for each severely injured victim, and CT scans and angiography are also used extensively. The SIC, together with treating teams, conducts repeated cycles of bedside reassessments on each patient in the ED, ICU, and OR during the initial 6–8 hours consisting of physical examination and review of the laboratory and imaging findings. Our protocol ensures that care is led by attendings experienced in major trauma who can provide quicker and better decision-making and thus save lives.

Identification and Communication

A special system has been developed for identifying, registering, and tracking patients that is activated in the event of an MCI where scores of casualties may be evacuated to different EDs. The system is connected to other hospitals as well as to the Ministry of Health, and all information is centrally shared and immediately accessible. Identification of victims is facilitated by using digital photos and Polaroid™ and obvious external signs such as birthmarks and tattoos. A crisis information center is set up for families staffed by a doctor, psychologists, nurses, social workers, a hospital spokesperson and police. The center can be reached by telephone, and the numbers are broadcast over the media and on the Internet. A nurse coordinator role is established; the nurse has direct access to the ED, trauma room, OR, ICU, and crisis center and is updated by the surgeons with all relevant patient information. The nurse in turn locates and informs the families of the condition and progress of their loved ones until the situation stabilizes.

A national system is also in place in Israel to prepare for extreme major disaster, such as earthquakes, when patients would be redirected to hospitals on the outskirts of Jerusalem for treatment; however, to date, our resources at HUH although heavily burdened have not been outstripped. This is in no small part due to the presence of a predetermined, well-defined, and rehearsed protocol with a definite chain of command whose effectiveness is achieved by a centrally coordinated effort centered on the SIC.

Challenges

- The surge in the inflow of injured victims presents a logistical challenge in terms of rapidly processing the casualties through the system and a medical challenge in providing the best possible trauma care to all victims [5]. This may be amplified by back-to-back attacks.
- First responders in the field are not all trained in advanced life support, and as a result, some severely injured victims are not brought to a level 1 trauma center [6].
- Following a terrorist attack, EMS crews are faced with the risk of second-hit explosions caused by additional attackers or devices, building collapse, and ignition of fuel aboard buses.
- Terrorist bombers have been infected by hepatitis B and HIV, so there is a risk of transmission to victims. All MCI victims should be immunized for hepatitis B.

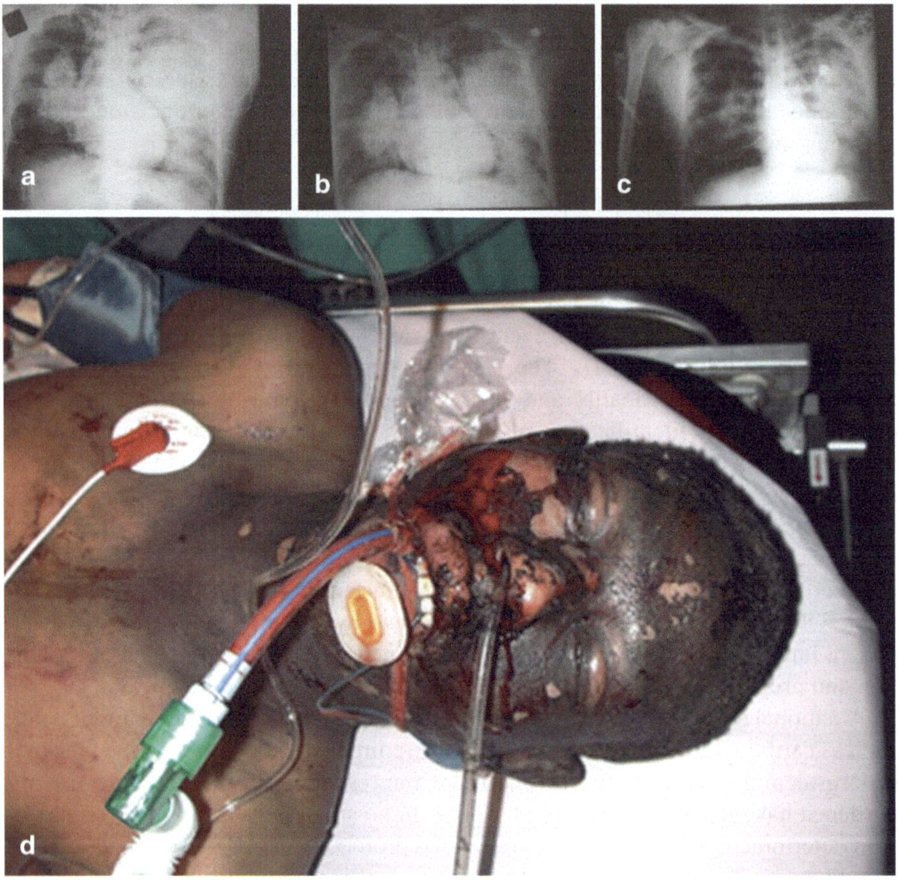

Fig. 26.4 Chest X-rays of a 21-year-old border policeman show development of blast lung injury (**a**–**c**). The man identified a terrorist at the entrance to a hospital and hugged him in order to prevent him entering. The border policeman blew up together with the terrorist. Note typical bilateral patchy lung infiltrates in a classic "butterfly appearance" consistent with blast lung injury (**b**). He also suffered from facial burns. Note blood inside the endotracheal tube, an indicator of severe primary blast lung (**d**)

- High index of suspicion in treating victims. With blast lung injury (Figs. 26.4 and 26.5), victims may walk into the emergency department without obvious external chest injury but bearing severe internal injuries including tearing, hemorrhage, contusions, and edema. There should be repeated examination and assessment of patients exposed to a blast for delayed presentation.

Lessons Learned

- Swift recognition of life-threatening injuries. External signs of injury, such as penetrating head and torso injury, and the number of body areas injured should guide prehospital and in-hospital triage for mass blast casualties of terror attacks.

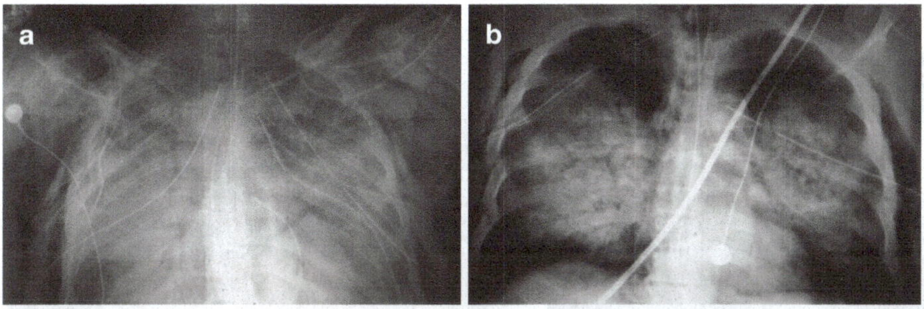

Fig. 26.5 Severe primary blast lung injury. Chest X-rays showing presence of multiple chest tubes inserted to treat severe primary blast lung (**a**, **b**)

Burns, open fractures, and amputations are significantly associated with death at the scene [7].

- Trauma education for doctors, nurses, as well as the new generation of medical school students and nurses significantly improves their management of trauma patients [8]. Students should be taught the pathophysiology of injury in patients suffering from primary, secondary, tertiary, and quaternary blast injury and be aware that bombing victims may sustain a combination of "the worst of both worlds" – multisite injuries from blast trauma caused by heavy particles as well as injury to isolated parts of the body from each particle at their site of entry, much like penetrating trauma. Students should also be aware of the implications for the physical setting of the incident on incidence and type of injury [4]. Mock disaster drills are integral to ingraining trauma preparedness, and HUH itself runs an annual drill to assure preparedness is at an optimum.
- Extensive use of CT scanners and angiography suites should be applied following an attack.
- Liberal use of chest drains to treat pneumothorax and to allow proper ventilation and oxygenation (see Fig. 26.5). Surgeons do not hesitate to use multiple chest drains.
- Liberal use of Foley catheters – can control bleeding/air leak (Fig. 26.6).
- Different modes of ventilation for blast lung injury – use independent lung ventilation, nitrous oxide, etc. [9].
- Creation of the roles of SIC and nurse coordinator.
- Do not chase after shrapnel – the majority retained in soft tissues becomes inert, and postponing exploration for and removal to a later stage after the initial chaos has subsided can still achieve excellent long-term results. The exception is in the case of infection, pain, and discomfort or where shrapnel is lodged in joints and bursae in order to prevent the development of destructive arthritis [10]. Computerized navigation-directed removal of foreign objects on MCI victims of terror attacks [11] has shown excellent results and within minimal operating time.
- Debriefings – held 12–18 hours after every MCI with the SIC, treating teams, department chairmen, nurses, administrative staff, hospital spokesperson, and EMS representatives.

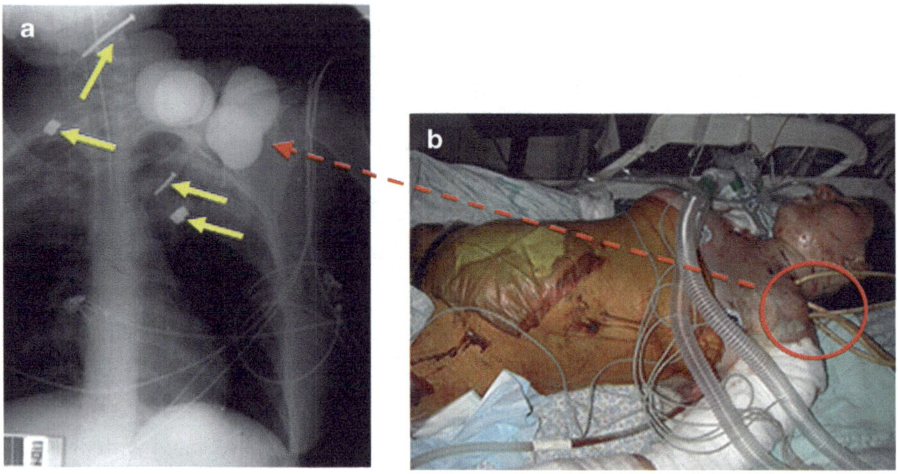

Fig. 26.6 Chest X-ray of a 19-year-old woman injured from multiple shrapnel in a suicide bombing attack (**a**). She suffered from profuse bleeding from her left upper chest and shoulder area due to shrapnel penetrating wounds reaching from the shoulder area to the lung. Note foreign bodies (arrows) and presence of four inflated Foley catheters (**b**)

References

1. Almogy G, Rivkind AI. Surgical lessons learned from suicide bombing attacks. J Am Coll Surg. 2006;202:313–9.
2. Almogy G, Rivkind AI. Terror in the 21st century: milestones and prospects—part II. Curr Probl Surg. 2007;44:566–619.
3. Rivkind AI, Blum R, Gershenstein I, Stein Y, Coleman S, Mintz Y, et al. Trauma care and case fatality during a period of frequent, violent terror attacks and thereafter. World J Surg. 2012;36:2108–18.
4. Almogy G, Belzberg H, Mintz Y, Pikarsky AJ, Zamir G, Rivkind AI. Suicide bombing attacks: update and modifications to the protocol. Ann Surg. 2004;239:295–303.
5. Hirshberg A. Multiple casualty incidents: lessons from the front line. Ann Surg. 2004;239:322–4.
6. Shamir MY, Rivkind A, Weissman C, Sprung CL, Weiss YG. Conventional terrorist bomb incidents and the intensive care unit. Curr Opin Crit Care. 2005;11:580–4.
7. Almogy G, Mintz Y, Zamir G, Bdolah-Abram T, Elazary R, Dotan L, et al. Suicide bombing attacks: can external signs predict internal injuries? Ann Surg. 2006;243:541–6.
8. Rivkind AI, Faroja M, Mintz Y, Pikarsky AJ, Zamir G, Elazary R, et al. Combating terror: a new paradigm in student trauma education. J Trauma Acute Care Surg. 2015;78(2):415–21.
9. Pizov R, Oppenheim-Eden A, Matot I, Weiss YG, Eidelman LA, Rivkind AI, et al. Blast lung injury from an explosion on a civilian bus. Chest. 1999;115(1):165–72.
10. Rhee JM, Martin R. The management of retained bullets in the limbs. Injury. 1997;28:S-C23-8.
11. Mosheiff R, Weil Y, Khoury A, Liebergall M. The use of computerized navigation in the treatment of gunshot and shrapnel injury. Comput Aided Surg. 2004;9:39–43.

Part IV

Surgical Management

Scope of the Problem and Operational Considerations: Logistics, Surge Capacity, Organizing a Response, Sustainment Issues, Resource Utilization

27

Brian J. Eastridge

Introduction

Mass casualty incident (MCI) events have the potential to overwhelm the capabilities of a regional trauma system. The challenge of explosive-associated MCI events is their inherent potential to inflict numerous casualties, each with the potential for multiple significant injuries. The threat of this scenario is further compounded by the fact that few providers or medical facilities have experience with events in which human and material resources can be rapidly overwhelmed. Several operational challenges impact the surgical response to MCI, including lack of information (or even disinformation), limited human resources, blood and blood product resuscitation resources, operating room availability, and materiel resources.

The most fundamental and important clinical element in the early phase of patient care after an explosive injury event is triage, which often needs to be performed at multiple tiers, including outside the emergency department, in relation to radiologic imaging, and for the use of an operating room. Triage must be performed by a provider with sufficient clinical expertise and administrative authority to make decisions. Injuries produced by an explosive agent are often multifactorial owing to device and environmental characteristics. Subcategories of explosive injury yield distinctly different spectra of injuries that must be surgically managed. The primary energy wave (blast wave) produces an incremental supersonic high-amplitude spike in pressure, which affects primarily air-filled viscera. These injuries often manifest as sequelae of pulmonary dysfunction. Secondary explosive injury caused by device fragmentation or secondary debris and tertiary explosive injury caused by physical displacement of the casualty inflict the majority of wounds that require surgical

B. J. Eastridge (✉)
Department of Surgery, Trauma and Emergency General Surgery, University of Texas Health Science Center at San Antonio, San Antonio, TX, USA
e-mail: eastridge@uthscsa.edu

D. W. Callaway, J. L. Burstein (eds.), *Operational and Medical Management of Explosive and Blast Incidents*, https://doi.org/10.1007/978-3-030-40655-4_27

management. Due to the nature of secondary explosive injury, casualties presenting for care after these events often have multiple penetrating injuries. In addition, it is important to note that injuries are often caused by more than one explosive mechanism, including quaternary crush, inhalation, and burns, further compounding the complexity of their management [1–3]. Although clinical care of explosive-related injury is founded upon the same basic principles as standard trauma management paradigms, it is incumbent upon the surgeon to also understand the principles of triage and potential limitations imposed by the casualty volume or complexity of injuries. Likewise, it is important to note that damage control strategies to control hemorrhage may serve a more prominent role so as to manage multiple casualties and optimize resource utilization. Supporting this assertion is evidence from recent contingency operations in which the most significant mechanism of injury was explosion. Analyses from these operations validate hemorrhage as the most substantial etiology of potentially preventable deaths, both prehospital and in the military medical treatment facility [4–6]. In fact, 24% of all casualties who died prior to reaching a medical treatment facility had potentially survivable wounds, of which 90% were associated with hemorrhage [5]. Of those who died after they reached a treatment facility, 51% had potentially survivable injury of which 80% were associated with a hemorrhagic cause [4].

The surgeon must be able to manage complex wounds and their sequelae that are well beyond the bounds of day-to-day practice. An editorial by Hirshberg published in 2004 summarizes and highlights:

> Terrorist bombings bring with them a host of new and vexing clinical problems.... What do you do with a hemodynamically stable, awake, and alert patient harboring dozens of small metal fragments in multiple body cavities, including the brain? How do you manage a "human remains shrapnel," a fragment of the suicide bomber's bone embedded in the chest of an asymptomatic patient? What if the suicide bomber was carrying a transmissible disease? Unexpected encounters with difficult clinical problems are a hallmark of MCIs. The answers must be learned from experience and rapidly disseminated to other surgeons facing the same challenges [7].

Trauma Systems

Effective functioning of the modern trauma system requires timely and structured cooperation, process, and communication across the continuum of care from the emergency medical services response through hospitalization. Optimizing performance of the trauma system requires a vision taken from the military mantra to "train like we fight." Utilizing resources, processes, and systems that would be integral to a disaster response on a daily basis produces the "muscle memory" to be proficient on "game day" basis. In addition, a critical requirement for successful performance during a mass casualty incident is carrying out realistic and relevant exercises and assessment of the mass casualty response plan before a real event. Regions with highly developed trauma systems are better prepared to respond to mass casualty events and wide-scale disasters—both natural and intentional [8–10]. Several studies have educed the association between the maturity of regionalized trauma systems and disaster readiness. Trauma system structures integrating EMS, evacuation assets, and tiered trauma centers through a robust and effective communication system have demonstrated the highest efficacy in MCI events [11]. The urban response plan in Israel manifests similar capabilities but is structured in three distinct tiers of graded requirement based upon incident magnitude, hospital capability, and surge capacity [12].

Triage

The effective triage of explosive MCI casualties must be performed by an experienced emergency physician/surgeon who is familiar with the capabilities of staff and resources available. Leadership capability is paramount for the triage officer, who must have a broad situational awareness as well as focused responsibility to make a decision on every patient. The classic triage categories of immediate, delayed, and expectant are a relative determination made by the triage officer based upon casualty volume and acuity balanced against resources in order to optimize outcomes for the greatest number of casualties.

Explosive injuries are characterized by a significant degree of tissue injury/loss, wound contamination, and a tendency to produce significant bleeding. The highest acuity casualties designated as emergent should be those with hemodynamic instability, particularly those with fragmentation injuries to the torso, due to the likelihood of a noncompressible hemorrhagic source being the source for their clinical deterioration. Therefore, minimizing unnecessary delays, specifically delays to operation in severely injured casualties, is a major goal of the triage process. In many systems, a "direct to the operating room" triage decision that bypasses the typical emergency department evaluation and resuscitation processes may best serve casualties at risk of further decompensation from obvious bleeding source(s).

Prioritization of surgical procedures, "the OR board," is a secondary triage capability for which the surgeon must take responsibility. This prioritization must be made relative to the casualty acuity within the context of the clinical operational scenario. A pragmatic approach has been proposed by Israeli trauma surgeons managing blast MCI casualties whereby procedures are performed based upon clinical urgency as follows:

- Surgical airway (cricothyroidotomy)
- Control of life-threatening hemorrhage in the torso or junctional regions
- Craniotomy for neurologically deteriorating brain injuries amenable to surgery

Notably, resource constraints suggest there is no indication for resuscitative thoracotomy in these circumstances. Secondary priority is subsequently assigned to casualties with non-exsanguinating hemorrhage, suspected visceral injury, and vascular injuries with limb-threatening ischemia. Tertiary priority is given to musculoskeletal injuries, soft tissue wound debridements, and burn care [12].

Logistics

Management of hospital resources is a critical element of the MCI response. Several recent civilian- and conflict-associated MCI events have provided a valuable perspective on the surgical resource allocations necessary for response. As a result of the Madrid train bombings in 2004, 198 casualties died and 2312 were injured. Of those injured, only 37 lifesaving procedures were performed on 34 patients. The majority of the operative resources (41%) were dedicated to the management of orthopedic injuries [13]. Lynn and colleagues evaluated logistic requirements in the context of current global terrorism events, largely blast-related. From this composite analysis, the authors concluded that 50% of MCI casualties will ultimately require surgery. However, only 2–4% of the most severely injured casualties require lifesaving resuscitative surgery for hemorrhage control or other emergent procedure [14, 15]. Another contemporary study utilized data from the Israeli Trauma Registry in order to develop clinical practice guidelines to support MCI preparedness. Results of the analysis of 325 explosive casualties from 32 events demonstrated that severely injured patients (ISS $\geq$ 16) constituted approximately one-third of the admissions and tended to arrive early in the event. Due to the propensity for life-threatening injuries in these casualties, operative services, particularly anesthesiology and surgical specialties (general/trauma, thoracic, cardiovascular), were noted to be in immediate demand during the earlier phase of the MCI response. The majority of procedures following a blast MCI were orthopedic and soft tissue procedures, which were expected to be continuous for extended periods depending upon the event magnitude [16]. Consequently, civilian evidence suggests that hospital contingency plans for MCI events should accommodate both surgical phases of the response.

Numerous case series from recent conflict in Iraq and Afghanistan have highlighted the propensity for wounding by explosive mechanisms. Likewise, the majority of operative procedures performed for explosive injuries were musculoskeletal (21.5%) and integumentary (22.6%). One-third of the musculoskeletal cases were associated with procedures for the management of long bone fractures. The majority of integumentary procedures (74%) were soft tissue debridements [17]. A study by Propper et al. evaluated three multiple casualty events managed at the US Air Force Theater Hospital in Balad, Iraq. Of the casualties treated, 48% required blood transfusion, including 8% who required massive transfusion (~18 units/casualty).

Of those casualties receiving blood, each received an average of 3.5 units pRBC and 3.8 units plasma. In contrast to civilian events, the battlefield experience demonstrated that 76% of patients required operation. Many casualties had simultaneous procedures and each casualty had ~3.8 procedures [18]. Another military study produced similar results. Evaluating casualties over a 1-year period, 415/539 (77%) MCI casualties required operative therapy for injuries. The number of casualties requiring blood was 135 (22%), although the mean RBCs transfused for any injured patient requiring blood was 6.3 units. Similar to previous studies, the number of massive transfusion casualties was 26 (4.6%). As blood and blood products are a particularly precious resources during MCI events, the authors sought to develop a reliable predictive index of blood product requirements for a multiple or mass casualty events. From their analyses, the average number of RBC units, inclusive of whole blood per patient (per patient index/PPI) for MCI events, was 1.4 [19].

Within the context of the blast mass casualty event, each casualty with a surgical requirement projects a cumulative resource requirement on the system. Depending upon available resources, surgeons managing explosive mass casualties must have a low threshold to exercise damage control surgery techniques, initially providing only temporizing lifesaving interventions in order to accommodate the casualty load within the system. As a consequence, the most severely injured surgical casualties may require interval damage control procedures.

Contemporary/Best Practice

A recent project conducted by the University Center for Disaster Preparedness and Emergency Response at Robert Wood Johnson University Hospital sought to develop best practice consensus on the management of explosive incidents. This work was funded under a grant supported by the US Army Telemedicine and Advanced Technology Research Center of the US Army Medical Research and Materiel Command. Findings of the panel associated with the surgical response to explosive MCI include the following [20]:

- Blast events are a special subset of mass casualty incidents that are characterized by the abrupt nature of an explosion, its physical results, and the complexity of the injuries sustained by casualties.
- All blast incidents should be considered terrorist events until proven otherwise. This has far-reaching implications for security at both the scene and the hospital, requiring a specific mindset and perspective that must be acquired and refined in responders and hospital staff.
- On-scene medical treatment should be limited to basic life support for the most seriously injured casualties. Only casualties requiring advanced life support and immediate treatment at trauma centers should be transported to hospitals as quickly as possible where they can receive appropriate treatment for their wounds.
- Emergency medicine physicians, surgeons, and other physicians, for the most part, know what to do to treat and save casualties; however, they need to understand the complexity of the multisystem and multidimensional injuries received in an explosion and the order in which to deal with them.
- Responders and hospitals need to incorporate as many processes and procedures required to deal with explosive incidents as possible into daily routine practices so that they are familiar with them should a mass casualty event occur.

Although not specifically delineated within this best practice consensus, a few additional noteworthy best practice tenets have emerged relative to recent study of the topic.

- Surgeons must approach the evaluation and management of explosive mass casualty injuries with a damage control philosophy, both in the context of resuscitation and operation.
- All MCI incidents start locally. Functionally effective trauma systems are the framework for MCI preparedness and response.

Conclusion

Inherent in their nature, explosion events have the potential to generate masses of significantly injured casualties through a number of different mechanisms. The most substantial causes of explosive injury mortality in the prehospital environment are severe tissue disruption, traumatic brain injury, and hemorrhage. As hemorrhage is the most significant etiology of potentially injury-preventable mortality, it is vital that the surgeon and trauma team be integrated into the hospital regional trauma system preparedness and response system plans. The trauma management capabilities of the local environment must be developed and consistently rehearsed through day-to-day clinical practice and through periodic disaster drills that are both realistic and relevant in order to develop the "muscle memory" to optimally support the contingency of a response to an explosion event. The surgeon must take a substantial leadership role, working alongside peers, to establish roles, triage process, and patient flow dynamics for response planning in the context of the local environment. Likewise, the MCI response team must understand the human resources, material assets, and hospital surge capacity available for response, both at the hospital and greater systemic levels.

Pitfalls

- Failure of trauma systems communications with component elements across the continuum of care leading to lack of information or misinformation
- Delays in declaring a mass casualty event associated with lag in resuscitation and surgical resources for MCI response
- Ineffective triage leading to delays in care
- Doing "too much operating"

References

1. Luks FI. Blast injuries--and the pivotal role of trauma surgeons. Acta Chir Belg. 2010;110:517–20.
2. Mathews ZR, Koyfman A. Blast Injuries. J Emerg Med. 2015;49:573–87.

3. Wolf SJ, Bebarta VS, Bonnett CJ, Pons PT, Cantrill SV. Blast injuries. Lancet. 2009;374:405–15.
4. Eastridge BJ, Hardin M, Cantrell J, Oetjen-Gerdes L, Zubko T, Mallak C, et al. Died of wounds on the battlefield: causation and implications for improving combat casualty care. J Trauma. 2011;71:S4–8.
5. Eastridge BJ, Mabry RL, Seguin P, Cantrell J, Tops T, Uribe P, et al. Death on the battlefield (2001-2011): implications for the future of combat casualty care. J Trauma Acute Care Surg. 2012;73:S431–7.
6. Blackbourne LH, Czarnik J, Mabry R, Eastridge B, Baer D, Butler F, et al. Decreasing killed in action and died of wounds rates in combat wounded. J Trauma. 2010;69(Suppl 1):S1–4.
7. Hirshberg A. Multiple casualty incidents: lessons from the front line. Ann Surg. 2004;239:322–4.
8. Kuhls D, Fildes J, Johnson M, Dort S, et al. Southern Nevada Trauma System uses proven techniques to save lives after 1 October shooting. Bull Am Coll Surg. 2018;103(3):39–46.
9. Wild J, Maher J, Frazee RC, Craun ML, Davis ML, Childs EW, et al. The Fort Hood Massacre: lessons learned from a high profile mass casualty. J Trauma Acute Care Surg. 2012;72:1709–13.
10. Force AMCDCBIT. Dismounted complex blast injury: report of the dismounted complex blast injury task force. 2011.
11. Bachman S, Demeter N, Lee G, Burke R, Valente TW, Upperman JS. The impact of trauma systems on disaster preparedness: a systematic review. Clin Pediatr Emerg Med. 2014;15:296–308.
12. Stein M. Urban bombing: a trauma surgeon's perspective. Scand J Surg. 2005;94:286–92.
13. Bolling R, Ehrlin Y, Forsberg R, Rüter A, Soest V, Vikström T, et al. KAMEDO report 90: terrorist attacks in Madrid, Spain, 2004. Prehosp Disaster Med. 2007;22:252–7.
14. Lynn M, Gurr D, Memon A, Kaliff J. Management of conventional mass casualty incidents: ten commandments for hospital planning. J Burn Care Res. 2006;27:649–58.
15. Kashuk JL, Halperin P, Caspi G, Colwell C, Moore EE. Bomb explosions in acts of terrorism: evil creativity challenges our trauma systems. J Am Coll Surg. 2009;209:134–40.
16. Einav S, Aharonson-Daniel L, Weissman C, Freund HR, Peleg K, Israel Trauma G. In-hospital resource utilization during multiple casualty incidents. Ann Surg. 2006;243:533–40.
17. Chambers LW, Green DJ, Gillingham BL, Sample K, Rhee P, Brown C, et al. The experience of the US Marine Corps' Surgical Shock Trauma Platoon with 417 operative combat casualties during a 12 month period of operation Iraqi freedom. J Trauma. 2006;60:1155–61; discussion 61-4.
18. Propper BW, Rasmussen TE, Davidson SB, Vandenberg SL, Clouse WD, Burkhardt GE, et al. Surgical response to multiple casualty incidents following single explosive events. Ann Surg. 2009;250:311–5.
19. Beekley AC, Martin MJ, Spinella PC, Telian SP, Holcomb JB. Predicting resource needs for multiple and mass casualty events in combat: lessons learned from combat support hospital experience in operation Iraqi freedom. J Trauma. 2009;66:S129–37.
20. Lacy CR, Ballagh R, Donovan CM, Bucher J. Management of explosive incidents: overview of the project and summary of best practices consensus statements of the expert panel. Ann Emerg Med. 2017;69:S1–3.

Combat Lessons Learned

28

Jacob R. Peschman and Donald H. Jenkins

Introduction

Lessons learned in the surgical management of combat-injured patients have been a staple of military medicine for centuries. These hard-fought and hard-learned lessons in the care of injury victims during military conflicts infallibly return home with the surgeons and their patients to change, almost invariably for the better, civilian surgical practice globally. To quote Evan Renz, a retired colonel who served in the US Army, "the only winner in war is medicine." While some of the advances are quite specific to combat mechanisms of injuries and wounding patterns such as complex dismounted blast injuries, many are not or are based on principles that can be applied for novel treatment of more conventional surgical problems. At the outset of the deployment to the combat theater of operations in September of 2001, coalition forces employed a previously non-battlefield-tested and rather unconventional concept, forward or mobile surgical teams sent to care for the injured rather than having the injured sent to them. These teams were small surgical teams, typically composed of surgeons, orthopedists, anesthesia providers, nurses, and medics, meant to be forward deployed closer to the location of the wounding with the intent to decrease the time from injury to initial surgical management [1]. This, for the first time, gave a role 2 military treatment facility (MTF) surgical capability (Fig. 28.1).

These forward surgical teams, employed by the medical branches of each service, were composed and outfitted differently, but their missions were the same: to

J. R. Peschman (✉)
Department of Surgery, The Medical College of Wisconsin, Milwaukee, WI, USA
e-mail: jpeschma@mcw.edu

D. H. Jenkins
Department of Surgery, Division of Trauma and Emergency Surgery, UT Health San Antonio, San Antonio, TX, USA

D. W. Callaway, J. L. Burstein (eds.), *Operational and Medical Management of Explosive and Blast Incidents*, https://doi.org/10.1007/978-3-030-40655-4_28

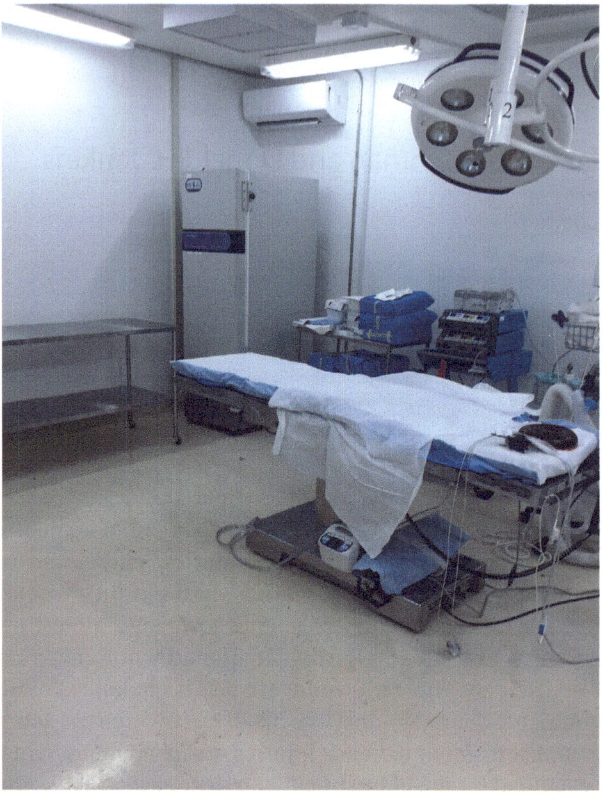

Fig. 28.1 Role 2 MTF operating room. (Photographer J. Peschman)

save lives and limbs using damage control and other nontraditional techniques. Therefore, badly injured casualties received abbreviated surgical care before being transported to the next level (echelon or role) of care by a different team capable of providing critical care in the back of a helicopter or ambulance. This was yet another untested concept but ultimately allowed delivery of a living, salvageable patient for definitive surgical management at the next-level MTF where more robust resources (e.g., CT scans, fluoroscopy, surgical subspecialists, etc.) awaited them [2]. The groups providing care quickly gained valuable experience, and it became apparent that those responsible for the design and implementation of these teams had fielded a highly capable and successful new system of combat casualty care.

Many lessons about the surgical care of blast injuries were learned by these forward teams and at the larger role 3 facilities that provided definitive care. Those lessons have been captured and informed by data. The outcomes are tracked in the Department of Defense (DoD) Trauma Registry (TR), allowing management strategies to be revised over time. This process and these lessons have become the backbone of the DoD Trauma System (DoDTS) Clinical Practice Guidelines (CPGs) [3]. It is with this background that the lessons learned over the past 17 years of combat surgery are outlined in the remainder of this chapter.

Lesson 1: Listen to the Civilian Surgeons, Use Your Tools, and Don't Do It All at Once

Damage control surgery (DCS) was designed in civilian trauma centers of the 1980s and 1990s. The DCS principles were meant to be employed in critical, unstable, injured patients and were guiding tenets in the development, composition, and equipping of the small surgical teams [4]. As a treatment paradigm, DCS had never been tested in combat. But the surgical teams sent to provide this care had this training and knowledge from their clinical work in military and/or civilian treatment and training facilities. The basic principles employed in DCS are to stop bleeding and contamination, debride dead tissue, and utilize techniques of temporary closure of body cavities (e.g., open abdomen). This results in an expeditious completion of an operation addressing what is life or limb threatening before bringing the patient for further resuscitation in a critical care (intensive care unit) environment to reverse the physiology of shock, hypothermia, and coagulopathy, the so-called lethal triad of injury. Civilian studies showed that definitive surgery in injured patient with this lethal triad had a 90% mortality whereas DCS had a 50% mortality [5]. This DCS technique was successfully employed without modification from civilian experience. A main part of the lesson here is that employing surgical techniques proven in civilian settings have the potential to be adopted, and adapted, for use in the military wounding scenarios. While many of the specific techniques for DCS will be covered in more detail in subsequent chapters of this text, several warrant immediate attention as their implementation in combat operations provided invaluable information for current strategies of surgical care of the blast-injured patient.

Part of the armamentarium in DCS is vascular shunting of blood vessels (Fig. 28.2). This has been shown in civilian settings to allow for maintenance of perfusion to injured limbs in patients at high risk of dying of the lethal triad at index operation followed by definitive surgical management at a later time when the patient is more stable, offering potentially a better outcome than primary amputation for

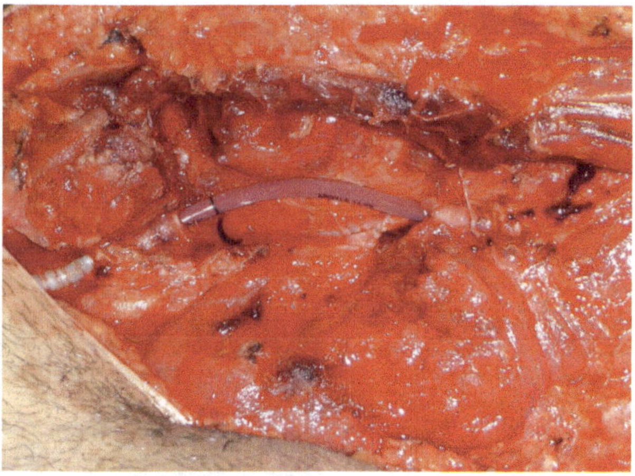

Fig. 28.2 Vascular shunt. (Photographer D. Jenkins)

many patients. For the first time, small surgical teams in forward facilities placed stabilizing shunts, and the casualty was evacuated to a higher role of care for definitive surgical vascular injury management. In some extreme cases, casualties with shunts did not have definitive surgical management until arrival in the continental United States. This aggressive shunting, never previously used in the combat-injured, was adopted quickly, and teams equipped to treat blast-injured patients with most complex injury patterns and long-segment vascular loss now had an additional option beyond amputation. Initial experience demonstrated that early viability in shunted extremities was 92% [6]. This supported shunting as a viable component of a core goal of vascular injury management and limb preservation. The Balad Vascular Registry was initiated early in the war and, in conjunction with the DoDTR, used to evaluate functional limb salvage [7]. It was apparent that arterial shunts were affiliated with limb salvage, including in injured combatants who also received tourniquets in the prehospital setting. The combination of vascular injury, tourniquet use, and vascular repair had not been practiced nor described prior to this current conflict. The basic tenets of vascular injury management were adopted and further adapted in the care of injured combatants and are a centerpiece of DoDTS CPGs [8].

Another key part of operative management of limb salvage following blast injury involves the use of other DCS concepts including use of external fixation for fractures and fasciotomies to prevent extremity compartment syndrome and its sequela. All of the techniques mentioned thus far have been incorporated into just-in-time, go-to-war training courses for surgeons. The combination of tourniquet use, external fixation, and fasciotomies is another unique combat injury management paradigm not seen before but has been quite successful in terms of limb salvage in this new pattern of complex blast injury. While a low number of external fixation fracture management patients have undergone definitive surgical management (internal fixation) in theater, there is robust, positive outcome data for this treatment regimen where definitive surgical management eventually occurs in role 4 or 5 (continental United States) (Fig. 28.3) [9–11].

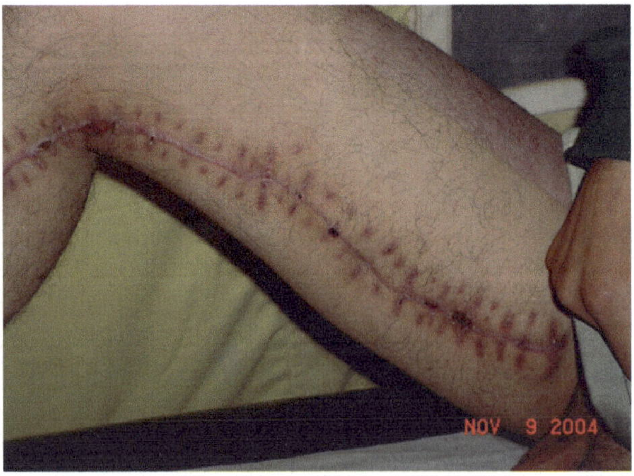

Fig. 28.3 Limb salvage outcomes. (Photographer D. Jenkins)

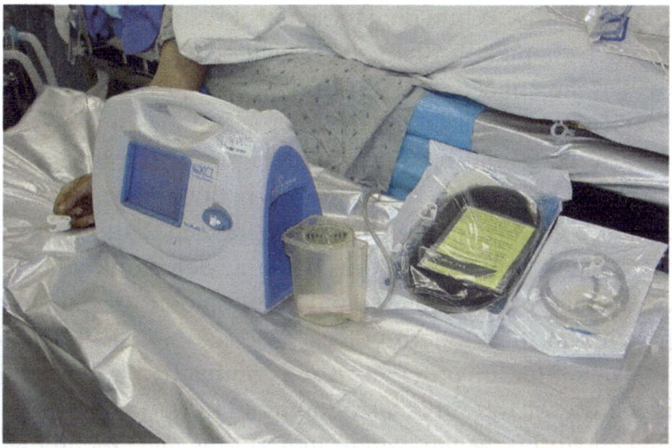

Fig. 28.4 Portable NWPT system. (Photographer D. Jenkins)

Another surgical management technique not previously employed for combat-injured patients was negative pressure wound therapy (NPWT) management. The long-standing military dogma that wounds suffered in combat should not be closed due to the exceptionally high infection/failure rate was taught to all surgeons going into combat until 2006. The use of NPWT was devised and employed in civilian settings for surgical management of wounds for trauma and non-trauma patients in order to promote earlier healing, decrease postsurgical wound complications, and decrease pain. When hostilities began in 2002, there was no thought about employing this wound management paradigm. The NPWT technique was novel, with little experience or data supporting its use, especially in military trauma. However, as the technique gained momentum and outcomes improved in civilian settings, NPWT made its way into the combat zone in 2004. Initially, NPWT utilization was confined to the host nation patients as there were no devices, supplies, plans, nor training to provide this care to the US combatants during transport along the continuum of care. Once simple, portable equipment became more widely available, the technique was transformative (Fig. 28.4). Lengths of stay, pain, the need for healing by secondary intent (natural ingrowth of tissue and skin), and skin grafting diminished in large blast wounds with significant defects that otherwise would have had limited treatment options. The rate of infection and failure to heal was shown to be diminishingly small if not nonexistent [12]. In addition, appreciation of the role of antibiotic therapy and special consideration for potential transmission of blood borne illnesses due to blast wounds from suicide bomber attacks have also improved infectious complication outcomes [13].

Lesson 2: Work Both Sides of the Drapes

Another major component of surgical management of blast injures is actually not the surgery itself but the resuscitation. Blast injuries represent a unique injury pattern, with components of penetrating and blunt trauma as well as thermal injury, making the resuscitation all the more important given the high risk of lethal coagulopathy. While damage control resuscitation (DCR) is covered extensively in another chapter in this text, it cannot be stressed enough how intrinsically intertwined the concept is with surgical care [14]. This includes the use of a hemostatic resuscitation, including the earlier use of plasma and platelets in a 1:1:1 ratio and/or the use of whole blood. Damage control improves survival in trauma, and these techniques have now been adopted in civilian trauma care. While not new in combat casualty care in terms of whole blood use, the deliberate use of whole blood to resuscitate combat casualties had not been employed since Vietnam. The first use of emergency release cold-stored whole blood for the resuscitation of combat-injured patients in the modern era was in October of 2001 (personal reflections), nearly 30 years after the previous use in combat by the US forces. Hand in hand with DCR is the use of thromboelastography (TEG), a laboratory technique to measure clotting capability of the patient in real time. The technique measures different aspects of the human clotting mechanics, including hyperfibrinolysis, and helps to guide targeted blood product resuscitation [15]. While early civilian use was mostly in transplant and cardiac surgery in the 1980s and 1990s, military adoption of TEG during recent conflicts has led to broad resurgence and interest in many civilian trauma systems.

Similar to early resuscitation, postsurgical management is immensely important and must always be on the mind of the surgeon caring for blast injuries. A unique problem is that the casualties cannot stay in the theater of operations. Casualties must be evacuated but often require ongoing resuscitation throughout this time. Thus, the US Air Force developed an advanced capability and employed teams of critical care experts including physicians, nurses, and respiratory therapists in Critical Care Air Transport Teams (CCATT). The first CCATT mission in the war took place in September 2001. Since, CCATT has transported with great success more than 30,000 [16].

Lesson 3: You Must Keep Learning from Your Successes and Failures

Lastly, as civilian trauma treatment has matured over the last 40 years with the development of emergency medical services (EMS), trauma centers, and systems, based upon lessons learned in Vietnam, the US DoD began the development of in-theater and global trauma system development in 2004. This included dedicated trauma surgeon leadership, development of a trauma registry (DoDTR), performance improvement in near-real time based upon outcomes, use of trauma nurse managers to monitor compliance with guidelines and gathering of data, conduct of trauma morbidity and mortality conferences, and inclusion of interfacility transfer care for review. None of this had ever been done in combat care and resulted in a dramatic change in combat casualty care management. CPGs, several previously cited in this chapter, were developed based upon these experiences, refined on a regular basis, and spread to the civilian community where applicable. Perhaps the most effective and unique aspect of this system development was the development of the weekly "Thursday teleconference" instituted in 2006. This teleconference includes care providers in the theater of combat providing initial care, the transporting teams, and the subsequent roles of care on several other continents. Patient care management decisions, subsequent developments and complications, and eventual outcomes are discussed by clinical care teams that in any prior conflict never had such opportunity. It allowed for near-real-time feedback to the initial care teams, modification and/or development of CPGs and correction of mistakes, and improved compliance with CPGs. Perhaps most importantly, subject matter experts and discipline leaders not currently deployed could capture and address issues to modify policy, training, and equipment for their respective services [17]. The DoDTS, informed by DoDTR, has authored, refined, published, and observed compliance with approximately 40 CPGs. The adoption of CPGs has undoubtedly improved outcomes, with publications showing decreased mortality by nearly 50% in massively transfused casualties following implementation of the DCR CPG [18]. The annual review and refreshment of these CPGs is regimented and unique; most civilian centers and systems do not frequently update such guidance nor determine compliance or success of such guidance. These include diagnosis and management of topics such as extremity compartment syndrome, amputation evaluation, burns, dismounted complex blast injury, pelvic fracture, urologic injury, vascular injury, and care of complex soft tissue wounds. Many of these have applicability in the civilian setting today. Unfortunately, based upon recent experiences, blast injury management especially must be understood in civilian trauma centers. The latest developments, still to be further elucidated, include retrograde endovascular balloon occlusion of the aorta (REBOA), ultrasmall surgical teams assigned to role 1 MTFs, use of whole blood in the prehospital setting, deployment of physicians in helicopter evacuation teams, and use of point of care testing in the prehospital setting. The National Defense Authorization Act 2017 calls for the formalization of the DoDTS and DoDTR, transfer of trauma injury management bilaterally between the DoD and civilian systems, research into improvements in injury management, and the worldwide development of a true DoDTS [19].

Conclusion

Implementing civilian damage control surgery and damage control resuscitation techniques in military conflicts has allowed us to learn from and refine techniques that are now returning to the civilian sector while improving outcomes of our patients. We are getting better. The DoDTS and DoDTR are models for creating evidence-based, data-informed, and experience-molded practices for improving the care of the complex poly-trauma associated with explosive incidents. We have many more combat blast victims surviving to live with the scars of war, and we have much more work to do. Douglas MacArthur is quoted as saying "The soldier above all others prays for peace, for it is the soldier who must suffer the deepest wounds and scars of war."

Pitfalls

- *Trying to do too much too soon can hurt your patient.* The civilian principles of damage control resuscitation and damage control surgery are just that, damage control, which is exactly what the critically injured blast victim needs. If your patient won't survive "definitive" care, it's not the time for it, and there are a multitude of techniques available to you to keep them alive with their limbs intact until they are including vascular shunting, external fixators, and negative pressure wound vacuum therapy.
- *Thinking surgical care takes place only on the operating table.* Damage control resuscitation is what the early blast-injured patient needs, of which damage control surgery is just a component. The goal is delivering a salvageable patient to definitive care, which means either correcting coagulopathy, even en route, or, at the very least, stopping it from getting worse. This takes real-time, proactive, two-way communication between the surgeon, the anesthesiologist, and the transport team.
- *Not learning from the past.* We can and should learn from every patient we treat to make the care we provide better for the next patient. This requires us to collect, analyze, and share techniques and outcomes to help advance the fields of medicine and surgery. Supporting trauma registries and research efforts is the only way to make sure the lessons of the past help the patients of the future.

References

1. Peoples GE, Gerlinger T, Craig R, Burlingame B. Combat casualties in Afghanistan cared for by a single Forward Surgical Team during the initial phases of Operation Enduring Freedom. Mil Med. 2005;170(6):462–8.
2. Kotwal RS, Howard JT, Orman JA, Tarpey BW, Bailey JA, Champion HR, et al. The effect of a golden hour policy on the morbidity and mortality of combat casualties. JAMA Surg. 2016;151(1):15–24.
3. Jenkins DH, Bailey JA. Origins and importance of the joint trauma system. J Trauma Acute Care Surg. 2016;81(5 Suppl 2 Proceedings of the 2015 Military Health System Research Symposium):S75–S6.
4. Rotondo MF, Schwab CW, McGonigal MD, Phillips GR 3rd, Fruchterman TM, Kauder DR, et al. 'Damage control': an approach for improved survival in exsanguinating penetrating abdominal injury. J Trauma. 1993;35(3):375–82; discussion 82–3.
5. Shapiro MB, Jenkins DH, Schwab CW, Rotondo MF. Damage control: collective review. J Trauma. 2000;49(5):969–78.
6. Rasmussen TE, Clouse WD, Jenkins DH, Peck MA, Eliason JL, Smith DL. The use of temporary vascular shunts as a damage control adjunct in the management of wartime vascular injury. J Trauma. 2006;61(1):8–12; discussion –5.

7. Clouse WD, Rasmussen TE, Peck MA, Eliason JL, Cox MW, Bowser AN, et al. In-theater management of vascular injury: 2 years of the Balad Vascular Registry. J Am Coll Surg. 2007;204(4):625–32.
8. Rasmussen T, Stockinger Z, Antevil J, White C, Fernandez N, White J, et al. Vascular Injury (CPG ID: 46) 2016. Available from: http://jts.amedd.army.mil/assets/docs/cpgs/JTS_Clinical_Practice_Guidelines_(CPGs)/Vascular_Injury_12_Aug_2016_ID46.pdf.
9. Kragh JF Jr, San Antonio J, Simmons JW, Mace JE, Stinner DJ, White CE, et al. Compartment syndrome performance improvement project is associated with increased combat casualty survival. J Trauma Acute Care Surg. 2013;74(1):259–63.
10. Peck MA, Clouse WD, Cox MW, Bowser AN, Eliason JL, Jenkins DH, et al. The complete management of extremity vascular injury in a local population: a wartime report from the 332nd Expeditionary Medical Group/Air Force Theater Hospital, Balad Air Base, Iraq. J Vasc Surg. 2007;45(6):1197–204; discussion 204–5.
11. Rasmussen TE, Clouse WD, Peck MA, Bowser AN, Eliason JL, Cox MW, et al. Development and implementation of endovascular capabilities in wartime. J Trauma. 2008;64(5):1169–76; discussion 76.
12. Leininger BE, Rasmussen TE, Smith DL, Jenkins DH, Coppola C. Experience with wound VAC and delayed primary closure of contaminated soft tissue injuries in Iraq. J Trauma. 2006;61(5):1207–11.
13. Saeed O, Tribble D, Biever K, Kavanaugh M, Crouch H. Infection Prevention in Combat-Related Injuries (CPG ID: 24) 2016. Available from: http://jts.amedd.army.mil/assets/docs/cpgs/JTS_Clinical_Practice_Guidelines_(CPGs)/Infection_Prevention_in_Combat-Related_Injuries_08_Aug_2016_ID24.pdf.
14. Holcomb JB, Jenkins D, Rhee P, Johannigman J, Mahoney P, Mehta S, et al. Damage control resuscitation: directly addressing the early coagulopathy of trauma. J Trauma. 2007;62(2):307–10.
15. Nylund CM, Borgman MA, Holcomb JB, Jenkins D, Spinella PC. Thromboelastography to direct the administration of recombinant activated factor VII in a child with traumatic injury requiring massive transfusion. Pediatr Crit Care Med. 2009;10(2):e22–6.
16. Ingalls N, Zonies D, Bailey JA, Martin KD, Iddins BO, Carlton PK, et al. A review of the first 10 years of critical care aeromedical transport during operation iraqi freedom and operation enduring freedom: the importance of evacuation timing. JAMA Surg. 2014;149(8):807–13.
17. Cannon JW, Hofmann LJ, Glasgow SC, Potter BK, Rodriguez CJ, Cancio LC, et al. Dismounted complex blast injuries: a comprehensive review of the modern combat experience. J Am Coll Surg. 2016;223(4):652–64 e8.
18. Eastridge BJ, Costanzo G, Jenkins D, Spott MA, Wade C, Greydanus D, et al. Impact of joint theater trauma system initiatives on battlefield injury outcomes. Am J Surg. 2009;198(6):852–7.
19. Jenkins DH, Winchell RJ, Coimbra R, Rotondo MF, Weireter LJ, Bulger EM, et al. Position statement of the American College of Surgeons Committee on Trauma on the National Academies of Sciences, Engineering and Medicine Report, A National Trauma Care System: integrating military and civilian trauma systems to achieve zero preventable deaths after injury. J Trauma Acute Care Surg. 2016;81(5):819–23.

Damage Control Surgery

29

Douglas M. Pokorny, John B. Holcomb, Jacob J. Glaser, Jennifer M. Gurney, and Matthew J. Bradley

Introduction

In 1945, the Bureau of Naval Personnel published the Damage Control Handbook in which they described “the capacity of a ship to absorb damage and maintain mission integrity…If the ship does not sink within a very few minutes after damage, she probably will survive for several hours” [1]. Naval damage control has four main foci: extinguish the fire, stop the flooding, repair machinery, and provide care to wounded personnel. Similarly, surgical damage control has four main foci that directly correlate: control hemorrhage, stop contamination, stabilize the patient’s metabolic disturbances, and perform definitive repairs. These principles are critical in the management of the complex polytrauma often associated with blast injuries.

D. M. Pokorny (✉)
Department of Surgery, Trauma, and Critical Care, University of Texas Health Science Center at San Antonio, San Antonio, TX, USA

J. B. Holcomb
Department of Surgery, UT-Health/Memorial Hermann Hospital, Houston, TX, USA

J. J. Glaser
Department of Trauma and Emergency Surgery, San Antonio Military Medical Center, San Antonio, TX, USA

J. M. Gurney
Department of Surgery, Joint Trauma System, US Army Institute of Surgical Research/San Antonio Military Medical Center, San Antonio, TX, USA

M. J. Bradley
Department of Surgery, Walter Reed National Military Medical Center, Bethesda, MD, USA

D. W. Callaway, J. L. Burstein (eds.), *Operational and Medical Management of Explosive and Blast Incidents*, https://doi.org/10.1007/978-3-030-40655-4_29

History of Operative Trauma

From Napoleon's surgeon Dominique Jean Larrey establishing the first field hospitals and battlefield triage [2] to Nicholas Senn and his innovative techniques for intestinal suturing after penetrating trauma, the military has always been closely tied to the advancement in care of the traumatically injured patient. The modern idea of emergency surgical stabilization became prominent in the early 1900s. J. Hogarth Pringle, of the aptly named "Pringle maneuver," described principles similar to damage control surgery in 1908 when discussing operative liver trauma [3, 4]. After the rapid exsanguination of his patients with significant hepatic lacerations, Dr. Pringle came to the conclusion that laparotomy, immediate control of the portal inflow, mass ligation of injured hepatic vessels, and well-placed packing were sufficient to salvage a patient. Additionally, he noted that the entire process needed to be completed swiftly in order to avoid the comorbid conditions associated with massive hemorrhage.

Despite Pringle's experiences, emphasis shifted in the 1940s toward definitive repair at the time of the initial exploration [5]. Postsurgical units at that time bore little resemblance to modern intensive care units, and perioperative care was limited. Patients underwent long, protracted operations with the thought that the best chance of surviving an injury was to correct all issues in a single surgery. As battlefield scenarios in the Vietnam War changed, a transition back to "abbreviated laparotomy" was observed. This approach was expanded upon in 1969 by Simmons et al., who examined the effects of major trauma on coagulopathy [6], and in 1983 by Stone et al. [7], who published a report in the Annals of Surgery regarding the management of patients that became coagulopathic in the operating room. Stone noted a substantial mortality advantage among patients packing with temporary closure over those who had definitive operations primarily.

In 1993, the phrase "damage control surgery" (DCS) was coined by Rotondo and Schwab [8] to describe the emerging comprehensive approach to the unstable trauma patient. In addition to correction of coagulopathy, Rotondo and colleagues also described the influence of hypothermia and acidosis on mortality. Now known as the trauma lethal triad, or "triad of death," attention was focused on rapid correction of these metabolic derangements in order to prevent the patients' rapid decline. This approach was refined over the years, and hundreds of other studies have been performed suggesting a mortality benefit using damage control principles. With greater emphasis on care of the traumatically injured, this was further extended into the control of neurologic, orthopedic, pelvic, and vascular injuries as well [9]. How best to apply the civilian damage control surgery principles into the military arena became a subject of great discussion in the late 1990s [10–12].

Damage control as a concept has expanded to all levels of care (Fig. 29.1). For example, at the point of injury, the main emphasis is now on hemorrhage control with compression and/or tourniquets. Rapid transport to surgical capability is paramount and should be standard of care [13]. Time-intensive therapies are avoided at the scene in order to facilitate reaching a higher level of care. Congruous to the adoption of DCS, our resuscitation strategies have transformed as well. Crystalloid

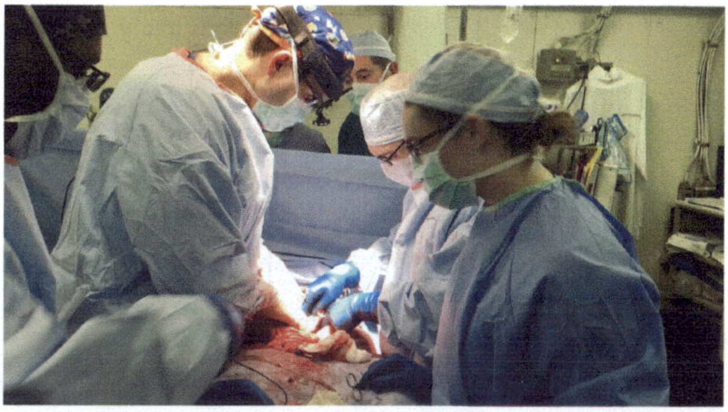

Fig. 29.1 Damage control laparotomy onboard USS Dwight D. Eisenhower (CVN-69)

resuscitation has been replaced by blood component therapy in balanced measures [14, 15]. Permissive hypotension has become widely accepted during resuscitation. Even now, the principles of damage control resuscitation (DCR) are evolving as whole blood transfusion, mobile blood banks, and tranexamic acid (TXA) return to favor. DCR and DCS have truly become one united field known simply as damage control (DC).

Physiology of Significant Trauma

Major trauma leads to significant metabolic effects (Fig. 29.2). Hemorrhage activates the coagulation cascade, and as bleeding continues, the body's native clotting factors are consumed. Non-blood product resuscitation further dilutes the pool of coagulation factors, worsening coagulopathy. As core temperature drops and hypothermia ensues, temperature-dependent enzyme reactions in the clotting cascade are also altered. This leads to decreased activation of platelets and increased fibrinolysis, thereby inhibiting the ability to form and maintain clot [8, 16].

The generation of thrombin is greatly affected during the acute phase of traumatic injury. In 2015, Rahbar et al. [17] described the effects of plasma colloid osmotic pressure (COP) on vascular permeability and coagulation. Plasma levels of four endothelial glycocalyx proteins were measured after significant traumatic injury and compared to healthy, non-injured subjects. While levels of all four proteins suggested increased shedding after traumatic injury, significant increases in syndecan-1 and hyaluronic acid were associated with decreased COP corresponding to increased cell permeability. Additionally, patients with decreased COP were found to have reduced peak thrombin generation time directly affecting coagulation.

Decreased circulatory volume leads to systemic hypoperfusion and diminished oxygen delivery. Cells are shunted to an anaerobic state promoting the creation of lactic acid. Progressive acidosis leads to further breakdown of plasma proteins and fibrinogen and additional loss of function of the coagulation factors; their activity can be reduced by as much as 50% at a pH of only 7.2 [18–21]. With the switch to anaerobic processes, there is a decrease in overall heat production in skeletal muscle due to a decreased metabolic rate leading to hypothermia. If not kept in check, the

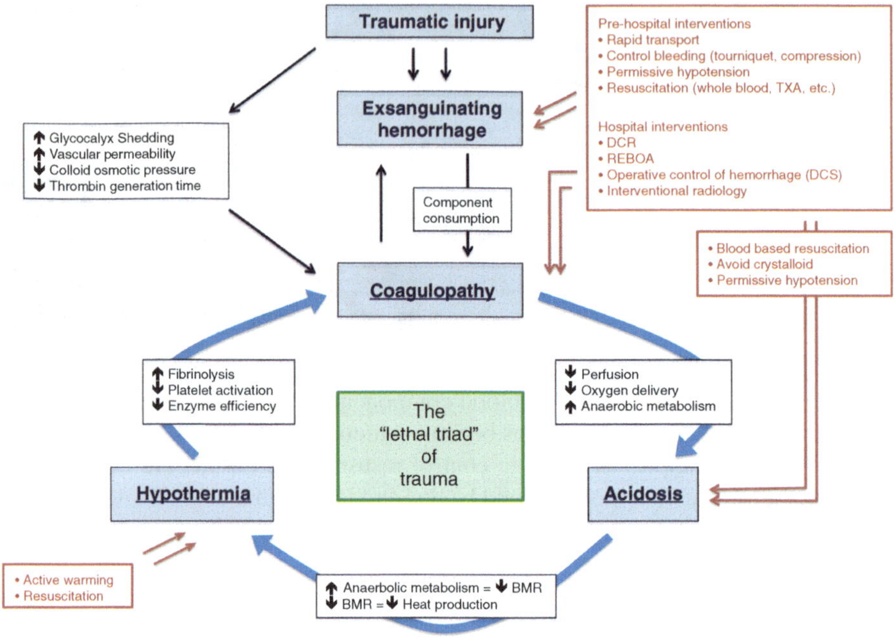

Fig. 29.2 If left uncorrected, acidosis, hypothermia, and coagulopathy form a "lethal triad" that will almost certainly result in mortality. Areas to intervene and correct the metabolic insults are shown in red (double arrows) above

"triad of death" will continue to fuel itself to a point where recovery is a near impossibility. The decision to follow a DC approach must be made early, after assessing the intraoperative trajectory of the patient's evolving physiology and the severity of their injuries [16, 22]. Waiting for metabolic failure is too late.

Indications for Damage Control

Absolute indications for DCS have diminished greatly with modern DCR (Table 29.1). Lower-volume blood-based resuscitation, greater attention paid to patient physiology, less significant bowel edema, and aggressive ICU care have all decreased the need for abbreviated procedures [23]. Harvin et al. instituted a quality improvement project analyzing their use of DCS at a high-volume level 1 trauma center [24]. The project consisted of a blinded method for staff to reflect on their departmental rates of damage control procedures and follow the outcome data of the patients involved. Analysis of their data demonstrated lower rates of damage control laparotomy in their facility (from 39% to 23%) with no difference in mortality or morbidity rate. Continued work in this area has led to even lower rates of DCS without an increase in complications.

Table 29.1 Modern situations in which to consider a DCS approach [24, 25]

Need for therapeutic packing to control hemorrhage
Continuous vasopressor and/or transfusion requirements
Prophylaxis of anticipated abdominal compartment syndrome
Need for a second-look operation
Persistent acidosis without continuing vasopressor support or transfusion requirement
Gross contamination at the time of exploration

Balanced Resuscitation

Damage control resuscitation is discussed in detail in another part of this text. Mention of recent shifts in practice to balanced blood component therapy and permissive hypotension, however, cannot be emphasized enough. Starting in World War I, there was significant utilization of whole blood. Between WWI and WWII, resuscitation in the US shifted slightly toward readily available agents such as dried plasma. By the 1960s, there was another shift from blood products or colloids to large-volume crystalloid agents [26]. Throughout the rest of the century, crystalloid reigned prevalent until the early 2000s when a resurgence of blood product resuscitation began. With experience on the battlefield and numerous studies to support its use, the term "balanced resuscitation" took hold, and the use of red cells, fresh frozen plasma, and platelets in an equal ratio (as close to 1:1:1 as possible) set the stage for DCR [14, 15, 27].

DCR continues to evolve as we learn (and return to) mechanisms for early hemorrhage control. Recently, there has been resurgence in the use of whole blood as an initial resuscitation choice not just on the battlefield but also in civilian centers. Preliminary data suggests that whole blood resuscitation is not only comparable to component therapy; it may in fact prove to be superior [28]. In addition, the availability of cold-stored, low-titer type O whole blood makes it a safe option even in the face of RhD-negative recipients with low chance of isoimmunization [29].

Complications of the Damage Control Approach

While retrospective studies have shown there is a mortality benefit associated with damage control surgery, no randomized, controlled trials have been performed. One recently planned trial, Based on Harvin's PI study discussed above, hopes to provide clarity to the situation and assess the necessity/utilization of DCS in the modern era of DCR [30].

With every day open, the patient's fascia retracts, musculature becomes less mobile, and adhesion forms. Reviewing complication rates among casualties at a single military institution over an 8-year period, Glaser et al. demonstrated a clear association between adherence to balanced resuscitation, reduced abdominal operations, and early fascial closure [31]. A percentage of patients will never be able to undergo primary closure of the fascia and will be left with a planned ventral hernia. A few options in this setting include skin grafting directly onto granulated bowel, grafting onto absorbable mesh, and skin closure over a biologic or synthetic mesh. Ultimately, the abdominal wall may be reconstructed at a much later date. For those patients that do remain open, there is an increased risk of enterocutaneous or enteroatmospheric fistula formation [32, 33]; this risk may be lessened or prevented by early bowel coverage. Attempts should be made to close the abdomen as soon as feasible; this may include the use of sequential closures with an absorbable mesh [34–37]. Additionally, a large number of DC patients have gross contamination of their peritoneal cavities which increases the risk of intra-abdominal abscess or wound infection.

In patients who remain open for greater than 8 days, the rate of morbidity increases [38]. Brenner et al. described the postoperative follow-up of 88 patients who underwent damage control surgery out to 7 years post injury and observed not only morbidities associated with the approach but also changes in quality of life. Overall infection rate of these patients (both intra-abdominal and superficial) and enteroatmospheric fistula rate were fairly high. The authors attributed this level of morbidity to the overall increase in survival among the severely injured patients [39].

A historic problem associated with DCS was abdominal compartment syndrome. In the era of massive transfusion with crystalloid solutions, bowel edema was a notable problem. This has been significantly decreased with the use of blood products in balanced ratios [40].

Clinical Approach to Damage Control for Blast Injuries

In blast injuries specifically, the emphasis is on rapid control of hemorrhage and contamination. Injuries commonly seen include extremity amputations, fragmentation injuries, "blast lung," pneumothorax, fractures, dermal burns, urogenital injuries, temporal bone fractures, internal hemorrhage or hollow viscus injury, traumatic brain injuries, and gross contamination with environmental debris [41, 42]. The utilization of improvised explosive devices (IEDs) in the modern war led to the identification of a special injury pattern known as the dismounted complex blast injury (DCBI). DCBI characteristically includes multiple extremity amputations (almost always both lower extremities and at least one upper extremity), complex pelvic orthopedic and vascular injuries, and urogenital/rectal injuries [43]. Patients should be expected to return to the operating room for frequent debridement and long, tedious operations.

Basic tenants of blast control parallel other trauma protocols. If the patient survives the incident, hemorrhage must be stopped or slowed through tourniquets, direct pressure, etc. Next, DCR with blood or blood products must be rapidly initiated simultaneous with establishing a secure airway. In the setting of extremity amputations and multiple tourniquets, intravenous (IV) access can prove difficult. Use of intraosseous (IO) devices or central venous catheters is often beneficial.

Adjuncts to care such as plain films, CT scan, or other supplemental data should not delay rapid control of hemorrhage. Once the patient has been stabilized, comprehensive imaging can be performed to evaluate for unseen injuries. Traumatically injured patients, specifically those with extremity amputations, are at high risk of deep venous thrombosis (DVT) and should be started on prophylactic dose anticoagulation as soon as possible. Additionally, although there is gross contamination of most wounds, empiric administration of broad-spectrum antibiotics is debated. Patients should be adequately debrided at their primary procedure to healthy-appearing tissue and treated with agents against skin flora (cephalexin, cefazolin, etc.) or topical antibiotics.

Extremity Trauma

As an explosive medium/casing breaks apart, pieces are thrown outward at high velocity with the blast wave. These pieces of shrapnel often lead to extensive soft tissue damage or extremity amputation and massive hemorrhage as they lacerate vasculature. A large portion of these injuries may be controlled with either direct pressure or application of a well-placed tourniquet. In the event of major vascular transection without amputation, shunting may temporarily restore blood flow to the limb until further repair can be performed [44]. Vasculature control should be obtained as distal as possible to minimize tissue loss and local ischemia. If a limb is deemed non-salvageable, amputation should be completed with debridement of all nonviable tissue at the primary operation [45].

Pelvic/Perineal Trauma

Pelvic and perineal blast injuries are complex and require careful attention during evaluation. Injuries to the pelvic ring and acetabular fractures can lead to significant hemorrhage. Rapid assessment of pelvic stability with anterior to posterior compression of the pelvis aids in determining the necessity of pelvic reduction. Commercially available binders are easily deployed and fairly effective in reducing pelvic volume/stabilizing the pelvis. However, a tightly wrapped blanket or sheet held with clamps will suffice. The most common mistake in using a pelvic binder or sheet is to center it too high; the device should be centered over the greater trochanter of the femur. Despite reduction in pelvic volume, exsanguinating hemorrhage is still possible.

After initiation of DCR and stabilization of pelvic structures, an extensive pelvic and perineal exam must be performed. Ongoing hemorrhage may require additional tourniquet placement. In cases of significant, uncontrolled hemorrhage from the pelvis or proximal femur, temporary ligation of the internal iliac arteries or femoral vessels may be performed. Avoid ligation of both internal iliac vessels as this may lead to significant perineal/gluteal soft tissue ischemia. Once the patient's hemorrhage is controlled and distal vasculature has been debrided/ligated, attempts should be made to revascularize or reperfuse the proximal trunks.

Perineal or pelvic penetrating wounds should raise concern for rectal injury. A digital rectal exam may reveal blood but is not a reliable test for injuries to the upper rectum. Rigid proctoscopy can be easily performed in the emergency room or operating room and is much more sensitive in detecting injuries. Evidence of blood in the rectum during proctoscopic exam in the presence of penetrating perineal or perianal wounds should be considered confirmation of penetrating rectal injury. In such cases, fecal diversion must be performed by stapling off the distal sigmoid colon at the peritoneal reflection and either creating a colostomy or leaving the patient in discontinuity until later procedures.

Injuries to the genitalia and bladder are also common in the setting of pelvic blast injuries (specifically DCBI). Primary procedures should preserve as much tissue as possible while focusing on hemorrhage control and urinary diversion. High-riding prostate on rectal exam, blood at the urethral meatus, or presence of a scrotal hematoma in the setting of perineal penetrating wounds should raise suspicion for a urethral injury [46]. A retrograde urethrogram should be performed to evaluate for an injury prior to Foley catheter placement. A retrograde cystogram may also be performed to evaluate the bladder. Extravasation of contrast intraperitoneally mandates exploration and repair. Extraperitoneal contrast extravasation may be managed with Foley catheter or suprapubic catheter decompression [47].

Thoracoabdominal Trauma

Laparotomy, if performed, relies upon proper DCR to optimize patient outcomes [48]. After rapid evacuation of hemoperitoneum, quickly pack the abdomen in all four quadrants. Properly inserted packs (tightly folded laparotomy pads) above and below the liver, in the splenic flexure, and the bilateral lower quadrants may slow any ongoing hemorrhage long enough to allow for exploration and control. In the presence of a great vessel injury, priority must be given to inflow and outflow control in order to prevent rapid exsanguination. Specific techniques for vascular control are discussed elsewhere in this text.

After rapid control of exsanguinating hemorrhage, the focus is shifted toward controlling contamination (Fig. 29.3). The small bowel is examined from the ligament of Treitz to the cecum looking for significant mesenteric hematomas, partial- or full-thickness injuries to the bowel wall, or areas of devascularization. The colon is then examined for similar findings along the ascending, transverse, descending, and sigmoid portions. If a significant injury is noted, it is addressed rapidly. Partial-thickness injuries or small full-thickness injuries in areas that otherwise appear viable should be debrided to clean edges and oversewn at the time of discovery. Full-thickness injuries encompassing more than 50% of the diameter of the bowel, when discovered during a true damage control procedure, are rapidly resected using a stapling device leaving the ends in discontinuity.

Once the patient's metabolic abnormalities have been addressed, they are no longer hemorrhaging, and they have no ongoing requirements for vasopressor support, they should be brought back to the operating room for repeat exploration.

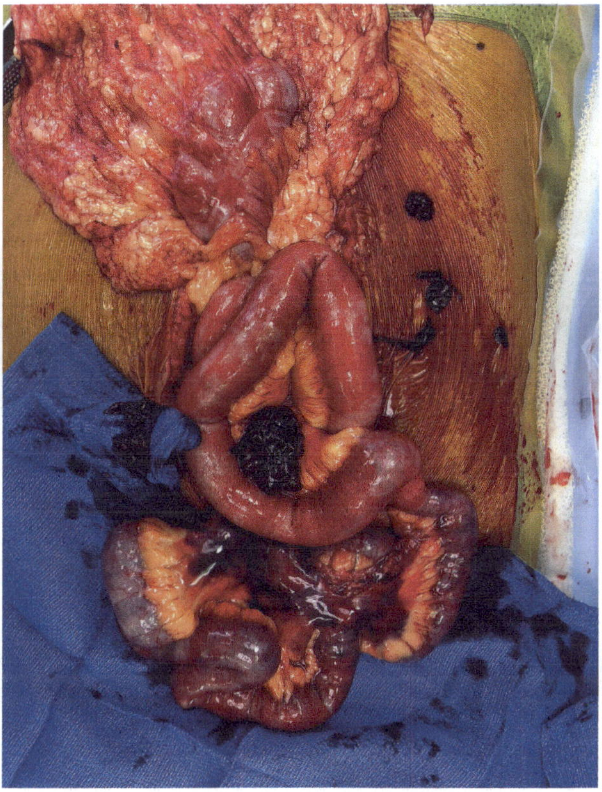

Fig. 29.3 Blunt mesenteric injury after high-speed MVC resulting in significant intraperitoneal hemorrhage and a 60-cm segment of devitalized bowel

Patients are typically ready after 6–12 hours of dedicated critical care and resuscitation but should not be delayed more than 24 hours before returning to the operating room.

Patients with significant thoracic injuries commonly present in extremis. Should a patient continue to worsen to a point where a pulse is no longer palpable or there is lack of a perfusing cardiac rhythm, then a left lateral thoracotomy should be performed [49]. If a perfusing cardiac rhythm returns, then aggressive balanced blood product resuscitation is continued, and the patient is transported to the operating room for exploration. If a rhythm does not return, then manual cardiac compression may be required.

Pulmonary injuries are also readily managed via the left anterior thoracotomy or clamshell incision. Bleeding emanating from the lung parenchyma can be addressed in multiple ways, but pulmonary tractotomy is highly efficient and easy to perform. After gently inserting a GIA stapler into the tract of the injury, it can be clamped and fired; while sealing the majority of the parenchyma, this also divides the tissue allowing it to be spread apart. Any ongoing bleeding can be ligated with suture. Eventual nonanatomic resection of the area may be required.

Figure 29.4 shows a combined thoracic and abdominal approach to a penetrating suprahepatic IVC injury.

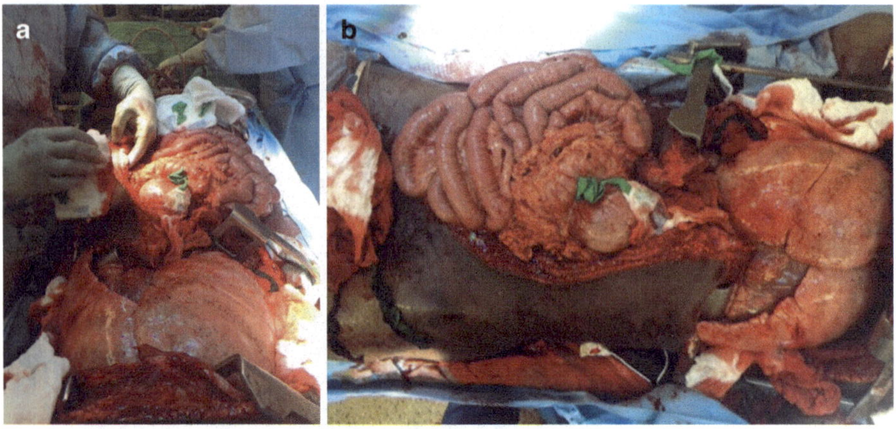

Fig. 29.4 (**a**, **b**) Combined thoracic and abdominal approach to a penetrating suprahepatic IVC injury

Special Considerations

After achieving rapid hemorrhage control and stopping contamination, it is important for the surgical team to reassess the situation. The extent of resuscitation, severity of injuries, time required to definitively repair the damage, availability of necessary resources, and overall trajectory of the patient must be integrated into the decision to forge on with the operation or commit to true DCS. In the event of a mass casualty incident (MCI), resources and personnel are limited. While patients may physiologically tolerate an extensive procedure, temporizing measures offer a team the ability to treat the most patients possible with the least amount of resources.

Multifaceted operating teams consisting of general or trauma surgeons and orthopedic surgeons are ideal when faced with these situations. One team is able to address vascular control of hemorrhage and abdominal/perineal injuries while the other team can simultaneously address the extremities. By working in concert, these teams facilitate quicker transition from operating room to intensive care or evacuation.

As mentioned previously, shunting of vasculature should be considered where definitive reconstruction is needed. Partial-thickness or small full-thickness injuries to bowel should be rapidly oversewn. Stapling of significant full-thickness bowel injuries or areas of devascularization will control contamination, but definitive reconstruction or ostomy formation should be delayed to secondary and tertiary operations. Soft tissue damage should be debrided to healthy, viable tissue and near amputations completed if the tissue appears nonviable. Plan to return to the operating room for at least three washouts of the soft tissue prior to closing any wounds. Pelvic orthopedic injuries should be stabilized with a sheet or binder temporarily until an external fixation device can be placed.

Conclusion

Damage control principles have drastically changed the face of trauma surgery. With a better understanding of the physiology of trauma, we have embraced concepts such as balanced blood product resuscitation containing minimal to no crystalloid solutions, whole blood use, permissive hypotension, and rapid metabolic correction in a critical care unit. Previously high mortality rates associated with significant trauma have decreased as we have embraced the concept of damage control as a whole. The initial approach involves two main goals: stop hemorrhage and control contamination. Hemorrhage must be rapidly and effectively controlled to avoid worsening the metabolic insults of hypothermia, acidosis, and coagulopathy; these will progress leading to near certain mortality. If the patient is rapidly corrected and improving in the operating room, then a definitive procedure may be considered at the time of the initial operation. However, if the patient continues to decline, ongoing resuscitation in an intensive care unit setting should be undertaken. This resuscitation of the unstable patient is best achieved using active warming, ongoing balanced blood product administration avoiding crystalloid solutions, and correction of metabolic abnormalities. Finally, if an abbreviated procedure is performed, the patient must return to the operating room in short-interval timing in order to definitively address their injuries. As evidenced by the sage wisdom of Lord Berkeley Moynihan (1865–1936) over a century ago, patient stabilization has always played a key role in treating trauma: "The modern operation is safe for the patient. The modern surgeon must make the patient safe for the modern operation."

Pitfalls

- Failure to rapidly achieve hemorrhage control and recognize a damage control situation
  - After initial control of hemorrhage and contamination, the surgeon must quickly decide whether to proceed with a definitive or abbreviated operation. Abbreviated operation using vascular shunts, external fixation, and stapling off bowel injuries is a safe approach primarily.
- Insufficient resuscitation
  - DCS and DCR go hand in hand—one relies upon the other to be successful. This includes avoiding failure in correcting the metabolic insult while in the ICU. If left uncorrected, acidosis, hypothermia, and coagulopathy form a lethal triad that will almost certainly result in mortality.
- Debride soft tissue to healthy, viable-appearing areas at the primary procedure with a plan to return for at least two additional washouts prior to closure or formalization.
  - Blast injuries tend to evolve with time, and viable-appearing tissue may be ischemic on takeback procedures.

References

1. Naval Damage Control Training Center (US); Bureau of Ships and the Naval Training School. Handbook of Damage Control. NavPers 16191, May 1945.
2. Brewer LA. Dominique Jean Larrey (1766–1842). Father of modern military surgery, innovator, humanist. J Thorac Cardiovasc Surg. 1986;92(6):1096–8.
3. Pringle JH. Notes on the arrest of hepatic hemorrhage due to trauma. Ann Surg. 1908;48(4):541–9.
4. Bhattacharya B. The pendulum of damage control laparotomy. SOJ Surg. 2015;2(1):1–2.
5. Sakran JV, Privette A. History of damage control. In: Papadakos PJ, Gestring ML, editors. Encyclopedia of trauma care. Berlin, Heidelberg: Springer; 2015.
6. Simmons RL, Collins JA. Coagulation disorders in combat casualties: I. acute changes after wounding, II. Effects of massive transfusion, III. Post-resuscitative changes. Ann Surg. 1969;169(4):455–82.
7. Stone HH, Strom PR, Mullins RJ. Management of the major coagulopathy with onset during laparotomy. Ann Surg. 1983;197(5):532–5.
8. Rotondo MF, Schwab CW, McGonigal MD. Damage control: an approach for improved survival in exsanguinating penetrating abdominal injury. J Trauma. 1986;26(8):738–43.
9. Wall MJ Jr, Soletro E. Damage control for thoracic injuries. Surg Clin North Am. 1997;77(4):863–78.
10. Holcomb JB, Helling TS. Military, civilian, and rural application of the damage control philosophy. Mil Med. 2001;166(6):490–3.
11. Holcomb JB, Champion HR. Military damage control. Arch Surg. 2001;136(8):965–7.
12. Mabry RL, Holcomb JB. United States Army rangers in Somalia: an analysis of combat casualties on an urban battlefield. J Trauma. 2000;49(3):515–28; discussion 528–9.
13. Holcomb JB. Transport time and preoperating room hemostatic interventions are important: improving outcomes after severe truncal injury. Crit Care Med. 2018;46(3):447–53.
14. Borgman MA, Spinella PC, Perkins JG. The ratio of blood products transfused affects mortality in patients receiving massive transfusions at a combat support hospital. J Trauma. 2007;63(4):805–13.
15. Holcomb JB, Jenkins D. Damage control resuscitation: directly addressing the early coagulopathy of trauma. J Trauma. 2007;62(2):307–10.
16. Brohi K. Damage control surgery [Internet]. London, UK. Trauma.org (US); 2000 [cited 2000 June 01]. Available from: http://www.trauma.org/index.php/main/article/368.
17. Rahbar E, Cardenas JC. Endothelial glycocalyx shedding and vascular permeability in severely injured trauma patients. J Transl Med. 2015;23:117.
18. Jana BA, MacLeod MD. Trauma and coagulopathy a new paradigm to consider. Arch Surg. 2008;143(8):797–801.
19. Dunn EL, Moore EE, Breslich DF. Acidosis-induced coagulopathy. Surg Forum. 1979:3047–73.
20. Meng ZH, Woberg AS, Monroe DM. The effect of temperature and pH on the activity of factor VIIa: implications for the efficacy of high-dose factor VIIa in hypothermic and acidotic patients. J Trauma. 2003;55(5):886–91.
21. Djaldetti MF, Fishman PB, Besler HC. pH induced platelet ultrastructural alterations: a possible mechanism for impaired platelet aggregation. Arch Surg. 1979;114(6):707–10.
22. Azim JB, Zangbar B. Improving mortality in trauma laparotomy through the evolution of damage control resuscitation: analysis of 1,030 consecutive trauma laparotomies. J Trauma Acute Care Surg. 2017;82(2):328–33.
23. Higa G, Friese R. Damage control laparotomy: a vital tool once overused. J Trauma. 2010;69(1):53–9.
24. Harvin JA, Kao LS. Decreasing the use of damage control laparotomy in trauma: a quality improvement project. J Am Coll Surg. 2017;225(2):200–9.

25. Roberts DJ, Bobrovitz N, Zygun DA. Indications for use of damage control surgery in civilian trauma patients: a content analysis and expert appropriateness rating study. Ann Surg. 2016;263(5):1018–27.
26. Fisher AD, Miles EA, Cap AP. Tactical damage control resuscitation. Mil Med. 2015;180(8):869–75.
27. Lanagan NR, Eckert M. Changing patterns of in-hospital deaths following implementation of damage control resuscitation practices in US forward military treatment facilities. JAMA Surg. 2014;149(9):904–12.
28. Spinella PC, Pidcoke HF. Whole blood for hemostatic resuscitation of major bleeding. Transfusion. 2016;56(suppl 2):S190–202.
29. McGinity AC, Zhu CS. Prehospital low-titer cold-stored whole blood: philosophy for ubiquitous utilization of O-positive product for emergency use in hemorrhage due to injury. J Trauma Acute Care Surg. 2018;84(6S):S115–9.
30. Harvin JA, Podbielski J. Damage control laparotomy trial: design, rationale and implementation of a randomized controlled trial. Trauma Surg Acute Care Open. 2017;2(1):e000083.
31. Glaser J, Vasuez M. Ratio-driven resuscitation predicts early fascial closure in the combat wounded. J Trauma Acute Care Surg. 2015;79(4 Suppl 2):S188–92.
32. Miller RS, Morris JA Jr, Diaz JJ Jr. Complications after 344 damage-control open celiotomies. J Trauma. 2005;59(6):1365–71.
33. Mayberry JC, Burgess EA, Goldman RK. Enterocutaneous fistula and ventral hernia after absorbable mesh prosthesis closure for trauma: the plain truth. J Trauma. 2004;57(1):157–62.
34. Jernigan TW, Fabian TC, Croce MA. Staged management of giant abdominal wall defects: acute and long-term results. Ann Surg. 2003;238(3):349–55.
35. Cothren CC, Moore EE, Johnson JL. One hundred percent fascial approximation with sequential abdominal closure of the open abdomen. Am J Surg. 2006;192(2):238–42.
36. Fox N, Crutchfield M, LaChant M. Early abdominal closure improves long term outcomes after damage-control laparotomy. J Trauma Acute Care Surg. 2013;75(5):854–8.
37. Hatch QM, Osterhout LM, Podbielski J. Impact of closure at the first take back: complication burden and potential overutilization of damage control laparotomy. J Trauma. 2011;71(6):1503–11.
38. Miller RS, Morris JA. Complications after 344 damage control open celiotomies. J Trauma. 2005;59(6):1365–71.
39. Brenner M, Bochicchio G, Bochicchio K. Long term impact of damage control laparotomy. A prospective study. Arch Surg. 2011;146(4):395–9.
40. Balogh Z, McKinley BA. Both primary and secondary abdominal compartment syndrome can be predicted early and are harbingers of multiple organ failure. J Trauma. 2003;54(5):848–59; discussion 859–61
41. Scott TE, Kirkman MH, Haque M, Gibb IE, Mahoney P, Hardman JG. Primary blast lung injury—a review. Br J Anaesth. 2017;118(3):311–6.
42. Ritenour AE, Wickley A, Ritenour JS. Tympanic membrane perforation and hearing loss from blast overpressure in Operation Enduring Freedom and Operation Iraqi Freedom wounded. J Trauma. 2008;64(2 Suppl):S174–8.
43. Gordon W, Talbot M. High bilateral amputations and dismounted complex blast injury (CPG ID:22). Joint Trauma System Clinical Practice Guidelines. 01 August 2016 from https://jts.amedd.army.mil/assets/docs/cpgs/JTS_Clinical_Practice_Guidelines_(CPGs)/High_Bilateral_Amputations_Dismnted_Cmplex_Blast_Injury_01_Aug_2016_ID22.pdf.
44. Inaba K, Aksoy H. Multicenter evaluation of temporary intravascular shunt use in vascular trauma. J Trauma Acute Care Surg. 2016;80(3):359–64.
45. Bumbasirevic M, Lesic A, Mitkovic M, Bumbasirević V. Treatment of blast injuries of the extremity. J Am Acad Orthop Surg. 2006;14(10 Spec No): S77–81.

46. Jezoir J, Hudak S, et al. Genitourinary (GU) Injury Management (CPG ID:42). Joint Trauma System Clinical Practice Guidelines. 06 March 2019 from https://jts.amedd.army.mil/assets/docs/cpgs/JTS_Clinical_Practice_Guidelines_(CPGs)/Genitourinary_(GU)_Injury_Trauma_Management_06_Mar_2019_ID42.pdf.
47. Shoobridge JJ, Niall MC. Contemporary management of renal trauma. Rev Urol. 2011;13(2):65–72.
48. Polk JD. Response to blast injuries: considerations for responders to intentional or unintentional blast incidents. J Emerg Med Services. 2012;21
49. Savitsky E, Eastridge B. Damage control surgery. In: Savitsky E, Eastridge B, editors. Combat casualty care: lessons learned from OEF and OIF. Frederick, MD: Office of the Surgeon General; 2012. p. 165–224.

Anesthesia Care in Blast Injury

30

David C. Asseff

Introduction

Providing anesthetic care for victims of blast injuries represents one of the potentially most complex and daunting clinical scenarios confronting the practitioner of anesthesiology. Clinical challenges arising from blast injuries requiring expert anesthetic care may include, but not necessarily be limited to, the management of hypovolemic shock and its resultant metabolic and coagulopathic derangements, organ injury due to blast effect, difficult airway management, blast-related lung injury, and burn injuries. Anesthesiologists' knowledge of physiology and pharmacology combined with their ability to resuscitate critically wounded patients puts them in a unique position among a team of caregivers to provide lifesaving treatment in a major explosion incident, be it in military or civilian settings [1].

Blast injury may be divided into four different phases, each producing a characteristic injury pattern. Primary blast injury results from direct effect on tissue to the blast overpressure wave, producing injury to air-filled structures, such as the lungs, hollow viscera of the GI tract, and the tympanic membranes [2]. Secondary blast injury, the most common cause of fatality in a blast event, is produced by impact of the patient with fragmentation and other projectiles set in motion by the blast, producing shrapnel wounds, penetrating and vascular trauma, and penetrating infectious biological fragmentation injuries [1, 2]. Tertiary blast injury is caused by impact of the victim's body being thrown against stationary objects or by structural collapse, producing blunt and penetrating trauma injuries, crush injuries and traumatic amputations, compartment syndrome, and closed head injury [2]. Lastly, quaternary injuries consist of all other explosion-related injuries such as thermal injury,

D. C. Asseff (✉)
Department of Anesthesiology, University of California, Davis, Sacramento, CA, USA
e-mail: dasseff@ucdavis.edu

D. W. Callaway, J. L. Burstein (eds.), *Operational and Medical Management of Explosive and Blast Incidents*, https://doi.org/10.1007/978-3-030-40655-4_30

exposure to toxins or radiation, asphyxiation, or exacerbation of chronic medical conditions [1, 2]. The immediate physiologic response to a blast wave can include a triad of bradycardia, apnea, and hypotension, mediated in part by the vagus nerve and specifically by pulmonary C fibers [3]. Hypotension may be the result of nitric oxide release by the injured lung and a decrease in systemic vascular resistance lasting several hours [3].

Injuries from blast mechanism may occur in a variety of settings, although the overwhelmingly predominant body of recent knowledge derives from the military medical experience treating combat casualties in the Iraq and Afghanistan conflicts. Blast injury events in the civilian world remain relatively rare, but some potential sources in the United States and elsewhere include industrial explosions (e.g., Texas City Refinery Explosion 2005, West Fertilizer Plant Explosion 2013), domestic mishaps (fireworks accidents), or acts of terrorism (e.g., Oklahoma City 1995, Atlanta Olympics 1996, Boston Marathon 2013, Madrid 2004, London 2005). There exist significant differences between blast injuries sustained in military theaters of war and civilian settings. Injured military personnel tend to be younger, healthy, and male, often wearing body armor, whereas civilian incidents cause more casualties of diverse age and gender groups and with greater prevalence of preexisting health conditions. For military personnel, improved body armor and enemy tactics have influenced the pattern of blast injuries encountered in theater, with relative protection of the torso while leaving extremities, facial, and neck regions exposed [4, 5]. This chapter will emphasize the military experience due to the larger body of available data and elaborate on anesthetic challenges relevant to the treatment of the most severe, complex blast injury mechanisms, as these treatment principles and lessons learned may also be applicable to potentially less complex injuries encountered in civilian settings.

Epidemiology

Injuries from blast mechanism have constituted the predominant proportion of combat casualties of twentieth century armed conflicts [6]. This trend has particular recent relevance relating to the treatment of combat casualties in the Iraq and Afghanistan conflicts where retrospective reviews suggest blast mechanisms are responsible for between 75% and 81% of injuries [6, 7]. Given the enemy's tendency to adopt asymmetric means of warfare against the US and coalition forces, such as the employment of improvised explosive devices (IEDs) and suicide/homicide bombers, findings from the study of military casualties from this era may be translatable to disaster preparedness and mass-casualty terror events in the civilian sector [7]. The dismounted complex blast injury (DCBI) is the most extreme and devastating pattern of such injury and is the focus of this section.

The DCBI is defined as "an explosion-induced battle injury sustained by a warfighter on foot patrol that produces a specific pattern of wounds" [8]. These injuries are characterized by high-energy wounds to the bilateral lower extremities (usually proximal transfemoral amputations) and/or upper extremity (usually involving the nondominant side), combined with open pelvic injuries and genitourinary and abdominal trauma [9]. In one retrospective review of the Combat Trauma Registry (JTTR) from September 2007 to December 2010, examining injury patterns and resource utilization in DCBI patients, it was observed that of 685 patients, 16% sustained at least one traumatic amputation, and of those patients suffering traumatic amputation, 57% sustained more than one amputation [10]. Of the patients with multiple extremity amputations, the most common pattern was bilateral transfemoral followed by bilateral transtibial amputations [10]. Another retrospective review of the JTTR between 1 January 2009 and 29 February 2012 of patients seen at the Camp Bastion Role 3 Hospital in Afghanistan demonstrated 457 patients injured by dismounted IED blast, with a median ISS of 10% and 30% of patients requiring massive transfusion [8]. The extremities and pelvis constituted the most frequently injured body region. Severe head and neck injuries were relatively uncommon in this cohort as were chest and abdominal injuries. Thirty-eight percent (172) of patients sustained limb amputations, and of these, 116 had two limbs affected. The lower limbs accounted for 96% of all amputated extremities. The overall incidence of pelvic fractures was 7.4%, with the overall incidence of open pelvic fracture being 5.3% [8]. Despite observed increases in severity of injuries caused by IEDs over the course of the Afghanistan and Iraq conflicts, the mitigation of mortality and paradoxical stability of survival rates may be credited to improved tactical combat casualty care, the far forward and individual use of tourniquets and rapid and aggressive resuscitation and hemorrhage control strategies involving a multidisciplinary approach [8–10], integral to which is the anesthesiologist or CRNA whose responsibilities in this setting include airway management; the appropriate administration of blood products; management and correction of acid–base derangements, coagulopathy, and hypothermia; and monitoring of physiologic and metabolic parameters as markers of resuscitative efficacy.

Anesthesia Considerations in Resuscitation and Stabilization

Massive Hemorrhage and Hypovolemic Shock

Massive hemorrhage and hypovolemic shock are frequently encountered complications of dismounted complex blast injury, and the treating surgeons, anesthesiologists, and resuscitative support staff must be prepared for implementation of massive transfusion and knowledgeable of trauma resuscitation protocols and the management of hypovolemic shock as well as its concomitant metabolic and coagulopathic derangements. Blast-injured patients often have significant injury burden and require large-volume transfusions (Fig. 30.1). Fleming et al. reported that DCBI casualties with a single extremity amputee patients were transfused a mean of 6.1 units of packed red blood cells, while multiple extremity amputees received a mean of 19.5 units of PRBCs during their resuscitative course [10]. Oh et al. review of 457 JTTR patients seen at Camp Bastion, Afghanistan, demonstrated similar requirements with 30% of DCBI casualties requiring a massive transfusion

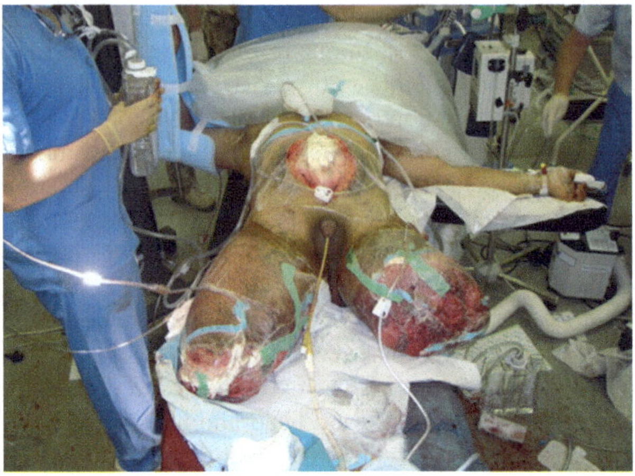

Fig. 30.1 Dismounted complex blast injury bilateral traumatic amputation

(defined as 10 or more units of PRBCs within a 24-h period) [8]. During the Iraq and Afghanistan conflicts between 2003 and 2012, 14% of patients admitted to Role 3 military treatment facilities received a transfusion of at least one blood product, and of these, 35% received a massive transfusion (10 units of PRBCs and/or whole blood within 24 h). By 2011, this proportion had reached 50% [11].

The incidence of complex blast trauma expedited the development of the principles of damage control resuscitation (DCR) as an extension of the strategy of damage control surgery in the treatment of trauma patients. The DCR principles emphasize temporizing early nonsurgical interventions that may reduce morbidity and mortality from trauma and hemorrhage. The major principles of DCR include hemorrhage control; repletion of blood volume with balanced blood product administration; the correction of coagulopathy, tissue hypoxia, acidosis, and hypothermia; and the restoration of normal physiology [11, 12]. Retrospective evidence from civilian and military trauma populations supports the administration of higher ratio plasma and platelets to red cells in patients requiring massive transfusion [11]. Massive transfusion at a 1:1:1 ratio has been associated with improved survival [13].

Among some of the central recommendations by the US DoD Joint Trauma System DCR Clinical Practice Guidelines are blood product with a focus on whole blood (e.g., stored whole blood or fresh warm whole blood), balanced ration blood product administration (i.e., PRBC, plasma and platelets in a 1:1:1 ratio), and use of hemostatic adjuncts such as cryoprecipitate and tranexamic acid. While less of an issue in civilian trauma centers with robust blood bank capability, the use of platelets in military forward deployed medical facilities is limited by the logistical constraints of their short storage life (5–7 days at 20–24 °C, with need for mechanical agitation). Cold-stored platelets can be stored under refrigeration for 3 days without agitation, are approved by the FDA for treatment of hemorrhage, and carry a reduced risk of bacterial growth as compared to room temperature-stored platelets. Cold-stored platelets in platelet additive solution retain function for 15 days. Low Titer Group O Whole Blood (LTOWB), collected either on site or through Armed

Forces Blood Program, can be stored refrigerated for 21–35 days [11]. In forward deployed environments, "walking blood banks," on-site collection from prescreened donors, have served to mitigate the logistical constraints associated with supplying blood components, particularly platelets for hemostatic resuscitation [11].

Additional adjunctive therapies include hypotensive resuscitation (excluding casualties with evidence of central nervous system injury) prior to surgical hemostasis whereby the casualty is maintained at a lower-target systolic blood pressure (90 mmHg) to minimize intravascular hydrostatic pressure, empiric administration of tranexamic acid (antifibrinolytic) within 3 h of injury in patients at high risk of hemorrhagic shock, and aggressive treatment of hypothermia through use of increased ambient resuscitative/operating suite temperature, warming blankets, and warmed fluid administration [11]. Rapid establishment of adequate intravascular access is paramount, as casualties may arrive from the field without adequate IV access. Intraosseous access can represent a useful adjunct to begin initial resuscitation but is not a substitute for large-bore venous access, which should be established either peripherally or preferentially by a large central vein as rapidly as possible by an experienced practitioner [14]. In a DCBI setting, femoral veins and surrounding anatomy may have been disrupted by the blast mechanism. In the absence of this or suspicion of a pelvic fracture, a femoral venous line is acceptable. Most patients will arrive from the field in cervical spine precautions, rendering placement of an internal jugular venous line difficult to impracticable. In most battlefield Role 2 or Role 3 settings, the subclavian approach to large bore central access has proven the preferred technique (Fig. 30.2).

The anesthesiologist assumes a critical role in the DCR continuum, serving as an expert in vascular access, shock physiology including hemorrhagic and reperfusion states, and the execution of DCR principles. This role is particularly important during the operative phase, and strict attention should be paid to hypothermia prevention, maintaining physiologic homeostasis, and anticipating pitfalls associated with complex blast pathophysiology.

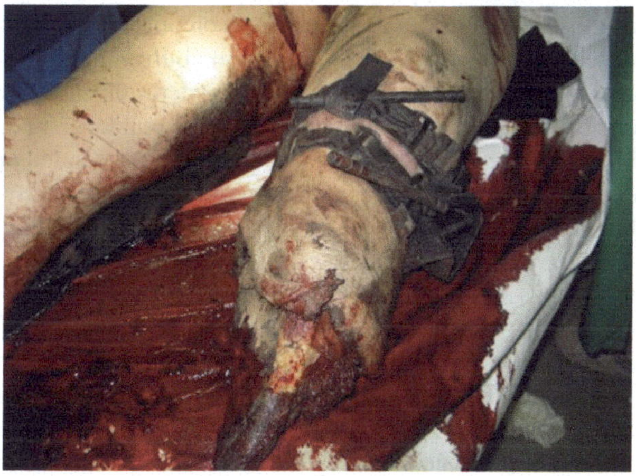

Fig. 30.2 Dismounted complex blast injury traumatic extremity amputation

Airway Management

Airway compromise has been estimated to represent the third leading major cause of potentially survivable death on the battlefield emphasizing the need for anesthesiologists and other practitioners of airway management to establish and maintain effective emergency airway stabilization practices [15–17]. Trauma airway management complicated by blast injury may pose formidable challenges to the anesthesiologist due to the potential for tissue destruction, anatomic distortion, and thermal injury produced by blast energy and secondary fragmentation from exposure to IEDs, mines, rocket-propelled grenades, or other types of explosives. Penetrating neck trauma and tissue disruption caused by blast injury can cause immediate life-threatening airway issues and devastating maxillofacial injuries which can further compound difficulty in management of these emergent airways [15]. A characteristic of blast trauma is that of high-velocity penetrating and blunt injury that produces massive tissue avulsion [15].

Modern combat body armor reinforced with ceramic plates has proven extremely effective at limiting penetrating injury to the torso, but current design leaves the extremities, face, and neck vulnerable to injury, resulting in a relatively high proportion of neck and facial injuries among combat casualties [4, 18]. The head, neck, and face, despite a relatively small percentage of total body surface area, have comprised a disproportionately high percentage of combat injuries in the Iraq and Afghanistan conflicts [5, 19]. A study by Brennan et al. on traumatic airway injury in Operation Iraqi Freedom (OIF) documents penetrating face and neck injuries rates at 46% and 31%, respectively, with blast mechanisms accounting for a combined 62% of those [19].

High-velocity blunt force and fragmentation injuries by blast mechanisms may present formidable challenges in airway management due to some of the following factors: potential for penetrating vascular injury to produce rapidly progressive edema, the degree to which even a relatively small degree of anatomic distortion may render normal anatomic landmarks significantly less recognizable, disruption of anatomically supportive bone and cartilage, and the presence of blood, secretions, or loose tissue in the upper airway potentially confounding traditional approaches to securing the airway [19]. The team confronted with such injuries must approach airway management, taking into consideration multiple factors, and formulate an effective management strategy in a very condensed period of time. The nature of blast injury is to create a high potential for associated upper airway injury with the expectation that tracheal intubation may prove difficult in a patient with oral-maxillofacial and/or neck injuries due to potential for obscured view of the vocal cords on direct laryngoscopy; the obscuring effect of blood, secretions, or tissue and/or bone fragments in the oral, pharyngeal, or laryngeal cavities; diminished neck mobility due to the possibility of cervical spine injury; potential for patient combativeness; and aspiration risk [20].

The airway must be evaluated as much as possible under the circumstances and time constraints. At a minimum, the LEMON assessment should be employed to the degree possible, whereby the practitioner evaluates external anatomic anomalies either preexisting or produced by injury and evaluates for thyromental distance, mouth opening, Mallampati score, and neck mobility [20]. Other valuable information obtained on exam consists of evaluating injury relative to anatomic zone. Zone 1 comprises the region from the clavicles to the cricoid cartilage, zone 2 from the cricoid to the angle of the mandible, and zone 3 from the angle of the mandible to the skull base. Zone analysis may help to predict potential injuries and help shape choice of approach with respect to airway management solutions [21]. Barak offers several scenarios associated with OMFS trauma that may adversely affect the airway: (1) posterior displacement of a fractured maxilla (nasopharyngeal obstruction); (2) bilateral fracture of the anterior mandible (posterior displacement of the tongue); (3) fractured or exfoliated teeth, bone fragments, vomitus, blood, secretions, or foreign bodies; (4) hemorrhage from distinct vessels or severe nasal bleeding; (5) soft tissue swelling and edema (delayed airway compromise); and (6) trauma to larynx and trachea, producing swelling and displacement of structures such as arytenoids, epiglottis, and vocal cords [20]. Assessment of the airway in the presence of these injuries and under conditions frequently encountered in battlefield hospitals may prove extremely challenging to even the experienced practitioner. A frequently offered, effective initial approach is the simple confirmation of phonation and verbalization during the primary trauma survey, with an intelligible and appropriate response indicating sufficient respiratory effort to generate voice and adequate cerebral perfusion consistent with a Glasgow Coma Scale score greater than 8 [19]. If the patient is conscious, then the administration of sedatives should be administered judiciously, if not altogether avoided, given the possibility of adverse effects upon spontaneous ventilation and airway patency [20]. If the patient is spontaneously breathing, then supplemental oxygen should be administered in order to optimize oxygenation and maximize "safe" apneic time [22]. In the absence of spontaneous ventilation, then all opportunities to deliver supplemental oxygen and prevent hypoxia should be pursued. These modalities may include supplemental oxygen through high-flow nasal cannula (apneic hyperoxygenation) [23], face mask, laryngeal mask airway, or jet insufflation [22]. If the patient is hypoxic, and preoxygenation is not possible, then ventilation should be pursued by the management team using what capabilities and equipment are at their disposal [20].

The choice of technique for definitive control of the airway will depend on a host of factors, taking into consideration the above elements together with the experience of the practitioner(s) and supporting personnel, conditions, and available equipment. While endotracheal intubation is a routine undertaking for anesthesiologists, this procedure should be approached with caution in the case of airway injury in the blast victim. Airway management in patients with maxillofacial trauma is complicated by injuries to routes of conventional intubation. Airway obstruction from hemorrhage, tissue prolapse, or edema may require emergent intervention to secure the airway [15]. Projectiles from secondary blast effect can transfix tissue and restrict mouth opening. Patients may also present with neck lacerations and open wounds to the airway [21]. Additionally, blast injuries carry a significant risk of burn injury to the airway. Recent combat experience has demonstrated a disproportionate distribution of burn injury toward anatomic regions unprotected by body armor, with burns accounting for 10% of combat-related injuries to the head and neck region and facial involvement present in 77% of all combat-related burn admissions [24].

One potentially devastating pitfall is the failure to recognize that an intact laryngeal inlet does not necessarily equate to an intact airway below the level of the vocal cords. Placement of an endotracheal tube by direct laryngoscopy could, in this instance, lead to advancement of the tip through the defect and creation of a false passage, producing obstruction, worsening of the tear, or pneumomediastinum [21]. The approach carrying possibly the least risk in these cases is that of instrumenting the trachea under direct visualization (i.e., bronchoscope confirmation) either with an awake patient or with spontaneous ventilation preserved after the induction of anesthesia [25]. However, while this approach carries with it many advantages, its practicability in the field hospital setting may be limited by its requirements for a cooperative patient, sufficient skill level of the operator, and availability of proper equipment. The confounding presence of blood, foreign bodies, or tissue fragments in the airway may also limit the utility of this method [21]. If conditions do not allow preservation of spontaneous ventilation and awake fiber-optic bronchoscopy, or if it becomes necessary to induce anesthesia and administer neuromuscular blockade prior to securing of the airway, then a suggested approach may consist of a rapid sequence induction together with a bronchoscope-assisted direct or video laryngoscopy approach [21]. With this technique, a tracheal tube is placed above the vocal cords under direct visualization followed by passage of a bronchoscope through the tube and into the trachea [25]. This allows for visual confirmation of the absence of a subglottic tear prior to delivery of the endotracheal tube into the airway. The video laryngoscope may also offer advantages in situations where neck mobility is limited due to concern for cervical spine injury or in patients with soft tissue swelling at the base of the tongue or where disruption of normal anatomy precludes identification of the epiglottis [20]. In the case of an actively bleeding upper airway, where visualization of the airway becomes difficult to impossible, time spent readying equipment, medications, and communication of the airway plan must simultaneously be used to apply supplemental oxygen and/or suction to the patient and optimizing conditions for instrumentation of the airway. If conscious, the patient may be placed in a position of comfort (use of gravity to divert blood and/or secretions away from the airway) with application of continuous suction (potentially self-administered in an awake and lucid patient) prior to the induction of anesthesia and ablation of respiratory drive.

The surgical airway is considered the option of last resort in airway management. However, in the patient with severe facial trauma, it may sometimes represent the best solution. If available, a qualified surgeon should be at the bedside during conventional airway management in blast victims. Performing a cricothyroidotomy or tracheotomy under local anesthesia can be a lifesaving procedure in patients falling under the "cannot intubate, cannot ventilate" branch of the difficult airway algorithm [20]. In general, airway injury from blast mechanisms can increase the complexity of management exponentially by the multitude of factors that have been addressed above. Multiple modalities and techniques exist with which to approach such management dilemmas.

Consideration of the following pitfalls in patients with penetrating airway injuries from a blast mechanism may assist the practitioner in the formulation of management strategies:

1. Ventilation: Use of positive pressure ventilation may risk exacerbating tissue plane disruption and produce tissue emphysema. Spontaneous ventilation should be preserved if possible, and supraglottic airways should be avoided in injuries distal to the vocal cords [20].
2. Intubation: Blind placement of an endotracheal tube runs the risk of the tube tip passing into a traumatic defect with placement outside the lumen of the airway. This is avoided by a fiber-optic, direct visual confirmation technique or a surgical airway [21]. Endotracheal intubation should be approached cautiously with avoidance of conventional oral intubation when the injury is distal to the vocal cords. Likewise, blind nasal intubation should also be avoided. Conventional fiber-optic intubation will likely prove difficult if not impossible when there is bleeding into the airway. Surgical airways are potentially very difficult in the presence of subcutaneous emphysema or an expanding hematoma [21].
3. Muscle relaxants in near or complete airway transection may ablate intrinsic muscle tone necessary to maintain airway integrity [20].
4. Burn injury to the airway may necessitate definitive airway management in the setting of blast injury. In combat blast injuries, thermal tissue damage may be disproportionately distributed to anatomic areas not protected by body armor. Johnson et al. reported in 2015 on analysis of the US Army Institute of Surgical Research Burn database. Inhalation injury was frequently seen (61%), and of all the military burn injuries contained in the database, 67.1% involved the face [24].

Blast-Related Lung Injury/ARDS

Blast-related lung injury may be the result of all phases of a blast mechanism from primary to quaternary [26]. Primary blast lung injury (PBLI) is defined as "radiological and clinical evidence of acute lung injury occurring within 12 h of blast wave exposure and not due to secondary or tertiary injury." The pathophysiology of PBLI is generally understood as follows: an initial autonomic response, followed by hemorrhage and parenchymal injury, then followed by an inflammatory phase [27]. The initial blast wave produces immediate tissue injury, characterized by rupture of alveolar capillaries and subsequent intrapulmonary hemorrhage and edema, analogous to pulmonary contusion from blunt chest trauma [28]. Furthermore, the presence of blood and free hemoglobin in the alveolar spaces is thought to lead to the formation of free radicals, edema, and an early inflammatory response with leukocyte accumulation and subsequent epithelial cell damage at 12–24 h, endothelial cell damage at 24–56 h, and edema formation typical of adult respiratory distress syndrome [28]. Other blast-related pulmonary sequelae may include pneumothorax and/or hemothorax, which may occur due to shearing forces of the detonation wave damaging peripheral alveoli (pneumothorax) and/or pulmonary vessels (hemothorax) [28]. Blast lung injury may also occur through secondary, tertiary, or quaternary mechanisms from injuries such as thoracic fractures (ribs, clavicles, scapulae, vertebrae), pulmonary contusions, pulmonary lacerations, crush injuries, and asphyxiation. Additionally, blast-related lung injury may be associated with factors less related to the mechanism of injury but rather with iatrogenic factors such as over-resuscitation and injurious mechanical ventilation [26].

Primary blast lung injury has been encountered globally as a result of military conflict, terrorist attacks, and industrial accidents, and identifying patients with PBLI can be challenging as they present with a mixed pattern of injury [27, 28]. Estimates of battlefield incidence of PBLI have been placed by one study between 6% and 11% of military casualties from the Afghanistan conflict who survived to reach a field hospital [27]. As is the case with primary blast injury, the incidence and severity of PBLI increase significantly with increasing proximity to the detonation. When injuries are sustained in an enclosed space, an enhancement and additive effect of blast waves is seen to occur when detonation overpressure reflects off surfaces such as walls or within vehicles, thus producing a significantly greater positive pressure phase (up to 20×) and thus increasing injury [27]. Upon receiving casualties from a blast event, elicitation of a history of distance from detonation epicenter or history of exposure within a confined space may be helpful in generating clinical suspicion. However, in practice, this information is often, in the immediate casualty receiving phase, difficult to obtain. Casualties with clinically significant PBLI will most likely manifest symptoms by the time of their arrival at a medical facility. Mild injury may not become apparent for several hours as the inflammatory response progresses [27]. Spontaneously breathing casualties will exhibit shortness of breath, possibly impaired gas exchange, and perhaps hemoptysis. Tachycardia, tachypnea, and cyanosis suggest increasing severity of injury. Hypoxia, if present, may not be evident initially but may develop over the first few hours in the post injury period [28]. Classic radiographic appearance of PBLI demonstrates interstitial and alveolar filling defects and air bronchograms in a perihilar "butterfly" infiltrate pattern, the result of pulmonary barotrauma [27, 29]. PBLI may not, however, always manifest radiographically in a "classical" appearance, with the picture complicated by lung contusion (tertiary blast injury) and penetrating fragments (secondary blast injury) [27].

Patients with multiple injuries are known to develop lung injury, and it is estimated that some degree of ARDS occurs in between 26% and 33% of combat casualties

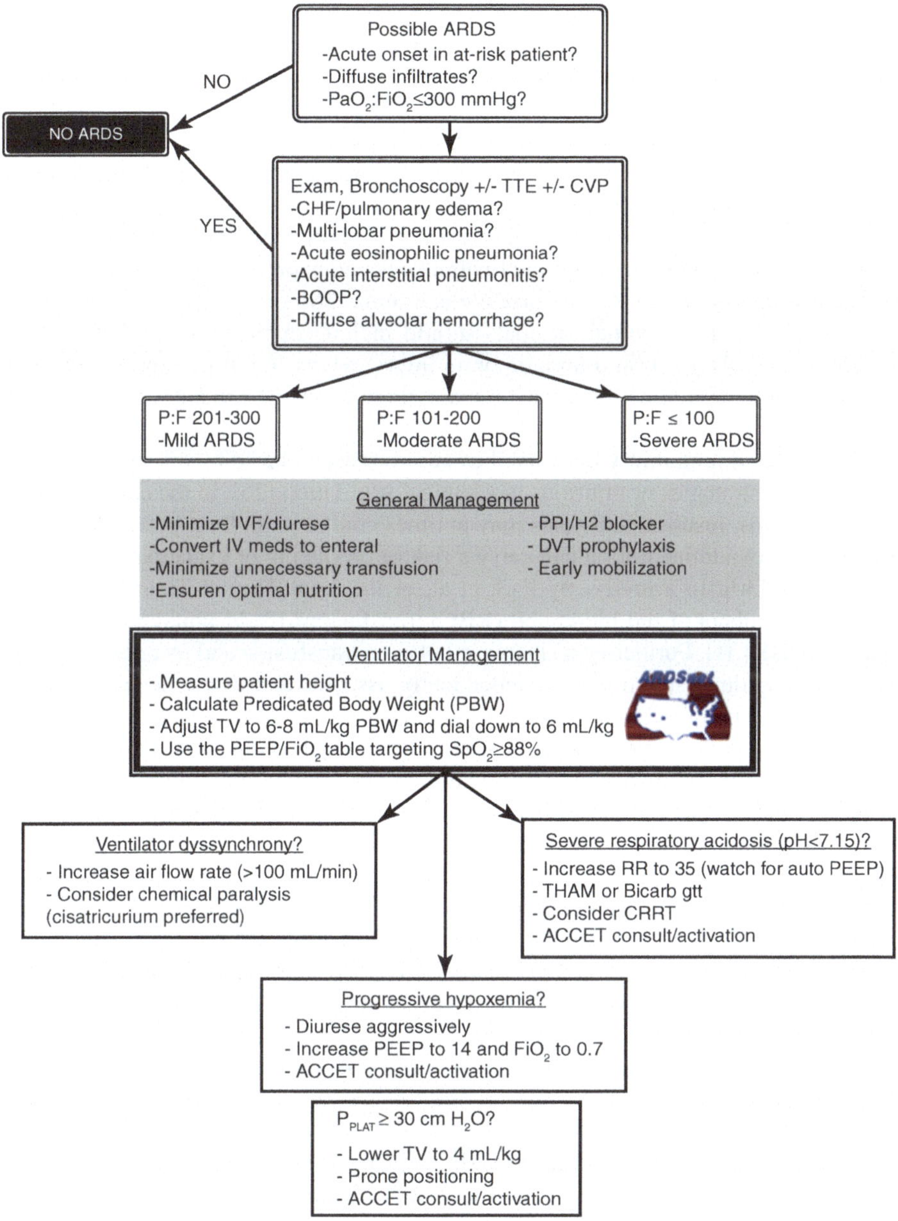

Fig. 30.3 ARDS diagnosis and treatment of acute respiratory failure CPG

[30]. Patients with severe blast injury will likely develop ARDS (Fig. 30.3) [27]. The management goals of patients with severe PBLI who manifest an ARDS picture should seek to balance the support of gas exchange without causing further injury to the patient's lungs [30]. Once ARDS has been established, the patient should be

placed on lung-protective ventilation settings according to the ARDSnet ventilator management protocol [30]. In patients with blast-related ARDS, by whatever mechanism, ventilation goals include:

1. Maintaining peak plateau pressures (Pplat) at or below 30 cm H_2O or peak inspiratory pressures (PIP) at or below 35 cm H_2O (where Pplat cannot be measured) in order to limit barotrauma [30].
2. Tidal volumes (VT) between 6 and 8 mL/kg of predicted body to minimize volutrauma and to maintain moderate to high peak end expiratory pressure (PEEP) to the ventilatory circuit to minimize atelectrauma [30].
3. Oxygenation and ventilation goals should include maintaining an SpO_2 ≥88–95% and a pH ≥7.3 (in traumatic brain injury, where ICP is of concern, this pH goal should be met with the $PaCO_2$ maintained at 35–40 mm Hg) [30].

Blast-related lung injury may also be caused or exacerbated by overly aggressive resuscitative strategies or injurious mechanical ventilation [26]. In the case of multi-trauma victims, resuscitative goals may at times conflict with lung-protective goals. Blood product administration can carry a risk of producing or exacerbating respiratory failure [30]. In a review by Park et al. of the Joint Theater Trauma Registry, moderate numbers of red blood cell (RBC) transfusions (2–14 units) increased the risk of ARDS [31]. Furthermore, increased plasma transfusion and increased crystalloid volume administered were independently associated with the development of ARDS [31]. Therefore, it is necessary for anesthesia practitioners engaged in the treatment of multi-injury blast victims to balance the benefits of DCR against the risk of ARDS. If hemorrhage is ongoing and blood volume replacement is required, blood products should not be withheld [30]. Conversely, in a patient in whom hemostasis has been achieved, and asymptomatic anemia or a mildly elevated International Normalized Ratio (INR) with normal viscoelastic studies (TEG/ROTEM), the risk of additional blood product may exceed any benefit. Ventilation strategies should reflect a balance for the need to maintain adequate oxygenation and CO_2 elimination and the limiting of barotrauma- and ventilator-associated lung injury in patients whose exposure to blast injury may render them susceptible to the development of ARDS.

Burn Injuries

During the recent conflicts in Iraq and Afghanistan, as referenced above, explosions have constituted the primary mechanism of injury, as high as 74% in one review [7]. Moreover, explosions were the leading cause of injury in burned combat casualties admitted to Brooke Army Medical Center (US Army burn center) during these conflicts (Fig. 30.4) [3]. Anesthetic challenges in burn patients can include airway management, alteration of drug pharmacokinetics, hypermetabolism, pain management issues, temperature control, and substantial blood loss [32]. Major burns cause large-scale tissue destruction and result in activation of a cytokine-mediated inflammatory response that produces dramatic pathophysiologic sequelae at sites local and distant from the burn. Systemic effects occur in two distinct phases, a burn shock

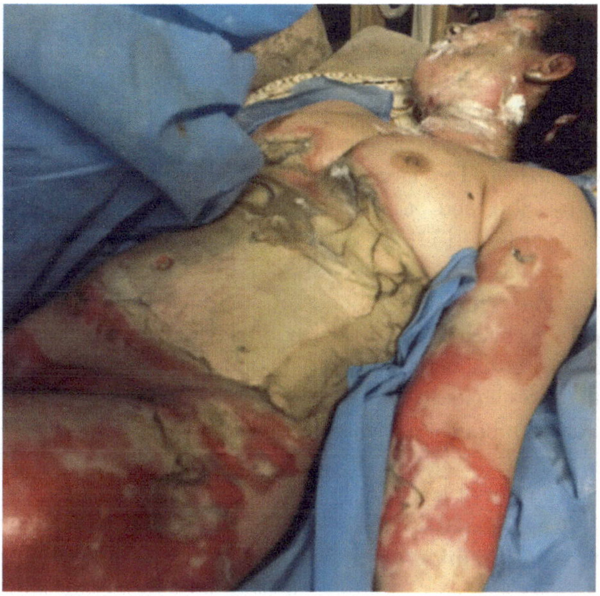

Fig. 30.4 Iraqi noncombatant burn injury victim

phase followed by a hypermetabolic phase [33]. Initial management recommendations of burn casualties at point of injury by Joint Trauma System Burn Care CPG include interrupting the burning process, addressing any life-threatening hemorrhage, airway compromise, or tension pneumothorax per tactical combat casualty care (TCCC) guidelines [34]. Primary and secondary surveys should be performed as for any trauma patient with identified injuries addressed as per standard trauma protocols. The tendency toward distraction by the appearance of burned tissues exists and should be avoided [34]. All burn patients should receive 100% supplemental oxygen (O_2) through a non-rebreathing mask on presentation [32]. As per primary trauma survey, a determination must be made as to the viability of the airway. Initial compromise of the airway in the burn patient is usually due to a low Glasgow Coma Score (GCS) and not the burn [32]. However, direct heat injury to the upper airway can produce marked edema of the face, tongue, epiglottis, and glottic opening resulting in airway obstruction [33]. Early tracheal intubation should be considered where any of the following findings are present: stridor, hypoxemia or hypercapnia, a GCS of 8 or less, deep facial burns, full-thickness neck burns, and oropharyngeal edema or over 40% TBSA [32, 34]. Use of a large endotracheal tube (ETT), preferably size 8, is recommended if inhalation injury is suspected as the larger diameter will facilitate subsequent bronchoscopy and pulmonary toilet and reduce the risk of later airway occlusion by blood, mucus, or debris [34]. Succinylcholine may be safely used in the first 24 h after a burn. Following this, it is contraindicated due to the risk of hyperkalemia leading to cardiac arrest. The ETT should be secured with cotton umbilical ties that can be adjusted as edema develops over the course of resuscitation [34]. For a patient in whom a long-range transport is necessary, consideration should be given to securing the ETT to a premolar tooth, particularly in patients with extensive facial burns [34].

Quantifying the magnitude of burn injury is established according to TBSA involved, depth of the burn, and the presence or absence of inhalational injury [33]. TBSA burned in adults can be estimated using the "rule of nines." The Lund–Browder chart more precisely accounts for the changing body surface area relationships with age [33]. Superficial burns should not be factored into the overall TBSA calculation. Two large-bore IV catheters should be established through unburnt skin if possible and baseline laboratory studies sent. Establishing central access may be necessary [32]. Patients with greater than 20% TBSA will likely require fluid resuscitation for the next 24–48 h [34]. There are varying approaches to fluid resuscitation, with the Parkland formula having common use in the United States. For patients greater than 40 kg, the JTS Burn Care CPG recommends use, if available, of a burn resuscitation decision support fluid calculator. In the absence of this system, the JTS CPG advocates use of the "Rule of 10's" (Rule of Tens) for initial resuscitation with hourly measurement of urine output as a measure of resuscitation:

- 10 ml/h of isotonic fluid (lactated Ringer's or PlasmaLyte) × % TBSA if patient weight is 40–80 kg.
- Add 100 ml/h for every 10 kg >80 kg.

Though guidelines recommend reevaluation of resuscitation efforts at 8–12 h, the anesthesiologist should be conducting hourly assessments utilizing hemodynamic parameters and urine output to monitor for potential over-resuscitation [34]. It is also crucial to recall that combat casualties with burns may often present with multisystem injury and that these associated injuries may increase fluid needs above and beyond standard burn resuscitation formulas [34]. Regardless which approach is employed, it should serve only as a guideline, and fluid resuscitation is titrated to physiologic endpoints [33].

Placement of an indwelling urinary catheter is mandatory, and resuscitation is titrated to maintain urinary output of 30–50 ml/h for patients >40 kg or 0.5–1.0 ml/kg/h [34]. Ventilatory management should follow the ARDS Network trial findings in burn patients with acute lung injury, with the administration of tidal volumes of less than or equal to 6 ml/kg ideal body weight and plateau airway pressures less than 30 cm H_2O in adults being recommended. The hypermetabolic state and increased carbon dioxide production of burn injury may dictate higher-than-normal ventilation rates [33].

Burns increase insensible heat loss. Burn casualties with injuries >20% TBSA are at high risk of hypothermia [34]. Additionally, patients with large burns reset their baseline temperature to 38.5 C. Thus, a patient with a core temperature of 37 C is relatively hypothermic [32]. Iatrogenic factors such as fluid resuscitation and exposure for surgical procedures can worsen hypothermia. Hypothermia prevention measures include active warming of the ambient temperature, warmed ventilation circuits, warming blankets, and warmed fluids. Of additional importance is the need to minimize the increase in basal metabolic rate caused by heat and evaporative water loss [32]. If possible, measure bladder pressures every 4 h in intubated patients with >20% TBSA burns. Persistent bladder pressures >20 mmHg may indicate abdominal compartment syndrome [34]. After approximately 24–72 h successful resuscitation is characterized by stabilizing hemodynamics and reduction of IV fluid rate to a maintenance level. Acid–base abnormalities should have normalized, hematocrit should reveal a dilutional anemia, and pulses should be present in all extremities [34].

A summary of the goals of anesthetic care for the burn patient as a result of blast injury includes the concepts of identifying and addressing life-threatening injuries as may be present; early securing of the airway in selected patients; establishment of adequate intravascular access; volume resuscitation based on extent of burn injury; fluid resuscitation formulas as guidelines and titration to physiologic endpoints; appropriate ventilatory management in burn patients with acute lung injury, blast-related, inhalational, or otherwise; and aggressive treatment of hypothermia.

Conclusion

Anesthetic management of blast injury presents one of the most formidable challenges that may confront the practitioner of anesthesia. Among the major challenges to be addressed are management of hypovolemic shock, prevention of tissue hypoxemia and acidemia, and mitigation of coagulopathy during resuscitation. In addition, the anesthesiologist will have significant roles in managing complex blast-induced airway injury and ventilator issues associated with blast-related lung injury and concomitant burns. Injury to the lower airway and lung parenchyma is part of the constellation of blast injury pattern and, combined with aggressive blood product administration, makes the development of ARDS in blast casualties highly likely.

Pitfalls

- Hemostatic resuscitation
  - Equation of a normal blood pressure with normovolemia
  - Failure to aggressively mitigate and reverse hypothermia
  - Failure to administer timely antifibrinolytic therapy
  - Failure to administer blood products in balanced proportion
- Airway management
  - Failure to adequately plan and train for potential anatomic disruption in blast injury emergent airway management
  - Failure to implement a focused airway management strategy emphasizing familiarity with and employment of a limited number of airway adjuncts versus reliance on a wider array of airway management implements with reduced familiarity
  - Failure to recognize need for surgical airway
  - Failure of early airway establishment in setting of blast thermal injury

- Ventilation
  - Failure to consider the presence of blast lung injury in DCBI and the subsequent pursuit of lung-protective strategies in initial ventilator management
  - Failure to consider risk to benefit ratio when administering blood product components in resuscitation of blast victims and consideration of risks associated with over-resuscitation and/or transfusion-related acute lung injury

References

1. Leissner K, Ortega R, Beattie WS. Anesthesia implications of burn injury. J Cardiothorac Vasc Anesth. 2006;20(6):872–80.
2. Lemonick DM. Bombings and blast injuries. Am J Clin Med. 2011;8(3):134–40.
3. Cancio LC, Sheridan RL, Dent R, Hjalmarson SG, Gardner E, Matherly AF, et al. Guidelines for burn care under austere conditions: special etiologies: blast, radiation, and chemical injuries. J Burn Care Res. 2017;38(1):e482–96.
4. Xydakis MS, Fravell MD, Nasser KE, Casler JD. Analysis of battlefield head and neck injuries in Iraq and Afghanistan. Otolaryngol Head Neck Surg. 2005;133:497–504.
5. Tong D, Beirne R. Combat body armor and injuries to the head, face, and neck region: a systematic review. Mil Med. 2013;178(4):421–6.
6. Schoenfeld AJ, Belmont PJ. Chapter 2: Traumatic combat injuries. In: Cameron KL, Owens BD, editors. Musculoskeletal injuries in the military. New York: Springer; 2016. https://doi.org/10.1007/978-1-4939-2984-9_2.
7. Belmont PJ Jr, McCriskin BJ, Sieg RN, Burks R, Schoenfeld AJ. Combat wounds in Iraq and Afghanistan from 2005 to 2009. J Trauma Acute Care Surg. 2012;73(1):3–12.
8. Oh JS, Tubb CC, Poepping TP, Ryan P, Clasper JC, Katschke AR, Truman C, Murray MJ. Dismounted blast injuries in patients treated at a role 3 military hospital in Afghanistan: patterns of injury and mortality. Mil Med. 2016;181(9):1069–74.
9. Andersen RC, Fleming M, Forsberg JA, Gordon WT, Nanos GP III, Charlton MT, Ficke JR. Dismounted complex blast injury. J Surg Orthop Adv. 2012;21(1):2–7.
10. Fleming M, Waterman S, Dunne J, D'Alleyrand JC, Andersen RC. Dismounted complex blast injuries: patterns of injuries and resource utilization associated with the multiple extremity amputee. J Surg Orthop Adv. 2012;21(1):32–7.
11. Cap AP, Pidcoke HF, Spinella P, et al. Joint Trauma System Clinical Practice Guideline. (JTS CPG) Damage Control Resuscitation (CPG ID:18) pp 1–24. jts.amedd.army.mil/index.cfm/PI_CPGs/cpgs.
12. Ball CG. Damage control resuscitation: history, theory and technique. Can J Surg. 2014;57(1):55–60.
13. Holcomb JB, Tilley BC, Baraniuk S, Fox EE, Wade CE, Podbielski JM, et al. Transfusion of plasma, platelets and red blood cells in a 1:1:1 vs a 1:1:2 ratio and mortality in patients with severe trauma: the PROPPR randomized clinical trial. JAMA. 2015;313(5):471–82.
14. Gordon W, Talbot M, Fleming M, et al. Joint Trauma System Clinical Practice Guideline. (JTS CPG) High Bilateral Amputations and Dismounted Complex Blast Injury (CPG ID:22) pp 1–10. jts.amedd.army.mil/index.cfm/PI_CPGs/cpgs.
15. Keller MW, Han PP, Galarneau MR, Brigger MT. Airway management in severe combat maxillofacial trauma. Otolaryngol Head Neck Surg. 2015;153(4):532–7.

16. Mabry RL, Edens JW, Pearse L, Kelly JF, Harke H. Fatal airway injuries during operation enduring freedom and operation Iraqi freedom. Prehosp Emerg Care. 2010;14(2):272–7. https://doi.org/10.3109/10903120903537205.
17. Walrath BD, Harper S, Barnard E, et al. Joint Trauma System Clinical Practice Guideline. (JTS CPG) Airway Management of Traumatic Injuries (CPG ID: 39) pp 1–7. jts.amedd.army.mil/index.cfm/PI_CPGs/cpgs.
18. Owens BD, Kragh JF, Wenke JC, Macaitis J, Wade CE, Holcomb JB. Combat wounds in operation Iraqi freedom and operation. J Trauma. 2008;64:295–9.
19. Brennan J, Gibbons MD, Lopez M, Hayes D, Faulkner J, Eller RL, Barton C. Traumatic airway management in operation Iraqi freedom. Otolaryngol Head Neck Surg. 2011;144(3):376–80.
20. Barak M, Bahouth H, Leiser Y, Abu El-Naaj I. Airway management of the patient with maxillofacial trauma: review of the literature and suggested clinical approach. Biomed Res Int. 2015;2015:1–9. https://doi.org/10.1155/2015/724032.
21. Mercer SJ, Lewis SE, Wilson SJ, Groom P, Mahoney PF. Creating airway management guidelines for casualties with penetrating airway injuries. J R Army Med Corps. 2010;156(4 Suppl 1):355–60. Review.
22. Practice Guidelines for Management of the Difficult Airway. An updated report by the American Society of Anesthesiologists Task Force on management of the difficult airway. Anesthesiology. 2013;118(2):251–270.
23. Gleason JM, Christian BR, Barton ED. Nasal cannula apneic oxygenation prevents desaturation during endotracheal intubation: an integrative literature review. West J Emerg Med. 2018;19(2):403–11.
24. Johnson BW, Madson AQ, Bong Thakur S, Tucker D, Hale RG, Chan RK. Combat-related facial burns: analysis of strategic pitfalls. 2015 American Association of Oral and Maxillofacial Surgeons. J Oral Maxillofac Surg. 2015;73:106–11.
25. Mercer SJ, Jones CP, Bridge M, Clitheroe E, Morton B, Groom P. Systematic review of the anaesthetic management of non-iatrogenic acute adult airway trauma. Br J Anaesth. 2016;117(S1):i49–59.
26. Mackenzie I, Tunnicliff B, Clasper J, Mahoney P, Kirkman E. What the intensive care doctor needs to know about blast-related lung injury. J Intensive Care Soc. 2013;14(4):303–12.
27. Scott TE, Kirkman E, Haque M, Gibb IE, Mahoney P, Hardman JG. Primary blast lung injury – a review. Br J Anaesth. 2017;118(3):311–6.
28. Smith JE. The epidemiology of blast lung injury during recent military conflicts: a retrospective database review of cases presenting to deployed military hospitals, 2003–2009. Philos Trans R Soc B. 2011;366:291–4. https://doi.org/10.1098/rstb.2010.0251.
29. Barnard E, Johnston E. Images in clinical medicine. Blast lung. N Engl J Med. 2013;368(11):1045.
30. Cannon JC, Pamplin J, Zonies D, Mason P, et al. Joint Trauma System Clinical Practice Guideline (JTS CPG) Acute Respiratory Failure (CPG ID:6) pp 1–14. jts.amedd.army.mil/index.cfm/PI_CPGs/cpgs.
31. Park P, Cannon J, Ye W, Blackbourne LH, Holcomb J, Beninati W, Napolitano LM. Transfusion strategies and development of acute respiratory distress syndrome in combat casualty care. J Trauma Acute Care Surg. 2013 Aug;75(2 Suppl 2):S238–46.
32. Bishop S, Maguire S. Anaesthesia and intensive care for major burns. Contin Ed Anaesth Crit Care Pain. 2012;12(3):118–22.
33. Bittner EA, Shank E, Woodson L, Martyn JA. Acute and perioperative care of the burn-injured patient. Anesthesiology. 2015;122(2):448–64.
34. Driscoll I, Mann-Salinas EA, Boyer N, et al. Joint trauma system clinical practice guideline. Burn Care (CPG ID:12) http://jts.amedd.army.mil/assets/docs/cpgs/JTS_Clinical_Practice_Guidelines_(CPGs)/Burn_Care_11_May_2016_ID12.pdf.

Vascular Injuries 31

William J. Parker, Robert W. DesPain, Matthew J. Bradley, and Todd E. Rasmussen

Introduction

Significant progress has been made in the management of severe vascular injury since Ambroise Pare's description of ligating the right carotid artery and jugular vein of a soldier who had suffered a bayonet injury [1, 2]. Despite advances in surgical techniques including experimentation with shunting, ligation remained the primary means for treating combat vascular injuries up until the mid-twentieth century [3–5]. Ligation was often performed out of necessity due to prolonged ischemic times and limitations with the surgical technology and experience at the time. Sentinel work from prominent military surgeons and improved surgical equipment helped drastically change the management paradigm for complex vascular injury from ligation and amputation to primary repair and limb salvage [6–11].

Severe explosive injury with a blast component was once thought to be almost exclusive to the combat setting. Unfortunately, more recent events in the civilian environment have underscored the importance of nonmilitary providers also needing to be familiar with the care of these types of casualties. For instance, inadequate training and lack of supplies prior to the Boston Marathon bombing led to the poor

W. J. Parker (✉) · R. W. DesPain
Department of General Surgery, Walter Reed National Military Medical Center, Bethesda, MD, USA
e-mail: William.j.parker70.mil@mail.mil

M. J. Bradley
Department of Surgery, Walter Reed National Military Medical Center, Bethesda, MD, USA

T. E. Rasmussen
Department of Surgery, Walter Reed National Military Medical Center, Bethesda, MD, USA

F. Edward Hebert School of Medicine, Uniformed Services University, Bethesda, MD, USA

D. W. Callaway, J. L. Burstein (eds.), *Operational and Medical Management of Explosive and Blast Incidents*, https://doi.org/10.1007/978-3-030-40655-4_31

experience with ineffective improvised tourniquets used during the event [12]. Moving forward, ongoing collaborative knowledge sharing between military and civilian trauma and trauma systems communities will be essential to improving the management of major vascular injury from explosive mechanisms. Given the inherent life- and limb-threating nature of major vascular injury, it is vital that providers apply a rapid and systematic approach to these injuries. The following is a description of the epidemiology, diagnosis, and advanced management of vascular injury as a result of blast/mass casualty incidents. A brief review of point of injury and immediate emergency care is provided to create a common understanding across the spectrum of care for vascular injuries.

Epidemiology

With the increase in global terrorism, there has been a commensurate rise in the number of blast incidents and complex blast injuries in both the military and civilian populations. In the United States Department of State 2016 Country Report on Terrorism, there were 11,072 acts of terrorism worldwide with 33,814 casualties and 25,621 deaths. Fifty-four percent of these terrorist incidents were related to bombings or explosives [13]. The morbidity and mortality from blast-related incidents vary significantly from year to year though vascular injury burden remains a significant challenge [14].

The Boston Marathon bombing and the Manchester Arena bombings can be used as examples of the type of injury patterns expected from civilian blast incidents. Of the 243 patients who were injured in the Boston Marathon bombing, 66 presented with at least one extremity injury. Of these patients, 29 had extremity exsanguination at the scene. There were 10 patients and 12 limbs with major vascular injuries identified [12]. In the 2017 Manchester Arena bombing, 7% of the children treated at a single pediatric hospital sustained a major vascular injury requiring operative intervention [15]. This is in stark contrast to the normal distribution seen at civilian trauma centers. In urban trauma centers, peripheral vascular injuries are present in less than 5% of admissions, and in rural trauma centers, they occur in 1% [16, 17]. This is likely even less in European centers, as ballistic injuries account for only 0.53% of all recorded trauma injuries in the UK [18].

The most robust data on complex blast injury leading to vascular injury can be found from experiences with the wars in Iraq and Afghanistan. Vascular injury is significantly more prevalent in these wars than that reported from previous US armed conflicts. Upward of 20% of battle injuries during the wars in Afghanistan and Iraq, those injuries severe enough to preclude service members from returning to combat, are classified as "hemorrhage control not otherwise specified," implying the presence of a major vascular injury [19]. A recent report of data abstracted from the US military's Joint Trauma System from 2002 to 2016 reported that vascular surgery comprised 6.5% of surgeries performed for battle injuries [20]. Previous military data on the current conflicts stated that approximately 65% of major vascular injury is secondary to an explosive mechanism with or without a penetrating component (i.e., secondary versus primary blast injury) [21].

The distribution of vascular injuries has also differed from that of previously reported experiences from armed conflict. Based on data from Afghanistan and Iraq, 70–80% of vascular injuries occurred in extremities, 10–15% in the cervical region, and 5–10% in the torso [22]. In a large single institution series from Walter Reed, vascular injuries of the upper extremities constituted 39% of injuries, 51% were in the lower extremities, 7% were in the neck, and 3% were in the pelvis. Approximately 37% of service members with major vascular injury had associated fractures [21]. This may not be reflective of the distribution of injury that would be seen in civilian blast injury casualties as most of the military casualties were wearing personal protective equipment.

Blast Injury Classification and Kinematics of Vascular Injury

The Department of Defense separates blast injury into five categories: primary, secondary, tertiary, quaternary, and quinary (described in Chap. 4). Major vascular injury in the setting of blast is most often of a penetrating mechanism from secondary blast injury. This is because debris and added fragments travel over a much greater distance than does the shock wave from the primary blast [23]. Penetrating mechanisms are generally classified as low velocity (<2500 ft/s) or high velocity (>2500 ft/s). Fragment injury from blast is typically low velocity; however, it can be high velocity depending on the explosive, projectile, and proximity to the blast. Significant trauma to a blood vessel from these projectiles or from associated blunt injury does not always result in hemorrhage. Primary, secondary, and tertiary blast effects can also produce intimal damage from acute deformation/angulation, thrombosis, or spasm. Thrombus may enlarge or propagate, while dissected intima can occlude distal blood flow. Displaced bone from a fracture or dislocation can also interrupt distal blood flow by tearing the vessel or via external compression [1]. As one can ascertain from their description, not all of these injury patterns are as obvious as external exsanguination from a bleeding vessel (i.e., hard signs of vascular injury), and many are subtler (i.e., soft signs of vascular injury) and require clinical diligence to detect.

Prehospital Considerations

Appropriate prehospital care is one of the most important factors impacting patient survival in the setting of major vascular injury. This fact coupled with the unique challenges presented by blast incidents and mass casualty events requires a systematic approach by emergency medical services caring for blast casualties. The operational and prehospital management of explosive incidents is discussed in other sections of this book; however, as related to the management of vascular injuries, a focus on rapid hemorrhage control, expeditious patient transport, and appropriate prehospital resuscitation can lead to improved patient outcomes. Initiatives from both the Department of Defense (i.e., Tactical Combat Casualty Care [TCCC]) and civilian trauma consensus (i.e., Tactical Emergency Casualty Care [TECC]) stress the importance of establishing scene safety and early hemorrhage control [24, 25].

Tourniquet use for exsanguinating hemorrhage has been debated as far back as the middle ages [26]. The dismissive opinion of tourniquets from World War II and Vietnam was the result of improper placement, which led to increased morbidity and mortality. This so-called "venous" tourniquet, causing ineffective arterial hemorrhage control and compartment syndrome, was largely due to the design of the standard issue World War II era tourniquet. However, purpose-designed tourniquet use during modern conflict has produced startlingly different results. The expanded use of tourniquets during the most recent military campaigns may, in part, be responsible for the increase in the incidence of major vascular injury presenting to a surgically capable combat treatment team as compared to previous US conflicts [27]. Relatedly, mortality from extremity hemorrhage has decreased from 9% in Vietnam to 2% during the recent wars [28]. This is most likely due to the widespread use and proper training on the use of tourniquets. In a review of two retrospective studies from a single military treatment facility in Iraq, 483 patients had indications for a tourniquet. Overall, survival was 87%, whereas mortality was 100% in the 10 patients without tourniquet application despite meeting the indications [28, 29].

Much has been made of the potential complications of tourniquet use, which include nerve palsy, limb ischemia, worsening hemorrhage, and compartment syndrome. In the previously mentioned review, one of the largest specifically reviewing the use of tourniquets in combat, morbidity from tourniquet use included nerve palsy and major limb shortening, which occurred in 1.5% and 0.4% of patients, respectively [28]. Data from the military trauma registry demonstrated that patients who had a tourniquet on for less than 2 hours had a fasciotomy rate of 28%, while those patients with a tourniquet in place for more than 2 hours had a fasciotomy rate of 36%. In the face of historical concern, there were no documented cases of amputation due to the implementation of a tourniquet [30].

Addressing major, non-extremity vascular injury in the field has proven extremely challenging. No published data documents a decrease in hemorrhage when a bleeding extremity is elevated, and such manipulation may result in the conversion of a closed fracture to an open one [1]. Novel approaches for field hemostasis including topical hemostatic agents, like kaolin clay-impregnated Combat Gauze, should be considered for significant external hemorrhage from locations not amenable to the placement of a tourniquet (i.e., the neck, torso, axilla, or groin) and in large wounds that would benefit from packing [24]. Placement of pelvic binders may be helpful in patients with evidence of hemorrhagic shock and suspicion of pelvic fracture (though this is difficult to diagnose in the prehospital setting). Novel and investigational approaches to prehospital temporary hemostasis for junctional and torso hemorrhage control devices include devices such as the resuscitative endovascular balloon occlusion of the aorta (REBOA) catheter, injection of intracavitary self-expanding foam, and application of the Abdominal Aortic Junctional Tourniquet (AAJT) [31].

Initial Assessment and Diagnosis

Initial assessment of the trauma patient should follow the standard sequence as prescribed by ATLS [32]. Increasingly, a patient with extremity trauma may present with a tourniquet placed in the prehospital setting. Adequacy of hemorrhage control should be quickly verified in the trauma bay/emergency department. Circulation should be efficiently assessed by the palpation of central and distal pulses. ATLS teaches that particular pulses correspond with a minimum systolic blood pressure: carotid (60–70 mm Hg), femoral (70–80 mm Hg), radial (90–100 mm Hg), and pedal (>100 mm Hg) [32]. While the accuracy of this teaching has been called into question, the general principle that radial, femoral, and then carotid pulses are lost sequentially and are evidence of profound hypotension is accurate [33]. It is important to note that resuscitation and rewarming may improve the pulse exam in the limb without a vascular injury but will have no effect in the limb with a vascular injury [1].

Unstable patients with evidence of hemorrhagic shock should proceed to whatever setting will provide definitive hemorrhage control as quickly as possible, which is most often the operating room. One of the most important goals of the circulation portion of the primary survey is to determine into which body cavity the patient is bleeding. This will determine the appropriate surgical incision or alternative therapy (i.e., angioembolization in the setting of pelvic fracture). This is essential for victims of explosive incidents who may have life-threatening hemorrhage in multiple body cavities.

As soon as possible, a history should be obtained from prehospital providers with information including the time of injury, proximity to the blast, the state in which the patient was found (i.e., found under or adjacent to significant rubble indicative of blunt trauma), and the amount of blood loss at the scene and during transport. History of claudication in the lower extremities or other cardiovascular comorbidities should be sought as well [1].

Initial physical examination should focus on the "hard signs" of vascular injury. These include pulsatile bleeding, expanding hematoma, palpable thrill, audible bruit, and occlusion (pulseless, pallor, paresthesia, pain, paralysis, and poikilothermy) [1]. Traditionally, hard signs of vascular injury are an indication to proceed with immediate operative exploration [34]. The US military Joint Trauma System (JTS) clinical practice guidelines also recommend expedited operative exploration for patients with hard signs of vascular injury [27].

The next step in the evaluation for vascular injury should be an exploration for "soft signs" of vascular injury. These "soft signs" of vascular injury include history of significant hemorrhage, injury proximity to major vessels (fracture pattern, dislocation, penetrating wound or blast injury), bruising or hematoma, or question regarding the presence or absence of a palpable pulse. The presence of any of these "soft signs" of vascular injury should prompt the performance of either an ankle-brachial index (ABI) or, more efficiently, an injured extremity index (IEI) [27]. The IEI is similar to the ABI and is calculated using a manual blood pressure cuff and a continuous wave Doppler. The first step is to determine the pressure at which the arterial Doppler signal returns in the injured extremity as the cuff is deflated; this is the numerator in the equation. Next, the cuff and Doppler are moved to the uninjured extremity, ideally an uninjured upper extremity, and again the pressure at which the arterial Doppler signal returns as the cuff is deflated is recorded as the denominator in the ratio [27]. It is important to note that the arterial pressure index/injured extremity index may not be useful in patients with preexisting advanced diabetes.

Beyond the index itself, the pressure should be within 20 mm Hg of the contralateral extremity, and an absolute pressure below 50–60 indicates limb-threatening ischemia [1]. In a preliminary study by Johansen and colleagues, a Doppler arterial pressure index (API) (the systolic AP in the injured extremity divided by the AP in an uninvolved arm) of less than 0.90 was found to have sensitivity and specificity of 95% and 97%, respectively, for major arterial injury. The negative predictive value for an API greater than 0.90 was 99% [35]. This initial study suggested that noninvasive vascular tests could be a highly sensitive substitute for arteriography to exclude vascular injury. These same investigators conducted a follow-up trial in which arteriography was performed in extremity of trauma victims only when the arterial pressure index was less than 0.9. They found that 16 of 17 limbs with an API less than 0.9 had positive findings on arteriography and seven underwent arterial reconstruction. Of the 83 limbs with an API greater than 0.9, follow-up duplex found five minor arterial lesions, but no major injuries [35]. A meta-analysis of the use of physical exam and arterial pressure index found that the post-test probability for major vascular injury with a normal physical exam and a normal arterial pressure index in combination was 0% [36]. Thus, an injured extremity index/arterial pressure index greater than 0.9 can reliably exclude major vascular injury and obviates the need for follow-on vascular imaging in the absence of symptoms.

Patients not meeting criteria for immediate operative exploration, but with positive "soft signs" of vascular injury, should proceed with some form of vascular imaging. In the past, catheter-based arteriography has been the mainstay of vascular imaging in this scenario. This has largely been replaced by multi-detector CT angiography (MDCTA) in both the military and civilian settings. A series of 635 patients was published from a level I urban trauma center. After appropriate selection with physical examination and in the absence of significant artifact, MDCTA achieved 100% sensitivity and specificity for clinically significant arterial injuries [37]. However, it is important to note that high-quality MDCTA is not available or nonexistent in certain settings, such as mass casualty incidents or austere combat environments. Perhaps more importantly, even if MDCTA is available, fragments from blast injury may cause significant artifact limiting the interpretation of such imaging. Angiography has its greatest utility in the setting of multiple penetrating wounds at various levels of the same extremity. When performed in a resource-limited environment, arteriography can be done via a cutdown on the femoral artery using a 19- to 21-gauge butterfly needle to inject contrast and standard digital x-ray to obtain static images. When in doubt, it is always acceptable to proceed with operative exploration to rule out major vascular injury [27].

Clinical Management

Nonoperative Management

Minimal vascular injuries are asymptomatic and often identified on imaging; these include intimal irregularities, small arteriovenous fistulae, focal spasm with minimal narrowing, and small pseudoaneurysms. Approximately 5–15% of these lesions will eventually become symptomatic, and this usually occurs early following injury. There is evidence that these asymptomatic lesions can be managed expectantly with good outcomes [38]. Operative therapy is required for thrombosis, ischemia, or an expanding/unresolved small pseudoaneurysm. Identification of these lesions should prompt consultation with a vascular surgeon with a long-term surveillance plan.

Operative Management

Resuscitative Thoracotomy/REBOA

At times, patients arriving to the trauma bay with major vascular injury to the torso may have such severe physiologic derangement that immediate proximal control is necessary. Two such methods for patients in extremis are the resuscitative thoracotomy (RT) and the resuscitative endovascular balloon occlusion of the aorta (REBOA) catheter. Generally agreed-upon indications for an RT applicable to major vascular injury include penetrating thoracic trauma with less than 15 minutes of prehospital CPR, penetrating non-thoracic trauma with less than 5 minutes of prehospital CPR, blunt trauma with less than 10 minutes of prehospital CPR, and patients with persistent severe hypotension (SBP less than 60 mm Hg) due to cardiac tamponade or hemorrhage from the thorax/abdomen/extremity/neck [39]. The military clinical practice guideline recommends the use of emergency thoracotomy for patients suffering penetrating trauma and CPR for less than 10 minutes and emphasizes the use of clinical judgment for blunt injury with the recognition of poor outcomes for this patient population. Perhaps most importantly, in a resource-limited environment (e.g., distance, capabilities, or MCI), an RT should only be performed if capabilities for follow-on damage control resuscitation and surgery exist [40].

REBOA was introduced as an alternative, or adjunct, to an RT for temporary aortic control of noncompressible intra-abdominal and retroperitoneal hemorrhage. Endovascular balloon occlusion of the aorta was first described by Hughes during the Korean War as an alternative method for proximal torso hemorrhage control [41]. Since then, several surgeons have used the technique with various devices and for different indications.

Building on Hughes' experience, and taking advantage of a modern revolution in endovascular devices, military surgeons today have proposed five specific steps for successful deployment of a REBOA catheter: arterial access, balloon selection and positioning, balloon inflation, balloon deflation, and sheath removal. The modern REBOA effort also describes three different anatomic aortic zones for balloon placement and inflation: zone I covers the descending thoracic aorta between the origin of the left subclavian and the celiac axis, zone II is between the celiac axis and the lowest renal artery, and zone III is the infrarenal abdominal aorta between the lowest renal artery and the aortic bifurcation [42].

In one of the first published series of the use of the REBOA catheter in trauma patients, Brenner et al. described four of six patients in hemorrhagic shock surviving, two from penetrating mechanisms and two after motor vehicle collisions [43]. Subsequent studies have also demonstrated the potential benefit of REBOA.

A retrospective review from two level I trauma centers compared the outcomes of REBOA to emergency resuscitative thoracotomy for noncompressible truncal hemorrhage. The study found that the REBOA group had an improved overall survival at 37.5% compared to the thoracotomy group at 9.7% [44].

Factors important to optimal outcomes in the implementation of REBOA are rapid arterial access and minimizing the occlusion time [45, 46]. It is important to note, though, that REBOA is not intended to address hemorrhage from vessels proximal to the origin of the left subclavian artery, cardiac tamponade, or large air embolism, and reliably ruling out proximal injuries may be difficult in victims of explosive incidents with polytrauma.

The Joint Trauma System recently developed a clinical practice guideline for use of REBOA in the deployed military combat setting. The recommended indications for the REBOA catheter are for patients in extremis secondary to hemorrhagic shock or traumatic arrest from blunt mechanisms or from penetrating injuries to the abdomen, pelvis, or junctional sites [47]. REBOA is certainly an important tool in the armamentarium of trauma surgeons, but its precise role is currently undergoing clinical study.

Damage Control Surgery/Temporary Vascular Shunting

The idea of damage control surgery was first published by Rotondo et al. in 1993, formally describing a surgical approach focusing on minimizing operative time with rapid surgical hemostasis and control of contamination, followed by aggressive resuscitation. This was with the goal to avoid the "lethal triad" of acidosis, hypothermia, and coagulopathy prior to proceeding with definitive surgical procedures [48]. Whether or not to initiate damage control strategies is largely based on the clinical judgment of the surgeon; however, some published parameters that suggest the need for damage control include decompensated hemodynamic shock (systolic blood pressure <70 mmHg), hypothermia <34 °C, transfusion >10 units of packed red blood cells (RBC), acidosis with pH <7.2, and coagulopathy with an INR of >2 [49]. Damage control surgery and resuscitation are both extensively covered in Chap. 29 of this book.

Specific to major vascular injury, damage control measures include primary amputation, ligation, or placement of a temporary vascular shunt. Temporary shunt placement for the initial management of proximal extremity vascular injury is associated with high rates of successful limb salvage, and shunt patency has been demonstrated for periods up to 12 hours [50]. One study reported that 22 of 23 proximal vascular shunts placed in a forward surgical unit in Iraq remained patent on arrival to a role 3 facility. In this study, the patients were able to undergo autologous vein reconstruction, and 100% of the patients survived their injuries with early limb preservation [50]. However, experience with shunt utilization without systemic anticoagulation for longer periods is limited, and the risk of distal embolization (i.e., blue toe or foot syndrome) and/or shunt thrombosis is increased when shunts are left in place beyond 12 hours [51]. The successful use of temporary vascular shunts in the civilian setting has also been demonstrated. In retrospective review of seven level I trauma centers from 2003 to 2015, the limb salvage rate with the use of temporary vascular shunts was 96.3% with a low rate of thrombosis (5.6%) [52].

Specific indications for the use of temporary vascular shunting include severely ill polytrauma patients requiring a damage control approach, mutilating extremity wounds, lack of surgical expertise, or the overwhelming arrival of trauma victims in a mass casualty incident (i.e., need for abbreviated operating techniques) [53]. Temporary vascular shunting has been shown to decrease the time to revascularization in the mangled extremity, decrease the incidence of compartment syndrome, and shorten hospital stay [54]. Intervals from 2 to 52 hours of shunt placement with successful revascularization have been reported, but every effort should be made to remove the shunt and revascularize by 12 hours [53]. In combined vascular and orthopedic injuries, common after blast injuries, shunts are often inserted to quickly restore flow, followed by lengthening of the bony fragments, subsequent shunt removal, and definitive vascular repair. Addressing the injuries in this fashion improves the vascular operative field and prevents disruption of a vascular repair from bony manipulation.

Regarding the technique of shunt placement, after proximal and distal control of the injured vessel is obtained and prior to shunt insertion, Fogarty catheter thrombectomy should be performed to ensure inflow and back bleeding followed by lavage with heparinized saline. The shunt can then be inserted distally first and then proximally. Silk ties can be used to secure the ends of the shunt to the vessel. The diameter of the shunt should be closely approximated to that of the artery, erring on the smaller side. Oversized shunts are to be avoided as they may result in intimal tears. Routine performance of decompressive fasciotomy is recommended to prevent compartment syndrome. In the immediate postoperative period, the need for systematic use of anticoagulant or antiplatelet medications has not been demonstrated. The patient should proceed to definitive vascular repair as soon as possible.

Many types of shunts are available: Javid® (Bard Peripheral Vascular Inc., Tempe, AZ, USA), Argyle® (Kendall Healthcare Products, Mansfield, MA, USA), Sundt® (Integra, Plainsboro, NJ, USA), and Pruitt-Inihara® (Horizon Medical, Santa Ana, CA, USA). While these prostheses have different shapes and designs, in practice, their performance is the same in terms of restoration of arterial flow and secondary arterial thrombosis [52, 53]. However, the Pruitt-Inihara is the only shunt to offer a side port for medication administration or angiography if indicated. Providers should be mindful of shunts getting snared and dislodged particularly with looped shunts. In the austere environment, intravenous tubing, red rubber catheters, nasoenteric tubes, or even chest tubes can all be fashioned as a shunt provided appropriate size matching.

Basic Tenants of Vascular Repair/Reconstruction

Basic principles of vascular trauma management include adequate exposure; proximal and distal control; vessel debridement to viable tissue; the creation of a tension-free anastomosis, repair, or shunt; and adequate coverage with viable tissue [27]. These principles need to be kept in mind through all aspects of operative care from preparation to closure. While vascular expertise should be sought when available, this is often not the case in resource-limited settings like forward military treatment facilities and during mass casualty incidents, both settings very likely needing to manage blast-injured patients. In fact, trauma surgeons with general surgery training perform the majority of complex vascular repairs of injured vessels with limb salvage rates being similar between general surgeons and vascular/cardiovascular surgeons (94% and 95%, respectively) [55]. For maximal success, the surgical team needs to prepare appropriately to address each one of the aforementioned vascular principles.

In the setting of vascular occlusion, if there is no evidence of bleeding in the limb and no intracranial or intracavitary hemorrhage, systemic unfractionated heparin should be administered [1]. When preparing and draping a patient with sterile technique, one needs to keep several factors in mind. The patient should be draped in a manner where proximal control can always be obtained. For isolated extremity injuries, this may involve the ipsilateral chest and shoulder for upper extremities and the lower torso up to the umbilicus for lower extremities [1]. Another important consideration is the potential need for access to autologous conduits (i.e., the greater saphenous vein in the lower extremities). While avoiding hypothermia is also an important consideration, limited preparation is often the exception rather than the rule for patients in hemorrhagic shock from major vascular injury, especially to the torso.

One should consider early consultation with a plastic surgeon, if available, for significant soft tissue defects for appropriate coverage of any definitive vascular repair. Desiccation or superficial infection in the inadequately covered repair leads to suture disruption and hemorrhage. With complex blast injury, this may require the rotation of regional muscle or local advancement of skin flaps. Complex myocutaneous flaps or free tissue transfer is inappropriate at the initial operation because they are time-consuming and can put the patient at risk for hypothermia. Vascular repairs can be temporarily covered by either cadaver skin graft, porcine xenograft, or even negative pressure wound therapy using a two-sponge (polyvinyl alcohol and polyurethane) system [56, 57].

Other factors are important to the optimal surgical management of major vascular injury in blast-injured patients. If bleeding continues as the patient is being brought to the operating room, a properly placed tourniquet, direct digital pressure, or Foley catheter balloon tamponade into the bleeding cavity can be applied for temporary control. Emergent settings are not the time to gather appropriate equipment necessary for vascular exposure and reconstruction. Premade kits should be assembled for use in the event of a major vascular injury [1].

If limb salvage is to be attempted, initiation of basic maneuvers including removal of tourniquet, exploration and control of the vascular injury, thrombectomy, and administration of heparinized saline through the inflow and outflow vessels are recommended. If an interposition graft is necessary, an autologous conduit is preferential to synthetic graft due to improved long-term patency and a reduction in the risk of secondary infection as compared to synthetic vascular conduits [58, 59]. However, in complex blast, multi-extremity-injured patients, there may not be autologous conduits available for reconstruction. Alternatives include prosthetic graft materials such as PTFE and Dacron or human umbilical vein. The military largely uses PTFE based on animal studies suggesting increased resistance to infection [60]. However, more recent data in vascular surgery literature suggests relative equivalency between these graft materials [61].

In a review of the US military trauma system trauma registry from March 2003 to April 2006, 15% of extremity bypass was performed with synthetic conduit, all of which were PTFE. Approximately half of these patients had vascular injury secondary to blast injury. Seventy-nine percent of the grafts stayed patent in the short term allowing for stabilization, transfer to a stateside facility, and elective revascularization with remaining autologous conduit. No patients required amputation because of prosthetic graft failure [62].

Management of Specific Vessels

- *Thoracic Aorta*: In a controlled setting, the proximal aorta and aortic arch are best approached through a median sternotomy. In the rare instance these highly lethal injuries arrive to a trauma facility, an anterolateral thoracotomy is necessary as these patients are hemodynamically labile. Extending the incision across the sternum ("clamshell" thoracotomy) is typically necessary for optimal exposure. The descending thoracic aorta is also approached through the left chest. If necessary, exposure can be improved by extension into the right chest or by surgically removing a rib. Single lung ventilation can also be helpful to optimize exposure. However, this can take valuable time away from addressing the injury and thus should be entertained after obtaining hemostatic control. Instead, intermittently pausing ventilation can be employed as an alternative. Aortic control proximal and distal to the injury must be obtained including isolation or control of any intercostal arteries in this segment. An adequate length of aorta must be debrided to allow placement of large caliber (20–26 mm) Dacron graft sewn end to end to the proximal and distal segments. In dire circumstances, a chest tube could be used as a shunt. Management of blunt injury to the thoracic aorta will be discussed later in this chapter.
- *Abdominal Aorta and Mesenteric Branches*: Blunt and penetrating injuries to the abdominal aorta present as a central, or zone I, hematoma usually with intraperitoneal hemorrhage especially in the case of penetrating injury. Generally, all zone I hematomas will warrant exploration, especially those that are rapidly expanding. An exception may be a small, non-expanding mesenteric hematoma at the base of the SMA. Zone I can be subdivided into two locations, supra- and infra-mesocolic. The hematoma should not be entered until proximal and distal control is obtained, blood products are available, and adequate intravenous or intraosseous access is established. A left medial visceral rotation provides excellent exposure for the length of the abdominal aorta. This approach involves medially mobilizing the colon, spleen, pancreas, and kidney. An option is to leave the kidney in situ to speed up the exposure; however, this maneuver still takes some time to perform. The supra-celiac aortic control through a window or division of the gastrohepatic ligament is a more rapid technique and can be especially beneficial in situations with active supra-mesocolic hemorrhage. Retracting the esophagus to the left and the liver to the right (sometimes assisted by dividing the left triangular ligament of the liver) as well as dividing the diaphragmatic crus improves exposure. Once a clamp is placed, a medial visceral rotation can be performed, and the clamp can be marched down to isolate the injury. Distal control can be obtained at the level of the distal aorta or iliac vessels. In a damage

control setting, a chest tube can be fashioned as a shunt for the aorta. This may also be a better option in the presence of gross fecal contamination instead of inserting a prosthetic graft or performing an extra-anatomic bypass. Upon entering a zone I hematoma, one may find injury to the celiac axis, its branches, or mesenteric vessels. Unless primary repair is possible, the celiac axis or any of its branches can be ligated if necessary due to the rich collateral blood flow in this region. One exception is that prior to ligation of the hepatic artery, a patent and uninjured portal vein should be ensured. Alternatively, all efforts should be employed to avoid ligation of the proximal superior mesenteric artery. This would likely result in ischemia to much of the small bowel. If ligation of the SMA at or close to its origin is required, it should be followed with a plan for immediate bypass. In cases where injury to the artery or vein is distal (i.e., beyond the middle colic artery or jejunal vein branches) or in which the patient's physiology is severely compromised, the vessels can be ligated.

- *Inferior Vena Cava*: The approach to the vena cava in the abdomen is through a right medial visceral rotation. Performing a full right-sided rotation will expose the cava, renal veins, common iliac veins, distal aorta, and iliac arteries. Mobilization of the liver is required to expose the retrohepatic vena cava; however, retrohepatic hematomas should not be disturbed if not expanding. Sponge sticks directly proximal and distal to the injury are helpful in obtaining temporary hemostasis. Once identified, the edges of the laceration can be grasped with intestinal Allis clamps or a Satinsky clamp. A running 4-0 Prolene can then be passed under the instruments. Attempts should be made to identify large lumbar veins feeding into the injured segment that may bleed as much as the main channel of the vena cava if not controlled. Repair of tangential injuries to the cava can be accomplished using lateral suture repair (i.e., running venorrhaphy). In instances where lateral repair will result in more than 50% narrowing, patch angioplasty or interposition graft should be employed. Options for grafting include prosthetic or autologous internal jugular, external iliac, or spiral saphenous vein graft. When an anterior and posterior IVC injury is present, the posterior injury can be repaired through the anterior laceration. Ligation of the infrarenal cava is acceptable as a damage control maneuver, although this carries a significant mortality risk and major morbidity in the form of decreased cardiac preload and significant lower extremity edema [63]. If unable to closely monitor the patient in the setting of an austere environment or mass casualty incident, then it is recommended to perform bilateral lower leg fasciotomies to reduce the risk for compartment syndrome. Suprarenal occlusion of the IVC is generally not compatible with survival and should be considered a measure of last resort.
- *Portal Vein*: Portal vein and hepatic artery injuries typically present as hematomas of the porta hepatis and should be explored after isolation of the hepatoduodenal ligament and application of a Pringle maneuver. Next, careful dissection of the porta is performed to determine which structures have been injured. Repair of the portal vein should be attempted using the technique of lateral venorrhaphy if possible. If a large segment of the portal vein is damaged, vein patch angioplasty or, in rare instances, interposition vein graft may be performed. Ligation

of the portal vein is an option of last resort and will result in hepatic ischemia, splanchnic congestion, and hypervolemia for several days.

- *Renal Vessels*: Injury to the renal pedicle (blunt or penetrating) is closely associated with injury to the parenchyma; isolated arterial injury is rare. Essential considerations in the management of renal artery injury are the warm ischemic time of 30–60 minutes and complexity of renal artery repair. These factors significantly limit the surgeon's options in resource-limited deployed settings or mass casualty incidents, other than ligation and nephrectomy. If arterial injury manifests as occlusion with renal ischemia, then it has been too late to restore flow and function to the kidney. Considering the warm ischemic time of the kidney, complex operations to maintain or reestablish perfusion in the renal artery are not recommended and should be abandoned in favor of nephrectomy in most cases. If presented with an isolated renal vein injury, ligation of the proximal left renal vein is well tolerated due to collateral drainage from the gonadal vein. Ligation of the right renal vein is not recommended.

  The method by which to approach an expanding or penetrating lateral retroperitoneal hematoma is controversial and case-specific. Isolation of the renal pedicle before exploring the hematoma is doctrine in many institutions and has the advantage of aortic isolation and definitive proximal control. However, from a practical standpoint, mobilization of the damaged kidney from a lateral to medial direction without hilar control may be faster.
- *Iliac Vessels*: Iliac artery injuries generally present as a lower retroperitoneal or pelvic hematoma with or without extremity ischemia. Exploration of the hematoma should be performed after proximal control is obtained at the infrarenal aorta and the contralateral iliac artery if possible. The infrarenal aorta can be approached directly through an incision in the peritoneum or via a right medial visceral rotation. The distal external iliac artery should be found as it exits the pelvis at the inguinal ligament at a point where it is free from the hematoma. When isolating the injury, the surgeon should be mindful of the intimate relationship of the iliac veins to their respective arteries to prevent an iatrogenic injury. One may need to open the hematoma to gain access to the internal iliac vessels. In an unstable patient or a patient where there is contamination of the field, shunt placement with definitive repair or reconstruction done at a later point is a good option. If the primary injury is to the internal iliac artery (hypogastric), it may be ligated. Bleeding from associated iliac veins may be severe and difficult to expose. Due to the anatomic relationship of the artery and vein on the right, the iliac artery may be divided if necessary to facilitate exposure and repair of the vein. This should be followed by immediate repair of the artery. Selective embolization of bleeding hypogastric artery or branches is an option, particularly in blunt trauma.
- *Carotid Artery*: Exposure of the carotid artery is through a generous incision coursing anterior to the sternocleidomastoid and facilitated by a roll under the shoulders, extension of the neck, and turning of the head away from the injury. The carotid is exposed proximal to the hematoma and controlled with an umbilical tape into a Rummel device (i.e., red rubber catheter). In the absence of

uncontrolled bleeding, there is no need to tighten the Rummel, but having it in place gives one this option and allows for securing the proximal end of a temporary shunt. If bleeding is encountered, the Rummel may be cinched or a clamp (angled DeBakey) slid proximal to the umbilical tape using it to pull the carotid up into the clamp, thereby avoiding injury to the vagus nerve. Back bleeding from the internal carotid artery is a favorable sign and can be controlled with a small clamp or a (3-Fr) Fogarty inserted into the lumen and inflated using a 1-cc syringe and three-way stopcock to maintain inflation. The external carotid artery is controlled with vessel loops or ligated. If the internal and common carotid arteries are controlled above and below the injury, a temporary shunt can be placed to maintain perfusion while the injury is identified and options considered. Regardless of whether a shunt is used, the mean arterial pressure should be kept above 90 mmHg during the repair to optimize cerebral perfusion. If no other life-threatening injuries are present, a small amount (50 u/kg) of systemic heparin is recommended along with generous flushing of the repair with heparinized saline to prevent platelet aggregation and clot formation. Ligation of the internal carotid artery is an acceptable damage control maneuver to stop hemorrhage but has an incidence of stroke up to approximately 50% [64, 65].

- *Jugular Vein*: The jugular vein can often be ligated with no consequence, though repair may be undertaken in a stable patient with limited concomitant injuries. Operative exposure of the jugular vein is the same as that described for the carotid artery.
- *Subclavian Artery*: Both proximal subclavian arteries and the innominate can be exposed through a full or mini sternotomy with supraclavicular extension. Alternatively, given the relatively posterior position of the left subclavian, a high (third intercostal space) anterolateral thoracotomy may be more frequently used. The innominate vein can be ligated and divided to facilitate exposure to the innominate artery. The mid and distal subclavian arteries on both sides can be exposed through a supraclavicular incision or combined supraclavicular/infraclavicular incisions. Resection of the clavicular head improves exposure. In an unstable patient, it is recommended that initial proximal control be obtained via thoracotomy as this will allow for more rapid control than use of the supraclavicular approach. Because of the technical challenges with exposure, the utility of temporary vascular shunts in this injury pattern is limited.
- *Axillary Artery*: Exposure of the axillary artery is via an infraclavicular incision along the deltopectoral groove. Splitting the pectoralis major and dividing the pectoralis minor will reveal the axillary vessels. Repair of the axillary artery most commonly involves an interposition graft using reversed saphenous vein. Shunt utilization can be very useful for injury to the axillary artery.
- *Brachial Artery*: The brachial artery is exposed through a medial incision in the upper arm in the groove between the bicep and triceps. The surgeon needs to be mindful of the median nerve as it is the most superficial, and therefore first, structure encountered upon entering the brachial sheath. The ulnar nerve runs posterior to the artery which is surrounded by paired deep brachial veins. Although it

may be possible to ligate the brachial artery below the origin of the deep (profunda) brachial artery and maintain a viable arm and hand, this proposition is based on intact collateral circulation. Unfortunately, collaterals from the shoulder and deep brachial artery are often damaged in the setting of penetrating blast wounds, and therefore, maintenance of flow through the brachial artery with a temporary shunt or vascular repair is advised. Ligation or primary amputation is an acceptable damage control maneuver if there is not time for shunting or the patient is in extremis.

- *Radial/Ulnar Arteries*: Most often, the hand has a dual arterial supply and therefore can tolerate ligation of either the radial or ulnar artery. As such, repair or reconstruction of an injury at this level is rare. Perfusion to the hand should be assessed with Doppler before and after occlusion or ligation, and if the absence of a signal persists, repair/reconstruction should be performed. Given the relatively small muscle mass of the hand and the degree of collateral circulation, ligation is most often tolerated understanding that if ischemia persists, evaluation and revascularization can be performed later.
- *Common Femoral, Profunda Femoris, and Superficial Femoral Artery*: Exposure of the common femoral and profunda femoris is obtained through a single longitudinal incision above the artery (2–3 cm lateral to the pubic tubercle), exposing the artery at the inguinal ligament. A key point in exposing the femoral artery is placing the incision proximal enough so that the abdominal wall and inguinal ligament can be identified first in a consistent and familiar location. Alternatively, proximal control can be obtained in the retroperitoneum (i.e., external iliac) through the proximal extension of this groin incision or by using a separate Gibson incision in the lower abdomen. Exposure of the superficial femoral is performed through a medial thigh incision and the adductors of the leg (i.e., adductor magnus). Exposure is facilitated by placing a lift or "bump" below the knee which allows the femoral artery, sartorius, and adductors to be suspended improving separation. When exposing the superficial femoral artery, it is important to recognize the femoral vein is intimately associated with, and possibly adherent to, the artery. Every attempt should be made to maintain flow into the profunda femoris artery, although the feasibility of this will depend upon the pattern of injury and the comfort level of the surgeon to perform a more complicated reconstruction. If patency of the superficial femoral artery can be confirmed, ligation of mid and distal profunda femoris injuries is acceptable as they lie deep in the thigh musculature and are not required for leg viability.
- *Popliteal Artery*: Vascular injuries in the popliteal space are exposed through a medial incision. The dissection is extended from above to below the knee and is facilitated by a lift or "bump" under the calf of the leg with the knee flexed. When exposing below the knee, this bump is placed under the thigh. Natural dissection planes exist in exposing the above-knee popliteal artery (i.e., popliteal space) apart from the need to divide the fibers of the adductor magnus that envelop the distal superficial femoral artery (Hunter's canal). Similarly, a natural dissection plane exists into the popliteal space from below the knee, but added exposure

should be accomplished by division of the gastrocnemius and soleus muscle fibers from the medial tibia. To completely expose the popliteal space, the medial attachments of the sartorius, semitendinosus, semimembranosus, and gracilis to the medial condyle of the tibia can be divided. When feasible, the pes anserinus should be reconstructed given its significant role in medial knee stabilization. If a damage control approach is necessary, a temporary vascular shunt is extremely helpful in this setting especially with a combined orthopedic injury.
- *Tibial Arteries*: Because of their distal location and redundant nature, isolated and sometimes multiple tibial artery injuries can be ligated without adverse outcomes. If one tibial artery is uninjured and patent to the ankle (i.e., an arterial signal at the ankle or foot), no additional tests or repair is required. Continuous wave Doppler exam of the foot is critical in the setting of tibial artery injuries and concern for viability of the foot. Temporary vascular shunts may be placed, recognizing a much lower success rate as compared to larger more proximal vessels. Reconstruction of a peroneal artery injury is rarely necessary, and ligation is adequate. Importantly, tibial reconstruction is technically more challenging and may therefore take longer to complete. Like other vascular repairs, tibial reconstruction should not be undertaken if the patient has other life-threatening injuries or is in extremis.
- *Extremity Venous Injury*: Many extremity venous injuries, especially small distal veins, can be ligated with no adverse effects because of collateral venous drainage. However, ligation of more proximal or watershed veins, or even axial veins when collaterals have been destroyed by soft tissue wounds, will result in venous hypertension and congestion. In such instances, an attempt should be made to repair the vein and restore venous outflow. Temporary shunts have been shown to be effective in restoring venous outflow in the femoral veins until formal repair can be accomplished.

Compartment Syndrome/Fasciotomy

The most common cause of preventable limb loss in extremity trauma is unrecognized compartment syndrome. It can be an extremely difficult problem to manage in the patient with major vascular injury as it may be a consequence of reperfusion injury and only clinically apparent in a delayed fashion [1]. One must be hypervigilant in preventing/treating compartment syndrome as even a technically perfect vascular reconstruction can end in catastrophe if compartment syndrome goes unrecognized.

Based on animal models, ideal reperfusion time is within 3 hours of vascular occlusion, and reperfusion greater than 6 hours from occlusion results in myonecrosis and Wallerian degeneration of the peripheral nerves [66]. Preemptive fasciotomy should be performed in patients with prolonged ischemia (ranging from >3–6 hours depending on overall patient status and clinical judgment), closed fractures, crush injury, or combined arterial and venous injury. If fasciotomy is not performed, compartment pressures should be measured in the operating room before termination of anesthetic. There is no consensus regarding the exact pressure indicative of compartment syndrome, but any pressure above 25 should heighten concern [1].

Endovascular Treatment, Blunt Thoracic Aortic Injury, and Blunt Cerebrovascular Injury

Endovascular management of nontraumatic vascular disease is being utilized with increasing frequency. However, for traumatic injury, endovascular therapy is used much more selectively. There will likely always be a place for the open surgical management of major vascular injury, especially in the setting of blast injury and mass casualty events. Endovascular techniques provide promise, though especially in areas that are difficult to access via open techniques.

The most common setting in endovascular therapy is employed in the thorax for blunt thoracic aortic injury. It is unclear how often this clinical entity would present itself in the setting of the blast-injured patient, but the overall incidence of blunt thoracic aortic injury is approximately 1–2% in patients that have been subjected to blunt thoracic trauma [67]. In the setting of blast injury, this would most likely be the result of tertiary injury (i.e., a crush injury forms local debris). The Society for Vascular Surgery has published guidelines for traumatic thoracic aortic injury in which they classify the degree of injury: Type I, intimal tear; Type II, intramural hematoma; Type III, pseudoaneurysm; and Type IV, rupture [68]. Features of blunt thoracic aortic injury on plain film radiograph include wide mediastinum (AP chest radiograph >8 cm and PA CXR >6 cm), abnormal aortic contour, left "apical cap," large left hemothorax, displacement of the left mainstem bronchus, deviation of nasogastric tube to the right, deviation of the trachea to the right/mainstem bronchus downward, or a wide paravertebral stripe [69]. The mainstay of imaging for patients suspected of having blunt thoracic aortic injury are CT angiography and transesophageal echocardiography [70]. Initial treatment involves medical management to control the change in pressure over time (dP/dt), thereby limiting the shear stress on the vessel wall. Patients either treated nonoperatively or those awaiting repair should be managed with beta-blockade with a goal heart rate less than 100 and a goal systolic blood pressure at around 100 mm Hg [71]. Type I injuries can be treated nonoperatively. Patients with Type II, III, or IV injuries and without hemodynamic compromise should undergo endovascular stent-graft placement, provided anatomic suitability. The endovascular approach has replaced the open technique as the primary method of repair due to the lower rates of mortality, spinal cord ischemia, and end-stage renal disease associated with endovascular repair [72].

Endovascular therapies have also been employed in the setting of cerebrovascular trauma, particularly in the setting of blunt cerebrovascular injury (BCVI). Blunt cerebrovascular injury is graded based on the scale established by Biffl et al. in 1999: grade I, luminal irregularity or dissection with less than 25% narrowing; grade II, dissection or intraluminal hematoma with > or equal to 25% luminal narrowing, intraluminal thrombus, or raised intimal flap; grade III, pseudoaneurysm; grade IV, occlusion; and grade V, transection with free extravasation [73]. While blunt cerebrovascular injury can present with traditional signs of vascular injury, it can also present with devastating neurologic consequences. Given the severe impact these injuries can have, screening criteria for a CT angiogram of the neck to evaluate for BCVI have been established: LeFort II or III facial fractures, mandibular fractures, basilar skull fractures, occipital condyle fractures, severe traumatic brain injury with a GCS <6, cervical spine fracture, subluxation or ligamentous injury, near hanging with anoxic brain injury, clothesline-type injury or seat belt abrasion with significant welling, pain, or altered mental status, scalp degloving, or major thoracic injuries [74]. Guidelines from the Western Trauma Association (WTA) recommend anticoagulation for injury grade I–IV for 7–10 days with CT angiography, while patients with grade V injuries should proceed immediately to endovascular treatment, most commonly stenting for the carotid artery and embolization for the vertebral artery. Patients with grade I–IV injuries that do not resolve on repeat imaging should either be placed on antiplatelet therapy for 3 months with repeat imaging or proceed to endovascular treatment [74]. Heparin was chosen for the guideline in the acute setting due to its rapid reversibility; however, there is data suggesting that there is no difference in injury healing, progression of injury grade, or incidence of stroke between antiplatelet and anticoagulation therapy [75]. Several hospitals have institutional-specific treatment algorithms that may vary from the WTA with regard to treatment with antiplatelet or anticoagulation and duration or frequency of interval follow-up imaging.

While endovascular treatment of injuries to the thoracic aorta is well accepted, endovascular treatment of abdominal major vascular injuries is not as well established [1]. No high-level data exists for the endovascular treatment of injuries to the abdominal aorta or the inferior vena cava; however, several case reports and series of the treatment of thrombotic injuries and contained hematomas exist [76, 77]. The benefits of angioembolization to branch vessels of the aorta and in the pelvis in the setting of severe fracture are well established including embolization to the renal artery, splenic artery, and internal iliac artery [1].

Endovascular treatment of extremity vascular injuries includes coil embolization, vasodilator infusion, and the use of covered and uncovered stents. Most common injuries treated acutely are subclavian and axillary artery injuries, largely due to the difficulty in open surgical exposure for these vessels. There is no consensus on the indications for endovascular treatment, no agreed-upon definitions of complications, and no established long-term follow-up plan for patients that have been treated. However, preliminary data suggests similar outcomes and perhaps shorter operative time for endovascular intervention for injuries to the thoracic outlet [78].

Conclusion

Major vascular injuries are challenging problems to manage even at level I trauma centers with nearly unlimited resources. Add on the challenges presented by the complex injury patterns seen in blast-injured patients and the resource strain presented by mass casualty incidents, and these problems can seem insurmountable. Focusing on data-supported interventions like prehospital hemorrhage control with tourniquets; damage control resuscitation and surgical techniques; rapid transport; efficient patient assessment with physical exam, Doppler, and imaging techniques;

the use of temporary venous shunts; prevention of compartment syndrome with the liberal use of fasciotomy; and the appropriate use of endovascular techniques can lead to excellent patient outcomes. With a thoughtful, systematic, and efficient approach from prehospital care to the operating room, medical care teams can maximize the number of lives and limbs saved.

Pitfalls

- Blast-injured patients can present with complex injury patterns including blunt and penetrating mechanisms in multiple body cavities; however, penetrating injury is most common and of the most relevance to major vascular injury.
- Tourniquet use saves lives, but only if commercially designed tourniquets are applied appropriately. Improperly placed improvised tourniquets can increase morbidity and mortality.
- In the setting of major vascular injuries, prehospital providers should focus on rapid external hemorrhage control and rapid transport to surgical capabilities. Prolonged attempts at intravenous access have been associated with poor outcomes.
- REBOA is a promising technique for proximal hemorrhage control in patients presenting in extremis; however, its precise indications are still being investigated, and there is still a place for resuscitative thoracotomy in appropriately selected patients.
- Appropriate preparation prior to embarking on surgical exploration is invaluable for avoiding disaster keeping in mind adequate exposure, proximal vascular control, and the potential need for autologous venous conduit.
- Do not perform definitive vascular reconstruction on patients more appropriate for damage control techniques. Live to fight another day.
- Temporary vascular shunting is an excellent alternative to primary amputation or ligation that can be used for limb preservation in damage control scenarios.
- Autologous venous conduit should be used preferentially for vascular reconstruction and bypass; however, in the blast-injured patient, these may not be available. PTFE conduits have been used with good rates of limb preservation.
- In the setting of major vascular injury, fasciotomy should be used liberally to avoid compartment syndrome, especially in the setting of prolonged ischemia, closed fractures, crush injury, and combined arterial and venous injury or the use of a temporary vascular shunt.
- For stable vascular injuries in difficult regions to reach anatomically, endovascular techniques should be considered where resources and expertise are available.

References

1. Moore E, Feliciano D, Mattox K. Trauma. 8th ed. New York: McGraw-Hill Education; 2017.
2. Key G, editor. The apologies and treatise of Ambroise Pare containing the Ayages made into divers places with many writings upon surgery. London: Falcon Education Books; 1957.
3. Tuffier. French surgery in 1915. Br J Surg. 1916;4(15):420–32.
4. Makins GH. On gunshot injuries to the blood-vessels, founded on experience gained in France during the Great War, 1914–1918. Bristol: John Wright and Sons; 1919. p. 109–11.
5. DeBakey ME, Simeone FA. Battle injuries of the arteries in World War II: an analysis of 2,471 cases. Ann Surg. 1946;123:534.
6. DeBakey ME. History, the torch that illuminates: lessons from military medicine. Mil Med. 1996;161:711–6.
7. Rich NM. Vascular Trauma in Vietnam. J Cardiovasc Surg. 1970;11:368–77.
8. Rich NM, Baugh JH, Hughes CW. Significance of complications associated with vascular repairs performed in Vietnam. Arch Surg. 1970;100:646–51.
9. Rich NM, Hughes CW. Vietnam vascular registry: a preliminary report. Surgery. 1969;65:218–26.
10. Hughes CW. Arterial repair during the Korean War. Ann Surg. 1958;147:155.
11. Rich NM, Baugh JH, Hughes CW. Acute arterial injuries in Vietnam: 1,000 cases. J Trauma. 1970;10:359.
12. King D, Larentzakis A, Ramly E. Tourniquet use at the Boston Marathon bombing. J Trauma Acute Care Surg. 2015;78(3):594–9.
13. National Consortium for the Study of Terrorism and Responses to Terrorism: annex of statistical information [Internet]. U.S. Department of State; 2018 [cited 24 July 2018]. Available from: https://www.state.gov/j/ct/rls/crt/2016/272241.htm.
14. Schenken B. Explosives incident report [Internet]. United States Bomb Data Center; 2016 [cited 19 July 2018]. Available from: https://www.atf.gov/explosives/docs/report/2016-explosives-incident-report/download.
15. Craigie R, Farrelly P, Santos R, Smith S, Pollard J, Jones D. Manchester Arena bombing: lessons learnt from a mass casualty incident. J R Army Med Corps. 2018:jramc-2018-000930.
16. Mattox K, Feliciano D, Burch J, Beall A, Jordan G, DeBakey M. Five thousand seven hundred sixty cardiovascular injuries in 4459 patients. Ann Surg. 1989;209(6):698–707.
17. Oller D, Rutledge R, Clancy T, Cunningham P, Thomason M, Meredith W, et al. Vascular injuries in a rural state: a review of 978 patients from a state trauma registry. J Trauma. 1992;32(6):740–6.
18. Davies MJ, Wells C, Squires PA, et al. Civilian firearm injury and death in England and Wales. Emerg Med J. 2012;29:10–4.
19. White JM, Stannard A, Burkhard GE, Eastridge BJ, Blackbourne LH, Rasmussen TE. The epidemiology of vascular injury in the wars in Iraq and Afghanistan. Ann Surg. 2011;253:1184–9.
20. Turner C, Stockinger C, Gurney C. Vascular surgery during U.S. combat operations from 2002–2016: analysis of vascular procedures performed to inform military training. J Trauma Acute Care Surg. 2018;85(1S Suppl 2):S145–53.
21. Fox CJ, Gillespie DL, O'Donnell SD, Rasmussen TE, Goff JM, Johnson CA, et al. Contemporary management of wartime vascular trauma. J Vasc Surg. 2005;41(4):638–44.
22. Clouse WD, Rasmussen TE, Peck MA, Eliason JL, Cox MW, Bowser AN, Jenkins DH, Smith DL, Rich NM. Current in theater management of wartime vascular injury: a report from Operation Iraqi Freedom. J Am Coll Surg. 2007;204(4):625–32.
23. Wolf S, Bebarta V, Bonnett C, Pons P, Cantrill S. Blast injuries. Lancet. 2009;374(9687):405–15.
24. The first responder guidance for improving survivability in improvised explosive device and/or active shooter incidents. Department of Homeland Security, Office of Health Affairs. June 2015.
25. Jacobs L, McSwain N, Rotondo M, Wade D, Fabbri W, Eastman A, et al. Improving survival from active shooter events. J Trauma Acute Care Surg. 2013;74(6):1399–400.

26. Welling D, McKay P, Rasmussen T, Rich N. A brief history of the tourniquet. J Vasc Surg. 2012;55(1):286–90.
27. Rasmussen T, Stockinger G, Antevil J, White C, Fernandez N, White J, et al. Vascular injury [Internet]. Joint Trauma System; 2016 [cited 20 July 2018]. Available from: http://jts.amedd.army.mil/assets/docs/cpgs/JTS_Clinical_Practice_Guidelines_(CPGs)/Vascular_Injury_12_Aug_2016_ID46.pdf.
28. Kragh J, Littrel M, Jones J, Walters T, Baer D, Wade C. Battle casualty survival with emergency tourniquet use to stop limb bleeding. J Emerg Med. 2011;41(6):590–7.
29. Kragh J, Walters T, Baer D, Fox C, Wade C, Salinas J. Survival with emergency tourniquet use to stop bleeding in major limb trauma. Ann Surg. 2009;249(1):1–7.
30. Kragh J, Dubick M, Aden J, McKeague A, Rasmussen T, Baer D, et al. U.S. military use of tourniquets from 2001 to 2010. Prehosp Emerg Care. 2014;19(2):184–90.
31. Cantle P, Hurley M, Swartz M, Holcomb J. Methods for early control of abdominal hemorrhage: an assessment of potential benefit. J Spec Oper Med [Internet]. 2018 [cited 20 July 2018];18:98–104. Available from: https://www.ncbi.nlm.nih.gov/pubmed/29889964.
32. American College of Surgeon Committee on Trauma. Advanced trauma life support for doctors. Chicago: American College of Surgeons; 2009.
33. Deakin C. Accuracy of the advanced trauma life support guidelines for predicting systolic blood pressure using carotid, femoral, and radial pulses: observational study. BMJ. 2000;321(7262):673–4.
34. Frykberg E, Dennis J, Bishop K, Laneve L, Alexander R. The reliability of physical examination in the evaluation of penetrating extremity trauma for vascular injury. J Trauma. 1991;31(4):502–11.
35. Johansen K, Lynch K, Paun M, Copass M. Non-invasive vascular tests reliably exclude occult arterial trauma in injured extremities. J Trauma. 1990;30(7):923.
36. deSouza I, Benabbas R, McKee S, Zangbar B, Jain A, Paladino L. Accuracy of physical examination, ankle-brachial index, and ultrasonography in the diagnosis of arterial injury in patients with penetrating extremity trauma: a systematic review and meta-analysis. Acad Emerg Med. 2017;24(8):994–1017.
37. Inaba K, Branco B, Reddy S, Park J, Green D, Plurad D, et al. Prospective evaluation of multidetector computed tomography for extremity vascular trauma. J Trauma. 2011;70(4):808–15.
38. Dennis J, Frykberg E, Veldenz H, Huffman S, Menawat S. Validation of nonoperative management of occult vascular injuries and accuracy of physical examination alone in penetrating extremity trauma. J Trauma. 1998;44(2):243–53.
39. Moore E, Knudson M, Burlew C, Inaba K, Dicker R, Biffl W, et al. Defining the limits of resuscitative emergency department thoracotomy: a contemporary Western Trauma Association perspective. J Trauma. 2011;70(2):334–9.
40. Emergency Resuscitative Thoracotomy [Internet]. Joint Trauma System; 2012 [cited 20 July 2018]. Available from: http://jts.amedd.army.mil/assets/docs/cpgs/JTS_Clinical_Practice_Guidelines_(CPGs)/Emergent_Resuscitative_Thoracotomy_11_Jun_2012_ID20.pdf.
41. Hughes CW. Use of an intra-aortic balloon catheter tamponade for controlling intraabdominal hemorrhage in man. Surgery. 1954;36:65–8.
42. Stannard A, Morrison JJ, Scott DJ, Ivatury RA, Ross JD, Rasmussen TE. The epidemiology of non-compressible hemorrhage in the wards in Iraq and Afghanistan. J Trauma Acute Care Surg. 2013;74:830–4.
43. Brenner M, Moore L, DuBose J, Tyson G, McNutt M, Albarado R, et al. A clinical series of resuscitative endovascular balloon occlusion of the aorta for hemorrhage control and resuscitation. J Trauma Acute Care Surg. 2013;75(3):506–11.
44. Moore L, Brenner M, Kozar R, Pasley J, Wade C, Baraniuk M, et al. Implementation of resuscitative endovascular balloon occlusion of the aorta as an alternative to resuscitative thoracotomy for noncompressible truncal hemorrhage. J Trauma Acute Care Surg. 2015;79(4):523–32.

45. Matsumura Y, Matsumoto J, Kondo H, Idoguchi K, Ishida T, Okada Y, et al. Early arterial access for REBOA is related to survival outcome in trauma. J Trauma Acute Care Surg. 2018;85:507.
46. Irahara T, Sato N, Moroe Y, Fukuda R, Iwai Y, Unemoto K, et al. Retrospective study of the effectiveness of Intra-Aortic Balloon Occlusion (IABO) for traumatic haemorrhagic shock. World J Emerg Surg. 2015;10(1):1.
47. Pasley J, Cannon J, Glaser J, Polk T, Morrison J, Brocker J, et al. Resuscitative endovascular balloon occlusion of the aorta (REBOA) for hemorrhagic shock [Internet]. Joint Trauma System; 2017 [cited 20 July 2018]. Available from: http://jts.amedd.army.mil/assets/docs/cpgs/JTS_Clinical_Practice_Guidelines_(CPGs)/REBOA_for_Hemorrhagic_Shock_06_Jul_2017_ID38.pdf.
48. Rotondo MF, Schwab CW, McGonigal MD, et al. "Damage control": an approach for improved survival in exsanguinating penetrating abdominal injury. J Trauma. 1993;35:375–82.
49. Rotondo MF, Zonies DH. The damage control sequence and underlying logic. Surg Clin North Am. 1997;77:761–77.
50. Taller JT, Kandar JP, Greene JA, Moore RA, Blankenship CL, Dabrowski P, Sharpe RP. Temporary vascular shunts as initial treatment of proximal extremity vascular injuries during combat operations: the new standard of care at echelon II facilities? J Trauma. 2008;65:595–603.
51. Rasmussen T, Clouse W, Jenkins D, Peck M, Eliason J, Smith D. The use of temporary vascular shunts as a damage control adjunct in the management of wartime vascular injury. J Trauma. 2006;61(1):8–15.
52. Inaba K, Aksoy H, Seamon M, Marks J, Duchesne J, Schroll R. Multicenter evaluation of temporary intravascular shunt use in vascular trauma. J Trauma Acute Care Surg. 2016;80(3):359–65.
53. Hornez E, Boddaert G, Ngabou U, Aguir S, Baudoin Y, Mocellin N, et al. Temporary vascular shunt for damage control of extremity vascular injury: a toolbox for trauma surgeons. J Visc Surg. 2015;152(6):363–8.
54. Hossny A. Blunt popliteal artery injury with complete lower limb ischemia: is routine use of temporary intraluminal arterial shunt justified? J Vasc Surg. 2004;40:61–6.
55. Shackford S, Kahl J, Calvo R, Shackford M, Danos L, Davis J, et al. Limb salvage after complex repairs of extremity arterial injuries is independent of surgical specialty training. J Trauma Acute Care Surg. 2013;74(3):716–24.
56. Ledgerwood A, Lucas C. Biological dressings for exposed vascular grafts. J Trauma. 1975;15(7):567–74.
57. Berger P, de Bie D, Moll F, de Borst G. Negative pressure wound therapy on exposed prosthetic vascular grafts in the groin. J Vasc Surg. 2012;56(3):714–20.
58. Klocker J, Bertoldi A, Benda B, Pellegrini L, Gorny O, Fraedrich G. Outcome after interposition of vein grafts for arterial repair of extremity injuries in civilians. J Vasc Surg. 2014;59(6):1633–7.
59. Mithcell F, Thal E. Results of venous interposition grafts in arterial injuries. J Trauma. 1990;30(3):336–9.
60. Schmitt D, Bandyk D, Pequet A, Towne J. Bacterial adherence to vascular prostheses. J Vasc Surg. 1986;3(5):732–40.
61. Ambler G, Twine C. Graft type for femoro-popliteal bypass surgery. Cochrane Database Syst Rev. 2018;2:CD001487.
62. Vertrees A, Fox C, Quan R, Cox M, Adams E, Gillespie D. The use of prosthetic grafts in complex military vascular trauma: a limb salvage strategy for patients with severely limited autologous conduit. J Trauma. 2009;66(4):980–3.
63. Sullivan P, Dente C, Patel S, Carmichael M, Srinivasan J, Wyrzykowski A. Outcome of ligation of the inferior vena cava in the modern era. Am J Surg. 2010;199(4):500–6.
64. du Toit D, van Schalkwyk G, Wadee S, Warren B. Neurologic outcome after penetrating extracranial arterial trauma. J Vasc Surg. 2003;38(2):257–62.

65. Reva V, Pronchenko A, Samokhvalov I. Operative management of penetrating carotid artery injuries. Eur J Vasc Endovasc Surg. 2011;42(1):16–20.
66. Burkhardt G, Spencer J, Gifford S, Propper B, Jones L, Sumner N, et al. A large animal survival model (Sus Scrofa) of extremity ischemia/reperfusion and neuromuscular outcomes assessment: a pilot study. J Trauma. 2010;69(Supplement):S146–53.
67. Dyer D, Moore E, Mestek M, Durham J, Heinig M, Bernstein S. Thoracic aortic injury: how predictive is mechanism and is chest CT a reliable screening tool? – a prospective study of 1000 patients. J Trauma. 1998;45(1):190.
68. Lee W, Matsumura J, Mitchell R, Farber M, Greenberg R, Azizzadeh A. Endovascular repair of traumatic thoracic aortic injury: clinical practice guidelines of the Society for Vascular Surgery. J Vasc Surg. 2011;53(1):187–92.
69. Woodring J, Dillon M. Radiographic manifestations of mediastinal hemorrhage from blunt chest trauma. Ann Thorac Surg. 1984;37(2):171–8.
70. Hiratzka L, Bakris G, Beckman J, Bersin R, Carr V, Casey D, et al. 2010 ACCF/AHA/AATS/ACR/ASA/SCA/SCAI/SIR/STS/SVM guidelines for the diagnosis and management of patients with thoracic aortic disease: a report of the American College of Cardiology Foundation/American Heart Association Task Force on Practice Guidelines, American Association for Thoracic Surgery, American College of Radiology, American Stroke Association, Society of Cardiovascular Anesthesiologists, Society for Cardiovascular Angiography and Interventions, Society of Interventional Radiology, Society of Thoracic Surgeons, and Society for Vascular Medicine. Circulation. 2010;121(13):e266–369.
71. Fabian T, Davis K, Gavant M, Croce M, Melton S, Patton J. Prospective study of blunt aortic injury. Ann Surg. 1998;227(5):666–77.
72. Murad M, Rizvi A, Malgor R, Carey J, Alkatib A, Erwin P. Comparative effectiveness of the treatments for thoracic aortic transaction. J Vasc Surg. 2011;53(1):193–199.e21.
73. Biffl W, Moore E, Offner P, Brega K, Franciose R, Burch J, et al. Blunt carotid arterial injuries: implications of a new grading scale. J Trauma. 1999;47(5):845.
74. Biffl W, Cothren C, Moore E, Kozar R, Cocanour C, Davis J, et al. Western Trauma Association critical decisions in trauma: screening for and treatment of blunt cerebrovascular injuries. J Trauma. 2009;67(6):1150–3.
75. Cothren C, Biffl W, Moore E. Treatment for blunt cerebrovascular injuries: equivalence of anticoagulation and antiplatelet agents. J Vasc Surg. 2009;50(5):1243.
76. Vernhet H, Marty-Ané C, Lesnik A, Chircop R, Serres-Cousiné O, Picard E. Dissection of the abdominal aorta in blunt trauma: management by percutaneous stent placement. Cardiovasc Intervent Radiol. 1997;20(6):473–6.
77. Castelli P, Caronno R, Piffaretti G, Tozzi M. Emergency endovascular repair for traumatic injury of the inferior vena cava. Eur J Cardiothorac Surg. 2005;28(6):906–8.
78. Sinha S, Patterson B, Ma J, Holt P, Thompson M, Carrell T, et al. Systematic review and meta-analysis of open surgical and endovascular management of thoracic outlet vascular injuries. J Vasc Surg. 2013;57(2):547–567.e8.

Management of Thoracoabdominal Blast Injuries

32

Stacy A. Shackelford

Introduction

The chest and abdominal regions are sensitive to the spectrum of blast injury mechanisms due to the close proximity of large air-containing organs susceptible to primary blast effects, multiple vital structures susceptible to secondary fragment wounds, and solid organs and bones susceptible to tertiary crush injuries.

Blast-related injury to thoracoabdominal structures occurs with variable frequency depending on the specific blast mechanism and presence or absence of protective gear worn. Data from the Department of Defense Trauma Registry for US military operations 2001–2016 demonstrates that explosions caused 44% of all injuries (including both battle and non-battle injuries). Among those injured by explosion, 14% sustained injury to the thorax and 19% injury to the abdominal region, of which the vast majority (73%) were polytrauma patients who sustained injuries to more than one body region. Of polytrauma injuries, 19% included wounds to the thorax, and 25% included wounds to the abdomen (Fig. 32.1). In general, the effect of body armor reduces the frequency and severity of injury to the torso, such that civilian or unarmored personnel subjected to blast injury may sustain a higher rate of thoracoabdominal injury.

Injury to multiple body regions occurs in 86% of civilian blast-injured patients [1]. In an analysis of civilians injured by explosions in Israel, the incidence of thoracoabdominal injury following blast was reported as 52%, with 15% suffering severe injury [2]. The study noted an even higher percentage reported for children injured by blasts [3]. Within the UK Joint Theater Trauma Registry, 21% of combat-related deaths after hospital arrival were associated with abdominal and pelvic

S. A. Shackelford (✉)
Joint Trauma System, Defense Health Agency, San Antonio, TX, USA
e-mail: stacy.a.shackelford.mil@mail.mil

D. W. Callaway, J. L. Burstein (eds.), *Operational and Medical Management of Explosive and Blast Incidents*, https://doi.org/10.1007/978-3-030-40655-4_32

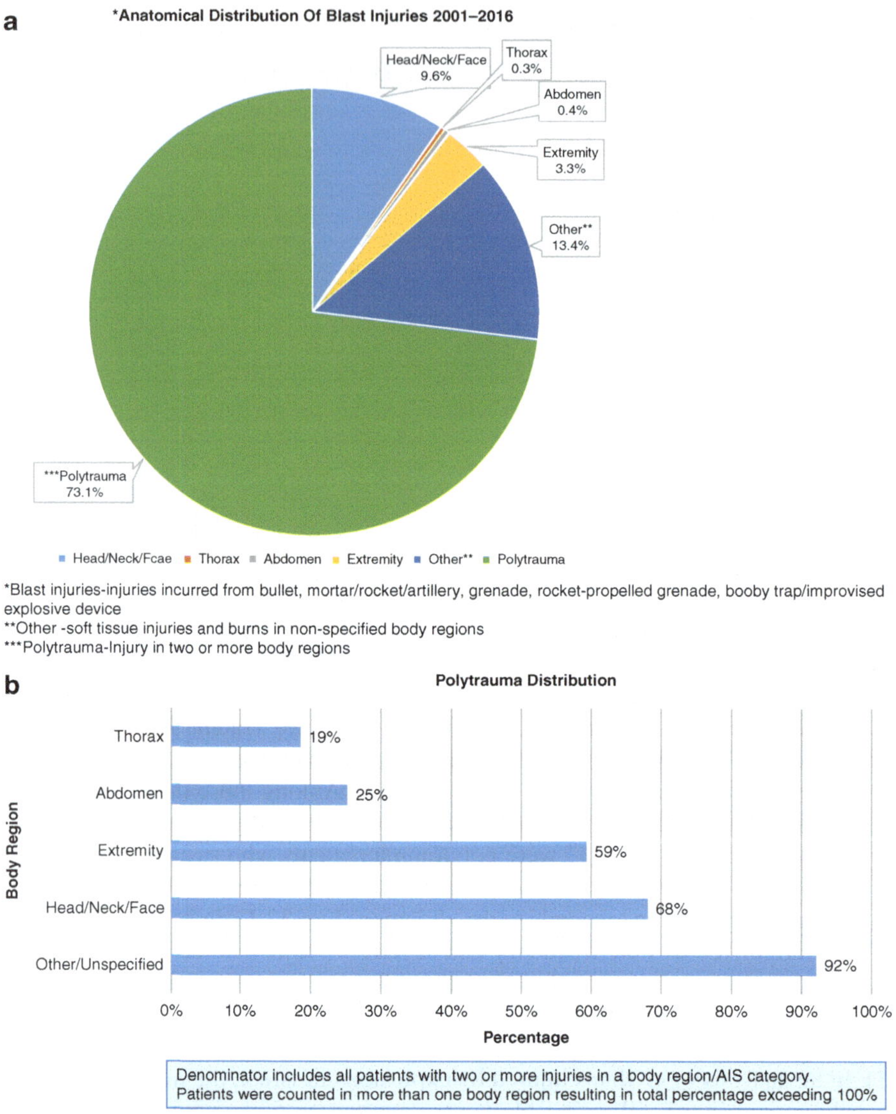

Fig. 32.1 Anatomic distribution of injury of blast-injured patients (**a**) and distribution of injuries in the subset of polytrauma patients (**b**) in the Department of Defense Trauma Registry

injuries combined with severe lower limb trauma [4]. Additionally, the presence of non-compressible torso hemorrhage is associated with increased mortality [5]. In particular, mediastinal injury predicts death with rare survivors from blast-related injury to the heart, thoracic aorta, pulmonary artery, pulmonary vein, or superior vena cava [6].

Blast Taxonomy and Thoracoabdominal Trauma

Primary blast injury affects air-filled organs in the chest and abdomen (Fig. 32.2). In the lungs this is manifested by pneumothorax, alveolar damage termed "blast lung," or potentially fatal air embolus. In the military, 7–11% of patients admitted to the hospital after explosion injury exhibit some degree of blast lung injury [7, 8]. Such injuries are managed by respiratory support with attention to lung-protective ventilator strategies when needed and chest tube placement when indicated for pneumothorax.

Air embolus is a dire emergency that may manifest with sudden hemodynamic collapse or in less severe cases with sudden respiratory distress or neurologic event. Air embolus associated with pulmonary trauma is caused by air drawn into the pulmonary venous circulation through a disruption of the vein that opens it to air through the bronchial system. In cases of hemodynamic collapse associated with chest injury, surgical treatment is immediate thoracotomy to the suspected side of injury with contralateral chest tube. Air embolus from the lung can be suspected based on the presence of lung laceration and possibly air bubbles visible within the coronary circulation. In such case, the hilum of the injured lung should be clamped, followed by open cardiac compressions, blood product transfusion, and ACLS resuscitation. If a spontaneous heartbeat and blood pressure are regained, the site of the broncho-venous fistula must be identified and ligated or resected prior to releasing the hilar clamp.

Blast wave effects on abdominal organs include rupture of the gastrointestinal tract, which can occur at any point along its length. Contusion or partial thickness injury to the bowel can also occur. And, as is typical of the blast effect on other soft tissues, necrosis can progress for several hours to days after injury, leading to delayed bowel perforation. The most common area of gastrointestinal perforation is the colon. Fortunately, primary blast injury of the intestine is quite rare, with the

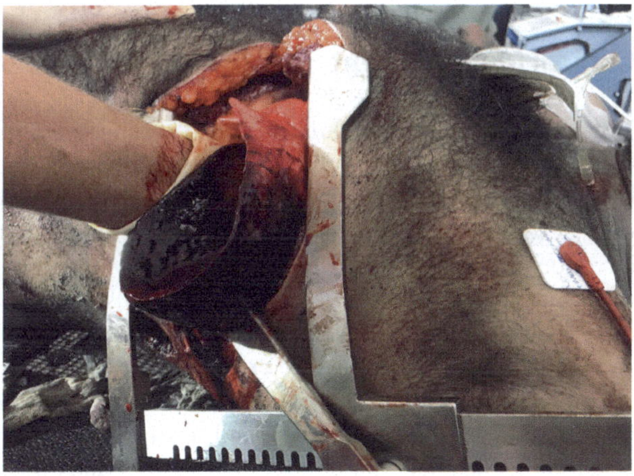

Fig. 32.2 Primary blast injury. Severe pulmonary contusion caused by blast injury with associated extensive extremity injuries

vast majority of blast-related bowel injuries caused by penetrating fragments [3]. High-order explosives, however, are characterized by a strong supersonic pressure wave and may inflict a greater amount of primary blast injuries. Additionally, blast exposure in a confined space may also result in a greater extent of primary blast injury [1].

Secondary blast effects result from fragments projected from the explosion and are the most frequent cause of injuries that require surgical intervention to the chest and abdomen. Explosive fragments are irregular in shape and size and lose energy rapidly with increasing distance from the detonation. Penetrating fragments may include metallic portions of the explosive device, metallic contents from improvised explosive devices (IED), dirt and debris from the terrain, or bone fragments from other victims or suicide bombers. Such fragments are frequently of relatively low velocity when striking the body; since the fragments vary in energy and composition, they will penetrate varying depths into body cavities. It is common to see numerous peppering wounds on the skin of the chest and abdomen caused by multiple fragments. Many such wounds may barely penetrate the skin; however, it is also common for a few such fragments to penetrate deeply into the body cavities threatening vital organs. In such cases, it is challenging to identify specific organ injuries.

Tertiary blast injuries result from blunt trauma from blast-related mechanisms such as being thrown through the air, vehicle rollover, or structural collapse. Combatants wearing protective gear may also present with blunt abdominal trauma where protected from fragmentation wounds, with energy transmitted to the body cavities from fragments striking the armor. Tertiary blast injury patterns to the torso are typical of injuries sustained by blunt trauma mechanisms such as fall or crush injuries and may include rib fractures, spine fractures, pulmonary contusion, solid organ abdominal injury, and pelvic fracture. In general, these injuries should be managed according to standard clinical practice guidelines. Open pelvic fractures are common in explosive incidents and are associated with lower extremity amputations and mortality [9].

Clinical Management

The complexity of clinical and surgical management increases when blunt trauma injuries are combined with the effects of penetrating trauma, multiple open wounds with massive contamination, and injury to multiple body regions (Fig. 32.3). For such severely injured patients who survive the initial resuscitation, devastating infectious complications are common. Early treatment with appropriate, broad-spectrum prophylactic antibiotics, meticulous and repeated wound debridement, early identification of infections, and transition to targeted therapeutic antibiotics and antifungals as indicated are critical to survival.

In hemodynamically stable patients, the initial treatment depends on the environment, overall casualty situation, and available diagnostic capabilities. In general, penetrating chest and abdominal fragment wounds in stable patients should not be aggressively explored, and initial treatments should proceed according to the results of chest X-ray, focused abdominal ultrasound for trauma (FAST), and abdominal

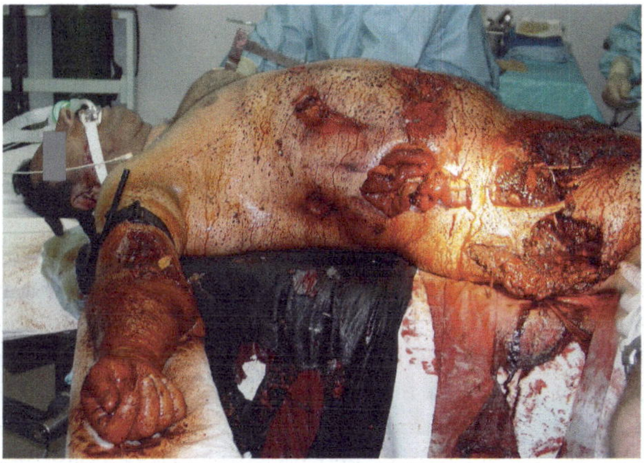

Fig. 32.3 Victim of improvised explosive device attack with multisystem trauma to extremities, chest, and abdomen

exam for peritonitis. A CT pan-scan of the head, neck, chest, abdomen, and pelvis should be considered for all hemodynamically stable blast-injured patients, even when the injury seems to be limited to a single body cavity. Commonly, fragments will be seen within the body cavities distant from the point of entry. Small fragments that are seen on CT scan to be located adjacent to vital structures without definite injury rarely require exploration. Although there is a theoretical risk of eroding into blood vessels over time, fragments should not be removed unless symptomatic, particularly if an invasive procedure is required to address. When diagnostic capabilities are limited, such as in austere environments or mass casualty events, a liberal approach to abdominal exploration may be the most expedient diagnostic and therapeutic maneuver when penetrating abdominal injury is suspected.

Bowel necrosis and perforation may occur even when no violation of the peritoneum is present [10]. Sections of perforated and necrotic bowel should be resected. In most cases, bowel continuity should be restored at the initial laparotomy. However, management of colorectal injuries in this setting remains controversial. Primary colon anastomosis or repair can be performed in select patients without associated injury, though the widespread acceptance of primary anastomosis for colorectal injuries, as adopted in the vast majority of civilian penetrating injuries, should be implemented with caution in blast injury. Factors associated with failure of colon repair or anastomosis in war-related injuries include concomitant pancreatic, splenic, renal, and diaphragm injuries, high ISS, and large transfusion requirements [11]. Damage control surgery with delayed anastomosis may improve the success rate for colon anastomosis [11]. Casualties with serious associated injuries may have a higher mortality rate with no fecal diversion compared to those treated with fecal diversion; however, there are no specific selection criteria for fecal diversion [11–14].

Chest and abdominal wall defects related to blast injury may be substantial. Large chest wall defects are frequently fatal at the point of injury. Prehospital treatment includes temporary closure of the chest wall defect with a chest seal and early initiation of positive pressure ventilation to overcome respiratory insufficiency. In these cases, chest tube placement at the earliest opportunity is important to prevent cardiopulmonary decompensation. In surgical settings, vacuum-assisted closure has been extensively utilized as a means to achieve temporary closure of both chest and abdominal wounds, to include complex and contaminated wounds and wounds with extensive loss of chest or abdominal wall. Eventual closure may be achieved using reconstructive techniques with a combination of component separation of the abdominal wall, prosthetic and biologic mesh closures, rotational flaps, and skin grafting [13].

When multiple fragment wounds are associated with hemodynamic instability, external hemorrhage must first be controlled, and subsequent evaluation should focus on rapid identification of potential bleeding sources. The clinician should rapidly obtain chest X-ray, FAST or extended-FAST exam, and pelvic X-ray to identify sources of massive hemorrhage, keeping in mind that injuries may result from any combination of blast wave and penetrating and blunt mechanisms. Chest tube placement is indicated for suspected or confirmed hemo- or pneumothorax. The indications to proceed to thoracotomy are no different than other types of penetrating trauma (massive hemorrhage with initial chest tube output greater than 1000–1500 ml or ongoing bleeding greater than about 250 ml/h). A high index of suspicion for pelvic fracture and intra-abdominal injury should be maintained whenever lower extremity amputation or near-amputation is present. Hemoperitoneum by FAST exam mandates laparotomy in all hemodynamically unstable victims of explosion. In such cases, resuscitative balloon occlusion of the aorta may also be considered once massive chest hemorrhage has been ruled out. Figure 32.4 shows a grenade blast victim who sustained multiple fragment wounds to the left side of his body and presented with hypotension, hemoperitoneum, and massive hematuria.

Explosive incidents can result in devastating multisystem trauma, and often, extensive extremity wounds are combined with injuries to the chest, abdomen, pelvis, eyes, and brain. Such an injury pattern is exemplified by the military dismounted complex blast injury [15] (Fig. 32.5) and may also occur in civilian settings such as land mine explosions or terrorist IED attacks. When destructive injuries or amputations to the lower extremities are present, immediate survival depends on external hemorrhage control with tourniquets, pelvic binder placement, and early resuscitation with blood products. Associated pelvic fractures occur in up to 40% of bilateral lower extremity amputations [16]. Particularly devastating are associated injuries to the external genitalia, anus, rectum, and sigmoid colon, and in such cases, early diverting colostomy is indicated. When proximal lower extremity amputations are present, particularly when combined with significant injuries to the perineum, a low threshold for abdominal exploration is an approach implemented by military surgeons to address simultaneously the need to assess intra-abdominal hemorrhage, obtain proximal control of external iliac vessels, perform preperitoneal pelvic packing, and create a diverting colostomy. Since such patients are typically treated initially in a damage control approach, the colon may simply be divided at the first operation with deferred stoma creation. In a study of combat blast victims,

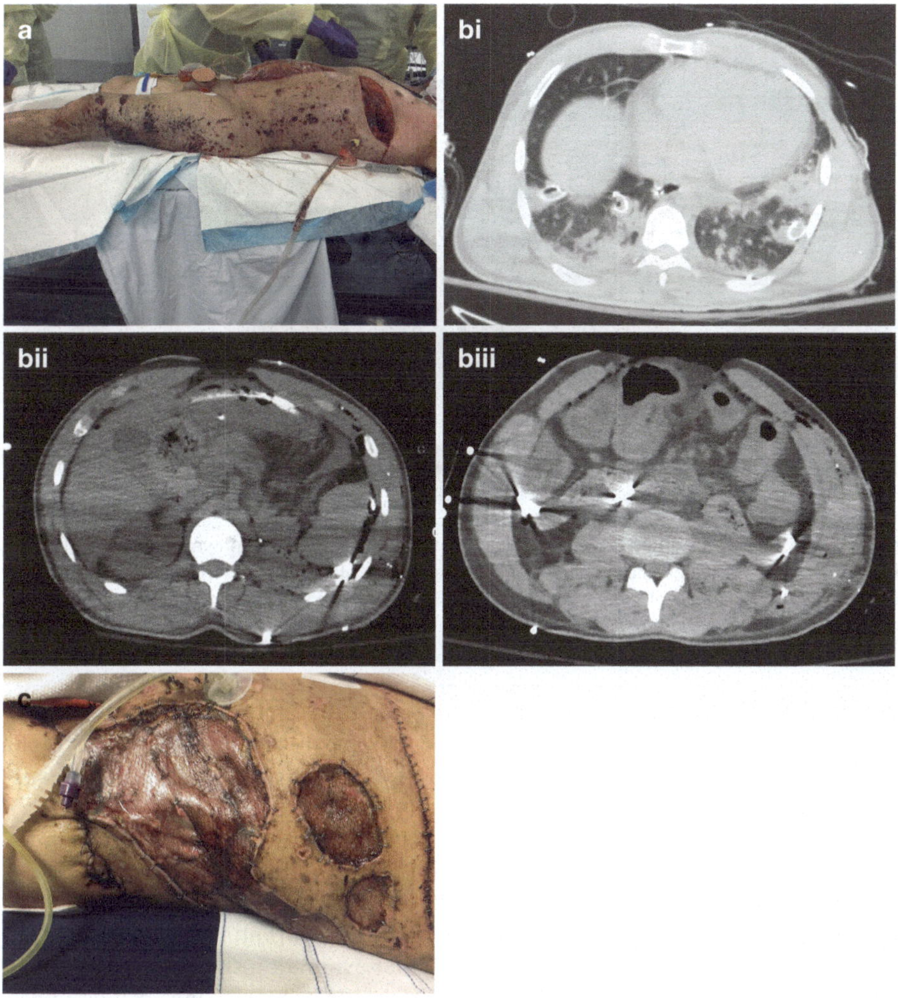

Fig. 32.4 (**a**) Multiple fragment wounds to left flank and thigh that presented with hemodynamic instability and hematuria. A laparotomy, splenectomy, and left nephrectomy were performed. During resuscitation, the patient developed cardiac arrest and received a resuscitative thoracotomy. Image shown is 1 day after injury illustrating multiple fragment wounds, laparotomy, and thoracotomy incisions. (**b**) Initial CT scan was obtained after initial laparotomy and demonstrated multiple lung lacerations and fragments throughout the abdomen. (**c**) Progressive necrosis and infection of skin and subcutaneous tissues required multiple debridements and eventual skin grafting

patients who underwent exploratory laparotomy for proximal vascular control alone, when no other incidental findings or occult injuries were identified, had a 98% incidence of massive transfusion, required a mean of 38 units of red blood cells, and had a 23% incidence of intra-abdominal complications [17]. This highlights not only the critical multisystem nature of such injuries but also

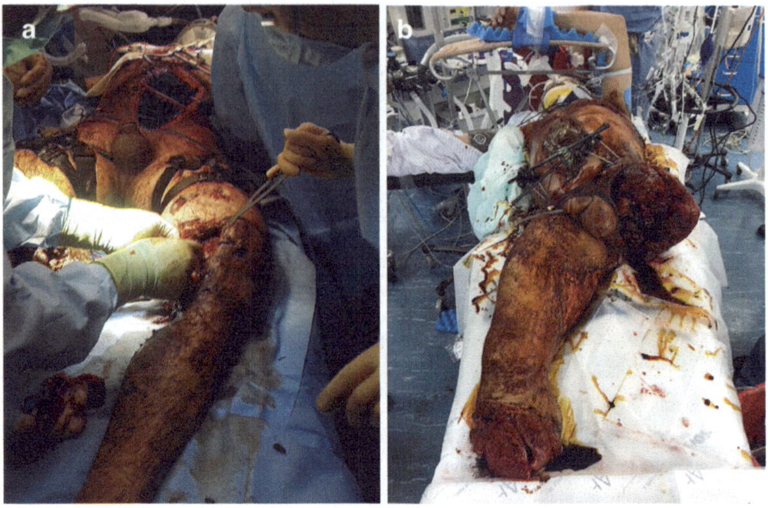

Fig. 32.5 Military dismounted complex blast injury from inprovised explosive device. (**a**) Day of injury with open abdomen and bilateral thigh tourniquets in place. (**b**) One week post injury, pelvic external fixation in place, abdomen remains open, and patient required a right above knee amputation due to large tissue loss posterior to the knee and progressive necrosis

the need for judicious use of laparotomy for proximal vascular control and consideration of alternatives to include the extraperitoneal approach to external iliac artery control as well as implementation of endovascular approaches to vascular control, when feasible.

Cautious and thorough physical examination is critical in victims of explosive incidents. At times, a single small fragment wound may seem innocuous. However, these wounds can be deadly. As an example, Fig. 32.6 illustrates a man who was struck by a fragment in a suicide bomb attack and sustained a small laceration to the lateral shoulder. Further evaluation showed that the fragment trajectory entered the mediastinum, and although avoiding serious injury to vital structures, it well demonstrates the need for vigilance and thorough evaluation. Often, multiple peppering wounds may cover large areas of the body. Figure 32.7 illustrates a child with multiple small peppering wounds to the chest and abdomen. Initial FAST exam was equivocal and subsequent CT scan demonstrated hemopericardium.

Not infrequently, a small fragment may be found within the abdominal cavity and seemingly within the bowel itself on CT scan (Fig. 32.8). If the patient is otherwise stable with benign abdominal exam, they should be observed in a location where serial abdominal exam can be performed. In such cases, exploratory laparotomy is indicated for peritonitis; however, the majority can be successfully managed nonoperatively.

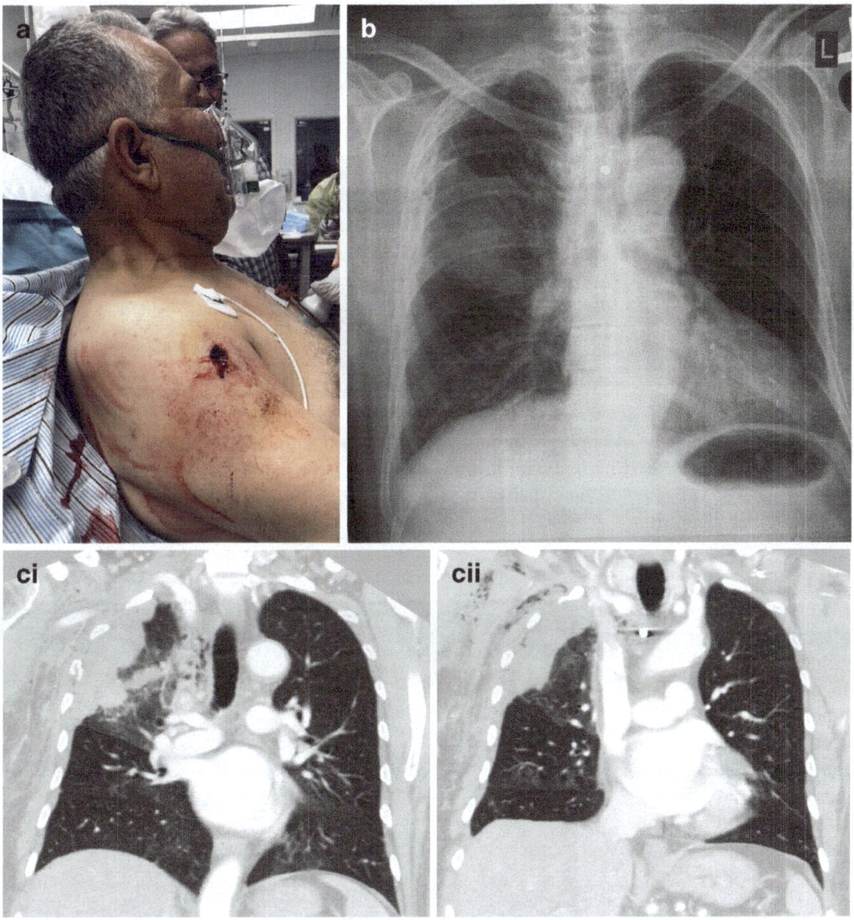

Fig. 32.6 (**a**) Fragment wound to right lateral shoulder from suicide bomb attack. (**b**) Chest X-ray demonstrates a small fragment in the central chest. (**c**) CT scan shows the fragment trajectory through the right axilla and right upper lobe into the mediastinum and lodged immediately anterior to the trachea with small pseudoaneurysm of the right upper lobe pulmonary artery. He was evaluated with bronchoscopy and clinical observation and did not require further intervention

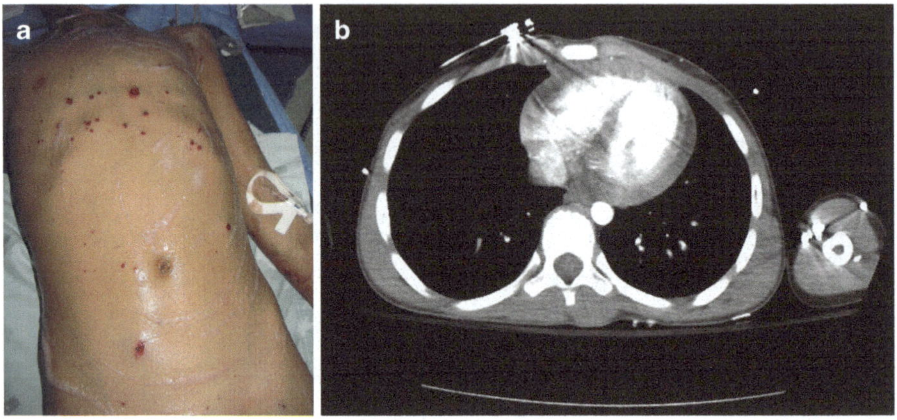

Fig. 32.7 (**a**) An 11-year-old male with multiple peppering wounds to the chest following a mine blast injury. He maintained hemodynamic stability, and FAST exam was initially equivocal. (**b**) Subsequent chest CT showed hemopericardium. He underwent sternotomy and repair of small right ventricular laceration

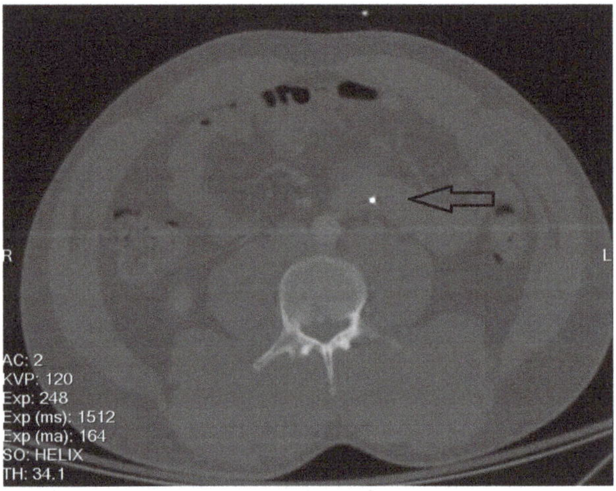

Fig. 32.8 Abdominal CT of blast injury victim with multiple peppering wounds from small fragments. One fragment appears to be located within the small intestine. The patient had no peritonitis and was observed for 24 h without further intervention

Conclusion

The spectrum of blast injuries affecting the chest and abdomen, from minor fragment wounds to massive multisystem trauma, will challenge decision-making. In stable patients, a thorough evaluation of all body cavities and watchful observation are appropriate. For the unstable patient with multiple injuries, early external hemorrhage control, balanced blood product resuscitation, and identification and control of torso hemorrhage are principles that are critical though not unique to blast injuries. However, the extent of multisystem blunt and penetrating trauma combined with the presence of severe contamination, progressive tissue necrosis, and devastating infections contributes to the multiple challenges of blast injury management.

Pitfalls

- Forgetting blunt trauma management (pelvic fracture, spine injury, or intra-abdominal injury may occur even without penetrating fragment wounds).
- Missing ongoing external bleeding from extremity or posterior wounds while concentrating on torso hemorrhage, particularly if the patient is covered for warming or if the wounds are hidden by surgical drapes during thoracotomy or laparotomy.
- Diffuse peppering wounds may look innocuous, while a single small fragment may pierce a vital organ. This may be difficult to localize when imaging studies are not readily available. When available, CT pan-scan should be obtained for all serious blast injuries.

References

1. Bala M, Rivking AI, Zamir G, Hadar T, Gertsenshtein I, Mintz Y, et al. Abdominal trauma after terrorist bombing attacks exhibits a unique pattern of injury. Ann Surg. 2008;248:303–9.
2. Rozenfeld M, Givon A, Shenhar G, Renert L, Peleg K. A new paradigm of injuries from terrorist explosions as a function of explosion setting type. Ann Surg. 2016;263:1228–34.
3. Thompson DC, Crooks RJ, Clasper JC, Lupu A, Stapley SA, Cloke DJ. The pattern of paediatric blast injury in Afghanistan. J R Army Med Corps. 2017;0:1–5.
4. Kerene DD, Penn-Barwell JG, Wood PR, Hunt N, Delaney R, Clasper J, et al. Died of wounds: a mortality review. J R Army Med Corps. 2016;162:355–60.
5. Eastridge BJ, Mabry RL, Seguin P, Cantrell J, Tops T, Uribe P, et al. Death on the battlefield (2001–2011): implications for the future of combat casualty care. J Trauma Acute Care Surg. 2012;73:S431–7.
6. Pearce AP, Bull AMJ, Clasper JC. Mediastinal injury is the strongest predictor of mortality in mounted blast amongst UK deployed forces. Int J Care Inj. 2017;48:1900–5.
7. Smith JE. The epidemiology of blast lung injury during recent military conflicts: a retrospective database review of cases presenting to deployed military hospitals, 2003–2009. Philos Trans R Soc Lond Ser B Biol Sci. 2011;366:291–4.
8. Aboudara M, Mahoney PF, Hicke B, Cuadrado D. Primary blast lung injury at a NATO Role 3 hospital. J R Army Med Corps. 2014;160:161–6.
9. Oh JS, Creighton CT, Poepping TP, Ryan P, Clasper JC, Katschke AR, et al. Dismounted blast injuries in patients treated at a role 3 military hospital in Afghanistan: patterns of injury and mortality. Mil Med. 2016;181:1069–74.
10. Velichkov NG, Losanoff JE, Kjossev KT, Katrov ET, Mironov MB, Losanoff HE. Delayed small bowel injury as a result of penetrating extraperitoneal high-velocity ballistic trauma to the abdomen. J Trauma. 2000;48:1335–42.

11. Vertrees A, Wakefield M, Pickett C, Greer L, Wilson A, Gillern S, et al. Outcomes of primary repair and primary anastomosis in war-related colon injuries. J Trauma. 2009;66:1286–93.
12. Duncan JE, Corwin CE, Sweeney WB, Dunne JR, Denobile JW, Perdue PW, et al. Management for colorectal injuries during Operation Iraqi Freedom: patterns of stoma usage. J Trauma. 2008;632:1043–7.
13. Plurad DS. Blast injury. Mil Med. 2011;176:276–82.
14. Glasgow SC, Steel SR, Duncan JE, Rasmussen TE. Epidemiology of modern battlefield colorectal trauma: a review of 977 coalition casualties. J Trauma Acute Care Surg. 2012;73(6 Supp;5):S5503–8.
15. Cannon JW, Hofmann LJ, Glasgow SC, Potter BK, Rodriguez CJ, Cancio LC, et al. Dismounted complex blast injuries: a comprehensive review of the modern combat experience. J Am Col Surg. 2016;223(4):652–64.
16. Cross AM, Davis C, Penn-Barwell J, Taylor DM, De Mello WF, Matthews JJ. The incidence of pelvic fractures with traumatic lower limb amputation in modern warfare due to improvised explosive devices. J R Nav Med Serv. 2014;100(2):152–6.
17. Hathaway E, Glaser J, Cardarelli C, Dunne J, Elster E, Safford S, et al. Exploratory laparotomy for proximal vascular control in combat-related injuries. Mil Med. 2016;181:247–52.

Genitourinary Injuries

33

Steven J. Hudak

Introduction

Genitourinary (GU) injuries, defined as injury to any structure or organ within the urinary, genital, or reproductive systems of men or women, are unique from injuries to all other body systems in that they are the only region or system which has the combination of the following attributes: low mortality when injured, innate sensitive/intimate nature of anatomy and function, and profoundly limited options for functional rehabilitation when tissues are lost. Thus, unlike those who sustain injuries to other body systems, the clinical care of men and women who sustain GU injuries begins at the time of injury and lasts for months, years, and beyond, depending on the severity of the initial injury and quantity of tissue lost. This long-term care is further challenged by the lack of standardized care pathways for complex genital trauma, the innate difficulty most clinicians have with discussing the effects of GU injuries on deeply private and intimate functions (i.e., urination, sexual activity, reproductive function), and the unfortunate lack of restorative care for those who sustain catastrophic loss of genital and/or reproductive organs.

Evolutions in modern warfare and combat casualty care have resulted in a relative increase in the proportion of casualties surviving with GU injuries after blast mechanisms. Thus, the objective of this chapter is to review contemporary military GU injury data; outline the early, intermediate, and long-term care of GU injuries; and offer pragmatic recommendations to improve the care of patients who sustain blast injuries to the GU system in peacetime and war.

S. J. Hudak (✉)
Department of Urology, UT Southwestern Medical Center, Dallas, TX, USA
e-mail: Steven.Hudak@utsouthwestern.edu

D. W. Callaway, J. L. Burstein (eds.), *Operational and Medical Management of Explosive and Blast Incidents*, https://doi.org/10.1007/978-3-030-40655-4_33

Historical Perspective

Severe blast injury sustained during the Civil War was uniformly fatal; thus, no information about GU injuries sustained during that era are available. During the twentieth century, battlefield injury data collection was not standardized, and thus the few publications pertaining to GU trauma from World War I, World War II, the Korean War, and the Vietnam War were based on the case series of individual surgeons and/or hospitals [1]. As a result, little is known about the evolution in blast-related GU injury care during this dynamic period in which innovations in medical and surgical care would see the mortality rate from combat injuries fall precipitously [2]. However, despite limitations in the data acquired across this large span of time, available data suggested that GU trauma was relatively rare overall (0.7–8% of all casualties) and that the frequency of injury to the external genitalia increased during World War II and the Vietnam War, where increased troop mobility elevated the risk of blast injury from explosive devices encountered while on foot [1, 3].

Another important shift in the distribution of GU injuries occurred by the end of the twentieth century. During the first Gulf War (1991), renal injuries had become even less common, and genital injuries were observed more frequently [4, 5]. While the true cause of this shift is not entirely clear, some authors hypothesized that Kevlar® body armor (the use of which had become widespread among US ground forces) afforded protection to internal urologic organs but not the more exposed external genitalia [4]. Detailed data on the initial and long-term management of blast-related GU injuries remained virtually nonexistent.

During the twenty-first-century US involvement in Iraq and Afghanistan, a number of factors converged which ultimately resulted in the frequency of blast-related GU injuries increasing to a level never before reported in the history of war. The high risk of mortality from dismounted complex blast injury (DCBI, defined as blast injury to a dismounted troop resulting in multiple extremity amputations, pelvic fractures, and extensive genital/perineal wounds [2]) was largely mitigated by advances in combat casualty care, thus improving the survival of complex blast injuries which in previous conflicts were uniformly fatal [2]. As a direct consequence, an unprecedented number of US service members (SMs) survived complex explosive polytrauma only to face the challenges of recovery from catastrophic blast-related GU injuries which in prior conflicts were not survivable. Given the increased frequency and unique complexity of GU injuries observed by military physicians during OIF/OEF, several investigators have queried Department of Defense data sources to report the epidemiology and clinical picture of GU injuries observed during this era [6–11].

In 2007, Paquette identified 98 GU injuries among 76 patients from a group of 2712 US SMs and coalition forces injured in Iraq (2.8%). Half of the patients were injured by explosions, and genital and/or urethral injuries comprised 55% of all GU injuries [10]. Later in the conflict, Serkin et al. published a report on 819 US SMs with 887 GU injuries, 90% of which were sustained in Iraq with the remainder sustained in Afghanistan. Explosive mechanisms injured 65.3% of the patients and genital injuries comprised 53% overall [11].

As strategic focus shifted toward Afghanistan, dismounted maneuvers were more common, placing SMs at risk for injury from ground-based explosive munitions resulting in an increased frequency of DCBI. Banti et al. were the first to report Department of Defense Trauma Registry (DoDTR) data after this shift occurred. They reviewed military electronic health records to confirm combat-related genital and/or urethral injury(ies) in 501 men among 890 SMs with GU injuries identified in the DoDTR. Explosive mechanisms predominated, and 96% of patients sustained concomitant non-GU injuries, most commonly limb amputation (36%), soft tissue injury (18%), and fractures (17%), thus illustrating the high complexity of explosive battlefield GU polytrauma [6].

After the formal conclusion of Operation Iraqi Freedom and Operation Enduring Freedom, Janak et al. published a comprehensive review of the DoDTR for GU injuries, representing the largest series of military GU injuries ever reported. During the 12 years analyzed, nearly 30,000 US SMs had injury codes available for review. Among them 1462 (5.3%) US SMs sustained 1 or more GU injuries. All but 20 were male and 75 of the SMs died of their wounds. Among the 1367 male survivors, 88.6% of injuries were sustained in battle, 74.1% were caused by an explosive mechanism, and 1000 (73.2%) had at least 1 injury to the external genitalia. GU injuries were classified as severe in 502 men (36.7%) [8].

Severe polytraumatic injury was common among male survivors of GU injury with 62.1% having an injury severity score (ISS) of 16 or higher. Comorbid injuries of interest included colorectal injury in 21.7%, pelvic fracture in 25.0%, traumatic brain injury in 40.2%, and extremity amputation(s) in 31.7%. Amputations of the lower extremities only were the most common (19.4%), but 3.4% of men sustained upper extremity amputation(s) only, and 8.9% had both upper and lower extremity amputations [8, 9]. Amputation level was through or above the knee in the majority of men with the combination of GU injuries and lower extremity amputation (300 of 387, 77.5%) [9]. Finally, men with severe GU injury had higher rates of ISS $\geq$ 16, colorectal injury, pelvic fracture, and lower extremity amputation [8], suggesting that the complexity of GU injury is a surrogate for overall injury severity.

The recently published reports on contemporary battlefield GU injury discussed above provide a robust account of the frequency and severity of GU injuries caused by blast mechanisms on the modern battlefield. While no previous studies have evaluated the long-term outcomes following GU injury in this setting, prospective evaluation of this large cohort of men is underway [8] and will hopefully provide much needed information on this topic.

Clinical Management of Casualties

Internal GU Injury: Kidney, Ureter, Bladder

As discussed above, injuries to the internal GU organs comprise the minority of combat GU injuries in contemporary conflicts. However, when blast mechanisms result in internal GU injury, management priorities are essentially no different than when similar injuries result from other penetrating or blunt mechanisms: hemostasis, urinary drainage/diversion, early reconstruction (if possible), and delayed reconstruction (when necessary). With the exception of high-grade renal injury, GU injuries are not immediately life-threatening; therefore, each of these principles must be followed in the context of overarching damage control and casualty evacuation principles.

Renal injuries, regardless of mechanism, are most often successfully managed with close observation and serial imaging [12, 13]. Rationale behind a nonoperative approach is that most renal injuries heal without consequence or less commonly require only endoscopic or angiographic procedures for delayed urinary extravasation or ongoing hemorrhage. Thus, the most likely outcome of avoiding exploration is renal preservation. Conversely, renal exploration most commonly results in nephrectomy [13]. Unfortunately, no series have specifically evaluated management strategies or outcomes after renal injury from blast mechanisms. Therefore, it is most reasonable to cautiously apply non-blast injury data to such patients, namely, observing stable renal injury patients, applying minimally invasive techniques when needed for hemorrhage or ongoing urinary extravasation, and exploring unstable patients, those with ureteropelvic junction disruption, and any other patients with concerning findings during laparotomy (expanding retroperitoneal hematoma, large retroperitoneal soft tissue defects, etc.). However, the trauma surgeon should tailor this approach to each patient based on the availability of local resources (i.e., angiography, urology) and the potential for prolonged infield care and/or distant aeromedical evacuation, taking a more aggressive surgical approach when resources are limited and/or a long delay to tertiary care is anticipated.

Ureteral injuries account for fewer than 3% of GU injuries and less than 1% of all injuries sustained in either civilian [14] or military [8] settings. When encountered, ureteral injuries are invariably associated with complex polytrauma [15] and thus are often undiagnosed until complications from urinary extravasation and/or obstruction occur. When recognized at the time of laparotomy, simple ureteral lacerations and transections without tissue loss should be primarily repaired over a stenting ureteral catheter [16]. When blast injuries result in more extensive ureteral loss, temporary urinary diversion can be achieved by externalizing a ureteral catheter or pediatric (5 to 8 Fr) feeding tube after advancing one end into the renal pelvis via the proximal ureteral defect, secured with a ligature at the level of the defect [16]. This straightforward, efficient maneuver prevents urinary extravasation and facilitates urinary collection until surgical resources and patient stability permit definitive ureteral reconstruction. Ureteral injuries diagnosed after abdominal closure are best treated percutaneously (drainage of the kidney *and* any associated urinoma) until the patient is fit for definitive reconstruction [16].

Bladder injuries account for approximately 5% of contemporary combat GU injuries [8]. Intraperitoneal bladder injuries should be closed in two layers (absorbable suture) and drained with a urethral catheter regardless of mechanism [16]. Extraperitoneal bladder injuries from explosive mechanisms are likely to be associated with complex pelvic polytrauma (open pelvic fracture, rectal and/or vaginal injury, bladder neck and/or urethral injury, extensive soft tissue loss, etc.) and thus should be also be repaired, in contrast to extraperitoneal injuries from blunt trauma which typically heal after 1–2 weeks of simple catheter drainage [16]. All patients with pelvic blast injury should have long-term urology follow-up as complex pelvic trauma can result in poor bladder compliance and/or urinary incontinence, even if the bladder seemed uninjured at the time of initial injury staging. Unfortunately, there are no published data which detail long-term bladder function after pelvic blast injury.

External GU Injury: Urethra and External Genitalia

In isolation, complex genital injury is not life-threatening. Therefore, genital injury management must adhere to damage control principles, while comorbid life-threatening injuries are initially staged and managed. Urinary drainage must be established as soon as possible [17]. If disfiguring genital injuries preclude successful passage of a transurethral catheter, a suprapubic cystostomy should be placed either percutaneously or in an open manner at the time of trauma laparotomy. A 16 French Foley or Malecot catheter placed through a small cystostomy in the anterior bladder wall, secured with an absorbable purse-string suture, and brought out through a separate stab incision in the lower abdomen provides prompt, safe bladder drainage. Concomitant bladder rupture is not uncommon and can be ruled out with plain film or CT cystography if not adequately evaluated intraoperatively.

Once urinary drainage is established, genital injuries should be irrigated with copious low-pressure saline solution, especially when blast mechanisms lead to extensive wound contamination. Any actively bleeding vessels can be ligated or fulgurated, although significant hemorrhage is rare given the small caliber of genital end arteries. Extensive debridement should be avoided at this time, given the difficult to replace nature of the genital structures (i.e., phallus, clitoris, testis). The genital wound can then be packed with moist gauze secured with a mesh undergarment while the patient is further resuscitated.

On secondary operative evaluation, comprehensive genital injury staging must be completed [18]. After dressing takedown, low-pressure irrigation is repeated, and each genital structure is examined. For males, this includes the paired corporal bodies, the pendulous and bulbar urethra, each testicle/spermatic cord, and the genital skin and soft tissue. The lithotomy position is helpful, especially when the wound extends toward the anorectal complex and posterior perineum. Each injured structure is assessed for continuity and viability. Corporal lacerations are closed with 2-0 polydioxanone suture. Urethral injuries are realigned over a Foley catheter and closed with 4-0 polydioxanone suture. Simple testicular lacerations are closed with 4-0 polyglactin suture after debriding any necrotic or protuberant seminiferous tubules. Large defects in the capsule of the testis (tunica albuginea) can be restored with a small graft of parietal tunica vaginalis, secured with 4-0 polyglactin suture [16]. Orchiectomy is appropriate for unilateral testicular injuries deemed non-salvageable. However, even a small remnant of the body of one testicle can maintain androgen function and thus preclude the need for long-term testosterone replacement. When orchiectomy is needed, the cord should be suture-ligated in two separate packets with 0 or 2-0 polyglactin suture. An attempt at sperm salvage can be considered if the abundant necessary resources are available [17, 19].

Once the deep genital structures are fully staged, the skin and soft tissue are assessed. Simple injuries can be closed in layers over one or several surgical drains. Blast injuries are usually contaminated with dirt and debris and may be associated with extensive tissue loss. Therefore, heroic attempts at full tissue coverage are not appropriate in the acute setting [18]. Rather, a vacuum-assisted wound dressing can be applied which simplifies wound care compared to traditional gauze dressings.

The interval of wound reevaluation will depend greatly upon the complexity of both the genital and comorbid injuries. Blast injuries with extensive contamination and questionable tissue viability may require daily or every-other-day reevaluation in the operating room [18]. With each examination under anesthesia, low-pressure wound irrigation is repeated and tissue viability is reassessed. Deep debridement of the glans penis, urethra, and corporal bodies should be avoided as the tissues are highly vascularized, resistant to infection, and difficult (if not impossible) to replace. However, clearly necrotic genital tissues should be debrided when necessary to prevent secondary infection. The vacuum-assisted dressing is then replaced and the cycle is repeated until the wound has stabilized and granulation tissue has formed.

Once the wound has stabilized and adequate granulation tissue has formed, genital reconstruction can ensue. A comprehensive discussion of reconstructive surgery after complex genital injury is beyond the scope of this chapter but has been summarized in a recent review [20]. There are, however, several broad principles which should be considered by trauma care teams. When the deep genital structures are preserved, split-thickness skin grafts (STSGs) are preferred for wound coverage and initial reconstruction. Thick (0.016″), non-meshed STSGs provide excellent cosmetic and functional outcomes for penile skin replacement, while thinner (0.010″) STSGs meshed 1:1.5 are preferred for scrotal and perineal reconstruction. Urethral injuries not addressed acutely or delayed complications of urethral injuries (such as stenosis or fistula) are repaired in one or more stages, depending on injury severity and degree of urethral, paraurethral, and perineal tissue loss.

Partial penile amputations should be circumferentially grafted to maintain a phallic shape as even a foreshortened phallus can maintain a male habitus, permit voiding from a standing position, and even provide erogenous sensation once healed. Complete penile loss is rare [8] but can be restored with either a radial artery-based forearm free flap [21] or pedicled flap from the anterolateral thigh [22]. Unfortunately, men with genital blast injury frequently have concomitant upper and/or lower extremity injury(ies) and/or amputation(s) [9], thus limiting potential flap donor sites. Additionally, outcome data after flap-based penile reconstruction in the blast-injured population are essentially nonexistent [21]. Penile allotransplantation is an investigational option for complete phallic replacement [23–25]. However, to date, there have been only four successful penile transplantations performed worldwide, three of which were performed for penile loss after iatrogenic or oncologic etiologies [23, 26]. Men who sustain penile blast injuries are profoundly different, both locally (due to the direct effects of the blast injury on the recipient urethral, corporal, and vascular beds) and systemically (due to the high prevalence of comorbid amputations, colorectal injury, traumatic brain injury, and prior blood transfusions) [8]. Thus, the future of penile transplantation for men with complex blast-related genital injury remains uncertain.

Beyond the obvious surgical needs created by GU blast injury, there are a multitude of long-term functional problems that complicate GU blast injury which necessitate long-term multidisciplinary care. These include erectile dysfunction (and other sexual problems for the patient and his/her sexual partner(s)), urinary obstruction and/or incontinence, infertility, hypogonadism, and mental health problems. Urology referral is mandatory even for patients in whom the acute injury was managed without urologist assistance as urologists are best equipped to manage the above problems either independently (i.e., urethral stricture, low testosterone, male factor infertility) or in collaboration with other specialists (i.e., gynecology, reproductive endocrinology, clinical health psychology, sexual health and intimacy counseling). Comprehensive post-GU injury care can help ensure survivors of complex GU blast injury maximize their functional recovery and long-term overall quality of life.

Conclusion

Improved survival after complex blast injury has led to unprecedented numbers of casualties surviving with complex GU injuries. A systematic approach to the evaluation, early surgical management, delayed surgical reconstruction, and long-term functional rehabilitation is essential to ensure GU functions are restored and quality of life is maximized.

Pitfalls
- Failing to adequately stage each GU structure following blast injury to the pelvis/perineum
- Overaggressive debridement of genital soft tissue after blast injury, resulting in excessive loss of unique, difficult to replace structures
- Failing to initiate the long-term multidisciplinary care required to restore urinary, sexual, and reproductive functions after GU blast injury

Conflict of Interest The author declares no conflicts of interest.

References

1. Hudak SJ, Morey AF, Rozanski TA, Fox CW Jr. Battlefield urogenital injuries: changing patterns during the past century. Urology. 2005;65(6):1041–6.
2. Cannon JW, Hofmann LJ, Glasgow SC, Potter BK, Rodriguez CJ, Cancio LC, et al. Dismounted complex blast injuries: a comprehensive review of the modern combat experience. J Am Coll Surg. 2016;223(4):652–64 e8. https://doi.org/10.1016/j.jamcollsurg.2016.07.009.

3. Wettlaufer JN, Weigel JW. Urology in the Vietnam war: casualty management and lessons learned. Washington, DC: Borden Institute, Office of the Surgeon General, US Army; 2005.
4. Thompson IM, Flaherty SF, Morey AF. Battlefield urologic injuries: the Gulf War experience. J Am Coll Surg. 1998;187(2):139–41.
5. Abu-Zidan FM, Al-Tawheed A, Ali YM. Urologic injuries in the Gulf War. Int Urol Nephrol. 1999;31(5):577–83.
6. Banti M, Walter J, Hudak S, Soderdahl D. Improvised explosive device-related lower genitourinary trauma in current overseas combat operations. J Trauma Acute Care Surg. 2016;80(1):131–4. https://doi.org/10.1097/TA.0000000000000864.
7. Hudak SJ, Hakim S. Operative management of wartime genitourinary injuries at Balad Air Force Theater Hospital, 2005 to 2008. J Urol. 2009;182(1):180–3. https://doi.org/10.1016/j.juro.2009.02.150.
8. Janak JC, Orman JA, Soderdahl DW, Hudak SJ. Epidemiology of genitourinary injuries among male U.S. service members deployed to Iraq and Afghanistan: early findings from the trauma outcomes and urogenital health (TOUGH) project. J Urol. 2017;197(2):414–9. https://doi.org/10.1016/j.juro.2016.08.005.
9. Nnamani NS, Janak JC, Hudak SJ, Rivera JC, Lewis EA, Soderdahl DW, et al. Genitourinary injuries and extremity amputation in operations enduring and iraqi freedom: early findings from the trauma outcomes and urogenital health (tough) project. J Trauma Acute Care Surg. 2016;81:S95. https://doi.org/10.1097/TA.0000000000001122.
10. Paquette EL. Genitourinary trauma at a combat support hospital during operation Iraqi freedom: the impact of body armor. J Urol. 2007;177(6):2196–9. discussion 9
11. Serkin FB, Soderdahl DW, Hernandez J, Patterson M, Blackbourne L, Wade CE. Combat urologic trauma in US military overseas contingency operations. J Trauma. 2010;69(Suppl 1):S175–8. https://doi.org/10.1097/TA.0b013e3181e45cd1.
12. Hadjipavlou M, Grouse E, Gray R, Sri D, Huang D, Brown C, et al. Managing penetrating renal trauma: experience from two major trauma centres in the UK. BJU Int. 2018;121(6):928–34. https://doi.org/10.1111/bju.14165.
13. Keihani S, Xu Y, Presson AP, Hotaling JM, Nirula R, Piotrowski J, et al. Contemporary management of high-grade renal trauma: results from the American Association for the Surgery of Trauma Genitourinary Trauma study. J Trauma Acute Care Surg. 2018;84(3):418–25. https://doi.org/10.1097/TA.0000000000001796.
14. McGeady JB, Breyer BN. Current epidemiology of genitourinary trauma. Urol Clin North Am. 2013;40(3):323–34. https://doi.org/10.1016/j.ucl.2013.04.001.
15. Pereira BM, Ogilvie MP, Gomez-Rodriguez JC, Ryan ML, Pena D, Marttos AC, et al. A review of ureteral injuries after external trauma. Scand J Trauma Resusc Emerg Med. 2010;18:6. https://doi.org/10.1186/1757-7241-18-6.
16. Morey AF, Brandes S, Dugi DD 3rd, Armstrong JH, Breyer BN, Broghammer JA, et al. Urotrauma: AUA guideline. J Urol. 2014;192(2):327–35. https://doi.org/10.1016/j.juro.2014.05.004.
17. Sharma DM, Bowley DM. Immediate surgical management of combat-related injury to the external genitalia. J R Army Med Corps. 2013;159(Suppl 1):i18–20.
18. Williams M, Jezior J. Management of combat-related urological trauma in the modern era. Nat Rev Urol. 2013;10(9):504–12. https://doi.org/10.1038/nrurol.2013.148.
19. Healy MW, Yauger BJ, James AN, Jezior JR, Parker P, Dean RC. Seminal vesicle sperm aspiration from wounded warriors. Fertil Steril. 2016;106(3):579–83. https://doi.org/10.1016/j.fertnstert.2016.05.028.
20. Hudak SJ. Complex genital trauma: lessons learned from operation Iraqi freedom and operation enduring freedom. Curr Trauma Rep. 2017;3(4):278–84. https://doi.org/10.1007/s40719-017-0106-y.

21. Garaffa G, Ralph DJ. Free flap phalloplasty for female to male gender dysphoria. J Sex Med. 2016;13(12):1942–7. https://doi.org/10.1016/j.jsxm.2016.10.004.
22. Gurjala AN, Nazerali RS, Salim A, Lee GK. World's first baby born through natural insemination by father with total phalloplasty reconstruction. Ann Plast Surg. 2016;76(Suppl 3):S179–83. https://doi.org/10.1097/SAP.0000000000000769.
23. Sopko NA, Tuffaha SH, Lough D, Brandacher G, Lee WPA, Bivalacqua TJ, et al. Penile allotransplantation for complex genitourinary reconstruction. J Urol. 2017;198:274. https://doi.org/10.1016/j.juro.2016.10.134.
24. Tuffaha SH, Cooney DS, Sopko NA, Bivalacqua TJ, Lough DM, Cooney CM, et al. Penile transplantation: an emerging option for genitourinary reconstruction. Transpl Int. 2017;30(5):441–50. https://doi.org/10.1111/tri.12928.
25. van der Merwe A, Graewe F, Zuhlke A, Barsdorf NW, Zarrabi AD, Viljoen JT, et al. Penile allotransplantation for penis amputation following ritual circumcision: a case report with 24 months of follow-up. Lancet. 2017;390(10099):1038–47. https://doi.org/10.1016/S0140-6736(17)31807-X.
26. Bateman C. World's first successful penis transplant at Tygerberg Hospital. S Afr Med J. 2015;105(4):251–2.

Management of Orthopedic Blast Injuries

34

Jason P. Welter and Brandon R. Horne

Introduction

With the prolonged combat operations in Iraq and Afghanistan spanning two decades, injury patterns and complexity have changed. Blast injuries account for up to 50–70% of all injuries incurred to both soldiers and civilians in the wartime setting [1–3]. With the advent of body armor, multiple extremity injuries and amputations are a predominate injury pattern. These severe extremity injuries are often accompanied by significant head and facial, lower abdominal, and genitourinary injuries [4]. Complex blast injuries are also being encountered with increasing frequency in terror attacks around the globe. Currently in Afghanistan, 70–80% of these injuries are incurred due to improvised explosive devices (IEDs), rocket-propelled grenades (RPG), land mines, rockets, and mortars [5]. Treatment of these complex injuries, many of which include severe soft tissue and bony injury, requires a team approach. Treatment most often consists of immediate hypotensive resuscitation, external and endovascular hemorrhage control modalities, damage control surgery to include an extensive and thorough irrigation and sharp debridement of open wounds, spanning external fixation for fractures, vacuum-assisted wound closure, and finally definitive repair or reconstruction [6]. Appropriate antibiotic and tetanus prophylaxis must also be administered [5]. Management of musculoskeletal injuries may include immediate amputation for nonviable limbs, initial reduction and external fixation, and the liberal use of fasciotomies to treat and, in some instances, prevent compartment syndrome [7]. Long-term complications such as infection, chronic pain, post-traumatic arthritis, heterotopic ossification, and PTSD still present significant problems that require long-term management. Although ongoing studies continue to collect data to help guide proper management of these injuries, recent studies suggest that good outcomes are possible.

J. P. Welter · B. R. Horne (✉)
Department of Orthopaedics, Wright-State University Boonshoft School of Medicine, Dayton, OH, USA

D. W. Callaway, J. L. Burstein (eds.), *Operational and Medical Management of Explosive and Blast Incidents*, https://doi.org/10.1007/978-3-030-40655-4_34

Pathophysiology of Blast Injury

There are four main mechanisms of blast injury that have been categorized as primary, secondary, tertiary, and quaternary. Primary blast injury to the body occurs as a result of the blast wave moving through an individual's body and interfacing with the body's air/fluid components. Traumatic amputations are rare but typically occur at the mid-shaft of long bones rather than through joint articulations [8]. Although not completely understood, this is thought to be due to the direct coupling of the blast wave into the tissues, resulting in axial stresses to the long bone. The blast wind to the flailing extremity completes the amputation [8, 9].

Secondary blast injury is related to lacerations, abrasions, and penetrating injury due to projectiles propagated from the primary blast. This can include shrapnel, nails, screws, nuts, bolts, or any other material intentionally embedded into the explosive device (primary fragmentation). Secondary fragmentation is related to local material that contacts the individual due to close proximity to airborne material from the blast such as glass, brick, stone, wood, or dirt (Fig. 34.1). Although the penetrating holes from secondary blast particles may be small, the zone of injury may involve a large surface area underneath the skin to include deep tissue, bone,

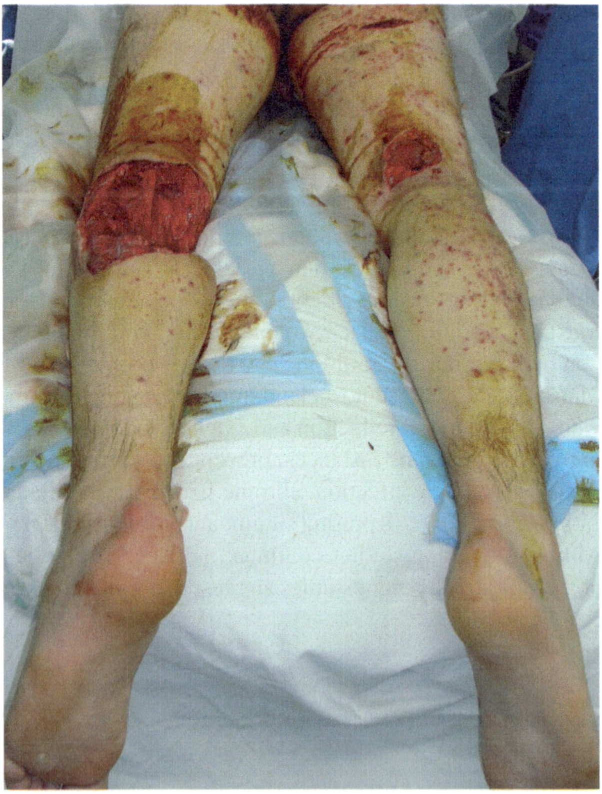

Fig. 34.1 Note small punctate wounds adjacent to larger wounds indicated entry points of dirt driven into the soft tissues from the blast

and joints [8]. These small wounds can contain bits of foreign material that can present an ongoing source of contamination if not properly addressed.

Tertiary blast injury occurs from the individual being propelled into the air and then forcefully coming into contact with a stationary object. This mechanism typically results in blunt force trauma and fracture [8]. Quaternary injury is the result of structural collapse often resulting in severe crush injury. These injuries can also involve significant burns from detonation devices or local fires secondary to explosions. A large combination of orthopedic-related injuries can result from tertiary and quaternary mechanisms, including crush injury, traumatic amputation, compartment syndrome, burns, rhabdomyolysis, and internal degloving (Morel-Lavallee) lesions [8].

Initial Antibiotic Infection Prophylaxis

Severe complex musculoskeletal wounds are the most common sites of injury related to blast events. Up to 15% of extremity blast injuries go on to develop osteomyelitis. Commonly and especially in the case of combat extremity blast injuries, infectious complications often involve multidrug-resistant bacteria [10]. It is notable that bacteria cultured from these contaminated wounds at the time of initial debridement do not correlate with those cultured at the time of infection [11]. The strongest recommendation regarding antibiotic administration related to musculoskeletal blast injuries calls for the antibiotic to be given as early as possible [11]. This involves the administration of a first-generation cephalosporin such as cefazolin within 1 hour. The currently recommended dose for a patient weighing between 81 and 160 kg is 2 g. Repeat dosing should be performed in the initial OR setting if OR time exceeds from 2 to 4 hours or if blood loss exceeds from 1500 to 2000 ml [11].

The routine administration of an aminoglycoside for Gustilo-Anderson grade 3 open fractures has recently become more controversial. A study by Patzakis et al. in 1974 found no significant difference with the use of an aminoglycoside antibiotic and a placebo in preventing infection in open fractures, and the use of a cephalosporin alone was significantly more efficacious than either [12]. Another study in 2007 reported that a large percentage of academic orthopedic surgery programs routinely used aminoglycoside antibiotics for prophylaxis in grade 3 open fractures due to the frequent culture of gram-negative organisms at the time of initial debridement, even though these organisms have been shown to not correlate with cultured microbes at the time of infection [13] This practice of adding aminoglycoside antibiotic administration is based on Gustilo's findings in his 1984 article demonstrating an increased incidence of gram-negative organisms in grade 3 open fractures. However, robust evidence for this recommendation is lacking [11].

The use of intravenous (IV) penicillin for antibiotic prophylaxis against clostridial species has also been commonly used for wounds grossly contaminated with dirt. This recommendation was based on a prominent 1989 study [14]. The serious consequences of such infections, including the historically high incidence of gas gangrene and its associated high mortality rate, once justified the common use of this antibiotic. However, due to recent advances in the expeditious and aggressive management of combat- and blast-related injuries, gas gangrene is very rarely seen. As such, the routine use of IV penicillin in the setting of musculoskeletal blast injuries has become controversial [11]. The use of locally administered antibiotics (topcially applied to the wound bed) has also recently gained popularity in the spine and joint reconstruction and, to a lesser extent, in the trauma literature. However, current evidence is lacking in regard to definitive recommendations on local administration, and further studies are ongoing [11].

Combat- and blast-related invasive fungal infections are another infectious consideration the surgeon must keep in mind. Invasive fungal infections have also been described in the civilian population related to blast injury involving agricultural accidents, natural disasters, and penetrating wounds with environmental debris. Risk factors for combat-related fungal infections include blast injuries occurring in the open, associated above-knee amputations, and large-volume blood transfusions. Diagnosis is confirmed by tissue-based histopathology or fungal cultures. Aggressive surgical debridement is the mainstay of treatment in combination with empiric antifungal therapy consisting of amphotericin B, voriconazole, or fluconazole [15].

Initial Surgical Management

A team approach should be utilized in the surgical management of the blast-injured patient [6]. Because the patient often has multiple organ system injuries, if possible, concurrent surgical procedures with general surgery, vascular surgery, plastic surgery, etc. should be considered in order to avoid prolonged operating room times, prolonged anesthesia, and excessive blood loss. This also facilitates expeditious throughput of patients in a mass casualty situation.

Initial management of musculoskeletal blast injuries focuses on determining the viability of the limb [7]. The spectrum of extremity blast injury can encompass fractures, amputations, crush injuries, burns, abrasions, lacerations, neurovascular injury, and compartment syndrome. Typically, orthopedic surgeons have used the classic Gustilo-Anderson classification system for open fractures (Table 34.1) [16]. However, this system was not originally developed to classify war wounds and massive soft tissue injuries often encompassing multiple extremities. Coupland developed a Red Cross classification of war wounds based on injuries seen and treated

Table 34.1 Gustilo and Anderson classification of open fractures

Grade 1	Puncture wound of less than 1 cm with minimal soft tissue injury
Grade 2	Wound is greater than 1 cm in length; moderate soft tissue injury; soft tissue coverage of bone is adequate with minimal bony comminution
Grade 3a	Extensive soft tissue damage; soft tissue coverage of the bone is adequate; includes massively contaminated and severely comminuted fractures
Grade 3b	Extensive soft tissue damage with periosteal stripping and bone exposure; severely contaminated with bony comminution; flap coverage is required to provide soft tissue coverage
Grade 3c	Associated with an arterial injury requiring repair for limb salvage

throughout the Soviet-Afghan War [17]. Wounds are scored by considering entry and exit sites, the presence of a cavity within the zone of injury, fracture, injury of a vital structure, and/or the presence of a metallic foreign body. The total number of wounds is recorded, although only the two worst wounds are scored (Table 34.2). Although this classification system is quite comprehensive, it has not reached widespread use [6].

Whether amputation or limb salvage is chosen, aggressive soft tissue sharp debridement and irrigation should be performed [5, 18]. It is important to recognize that the zone of injury may extend far beyond what is immediately visible to the surgeon (Fig. 34.2a, b) [5]. This may necessitate extended incisions to fully visualize and assess soft tissue injuries and possible occult traumatic arthrotomies. It is also important to recognize that the injury incurred to the tissues is an evolving process.

Table 34.2 Red Cross EXCFVM wound scores [17]

E (entry)	Entry wound maximum dimension (cm)
X (exit)	Exit wound maximum dimension (cm)
C (cavity)	Wound cavity admits two fingers: C0 = no C1 = yes
F (fracture)	F0 = no fracture F1 = fracture without comminution F2 = fracture with comminution
V (vital structure)	Breach of dura, pleura, peritoneum, or major vessel injury: V0 = no breach V1 = breach
M (metallic body)	M0 = no metallic body M1 = one metallic body M2 = more than one metallic body

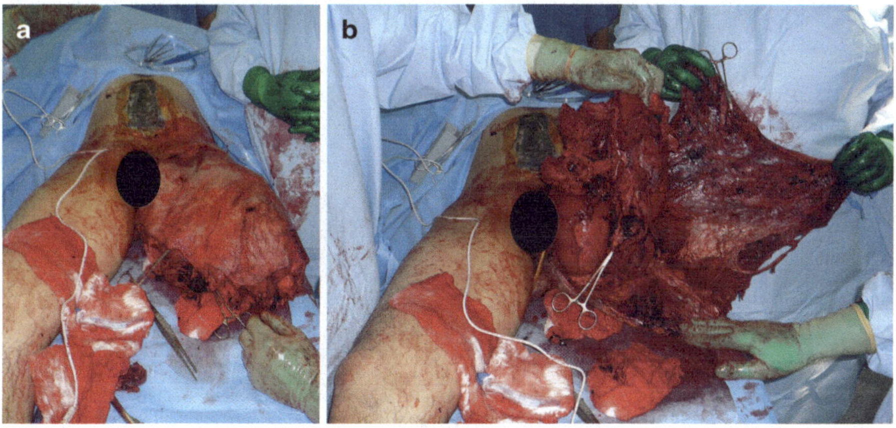

Fig. 34.2 (**a**) Appearance of blast injury with traumatic amputation showing general appearance at presentation. (**b**) The same wound showing significantly large zone of injury than initially apparent. This ultimately required hip disarticulation

As such, this may require multiple trips to the operating room for serial debridement due to the evolving nature of the soft tissue envelope [5, 18]. Grossly contaminated and necrotic tissue should be sharply debrided. Questionable tissue may be left if a return to the OR can be reliably planned to assess for the evolution of necrosis or viability. Copious irrigation with saline with high volume and low flow should be performed. Cystoscopy tubing is preferable to jet irrigation that may push contamination deeper into the tissues. Various different irrigation solutions (castile soap, Betadine, chlorhexidine, Dakin's, antibiotic solution) have been tried; however studies suggest standard saline is likely best. In situations where resources are limited, potable water can be used as a last resort [19, 20]. Bone fragments without soft tissue attachments should be removed from the wound. An exception to this would be large osteoarticular fragments that can be cleaned of gross contamination.

Fasciotomies should be performed to treat impending compartment syndrome. In case of delays due to an injury that occurs in a remote environment, prolonged aeromedical transport to a higher level of care, or with limb revascularization, prophylactic fasciotomies should be strongly considered [7]. However, indiscriminately compartment releases should be avoided as there can be significant morbidity associated with fasciotomies.

If amputation has already occurred or is the decided path of definitive treatment of the injury, it is important to avoid immediate primary closure [6]. Negative pressure vacuum-assisted wound closure devices should be used until the wound is ready for either definitive primary closure or soft tissue reconstruction [6, 21]. It is important to maintain as much viable skin and soft tissue as possible to allow for the greatest length amputation stump as possible. Guillotine amputation stumps should always be avoided [18]! Guillotine amputations result in a retraction of the soft tissues often necessitating revision of the bone cut at a higher level to obtain stump closure (Fig. 34.3). It should also be recognized that traumatic amputations or extremity injuries that go on to require amputations often require atypical soft tissue flaps for closure, again necessitating the need to be judicious with skin and soft

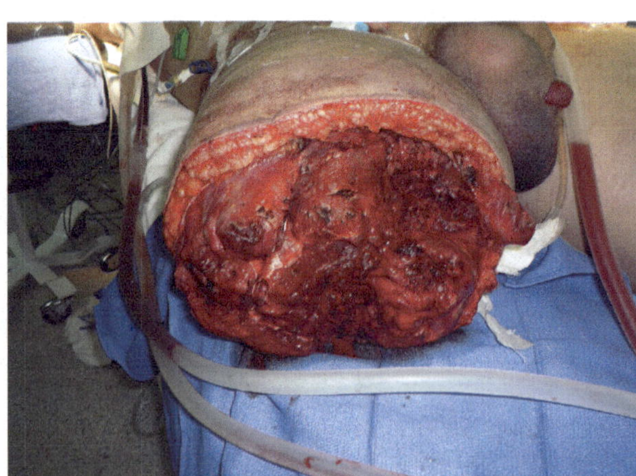

Fig. 34.3 Example of retraction of the soft tissues after open circular (guillotine-type) amputation

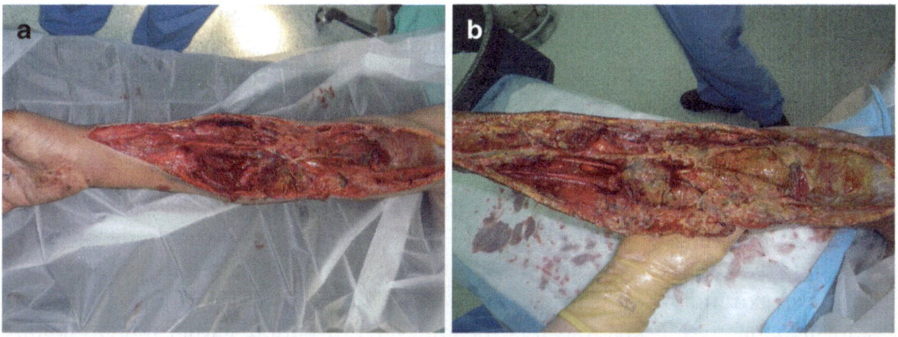

Fig. 34.4 (**a**) Example of evolution of tissue necrosis over the course of 48 hours between operative interventions. (**b**) Appearance of the same wound approximately 48 hours later

tissue retention if viable. In cases where bone is fractured proximal to the level of the traumatic amputation, an attempt should be made to treat the fracture rather than amputating at the higher level to maintain length.

Splinting the amputated limb can help stabilize the injured limb for transport, aid in pain control, and help protect the injured soft tissues. If a limb salvage approach is to be used, fracture stabilization with either an external fixator device, skeletal traction, or splint application is performed [5, 6, 18]. External fixator devices are excellent in these scenarios as they provide excellent stability, can be used for extended periods or even definitive fixation if required, facilitate wound management, and simplify patient transport (as opposed to traction) [7]. There are commercially packaged sterile external fixator systems available which allow for application in austere environments without the aid of fluoroscopy, additional surgical instruments, or power drills.

Segmental bone loss can temporarily be filled with antibiotic cement spacers or beads [6, 18]. Vacuum-assisted wound closure devices are again used for initial management and coverage of soft tissue wounds. Loosely reapproximating tissue over deep vacuum-assisted dressings can help prevent retraction of the soft tissue envelope, while still facilitating drainage. Repeat debridement should be performed every 24–48 hours until the soft tissue envelope has been deemed stable and contamination free. Tissue necrosis and onset of early infection can continue to evolve over several days post-injury (Fig. 34.4a, b). Antibiotic coverage should continue until definitive wound closure has occurred. The duration of antibiotic administration after wound closure is controversial with recommendations ranging from 24 up to 72 hours [10, 11].

Definitive Limb Reconstruction

Once the patient's soft tissue envelope has been thoroughly and completely debrided of all nonviable tissue and bony injuries have been preliminarily stabilized, a plan toward definitive limb reconstruction can be initiated. This often requires a multidisciplinary approach to include the orthopedic surgeon, plastic surgery, and possibly vascular surgery [18]. The reconstruction ladder begins with the simplest procedures being performed first, such as direct delayed primary closure, secondary closure, split-thickness skin grafting, or full-thickness skin grafting [5, 18]. If there is a significant soft tissue defect, depending on its characterization and severity, a number of local and soft tissue free flaps can be performed to obtain wound closure. Latissimus dorsi and rectus abdominis vascularized muscle flaps have greatly contributed to improved outcomes in reconstruction of extremity blast injuries [5]. Early coverage of open fractures within 7–10 days post-injury greatly reduces infection risk [1]. There is a growing trend toward more upper extremity limb salvage than lower extremity limb salvage, an increase in the use of perforator flaps and fasciocutaneous free tissue transfers for limb reconstruction, earlier time to definitive flap reconstruction, and > 95% flap success rate [2]. In some cases, acute shortening of a limb can facilitate wound closure without flaps [18].

Definitive management of fractures secondary to extremity blast injuries is often a complex process requiring multiple procedures. These fractures are often characterized by severe comminution and/or segmental bone loss. The severe nature of the surrounding soft tissue injury which often includes regional soft tissue loss, reduced local vascularity, regional scarring, and high propensity for local infections creates a challenge for the orthopedic surgeon to get these injuries to heal [18]. After initial management with an antibiotic cement spacer or beads accompanied by provisional external fixation and/or splinting, these fractures often require some form of bone grafting in conjunction with definitive internal fixation. Placement of an initial cement spacer creates a highly vascularized pseudomembrane that is rich in osteoinductive signaling factors [18, 22]. Bone grafting options include autograft harvested from the iliac crest or femoral intramedullary bone graft harvested via a reamer/irrigator/aspirator (RIA). Both of these options have their associated advantages and disadvantages [23]. Autologous bone graft is advantageous because it is osteoconductive, is rich in osteoinductive signaling factors, and contains high concentrations of osteogenic cells [23]. These bone graft characteristics are critical with complex extremity blast injuries as the local bone and soft tissue associated with these injuries is often devoid of these properties [18]. Vascularized structural grafting has gained in popularity and is best suited for upper extremity defects [24]. Another option for bone defects that exceed 8 cm in length is distraction osteogenesis via the use of either an external fixator or an intramedullary device [21, 25]. Drawbacks of using an external fixator frame are the prolonged amount of time required to wear the frame during correction of the deformity. The external frame also limits access to the surrounding soft tissues if associated wound coverage procedures are required [21, 26].

If the limb is found to be unsalvageable, treatment should proceed expeditiously to amputation. It is imperative to apply sound surgical principles of amputation such as maintenance of bone length, appropriate myodesis, preservation of soft tissue and skin flaps to allow for tension-free soft tissue closure, and proper management of neurovascular structures. This will maximize the functional potential for the patient during the rehabilitative phase [18]. There is recent evidence to suggest that targeted muscle reinnervation may reduce phantom limb pain and painful neuroma formation and aid in the use of bioprosthetics [27].

Conclusion

Extremity blast injuries are complex injuries that often require a multidisciplinary treatment approach. Involvement of more than one extremity is common. Often, multiple surgical procedures are required in both the initial phase and the definitive phase of management. Extensive research and data collection have occurred over the course of the Iraq and Afghanistan conflicts. This information has helped to guide updated treatment recommendations, improving outcomes. Whether limb salvage or amputation is performed, good outcomes can be obtained for the patient. Surgeon experience should guide which treatment path to take for each individualized patient. Extremity reconstruction is a long process that can span years. Additionally, psychiatric conditions such as PTSD, anxiety, and/or depression should be identified and treated appropriately. Continued research is still needed and ongoing in the treatment of heterotopic ossification, infection prevention and treatment, treatment of post-traumatic arthritis, and identification of risk factors for long-term complications in amputees and limb salvage patients.

Pitfalls

- Do not underestimate the zone or extent of injury.
- Avoid open guillotine-type amputations. Retain as much viable tissue/bone as possible to preserve length.
- Compartment syndrome is common. Fasciotomies should be performed liberally and appropriately. Avoid prophylactic fasciotomies unless tactical situation dictates.
- Early and aggressive sharp surgical debridement of wounds coupled with appropriate early antibiotic therapy can reduce infections. Avoid early closure of wounds!

References

1. Covey DC. Blast and fragment injuries of the musculoskeletal system. J Bone Joint Surg Am. 2002;84:1221–34.
2. Cernak I, Savic J, Ignjatovic D, Jevtic M. Blast injury from explosive munitions. J Trauma. 1999;47:96–103.
3. Savic J. Primary blast injuries. Vojnosanit Pregl. 1991;48:489–98.
4. Dismounted Complex Blast Injury Task Force: Dismounted Complex Blast Injury: Report of the Army Dismounted Complex Blast Injury Task Force. Available at: http://www.dtic.mil/dtic/trt/fulltext/u2/a550676.pdf. Accessed 20 July 2018.
5. Bumbasirevic M, Lesic A, Mitkovic M, Bumbasirevic V. Treatment of blast injuries of the extremity. J Am Acad Orthop Surg. 2006;10(14):S77–81.
6. Covey DC. Combat orthopaedics: a view from the trenches. J Am Acad Orthop Surg. 2006;10(14):S10–7.
7. Pollack P. Wound management, evacuation key in treating battlefield injuries. Available at: https://www.aaos.org/AAOSNow/2007/Jul/research/research3. Accessed 23 July 2018.

8. Born CT, Briggs SM, Ciraulo DL, Frykberg ER, Hammond JS, Hirshberg A, et al. Disasters and mass casualties: II. Explosive, biologic, chemical, and nuclear agents. J Am Acad Orthop Surg. 2007;15(8):461–73.
9. Hull JB, Cooper GJ. Pattern and mechanism of traumatic amputation by explosive blast. J Trauma. 1996;40:S198–205.
10. Murray CK, Obremskey WT, Hsu JR, Andersen RC, Calhoun JH, Clasper JC, et al. Prevention of infections associated with combat-related extremity injuries. J Trauma. 2011;71(2, suppl 2):S235–57.
11. Bible JE, Obremskey WT. Antibiotic prophylaxis in orthopaedic trauma. Available at: https://www.aaos.org/OKOJ/vol10/issue10/TRA045. Accessed 20 July 2018.
12. Patzakis MJ, Harvey JP Jr, Ivler D. The role of antibiotics in the management of open fractures. J Bone Joint Surg Am. 1974;56(3):532–41.
13. Lavelle WF, Uhl R, Krieves M, Drvaric DM. Management of open fractures in adult patients: current teaching in ACGME accredited residency programs. J Surg Orthop Adv. 2007;16(3):111–7.
14. Robinson D, On E, Hadas N, Halperin N, Hofman S, Boldur I. Microbiologic flora contaminating open fractures: its significance in the choice of primary antibiotic agents and the likelihood of deep wound infection. J Orthop Trauma. 1989;3(4):283–6.
15. Tribble DR, Rodriguez CJ. Combat-related invasive fungal wound infections. Curr Fungal Infect Rep. 2014 Dec 1;8(4):277–86.
16. Gustilo RB, Anderson JT. Prevention of infection in the treatment of one thousand and twenty-five open fractures of long bones: retrospective and prospective analyses. J Bone Joint Surg Am. 1976;58:453–8.
17. Coupland RM. The red cross classification of war wounds: the E.X.C.F.V.M. scoring system. World J Surg. 1992;16:910–7.
18. Fleming ME, Watson JT, Gaines RJ, O'Toole RV. Evolution of orthopaedic reconstructive care. J Am Acad Orthop Surg. 2012;20(suppl 1):S74–9.
19. Anglen JO. Wound irrigation in musculoskeletal injury. J Am Acad Orthop Surg. 2001;9(4):219–26.
20. FLOW Investigators. A trial of wound irrigation in the initial management of open fracture wounds. N Engl J Med. 2015;373(27):2629–41.
21. Pollak AN, Ficke JR. Extremity war injuries: challenges in definitive reconstruction. J Am Acad Orthop Surg. 2008;16(11):628–34.
22. Karger C, Kishi T, Schneider L, Fitoussi F, Masquelet AC. Treatment of posttraumatic bone defects by the induced membrane technique. Orthop Traumatol Surg Res. 2012;98(1):97–102.
23. Sagi HC, Young ML, Gerstenfeld L, Einhorn TA, Tornetta P. Qualitative and quantitative differences between bone graft obtained from the medullary canal (with a reamer/irrigator/aspirator) and the iliac crest of the same patient. J Bone Joint Surg Am. 2012;94(23):2128–35.
24. Ring D, Jupiter J, Toh S. Transarticular bony defects after trauma and sepsis: arthrodesis using vascularized fibular transfer. Plast Reconstr Surg. 1999;104:426–34.
25. Oh CW, Song HR, Roh JY, Oh JK, Min WK, Kyung HS, et al. Bone transport over an intramedullary nail for reconstruction of long bone defects in tibia. Arch Orthop Trauma Surg. 2008;128(8):801–8.
26. Paley D. Problems, obstacles, and complications of limb lengthening by the Ilizarov technique. Clin Orthop Relat Res. 1990;250:81–104.
27. Bowen JB, Wee CE, Kalik J, Valerio IL. Targeted muscle reinnervation to improve pain, prosthetic tolerance, and bioprosthetic outcomes in the amputee. Adv Wound Care. 2017;6(8):261–7.

Reconstructive Plastic Surgery for Blast and Burn Injuries

35

Edward J. Caterson and Justin C. McCarty

Introduction

The principles of reconstruction in burn and blast injuries are rooted in the history of plastic surgery as a specialty. In the early twentieth century, Sir Harold Gillies, viewed as the father of modern plastic surgery, performed complex reconstructions for soldiers injured in World War 1 by burn and blast injuries [1]. Blast injuries are a unique type of trauma in the extent and multiplicity of injuries that can occur in each individual patient coupled with the increased risk for infectious complications secondary to wound contamination from fragmentation. The dynamic sequence for successful reconstruction depends on patient resuscitation from the acute insult, early and frequent wound debridement, fracture repair/stabilization, repair of any vascular compromise, and soft tissue coverage, hinging on a collaborative multidisciplinary approach involving trauma, orthopedic, vascular, and plastic surgery teams. In the modern era, the most common causes of blast injuries globally are terrorist attacks, with 54,000 deaths and injuries from 11,800 incidents in 2008 alone [2].

The training pathway for plastic and reconstructive surgeons results in surgeons who can operate from the "head to the toe." Plastic surgeons develop a thorough knowledge of normal anatomy and anatomical relationships that enables them to approach complex injuries for which there is not a set template for repair. This full-body management additionally means that plastic surgeons' work crosses, and is integrative of, multiple different specialties.

E. J. Caterson (✉)
Division of Plastic and Reconstructive Surgery, Brigham and Women's Hospital, Boston, MA, USA
e-mail: ecaterson@partners.org

J. C. McCarty
Center for Surgery and Public Health, Brigham and Women's Hospital, Boston, MA, USA

D. W. Callaway, J. L. Burstein (eds.), *Operational and Medical Management of Explosive and Blast Incidents*, https://doi.org/10.1007/978-3-030-40655-4_35

This chapter discusses the role of the plastic surgeon in managing burn and blast injuries via the lens of the experience of the author's institution, Brigham and Women's Hospital, during the Boston Marathon bombing. This mass casualty incident resulted in 3 dead on the scene and 281 total injured patients from the explosion of two pressure cooker improvised explosive devices (IEDs) near the finish line of the race [3]. There were 127 major limb injuries, and of these 31 were major exsanguinating extremity wounds frequently complicated with heavy contamination [4, 5]. The IED detonation resulted in a predominance of lower extremity injuries from its ground-level location and high fragmentation burden from component projectiles. There was a localized thermal radius resulting in some burns. However, the heavy contamination of wounds from street-level dust, garbage, and biologic material, including human debris causing fragmentation injury, created more clinical impact. The distribution of injuries for patients admitted to the hospital predominantly included injuries to the lower extremities, though as is the nature of blast injuries, many patients had multiple injuries to various parts of their body. Surgical response to this type of explosive mass casualty incident requires many of the same principles learned on the battlefield, while also exposing the differences between civilian and military burn and blast injuries.

Brief Overview of Soft Tissue Blast Injury

The types and patterns of injuries to bone and soft tissue in blasts are dictated both by the type of explosive device and the proximity to the epicenter of the explosion [6]. The categories of injury that occur in blast injuries are classified as primary, secondary, tertiary, quaternary, and quinary (Table 35.1) [7]. In the Marathon bombing, there were a significant number of individuals injured via the shock wave (primary blast injury) and had ruptured tympanic membranes, often described as occurring in up to half of patients injured in explosions, and concussions [8, 9]. However, the degree of primary blast injury that occurred was less than that seen in the military and terrorist attacks in the Middle East due to the difference in munitions used by the assailant [9]. During the Marathon bombing, the largest source of morbidity and mortality, requirement for hospitalization, and operative procedures arose from device and biologic fragmentation (secondary blast injury). The extent of contamination of wounds in the Marathon bombing was significant and included fragmentation of human bone and soft tissue causing injury to other victims. The wound contamination that occurred is the "rule rather than the exception" in blast injuries resulting from the blast advancing contamination beyond the margins of the visible wound [10]. The power of the explosive device used primarily dictates the extent of acceleration/deceleration injury that occurs (tertiary blast injury). Burning and toxic exposure (quaternary blast injury) was not significant in the bombing as the device used was not incendiary in nature. The degree of quinary blast injury from contamination radiation contamination or toxic metal exposure did not play a large role at the Marathon bombing.

Table 35.1 Department of Defense classification of blast injuries

	Definition and causative agent	Common injuries	Boston Marathon experience
Primary	Blast wave/overpressure injury Direct tissue damage from shock wave Air-filled organs at highest risk	Tympanic membrane (TM) rupture Blast lung Hollow viscera perforation/hemorrhage Ocular globe injuries Concussion	+++ TM rupture
Secondary	*Primary fragments* → from exploding device *Secondary fragments* → from the environment (rocks, glass, biologic material including human)	Lacerations Penetrating injury Soft tissue injury including amputations Ocular injury	+++ lower extremity injuries +++ human to human contamination
Tertiary	Acceleration/deceleration of body onto nearby objects or objects onto individual	Blunt trauma Traumatic amputation Crush injury	Minimal
Quaternary	Burning components and toxic exposure	Burns Inhalational injury	Minimal
Quinary	Clinical consequences of post detonation environmental contaminants (bacteria, metals, radiation)	Radiation Sepsis	Minimal

Collaborative Team Approach to Management

When a patient survives past the initial blast and burn trauma, the view of those treating the patient should be that these patients will have to manage a lifetime with their injuries. The choices that the treatment team makes during the acute period affect the patients for the rest of their lives [11]. Studies of patients who suffer a burn injury has shown that even 10 years after the burn, patients have low heat sensitivity, affect, body image, and often do not return to work, supporting the conclusion that burns, and likely blast injuries which share many injury characteristics, are chronic conditions [11–13]. The patients may suffer various unique functional deficits secondary to their injury. It is this chronicity that reinforces the importance of the early team approach to management of these patients. The patients treated at the author's institution, as well as neighboring hospitals, after the Marathon bombing were all managed collaboratively by trauma, orthopedic, vascular, and plastic surgery (Fig. 35.1) [14, 15]. At Brigham and Women's Hospital, the plastic surgery service performed the most operations of any of these services and accounted for the most hospital days for the patients, reflecting the complexity of managing these

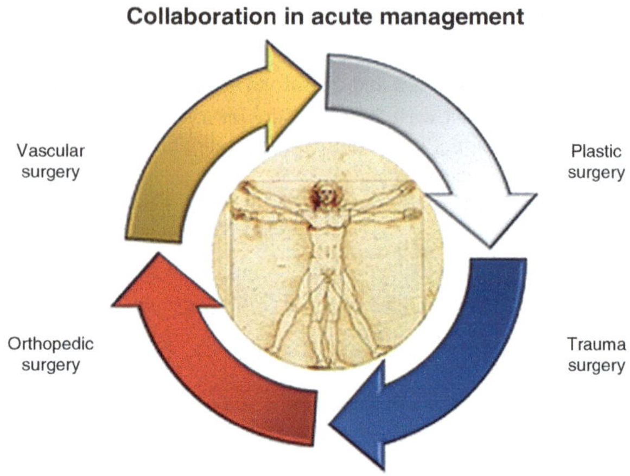

Fig. 35.1 Early and frequent collaboration between services is key to achieving good outcomes in burn and blast injuries given the complexity of injuries that occur

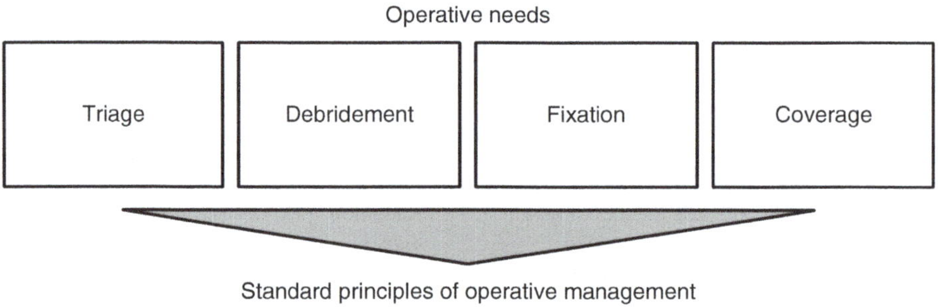

Fig. 35.2 The standard principles of operative management for burn and blast injuries follow the sequence of initial triage and prioritization of life- and then limb-threatening injuries, debridement of devitalized and contaminated tissue, fixation, and adequate tissue coverage of the injury

injuries. This interplay between teams allows for each specialty to play to their strengths in order to attain the best outcome for the patient.

Beyond the surgical teams, early involvement of social work and physical and occupational therapy specialists can help patients to adjust and adapt to their injuries [16]. Just as these patients require complex surgical care for their wounds, they require equally high-level care in their rehabilitation to aid in management of pain, stress disorders, and other deficits following the injury [17].

Initial Management of Blast Injuries

The principles of trauma, as described in earlier chapters, continue to play a key role in management of blast injury reconstruction. Adherence of these principles is key to the success of reconstructive procedures. This requires a multidisciplinary collaborative approach beginning early in the patient's hospitalization to increase the likelihood of optimal outcomes (Fig. 35.2). The components of reconstruction include fracture stabilization, evaluation and repair of injured vascular structures, an emphasis on aggressive early and serial debridement, and soft tissue coverage once the wound bed is clean of contamination [10].

It is accepted that all blast-injured patients should have early broad-spectrum antibiotic administration to reduce the risk of infection. But the most important component in infection prevention is adequate source control via early and serial debridement of devitalized and contaminated tissue [18]. The importance of adequate tissue debridement is paramount to the success of any reconstruction [19]. In the case of blast injuries, the secondary blast injury results in more extensive contamination of wounds than is typically seen in injuries from other forms of trauma as the blast pressure forces result in transfer of high kinetic energy, pushing fragments deep into tissues and disrupting fascial planes [20, 21]. This level of kinetic injury transfer also results in occult tissue damage and requires the exploration and debridement of injuries with openings less than 2 cm. Taken within the context of each individual case, other indications for operative debridement include all wounds associated with fractures or traumatic arthrotomy, those penetrating fascia, pleura, peritoneum, and vascular structures [19].

In ideal circumstances, initial debridement should occur early, with guidelines supporting that patients with open fractures should have operative debridement within 6 hours of injury. This ideal timing must be adjusted when other major injuries have occurred which take precedence. Wounds further may require take-back to the operating room as frequently as every 24 hours. In the Boston Marathon bombing, many of the patients underwent multiple serial debridements before they underwent their final reconstructive procedure.

The extent of debridement is guided by the patient's physiologic status and the likelihood of wound salvage. Debridement should proceed in an organized fashion, removing all foreign material and nonviable tissue, including all nonviable skin, subcutaneous tissue, fascia, and muscle via sharp excision. Determination of muscle viability during the procedure is best elucidated via its consistency and contractility. Bone fragments that lack their periosteum or soft tissue attachments should also be debrided. Wounds should then be irrigated with warm sterile fluid. Most often this can be normal saline, though in recent years 0.0125% Dakin's solution has been increasingly used because of its antifungal and antibacterial properties [10, 19]. A benefit of early involvement of a plastic surgeon in the care of the patient at the stage of first debridement is their ability to recognize reconstruction options stemming from "spare parts" surgery [22]. Spare parts reconstruction involves recognizing injuries that are in themselves non-salvageable but could be used as a source for reconstruction to provide wound coverage to other injuries via immediate tissue transplantation. The example demonstrating this principle from the Marathon bombing comes from a patient who had a non-salvageable foot from his injuries but was further at risk of needing an above-the-knee amputation due to more proximal injuries (Fig. 35.3). Patients who use prosthetic with an above-the-knee amputation expend significantly more energy ambulating and are slower than patients who undergo below-the-knee

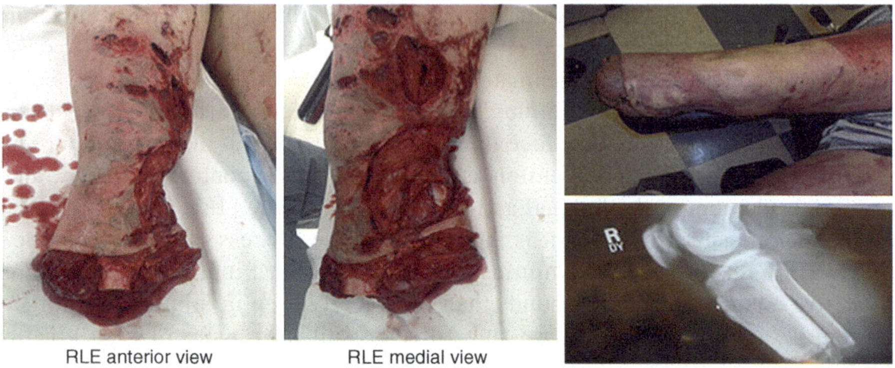

Fig. 35.3 This patient had traumatic amputation of his lower extremity and was at risk of needing an above-knee amputation. His foot which had been amputated in the explosion was used as "spare part" to provide tissue coverage to enable the patient to have a more functional below-knee amputation

amputations [23]. In this case, surgeons used the foot as a composite graft to provide wound coverage for the exposed tibia and the patient, allowing the patient to eventually be fitted with a prosthetic for his below-knee amputation.

Bridges and Adjuncts to Definitive Reconstruction

Negative-pressure wound therapy (NPWT) allows for temporary coverage of complex wounds, and there is increasing experience in its use for blast injuries [24, 25]. NPWT reduces edema in the wound, increases granulation tissue and promotes angiogenesis, and contracts the wound surface area [10]. NPWT can be further augmented with antibiotic delivery mechanisms and addition of silver to the porous sponges to decrease bacterial load and potentially infection rates [26]. However, there is limited evidence to definitively show the significant benefit of these adjuncts to NPWT on clinical outcomes such as infection rate, wound closure, and limb salvage [27, 28]. NPWT reduces the risk of infection and can simplify the reconstruction needed it can increase the take rate of skin grafts, skin substitutes, and composite grafts and allow fast graft incorporation, but it does not preclude the need for providing definitive soft tissue coverage [28, 29].

There are multiple *dermal substitutes* available that can be used to provide coverage of de-epithelized wounds. Full review of all available dermal substitutes and their properties is beyond the scope of this chapter. However, examples include a bilayer acellular dermal matrix which acts as a scaffold for tissue ingrowth and a bilayered living tissue-engineered cellular matrix of bovine type 1 collage with human neonatal foreskin fibroblasts [30]. Within the context of trauma, the materials are most prominently used in burn wounds after excision and grafting and are contraindicated in infected wounds. There is observational level III data to support their use in blast injury patients to provide dermal coverage early in the process [30, 31].

It is important to note that they should not be used as substitute for adequate debridement of devitalized or infected tissue. The example from the Marathon bombing involved a patient who had early Apligraf application but quickly developed a pseudomonal infection due to the wound bed not being debrided adequately prior to graft placement, thus, reinforcing the importance of adequate source control with sequential debridement prior to even the simplest of reconstructive attempts.

Reconstruction

The approach to the reconstruction of blast and burn injuries should follow the same principles as those applied to other types of reconstruction in trauma. The caveat being that this must be tailored to each individual patient, and the timing of reconstruction may vary from what is recommended in other types of trauma. The traditional teaching when initially approaching an individual case is to begin at the simplest level of reconstruction and work up from the reconstructive ladder. At the first rung is wound closure via secondary intention. Working up the ladder, the next steps are primary closure, split-thickness skin graft, local skin flaps, pedicle flaps, and finally free flaps. In blast injuries, it is often more appropriate to apply the reconstructive ladder, a term referring to the ability of the surgeon to decide to ascend directly to the appropriate level of treatment to meet the individual patient's needs [32–34].

The timing of reconstruction is a complex decision in victims of blast trauma. Traditional orthopedic trauma teaching espouses that fractures with open wounds should have soft tissue coverage within 72 hours, a guideline rooted in the seminal work of Godina in 1973 [35]. These recommendations primarily were made with traditional trauma patients and do not always generalize to the blast and burn injuries with their heavier contamination [36]. Depending on the individual case scenario, it may be more important to delay reconstruction and soft tissue coverage until adequate debridement and wound stabilization have occurred.

For complex extremity wounds from blast injuries, the competing choices are amputation versus limb salvage [37]. Early involvement of the reconstructive plastic surgeon may increase the limb salvage rate [14]. It is important to properly select patients for limb salvage. However, there are no definitive criteria for amputation versus salvage that apply to all potential scenarios. Multiple scoring systems are available, including Mangled Extremity Severity Score (MESS); the Limb Salvage Index (LSI); the Predictive Salvage Index (PSI); the Nerve Injury, Ischemia, Soft-Tissue Injury, Skeletal Injury, Shock, and Age of Patient Score (NISSSA); and the Hannover Fracture Scale-97 (HFS-97) for ischemic and nonischemic limbs [38, 39]. While these multiple scoring systems exist and can inform the surgeon's decisions, none are capable of providing definitive guidelines for the surgeon on which limbs should be salvaged and to what degree functional recovery to be expected.

Overall, risk factors for amputation put forth by the American College of Surgeons Committee on Trauma include [40]:

- Gustilo III-C injuries (comminuted, open tibial fractures with vascular disruption)
- Sciatic or tibial nerve or two of the three upper extremity nerves, anatomically transected
- Prolonged ischemia (greater than 4–6 hours)/muscle necrosis
- Crush or destructive soft tissue injury
- Significant wound contamination
- Multiple/severely comminuted fractures/segmental bone loss
- Old age/severe comorbidity
- Lower versus upper extremity
- Apparent futility of revascularization/failed revascularization

This complex choice in management is further complicated by evidence from the Lower Extremity Assessment Project (LEAP) study in 2010 which showed that functional outcomes between those undergoing salvage and those who underwent amputation were not significantly different [41]. It must be reinforced that the sequelae of the injury and reconstruction choices will become part of the chronic condition with which the patient will live.

In the case of primary amputation, there are reconstructive procedures that can improve the patient's long-term outcomes. In addition to the use of spare parts surgery to minimize the extent of amputation required, as discussed previously, recently developed adjuncts to limb amputation are the Ewing amputation and targeted muscle reinnervation. The Ewing amputation enables patients to have significantly increased proprioception of their prosthetic leg as well as being able to better interface with robotic prosthetics and have a near-normal gait [42, 43]. Targeted reinnervation transfers transected peripheral nerves in the amputated extremity to recipient motor nerves of residual muscle. This technique can help prevent the peripheral neuropathy and phantom limb pain that otherwise often accompanies extremity amputation as well as increases control of advanced myoelectric prosthetics [44]. Regardless of whether limb salvage or amputation is performed, adequate soft tissue coverage is essential in these cases [10]. The choice of soft tissue coverage is dictated by the location of the zone of injury and donor site availability [10]. Additionally, whether the optimum flap is free versus pedicled or muscle versus fasciocutaneous is controversial [45]. A collaborative team approach that thus takes in all available clinical and technical factors is important to make the proper choice in reconstruction. It is not just in limb salvage that soft tissue coverage is essential. Free flap reconstruction can also provide coverage of the amputation stump to facilitate prosthetic fitting (Fig. 35.4).

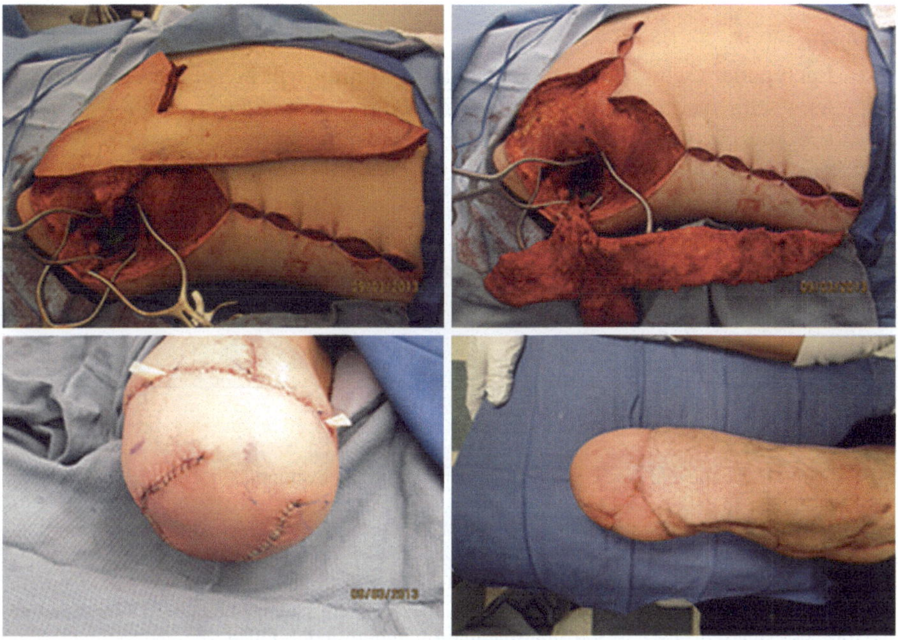

Fig. 35.4 This patient lacked sufficient tissue to undergo a traditional below-knee amputation. The plastic surgery team performed a free flap procedure to provide tissue coverage for the amputation stump

The highest level on the reconstructive ladder is a vascularized composite allograft (VCA) transplant. In blast injuries this could mean an upper extremity transplant or, if there is significant damage to the craniofacial skeleton, a face transplant [46, 47]. These procedures are performed only in select centers throughout the world typically when other reconstructive options are either exhausted or not feasible for the given injury.

Conclusion

Blast and burn injuries are complex and require a collaborative multidisciplinary approach to ensure the best long-term functional outcomes for patients. There are no set rules for reconstruction of blast injuries as no two cases are the same, but there are a set of underlying principles that guide the reconstructive surgeon. This chapter provides a brief overview of the reconstruction of blast injuries, while a full description of the nuances requires a dedicated text, and teams should involve experienced plastic surgeons early in the care of these patients.

Pitfalls

- Each patient who suffers a burn and blast injury will present unique challenges for reconstruction. While the operative principles remain the same (i.e., initial triage, debridement, fixation, and tissue coverage), surgeons must be able to adapt and innovate during the response.
- Performing reconstruction before devitalized and contaminated tissue adequately debrided.
- Not involving reconstructive surgeons early in the collaborative management of these complex burn and blast patients.

References

1. Hauben DJ, Sonneveld GJ. The influence of war on the development of plastic surgery. Ann Plast Surg. 1983;10(1):65–9.
2. Office of the Director of National Intelligence. 2008 report on terrorism. Washington, DC: National Counterterrorism Center; 2008.
3. After action report for the response to the 2013 Boston Marathon bombings. Massachusetts Emergency Management Agency http://www.mass.gov/eopss/docs/mema/after-action-report-for-the-response-to-the-2013-boston-marathon-bombings.pdf12/2014.
4. King DR, Larentzakis A, Ramly EP, Boston Trauma C. Tourniquet use at the Boston Marathon bombing: lost in translation. J Trauma Acute Care Surg. 2015;78(3):594–9.
5. Biddinger PD, Baggish A, Harrington L, d'Hemecourt P, Hooley J, Jones J, et al. Be prepared – the Boston Marathon and mass-casualty events. N Engl J Med. 2013;368(21):1958–60.
6. Emergency War Surgery. 4th United States Revision. Office of the Surgeon General, US Department of Defense; 2013.
7. Taxonomy of injuries from explosive devices. Medical Research for Prevention, Mitigation, and Treatment of Blast Injuries. Washington, DC: Department of Defense; 2006.
8. Ritenour AE, Baskin TW. Primary blast injury: update on diagnosis and treatment. Crit Care Med. 2008;36(7 Suppl):S311–7.
9. Ritenour AE, Blackbourne LH, Kelly JF, McLaughlin DF, Pearse LA, Holcomb JB, et al. Incidence of primary blast injury in US military overseas contingency operations: a retrospective study. Ann Surg. 2010;251(6):1140–4.
10. Sheean AJ, Tintle SM, Rhee PC. Soft tissue and wound management of blast injuries. Curr Rev Musculoskelet Med. 2015;8(3):265–71.
11. Stavrou D, Weissman O, Tessone A, Zilinsky I, Holloway S, Boyd J, et al. Health related quality of life in burn patients – a review of the literature. Burns. 2014;40(5):788–96.
12. Chin TL, Carrougher GJ, Amtmann D, McMullen K, Herndon DN, Holavanahalli R, et al. Trends 10 years after burn injury: a Burn Model System National Database study. Burns. 2018;44(8):1882–6.
13. Wasiak J, Lee SJ, Paul E, Mahar P, Pfitzer B, Spinks A, et al. Predictors of health status and health-related quality of life 12 months after severe burn. Burns. 2014;40(4):568–74.
14. Caterson EJ, Carty MJ, Weaver MJ, Holt EF. Boston bombings: a surgical view of lessons learned from combat casualty care and the applicability to Boston's terrorist attack. J Craniofac Surg. 2013;24(4):1061–7.
15. Kim PS, Malin E, Kirkham JC, Helliwell LA, Ibrahim AM, Tobias AM, et al. The Boston marathon bombings: the early plastic surgery experience of one Boston hospital. Plast Reconstr Surg. 2013;132(5):1351–63.

16. Melcer T, Pyo J, Walker J, Quinn K, Lebedda M, Neises K, et al. Rehabilitation and multiple limb amputations: a clinical report of patients injured in combat. J Rehabil Res Dev. 2016;53(6):1045–60.
17. Sayer NA, Cifu DX, McNamee S, Chiros CE, Sigford BJ, Scott S, et al. Rehabilitation needs of combat-injured service members admitted to the VA Polytrauma Rehabilitation Centers: the role of PM&R in the care of wounded warriors. PM R. 2009;1(1):23–8.
18. Murray CK, Obremskey WT, Hsu JR, Andersen RC, Calhoun JH, Clasper JC, et al. Prevention of infections associated with combat-related extremity injuries. J Trauma. 2011;71(2 Suppl 2):S235–57.
19. Erdle NJ, Verwiebe EG, Wenke JC, Smith CS. Debridement and irrigation: evolution and current recommendations. J Orthop Trauma. 2016;30 Suppl 3:S7–S10.
20. Bakhach J, Abu-Sitta G, Dibo S. Reconstruction of blast injuries of the hand and upper limb. Injury. 2013;44(3):305–12.
21. Weil YA, Mosheiff R, Liebergall M. Blast and penetrating fragment injuries to the extremities. J Am Acad Orthop Surg. 2006;14(10 Spec No.):S136–9.
22. Lin CH, Webb K, Neumeister MW. Immediate tissue transplantation in upper limb trauma: spare parts reconstruction. Clin Plast Surg. 2014;41(3):397–406.
23. Jeans KA, Browne RH, Karol LA. Effect of amputation level on energy expenditure during overground walking by children with an amputation. J Bone Joint Surg Am. 2011;93(1):49–56.
24. Hinck D, Franke A, Gatzka F. Use of vacuum-assisted closure negative pressure wound therapy in combat-related injuries – literature review. Mil Med. 2010;175(3):173–81.
25. Pollak AN, Powell ET, Fang R, Cooper EO, Ficke JR, Flaherty SF. Use of negative pressure wound therapy during aeromedical evacuation of patients with combat-related blast injuries. J Surg Orthop Adv. 2010;19(1):44–8.
26. Rispoli DM, Horne BR, Kryzak TJ, Richardson MW. Description of a technique for vacuum-assisted deep drains in the management of cavitary defects and deep infections in devastating military and civilian trauma. J Trauma. 2010;68(5):1247–52.
27. Putnis S, Khan WS, Wong JM. Negative pressure wound therapy – a review of its uses in orthopaedic trauma. Open Orthop J. 2014;8:142–7.
28. Liu X, Zhang H, Cen S, Huang F. Negative pressure wound therapy versus conventional wound dressings in treatment of open fractures: a systematic review and meta-analysis. Int J Surg. 2018;53:72–9.
29. Stannard JP, Singanamala N, Volgas DA. Fix and flap in the era of vacuum suction devices: what do we know in terms of evidence based medicine? Injury. 2010;41(8):780–6.
30. Hughes OB, Rakosi A, Macquhae F, Herskovitz I, Fox JD, Kirsner RS. A review of cellular and acellular matrix products: indications, techniques, and outcomes. Plast Reconstr Surg. 2016;138(3 Suppl):138S–47S.
31. Liu Y, Panayi AC, Bayer LR, Orgill DP. Current available cellular and tissue-based products for treatment of skin defects. Adv Skin Wound Care. 2019;32(1):19–25.
32. Janis JE, Kwon RK, Attinger CE. The new reconstructive ladder: modifications to the traditional model. Plast Reconstr Surg. 2011;127(Suppl 1):205S–12S.
33. Knobloch K, Vogt PM. The reconstructive clockwork of the twenty-first century: an extension of the concept of the reconstructive ladder and reconstructive elevator. Plast Reconstr Surg. 2010;126(4):220e–2e.
34. Gottlieb LJ, Krieger LM. From the reconstructive ladder to the reconstructive elevator. Plast Reconstr Surg. 1994;93(7):1503–4.
35. Godina M. Early microsurgical reconstruction of complex trauma of the extremities. Plast Reconstr Surg. 1986;78(3):285–92.
36. Ninkovic M, Voigt S, Dornseifer U, Lorenz S, Ninkovic M. Microsurgical advances in extremity salvage. Clin Plast Surg. 2012;39(4):491–505.
37. Hansen ST Jr. The type-IIIC tibial fracture. Salvage or amputation. J Bone Joint Surg Am. 1987;69(6):799–800.

38. Ly TV, Travison TG, Castillo RC, Bosse MJ, MacKenzie EJ, Group LS. Ability of lower-extremity injury severity scores to predict functional outcome after limb salvage. J Bone Joint Surg Am. 2008;90(8):1738–43.
39. Schiro GR, Sessa S, Piccioli A, Maccauro G. Primary amputation vs limb salvage in mangled extremity: a systematic review of the current scoring system. BMC Musculoskelet Disord. 2015;16:372.
40. Management of Complex Extremity Trauma: American College of Surgeons Committee on Trauma. Available from: https://www.facs.org/~/media/files/quality%20programs/trauma/publications/mancompexttrauma.ashx.
41. Higgins TF, Klatt JB, Beals TC. Lower Extremity Assessment Project (LEAP) – the best available evidence on limb-threatening lower extremity trauma. Orthop Clin North Am. 2010;41(2):233–9.
42. Clites TR, Carty MJ, Ullauri JB, Carney ME, Mooney LM, Duval JF, et al. Proprioception from a neurally controlled lower-extremity prosthesis. Sci Transl Med. 2018;10(443):eaap8373.
43. Clites TR, Herr HM, Srinivasan SS, Zorzos AN, Carty MJ. The ewing amputation: the first human implementation of the agonist-antagonist myoneural interface. Plast Reconstr Surg Glob Open. 2018;6(11):e1997.
44. Bowen JB, Ruter D, Wee C, West J, Valerio IL. Targeted muscle reinnervation technique in below-knee amputation. Plast Reconstr Surg. 2019;143(1):309–12.
45. Sabino J, Polfer E, Tintle S, Jessie E, Fleming M, Martin B, et al. A decade of conflict: flap coverage options and outcomes in traumatic war-related extremity reconstruction. Plast Reconstr Surg. 2015;135(3):895–902.
46. Caterson EJ, Diaz-Siso JR, Shetye P, Junker JP, Bueno EM, Soga S, et al. Craniofacial principles in face transplantation. J Craniofac Surg. 2012;23(5):1234–8.
47. Pomahac B, Bueno EM, Sisk GC, Pribaz JJ. Current principles of facial allotransplantation: the Brigham and Women's Hospital Experience. Plast Reconstr Surg. 2013;131(5):1069–76.

Pediatric Blast Injuries

36

A. Francois Trappey and Jeremy W. Cannon

Introduction

Over the past century, a number of blast events have involved children, starting with the massive explosion in Halifax Harbor in 1917 through the Boston Marathon bombing in 2013 [1–4]. In fact, because of Dr. Ladd's involvement in caring for injured children in Halifax, that devastating event has become an important part of the lore surrounding the birth of pediatric surgery. Since then, fireworks injuries, civilian terror incidents, and modern warfare have all led to the further characterization of the unique aspects of pediatric physiology, management, and outcomes following a blast event. Children, especially very young children, consistently have worse outcomes than their adult counterparts after exposure to a blast [5–8]. Thus, there appears to be an ongoing gap in knowledge and training regarding care for the youngest patients. Optimizing survival for these young victims requires a detailed understanding of the common injury patterns, appreciation of the physiologic response of children to blast injuries, and availability of the resources and supplies needed to manage critically injured children [9]. In this chapter, we advance the discussion from the emergency department section. We will discuss the epidemiology of pediatric blast injuries, review pediatric-specific anatomy and physiology relevant to blast injuries, and describe specific injury patterns and their management.

A. F. Trappey
Department of Pediatric Surgery, McGovern Medical School, University of Texas Health Science Center at Houston, Houston, TX, USA

J. W. Cannon (✉)
Division of Traumatology, Surgical Critical Care & Emergency Surgery, Perelman School of Medicine at the University of Pennsylvania, Philadelphia, PA, USA

Department of Surgery, Uniformed Services University, Bethesda, MD, USA
e-mail: jeremy.cannon@uphs.upenn.edu

D. W. Callaway, J. L. Burstein (eds.), *Operational and Medical Management of Explosive and Blast Incidents*, https://doi.org/10.1007/978-3-030-40655-4_36

Epidemiology

Pediatric blast injuries can be divided into those resulting from high- and low-energy ordinance. The most common injuries in the United States are overwhelmingly secondary to low-energy blasts from civilian small ordinance, such as fireworks. High-energy blast mechanisms usually occur in the setting of either civilian terror events or combat.

Fireworks Injuries

Inappropriate use of any type of firework can lead to severe injury – indeed, every type of legally available firework has been implicated in either injury or death [10]. A study by Billrock et al. analyzing data available through the US Consumer Product Safety Commission estimated that greater than 130,000 patients under 20 years of age received treatment in emergency departments for nonfatal firework-related injuries between 1990 and 2014 [11]. Nearly half of all firework-related injuries reported from June to July 2014 in their study occurred in patients under 20 years of age. A single-institution descriptive study from Children's Mercy in Kansas city revealed that 95% of children injured by fireworks are injured during the 3 weeks surrounding Independence Day [12]. This problem is not unique to celebrations in the United States as reports of blast events during celebrations are present in the international literature as well [13, 14].

No matter the country of origin, injuries are more likely to occur in males and the primary handler of the firework [11, 13, 14]. In the United States, males are three times more likely than females to be injured [11]. Injuries are most likely to the hand (30%), head and neck (22%), and eye (21%) and include most commonly burns, abrasions/contusions, and lacerations. Lower extremity injuries are more prevalent in children aged 0–9 than older children [11]. Unsurprisingly, firecrackers are the most commonly implicated firework; however, injuries due to sparklers are the most common in younger children. Injures are usually secondary to firework explosion; however young children are more likely to be struck by the firework than to be involved in the blast itself [11]. The vast majority of injuries, however, is minor with >90% of patients able to be discharged directly from the emergency department (ED).

Legislation and advocacy have the potential to decrease these entirely preventable events. During the 25 years of the Billrock study, the incidence of pediatric fireworks injuries decreased by 30% [11]. Although the overall incidence of fireworks injuries is decreasing, the rate of inpatient admission is significantly increasing, indicating that when injuries do occur, they are more severe than in times past [15]. Though fireworks laws have become less stringent over time, a strong recommendation is given by the American Academy of Pediatrics to restrict use to demonstration professionals [16] . They recommend families enjoy professional shows rather than participate in private festivities [16].

Civilian Terror Incidents

Children have been increasingly exposed to civilian terror events around the world including the Jerusalem bombings, Oklahoma City bombing, Madrid train bombings, and Boston Marathon bombing, among others [4, 17–19]. The majority of persons injured in these events are adults. Yet, the presence of multiple day care centers within proximity to the Alfred P. Murrah Federal Building in Oklahoma City lead to a large number of pediatric injuries. Unfortunately, this incident contributed a robust description of pediatric injury patterns as a result of high-energy blast.

Overall 66 children were victims of the incident in Oklahoma City with 40 treated and released. Among this population, the injury patterns resembled those of the adults injured on that day [20]. Tympanic membrane perforations were extremely common in children, with 25/30 patients from one of the nearby day care centers affected. Seven pediatric patients were hospitalized, and all required admission to the PICU and surgical management. Nineteen children died immediately after the blast. Among the mortalities and the severely injured, head injuries predominated, with severe skull fractures and partial or total cerebral evisceration common [20]. Also common were severe, multiple, orthopedic injures, including traumatic amputations [20]. A retrospective analysis of the Bath School bombing of 1927, an explosive attack with many similarities to the Oklahoma City bombing, reveals a similar injury pattern in children, where injuries to the face, head, and neck predominated [21].

Another detailed assessment of pediatric injuries after terrorist action was recently published from the Israel National Trauma Registry. Ahronson-Daniel et al. compared injury patterns among terror-injured versus non-terror-injured children in the Israel National Trauma Registry from October 2000 to December 2001 [22]. At that time, terror acts against civilian children became the second leading cause of death for children in Israel [23]. Terror-related injuries in children were mostly due to explosion (67%) and resulted in multiple injuries in 65% compared to 65% rate of solitary injury in non-terror trauma victims. The rate of penetrating injury was 54% in terror-related incidents versus 9% in non-terror victims. In the Israeli experience, the majority of explosive devices was packed with projectile foreign bodies that inflicted devastating secondary blast injuries [22]. Burns as a result of terror-related incidents were usually accompanied by penetrating injuries and were more severe. These injury patterns translated into a doubling in OR utilization in terror-injured children versus non-terror injured as well as higher ICU utilization and longer hospital stays [22].

Another series from the Israel National Trauma Registry by Jaffe et al. compared injury patterns among children, adolescents, and adults after terror explosions [24]. Though not statistically significant, there was a suggestion that infants and toddlers were more likely to sustain blunt injuries and less likely to sustain penetrating injury and that infants and toddlers were less likely to sustain injuries to multiple body regions [24]. Injuries among children were more likely to be severe compared to adults (27% vs 12% with ISS 16–24), and children were more likely to have traumatic brain injury (35% vs 20%, $p = 0.012$) and less likely to have open wounds compared to adults [24].

Combat Blast Injuries

Strategies utilizing explosive devices to cause death/injury from blast have become commonplace in the modern battlespace. The IED has become a weapon of choice of violent extremist organizations, and children are frequently collateral casualties. The experience of treating these casualties is now becoming well documented from US and European military treatment facilities from the conflicts in Iraq and Afghanistan. In an analysis of civilian blast injuries from the JTTR, 1822 patients under age 20 were treated between 2002 and 2010 [6]. IED was the most common blast mechanism across age groups [6]. Most patients were male and greater than 70% had more than one affected body region. Burns and extremity/pelvic injuries were the most common (70% and 50%, respectively) overall, while burns and head and neck injuries were the most common for those less than 15 years old. Chest injuries were the least common, although when present, they tended to be severe (92% with a chest injury had a Chest AIS 3–6) [6]. This is similar to findings in one series of adult victims of civilian terror incidents in Madrid, where the presence of chest injury indicates a high burden of injury [18].

Overall, Edwards et al. found a mortality of 7.8% for children compared to a documented approximately 3% mortality rate for US military casualties [6]. In a subsequent analysis, younger children (less than 3 years) required more neurosurgical interventions, while older children required more interventions for extremity injuries including repeated debridement [25]. A review of neurosurgical cases from the Craig Joint Theater Hospital from 2007 to 2009 reveals that the most common neurosurgical procedure performed on children during that time was craniotomy/craniectomy for penetrating cranial injury secondary to blast in the majority of cases [26]. Pediatric patients presenting with vascular injury to facilities recorded in the JTTR were most likely to be injured by blast (58%), and these patients had a higher incidence of chest trauma (23%) (although chest injuries are not broken down by mechanism) than in other series with a high risk ratio for mortality in those with torso injuries [27].

These patterns of injury are consistent among reports from coalition partners, who describe a similarly high mortality rate for blast-injured children. There seems to be a preponderance of lower extremity injury and more severe head injury in younger children compared to older children and adults [28–30]. The civil war in Syria has also produced a large number of pediatric casualties. Though the use of conventional weapons is more common in this conflict as compared to Iraq and Afghanistan, fragmentation injury is the most common mechanism (51%) seen at an Israeli Role 1 facility and extremity and head/cervical spine injuries the most common anatomic sites [31].

These children, injured as collateral casualties, consume a large portion of deployed resources. In a retrospective review of all patients admitted to combat support hospitals and forward surgical teams in Iraq and Afghanistan, Borgman et al. demonstrated that, while pediatric patients only represented 5.8% of admissions, they represent 11% of all bed days. Borgman et al. suggest these numbers may underestimate the actual number of children treated due to a lag in capturing all patients admitted at the beginning of the conflict.

Physiology and Pediatric Vulnerabilities

Children present with unique vulnerabilities to blast injury secondary to multiple aspects of their developing/juvenile anatomy, physiology, and behavior [9]. Many of these qualities make children more vulnerable to injuries of any mechanism. Table 36.1 demonstrates pediatric-specific vulnerabilities by blast mechanism.

Table 36.1 Pediatric vulnerabilities following a blast event

Blast Mechanism	Head/C-spine	Face/Eyes	Chest	Abdomen	Extremity
Primary – Blast wave (over–/under pressure) effects	bTBI difficult to assess in preverbal children. Long-term effects unknown Softer/immature calvaria – Potential mechanism for increased "skull-capping" type injuries Increased head size relative to body		Increased susceptibility to vagal response Increased chest/mediastinal compliance	Difficulty assessing abdomen in preverbal children – Possible delay in diagnosis of blast bowel injury	
Secondary – Ballistic/penetrating effects	Increased head size relative to body – Klimo et al. describe high incidence of penetrating skull injury after blast	Children usually attentive during displays such as fireworks Common to have eye injury			Short stature School-age children more likely to get an amputation – Curiosity/lack of situational awareness
Tertiary – Blunt trauma as a result of displacement of victim or surroundings	Lower overall mass		Increased chest/sternal compliance. Theoretical increased risk of blunt injury to mediastinal structures		Short stature School-age children more likely to get an amputation – Curiosity/lack of situational awareness
Quaternary – Burns/thermal injury/toxic inhalation			Increased minute ventilation		
Quinary – Radiation/toxic biochemical exposure			Increased minute ventilation		

In the case of fireworks and unexploded ordinance and/or landmines (all preventable blast injuries), a lack of awareness of potential danger may contribute to some of the observed injuries. This is demonstrated by the pattern of injuries associated with fireworks by age. School-age children and teens are more likely to be injured by firecrackers and illegal fireworks as the handler than younger children/infants. Younger children have limited mobility and are thus more likely to suffer primary blast injuries from fireworks [11]. This low situational awareness and poor mobility may explain some of the wartime observations as well, whereas school-age children are more likely to suffer primary, secondary, and tertiary blast injuries [25]. Furthermore, the high incidence of face/eye injuries in younger patients likely results from curiosity.

Children are clearly more susceptible to head injury than their adult counterparts secondary to relatively large head size compared to the rest of the body (Fig. 36.1) [17, 20, 32, 33]. A thorough review of anatomic and physiologic differences between adults and children with TBI was recently published by Figaji [33]. As with head-injured children from mechanisms other than blast, preverbal children can present a challenge regarding mental status assessment. It is unknown how primary blast TBI affects the developing brain and the effect that surgical decompression has on

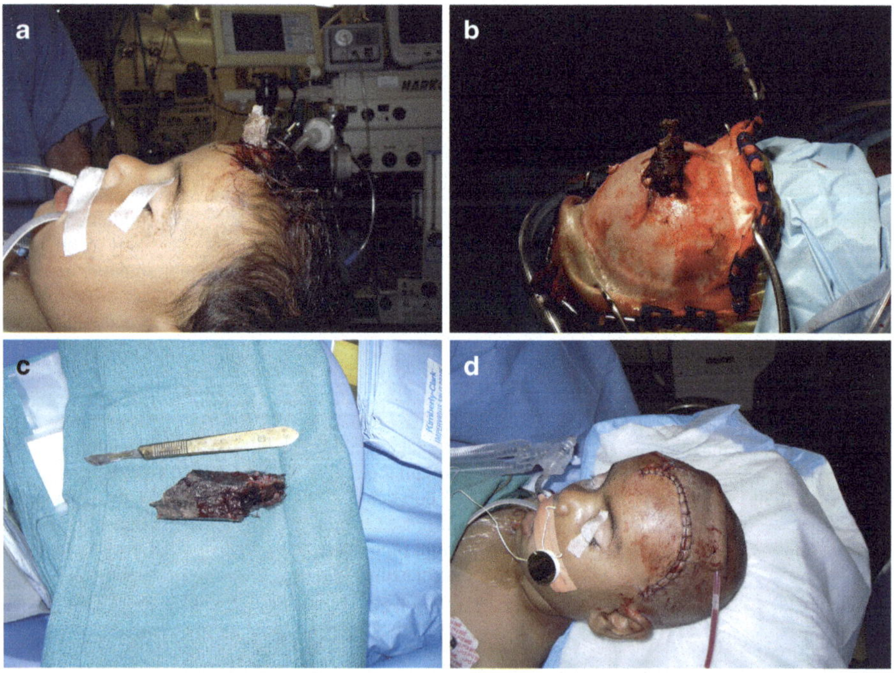

Fig. 36.1 Pediatric patient with a secondary blast injury resulting in a penetrating brain injury (**a**). The fragment was directly adjacent to the sagittal sinus (**b**), but upon careful exposure and removal of the fragment (**c**), the sinus was found to be uninjured. The patient's cranial defect was repaired (**d**), and she had a full recovery

outcomes compared to adults, though some posit that children may have a greater capacity for neurologic recovery after TBI than adult counterparts; however, data to support this hypothesis are lacking [33].

The pediatric chest presents specific vulnerabilities as well that can be assumed based on anatomy/physiology and epidemiologic observation. From a pulmonary standpoint, there is no indication that children are more susceptible to primary lung blast injury than adults. As above, when a child has injuries to the chest, they are more likely to be severely ill at presentation. Children are likely more susceptible to quaternary injury (toxic inhalation) secondary to increased minute ventilation [17]. Given the decreased musculature and increased compliance of the pediatric chest wall and sternum, children may be at increased risk for cardiac or pulmonary contusion from either primary or tertiary blast effect. The mediastinal structure is less robust in children, and hemodynamically significant shift due to tension from hemo- or pneumothorax may occur at lower pressures [34]. In some cases, death from primary blast results from a robust vagal response leading to bradycardia, hypotension, and apnea. Infants and young children may be more especially vulnerable to this mode of death due to an immature sympathetic drive [17, 35]. Clinicians should be highly suspicious if an infant or young child presents with bradycardia as this represents an inappropriate response to injury. This lack of compensatory drive may precede rapid circulatory collapse.

Gastrointestinal injury can be caused by all blast mechanisms. While the need for laparotomy seems to be less than adult counterparts, blast-injured children, especially preverbal children, may be more difficult to examine and therefore present a unique clinical challenge.

Extremity injuries and burns seem to be especially prevalent in children. This may be secondary to short stature. Children aged 4–9 were more likely to get an amputation in the series published by Edwards et al. [25]. This may be due to increased mobility and lack of situational awareness in this age group.

Rapid Assessment of the Blast-Injured Child

Children who are injured as a result of blast may present across a broad spectrum of acuity. Preparation for assessing a blast-injured child would ideally begin as soon as possible. Information regarding the type of explosive, number of injured people at the scene and their ages, proximity of victims to the blast, blast setting (open or closed space), and prehospital vital signs and possible injuries can be helpful to prepare the trauma team for triaging and resuscitating casualties. This information that can help with assuring the appropriate resources, especially pediatric-specific resources, are immediately available. When appropriate, pediatric specialists, including pediatric-trained nursing staff, and subspecialists may be invaluable in the initial assessment and disposition of pediatric trauma patients [36]. This is especially true of infants and young children.

Given the differences in hemodynamic parameters by age, a simplified method for identifying hemodynamic instability has been developed in children. The shock index (heart rate divided by blood pressure) pediatric age-adjusted (SIPA) has been shown to identify the sickest children presenting to a trauma center after trauma. A SIPA >1.22 in children 4–6 years old, >1 in 6–12 year olds, and > 0.9 in children greater than 13 years of age predicts higher injury severity [37, 38].

A Broselow™ tape can be another invaluable tool in the initial evaluation and resuscitation in children and will estimate, based upon height, needs from endotracheal and chest tube sizing to weight-based (estimated ideal body weight) dosing recommendations for medications commonly utilized during resuscitations [39]. The ability to rapidly obtain recommendations for weight-based dosing and intervention is a necessity. Thus, during the evaluation of a pediatric trauma patient, the Broselow™ tape provides readily available information and can greatly reduce cognitive loading.

In general, clinicians should adhere to ATLS principles. It is important to approach multiple-injured children in a systematic fashion. It is important to remember that a patient may have been injured by any of the five mechanisms related to blast. Specifically, there may be both blunt and penetrating injuries present. Small external wounds may be the only sign of devastating internal injury in a hemodynamically unstable child. The use of plain films and FAST in the resuscitation area can help to focus on specific injuries. In stable children, the use of CT imaging should be based on symptoms, exam, and laboratory evaluation.

For children without life-threatening injuries but who have a tympanic membrane rupture, we extrapolate recommendations posited by DePalma et al. [9]. Because traumatic tympanic membrane rupture may predict risk for late manifestations of primary blast injury to various body systems, an observation period with charted oxygen saturations for 6–8 hours is recommended. It should be noted that, while the majority of patients with severe primary blast injury will also have tympanic membrane rupture, it is possible to have severe primary blast injury without this finding [9].

Characterization, Diagnosis, and Treatment of Specific Injuries

Head Injury

Evaluation of children suspected of having head injury after blast should begin with a history of the blasting mechanism. Calculation of the child's GCS during ATLS primary survey should be a priority, and patients with a GCS less than 8 should have their airway secured. Gross assessment of motor and sensory functions should be performed if time allows. For children without obvious clinical sign of head injury, recommendations from PECARN regarding subsequent evaluation by CT scan can be extrapolated to this population given the caveat that blast mechanism was not included in this study cohort [40].

As soon as clinically able, hemodynamically stable children with severe TBI or who meet criteria based on recommendations of PECARN should undergo head CT. Patients with severe TBI who are intubated should be kept normocapnic. There are no data to support hyperventilation in children, especially in the setting of possible concomitant blast lung injury.

Early neurosurgical evaluation is recommended, if available, for children with depressed GCS or with intracranial bleeding seen on head CT. Pediatric neurosurgical support may not be available in austere locations, and adult neurosurgeons or general/trauma surgeons with appropriate training may be required to perform stabilization and damage control [26].

The benefits of neuromonitoring and decompressive craniotomy/craniectomy in children with head injury are still unclear due to limited prospective data [33, 41–43]. Generally, however, the data supports ICP monitoring and decompression for medically refractory increased ICP in children with severe head injury [44]. This may be especially true in penetrating head injury [26, 45]. There are no data regarding the surgical management of pediatric patients with predominantly primary blast TBI.

Adult wartime experience with predominantly blast-injured soldiers suggests a high rate of neurological improvement over time for those patients who underwent early decompressive surgery [46, 47]. These data do not include early deaths (those that died prior to reaching the hospital). Early resuscitation on the battlefield and the use of body armor, including sophisticated armored helmets, limit the extrapolation of these data to children.

Operative battlefield experience in pediatric traumatic brain injury is mostly due to penetrating (secondary) blast injury [26]. These authors report that the operative principles include wound washout, debridement of devitalized tissue, removal of foreign bodies, removal of hematoma, and hemostasis [26]. Results of operative management of these patients are generally favorable; however, there is an intrinsic selection bias in that patients who made it to rear-echelon care with neurosurgical support may have been more likely to survive regardless of treatment. Quality of life for children after decompressive craniotomy/craniectomy for TBI is generally favorable, but rates of return to normal academic performance are low [44].

Eye Injury

As above, eye injury as a result of blast is fairly common. No pediatric-specific literature exists regarding stabilization and treatment of these injuries. Some injuries may be isolated, while patients with other severe injuries may have eye injuries in conjunction. A careful history, especially from bystanders, should be obtained. In patients with high clinical suspicion of ocular injury, a convex shield (metal or plastic) should be placed to protect the eye from further injury, and precaution should be taken to keep from putting pressure on that eye. Physical exam should focus on evaluation for surgical emergencies such as globe rupture, chemical burns, or orbital compartment syndrome [48]. Visual acuity should be assessed if possible. Practitioners experienced in the visual acuity assessment of preverbal children may be required. CT scan of the head, face, and orbit should be obtained if penetrating eye or orbital injury is suspected to guide surgical therapy. Early ophthalmologic evaluation is imperative.

Chest Injury

Though the chest is the least likely body region to be injured in children based on wartime data, chest injuries in these patients and in adult victims of civilian trauma indicate a high injury burden [18, 49, 50]. Rapid assessment of the chest should begin during the primary survey. In hemodynamically unstable children or those that are obtunded, visual inspection and palpation of the chest wall for injury should be accomplished and treatment of suspected hemo-/pneumothorax accomplished rapidly. Selection of an appropriately sized chest tube for smaller children can be guided by a Broselow™ tape. Plain film of the chest can be obtained as a supplement to physical exam during the primary survey. Cardiac FAST to assess for pericardial fluid should also be accomplished. Further imaging of the pediatric chest with cross-sectional imaging should be based upon hemodynamic stability, history (including suspected blasting mechanism), physical exam, and chest X-ray [51]. Stable patients with suspicion for secondary blast injury should undergo CT to characterize position and trajectory of penetrating fragments to guide subsequent therapy.

Primary lung blast injury as a result of the blast wave traversing the multiple air-fluid interfaces present in the chest/lung may present as respiratory distress, dyspnea, or hemoptysis [17, 35]. CXR may demonstrate "batwing" central opacities [9, 35]. While no characterization specific to pediatric patients exists, its presentation should be similar to that of adults. In patients with suspected primary pulmonary blast injury, crystalloids should be minimized. Treatment for this condition is largely supportive with lung protective ventilation in those patients requiring intubation. Extracorporeal lung support has been utilized with some success in small series of adults after chest trauma, including some civilian blast injuries [52]. This series included some patients with head injuries who underwent ECLS without heparin or after demonstration of stable intracranial bleeding [52]. Given the clinical success of this salvage modality in children, it would be theoretically beneficial.

Thoracotomy is rarely needed in pediatric patients with blast injuries to the chest [25]. The indications for thoracotomy for children with hemorrhage from a chest injury are based loosely on adult indications (15–20 mL/kg blood upon initial placement or 2–3 mL/kg bloody output over 2–3 hours) [34]. Thoracotomy for aerodigestive or mediastinal vascular injury as a result of penetrating injury would have similar indications to non-blast mechanisms.

Abdominal Injury

The requirement for laparotomy as a result of blast is common [25]. It is unclear what proportion of patients undergoing laparotomy after blast is injured by primary blast injury versus secondary or tertiary effects. Regarding primary blast effects, the cecum and terminal ileum seem to be the most likely injured segments of bowel in animal models and in observational study [53]. Primary blast injury to the bowel can create scattered areas of mural hematoma that can progress to necrosis and perforation. Rarely, blast injury to the bowel can perforate primarily. Solid organ injury secondary to primary blasting mechanism is also rare (likely owing to a lack of gas-fluid interface) [53]. It is unknown how the relatively smaller size of the pediatric torso affects these injury patterns.

Indications for abdominal exploration in blast-injured children mirror those of non-blast-injured patients. Hemodynamic instability with evidence of penetrating abdominal injury should warrant emergent exploration. For pediatric patients with hemodynamic instability and no evidence of abdominal penetration, but who have other concerning history or physical findings, FAST exam has been shown to be specific for intra-abdominal fluid and can be used to guide therapy when positive. Low sensitivity for intra-abdominal fluid, however, means a negative FAST examination in children in whom intra-abdominal injury is suspected should not be reassuring and should prompt further workup [54]. Abdominal plain film to assess for free air or pelvic fracture plus diagnostic peritoneal lavage can be helpful in this situation and can help prioritize abdominal exploration versus a continued search for the source of instability.

In hemodynamically stable children without evidence of penetrating abdominal injury, the need for further imaging should be guided by history, physical exam, and laboratory examination. While most pediatric literature calls for a decrease in the use of CT scan for children citing a small but real increase in risk of malignancy over time, we suggest a liberalization of its use in patients with a history of significant blast mechanism and in whom abdominal exam may be unreliable or unavailable (e.g., patients who are ventilated). Otherwise, the use of CT should be restricted to those who have abdominal pain, an increase in liver enzyme levels, a urinalysis positive for microscopic blood, or elevated lipase [34]. Indication for operation based on CT findings would be similar to other mechanisms of injury.

The use of CT scan after urgent surgery for trauma is controversial [55–57]. There is emerging evidence, however, supporting the use of CT after damage control surgery to complete diagnostic workup for severely injured patients [56, 57]. Again, there is a lack of data to support the routine use of CT in children who have undergone urgent surgery in order to complete their workup; however, given the complexity of blast injury, we think the use of postoperative CT scan for blast-injured children is a prudent adjunct to surgical exploration.

Extremities and Bony Pelvis

Injuries to the extremity due to blast mechanism again depend on the ordinance. Fireworks injuries to the hands are extremely common and can include burns/abrasions, fractures, and amputations [58]. There is a high association with ophthalmologic injury, so patients with fireworks injuries to the hand should have an ophthalmologic evaluation [58].

High-energy blast mechanisms may lead to large amounts of tissue loss or amputation. Other than burns and superficial wounds, the extremities/pelvis is the most likely body region injured in children who are combat collateral casualties [6].

Prehospital and inhospital use of tourniquets should be utilized to temporize hemorrhage as a result of extremity trauma. Tourniquet use in children injured as combat collateral casualties demonstrated similar efficacy as in adults when used appropriately [59]. Sources of life-threatening junctional or truncal injuries can then be addressed.

To our knowledge, there are no studies looking at the use of pelvic binders in children. It seems reasonable to place a pelvic binder on an older child or teenager who is hypotensive with an unstable pelvis. If a commercially available product is too large, a bedsheet can be utilized similarly for smaller children.

Once life-threatening injury has been addressed, extremities must be evaluated for vascular injury or fracture. In the series by Villamaria et al., the majority of vascular injuries (66%) seen in combat-injured children was to the extremity [27]. The remainder of observed vascular injuries was to the torso and neck. Compared to vascular injuries to the torso, vascular injuries to the extremity carry a lower risk of mortality and are able to be treated with a 95% rate of limb salvage [27].

Splints should be used to stabilize obvious fracture to decrease pain and bleeding. Again, liberal use of plain film should be utilized if underlying fracture is suspected based on history or physical exam. Open fractures should receive appropriate and timely antibiotics upon presentation. Damage control principles for severe open limb fractures should be utilized [60]. Limb salvage in young patients should be sought. Fracture stabilization utilizing wound spanning external fixation should be followed by debridement as necessary. Concomitant vascular injury can then be addressed and soft tissue coverage arranged as necessary. Wounds should be debrided and washed out serially until clean. Definitive reconstruction may require pediatric or trauma orthopedic specialty care.

Unstable pelvic fractures in blast-injured children with associated hemorrhage should be treated with pelvic stabilization, pre-peritoneal packing, and/or angioembolization similar to the treatment for adults with similar injuries. There are some data to support this treatment in older children and teens [61]. Otherwise, in younger children, the use of angioembolization will depend on available resources and expertise in small vessel access [62]. In cases where these resources are unavailable, damage control principles including pelvic packing should be applied and operative therapy/vessel ligation utilized as necessary.

Spine

Pediatric spine injury with low-energy civilian ordinance and fireworks is understandably exceedingly rare. Spine injury as a result of civilian terror events is also rare. Of the hospitalized victims of terror events in Israel from 2000 to 2005, spine injuries were only present in 2% of 0–10 year olds and 4–5% for children and adults greater than 10 years of age [24]. Of those victims of a civilian terror event who present with a deficit consistent with a cervical spine injury (including children), the vast majority of these injuries is due to secondary (penetrating) blast injury [63].

However, spine injury among combatant victims of high-energy blast are very common with injuries usually occurring in the lumbar and thoracic spine secondary to compressive loading from below [64]. The high rate of adult spine injury from predominantly high-energy blast mechanism during recent conflicts is not observed in children [64]. In a small series of pediatric neurosurgical cases from the conflict in Afghanistan, no spine surgeries were performed for pediatric blast victims [26]. The lack of spine injuries is fairly consistent between series though this may be a failure of reporting [20].

Blunt cervical spine injury in civilian mass terror incidents, especially in children, is rare. The majority of the injuries that result in neurologic deficit is due to secondary (penetrating) blast effect and is immediate and nonreversible [63]. One study reports that application of a collar in the field can take several minutes, possibly delaying other life-saving therapy, especially in the setting of penetrating c-spine injury [63, 65]. Therefore, in children, delay of transport for application of a cervical collar is not recommended, especially if the collar is inappropriately sized or delays other field care such as application of tourniquets or pelvic binders. For children who present with a cervical collar after high-energy blast, the neck needs to be inspected early for penetrating injury. Spinal precautions should be utilized until the child can be examined and cleared by neurological exam or is able to undergo skeletal series or CT scan of the spine. Otherwise, guidance provided for imaging and clearance of the pediatric c-spine should be utilized [66].

External/Burns

Burns are the third leading injury related to fireworks in the United States and are more common in some series as a result of fireworks misuse in the developing world [11, 13]. While most burns related to fireworks are not life-threatening, they do have significant potential for morbidity (especially to the face, eyes, and hands).

Pediatric victims of high-energy blast mechanism with resultant burns have increased odds for mortality [6]. For pediatric blast victims in a warzone, 30% TBSA burns correlate with about a 30% chance of mortality [6]. The percent TBSA may correlate with proximity to the blast and may, thus, be a surrogate for other injury. The increased mortality for burned children in austere environments may represent a combination of a lack of resources, specialty training, or poor indigenous nutrition or a combination of factors and has been previously reported [6, 8].

In the case of pediatric victims of blast injury who present with burns, the initial evaluation and resuscitation should, again, take a protocolized approach to ruling out other sources of life-threatening injury. Burn injury can be very distracting and should be de-prioritized. We refer readers to the USAISR burn care clinical practice guideline that has a comprehensive treatment algorithm as well as a section on the care of burned children [67]. Children with signs of airway burns/edema must have their airway assessed and rapidly controlled as the small airway can occlude without much warning with ongoing resuscitation.

Conclusion

Pediatric patients present with a unique pattern of injury following exposure to a blast. Although most pediatric blast injuries are from low-energy devices (e.g., fireworks), civilian terror events and combat operations often result in high-energy pediatric blast injuries. Such high-energy mechanisms present special challenges to care teams that may not routinely care for pediatric patients. Adhering to pediatric-specific ATLS principles and employing guides such as the Broselow™ tape for medication dosing simplify the approach to the severely injured child. Understanding common patterns of injury and their appropriate management will further optimize the outcome of blast-injured children.

Pitfalls

- Failure to identify severely injured pediatric patients after a blast event
- Not identifying the patient's weight with appropriate medication doses and device sizes using a standardized measurement system such as a Broselow™ tape
- Unfamiliarity with common injury patterns in pediatric patients with blast injury
- Underutilization of imaging to identify critical injuries

References

1. Hendrix S. Two ships collided in Halifax Harbor. One of them was a floating, 3,000-ton bomb. 2017 [cited 2018 04/30/2018]. Available from: https://www.washingtonpost.com/news/retropolis/wp/2017/12/06/two-ships-collided-in-halifax-harbor-one-of-them-was-a-3000-ton-floating-bomb/?noredirect=on&utm_term=.ffb07dff2dbc.
2. Gillis DA, Lewis SD, Little DC. The Halifax explosion and the birth of a surgical specialty-myth or reality. J Pediatr Surg. 2010;45(5):855–8.
3. Nakayama DK. William Ladd before the Halifax explosion. J Pediatr Surg. 2017;52(12):2093–6.
4. Gates JD, Arabian S, Biddinger P, Blansfield J, Burke P, Chung S, et al. The initial response to the Boston marathon bombing: lessons learned to prepare for the next disaster. Ann Surg. 2014;260(6):960–6.
5. Matos RI, Holcomb JB, Callahan C, Spinella PC. Increased mortality rates of young children with traumatic injuries at a US army combat support hospital in Baghdad, Iraq, 2004. Pediatrics. 2008;122(5):e959–66.
6. Edwards MJ, Lustik M, Eichelberger MR, Elster E, Azarow K, Coppola C. Blast injury in children: an analysis from Afghanistan and Iraq, 2002–2010. J Trauma Acute Care Surg. 2012;73(5):1278–83.
7. Borgman M, Matos RI, Blackbourne LH, Spinella PC. Ten years of military pediatric care in Afghanistan and Iraq. J Trauma Acute Care Surg. 2012;73(6 Suppl 5):S509–13.
8. Borgman MA, Matos RI, Spinella PC. Isolated pediatric burn injury in Iraq and Afghanistan. Pediatr Crit Care Med. 2015;16(2):e23–7.
9. DePalma RG, Burris DG, Champion HR, Hodgson MJ. Blast injuries. N Engl J Med. 2005;352(13):1335–42.
10. Berger LR, Kalishman S, Rivara FP. Injuries from fireworks. Pediatrics. 1985;75(5):877–82.

11. Billock RM, Chounthirath T, Smith GA. Pediatric firework-related injuries presenting to United States Emergency Departments, 1990–2014. Clin Pediatr (Phila). 2017;56(6):535–44.
12. Smith GA, et al. The rockets' red glare, the bombs bursting in air: fireworks-related injuries to children. Pediatrics. 1996;98(1):1–9.
13. Vaghardoost R, Ghavami Y, Sobouti B, Mobayen MR. Mortality and morbidity of fireworks-related burns on the annual last wednesday of the year festival (charshanbeh soori) in Iran: an 11-year study. Trauma Mon. 2013;18(2):81–5.
14. Bagri N, Saha A, Chandelia S, Dubey NK, Bhatt A, Rai A, et al. Fireworks injuries in children: a prospective study during the festival of lights. Emerg Med Australas. 2013;25(5):452–6.
15. Myers J, Lehna C. Effect of fireworks laws on pediatric fireworks-related burn injuries. J Burn Care Res. 2017;38(1):e79–82.
16. American Academy of Pediatrics: Committee on Injury and Poison Prevention. Fireworks-related injuries to children. Pediatrics. 2001;108(1):190–1.
17. Hamele M, Poss WB, Sweney J. Disaster preparedness, pediatric considerations in primary blast injury, chemical, and biological terrorism. World J Crit Care Med. 2014;3(1):15–23.
18. Gutierrez de Ceballos JP, Turégano Fuentes F, Perez Diaz D, Sanz Sanchez M, Martin Llorente C, Guerrero Sanz JE. Casualties treated at the closest hospital in the Madrid, March 11, terrorist bombings. Crit Care Med. 2005;33(1 Suppl):S107–12.
19. Leibovici D, Gofrit ON, Stein M, Shapira SC, Noga Y, Heruti RJ, et al. Blast injuries: bus versus open-air bombings--a comparative study of injuries in survivors of open-air versus confined-space explosions. J Trauma. 1996;41(6):1030–5.
20. Quintana DA, Parker JR, Jordan FB, Tuggle DW, Mantor PC, Tunell WP. The spectrum of pediatric injuries after a bomb blast. J Pediatr Surg. 1997;32(2):307–10; discussion 310–1.
21. Kim D, Mosher BD, Morrison CA, Parker-Lee C, Opreanu RC, Stevens P, et al. A modern analysis of a historical pediatric disaster: the 1927 Bath school bombing. J Surg Res. 2010;163(2):309–16.
22. Aharonson-Daniel L, Waisman Y, Dannon YL, Peleg K, Members of the Israel Trauma Group. Epidemiology of terror-related versus non-terror-related traumatic injury in children. Pediatrics. 2003;112(4):e280.
23. Amir LD, Aharonson-Daniel L, Peleg K, Waisman Y, Israel Trauma Group. The severity of injury in children resulting from acts against civilian populations. Ann Surg. 2005;241(4):666–70.
24. Jaffe DH, Peleg K. Terror explosive injuries: a comparison of children, adolescents, and adults. Ann Surg. 2010;251(1):138–43.
25. Edwards MJ, Lustik M, Carlson T, Tabak B, Farmer D, Edwards K, et al. Surgical interventions for pediatric blast injury: an analysis from Afghanistan and Iraq 2002 to 2010. J Trauma Acute Care Surg. 2014;76(3):854–8.
26. Klimo P Jr, Ragel BT, Scott WH Jr, McCafferty R. Pediatric neurosurgery during Operation Enduring Freedom. J Neurosurg Pediatr. 2010;6(2):107–14.
27. Villamaria CY, Morrison JJ, Fitzpatrick CM, Cannon JW, Rasmussen TE. Wartime vascular injuries in the pediatric population of Iraq and Afghanistan: 2002-2011. J Pediatr Surg. 2014;49(3):428–32.
28. Thompson, D.C., Crooks RJ, Clasper JC, Lupu A, Stapley SA, Cloke DJ. The pattern of paediatric blast injury in Afghanistan. J R Army Med Corps, 2017 Oct 21 [Epub ahead of print].
29. Arul GS, Reynolds J, DiRusso S, Scott A, Bree S, Templeton P, et al. Paediatric admissions to the British military hospital at Camp Bastion, Afghanistan. Ann R Coll Surg Engl. 2012;94(1):52–7.
30. Pannell D, Poynter J, Wales PW, Tien H, Nathens AB, Shellington D. Factors affecting mortality of pediatric trauma patients encountered in Kandahar, Afghanistan. Can J Surg. 2015;58(3 Suppl 3):S141–5.
31. Bitterman Y, Benov A, Glassberg E, Satanovsky A, Bader T, Sagi R. Role 1 pediatric trauma care on the Israeli-Syrian border-first year of the humanitarian effort. Mil Med. 2016;181(8):849–53.
32. Kissoon N, Dreyer J, Walia M. Pediatric trauma: differences in pathophysiology, injury patterns and treatment compared with adult trauma. CMAJ. 1990;142(1):27–34.

33. Figaji AA. Anatomical and physiological differences between children and adults relevant to traumatic brain injury and the implications for clinical assessment and care. Front Neurol. 2017;8:685.
34. Vogel AM, Edwards MJ. Trauma resuscitation and initial evaluation. In: Pediatric surgery - not a textbook: Unbound(R) Medicine. American Pediatric Surgical Association; 2018. https://www.pedsurglibrary.com/apsa.
35. Ritenour AE, Baskin TW. Primary blast injury: update on diagnosis and treatment. Crit Care Med. 2008;36(7 Suppl):S311–7.
36. McKechnie PS, Wertin T, Parker P, Eckert M. Pediatric surgery skill sets in Role 3: the Afghanistan experience. Mil Med. 2014;179(7):762–5.
37. Linnaus ME, Notrica DM, Langlais CS, St Peter SD, Leys CM, Ostlie DJ, et al. Prospective validation of the shock index pediatric-adjusted (SIPA) in blunt liver and spleen trauma: an ATOMAC+ study. J Pediatr Surg. 2017;52(2):340–4.
38. Acker SN, Ross JT, Partrick DA, Tong S, Bensard DD. Pediatric specific shock index accurately identifies severely injured children. J Pediatr Surg. 2015;50(2):331–4.
39. Lubitz DS, Seidel JS, Chameides L, Luten RC, Zaritsky AL, Campbell FW. A rapid method for estimating weight and resuscitation drug dosages from length in the pediatric age group. Ann Emerg Med. 1988;17(6):576–81.
40. Kuppermann N, Holmes JF, Dayan PS, Hoyle JD Jr, Atabaki SM, Holubkov R, et al. Identification of children at very low risk of clinically-important brain injuries after head trauma: a prospective cohort study. Lancet. 2009;374(9696):1160–70.
41. Pechmann A, Anastasopoulos C, Korinthenberg R, van Velthoven-Wurster V, Kirschner J. Decompressive craniectomy after severe traumatic brain injury in children: complications and outcome. Neuropediatrics. 2015;46(1):5–12.
42. Davidson GH, Maier RV, Arbabi S, Goldin AB, Rivara FP. Impact of operative intervention delay on pediatric trauma outcomes. J Trauma Acute Care Surg. 2012;73(1):162–7.
43. Weintraub D, Williams BJ, Jane J Jr. Decompressive craniectomy in pediatric traumatic brain injury: a review of the literature. NeuroRehabilitation. 2012;30(3):219–23.
44. Beuriat PA, Javouhey E, Szathmari A, Courtil-Tesseydre S, Desgranges FP, Grassiot B, et al. Decompressive craniectomy in the treatment of post-traumatic intracranial hypertension in children: our philosophy and indications. J Neurosurg Sci. 2015;59(4):405–28.
45. DeCuypere M, Muhlbauer MS, Boop FA, Klimo P Jr. Pediatric intracranial gunshot wounds: the Memphis experience. J Neurosurg Pediatr. 2016;17(5):595–601.
46. Bell RS, Mossop CM, Dirks MS, Stephens FL, Mulligan L, Ecker R, et al. Early decompressive craniectomy for severe penetrating and closed head injury during wartime. Neurosurg Focus. 2010;28(5):E1.
47. DuBose JJ, Barmparas G, Inaba K, Stein DM, Scalea T, Cancio LC, et al. Isolated severe traumatic brain injuries sustained during combat operations: demographics, mortality outcomes, and lessons to be learned from contrasts to civilian counterparts. J Trauma. 2011;70:11–6; discussion 16–8.
48. Morley MG, Nguyen JK, Heier JS, Shingleton BJ, Pasternak JF, Bower KS. Blast eye injuries: a review for first responders. Disaster Med Public Health Prep. 2010;4(2):154–60.
49. Edwards MJ, Lustik M, Burnett MW, Eichelberger M. Pediatric inpatient humanitarian care in combat: Iraq and Afghanistan 2002 to 2012. J Am Coll Surg. 2014;218(5):1018–23.
50. Avidan V, Hersch M, Armon Y, Spira R, Aharoni D, Reissman P, et al. Blast lung injury: clinical manifestations, treatment, and outcome. Am J Surg. 2005;190(6):927–31.
51. Yanchar NL, Woo K, Brennan M, Palmer CS, Zs Ee M, Sweeney B, et al. Chest x-ray as a screening tool for blunt thoracic trauma in children. J Trauma Acute Care Surg. 2013;75(4):613–9.
52. Ried M, Bein T, Philipp A, Müller T, Graf B, Schmid C, et al. Extracorporeal lung support in trauma patients with severe chest injury and acute lung failure: a 10-year institutional experience. Crit Care. 2013;17(3):R110.
53. Owers C, Morgan JL, Garner JP. Abdominal trauma in primary blast injury. Br J Surg. 2011;98(2):168–79.

54. Scaife ER, Rollins MD, Barnhart DC, Downey EC, Black RE, Meyers RL, et al. The role of focused abdominal sonography for trauma (FAST) in pediatric trauma evaluation. J Pediatr Surg. 2013;48(6):1377–83.
55. Weis JJ, Cunningham KE, Forsythe RM, Billiar TR, Peitzman AB, Sperry JL. The importance of empiric abdominal computed tomography after urgent laparotomy for trauma: do they reveal unexpected injuries? Surgery. 2014;156(4):979–85.
56. Matsushima K, Inaba K, Dollbaum R, Khor D, Jhaveri V, Jimenez O, et al. The role of computed tomography after emergent trauma operation. J Surg Res. 2016;206(2):286–91.
57. Mendoza AE, Wybourn CA, Charles AG, Campbell AR, Cairns BA, Knudson MM. Routine computed tomography after recent operative exploration for penetrating trauma: what injuries do we miss? J Trauma Acute Care Surg. 2017;83(4):575–8.
58. Moore RS Jr, Tan V, Dormans JP, Bozentka DJ. Major pediatric hand trauma associated with fireworks. J Orthop Trauma. 2000;14(6):426–8.
59. Kragh JF Jr, Cooper A, Aden JK, Dubick MA, Baer DG, Wade CE, et al. Survey of trauma registry data on tourniquet use in pediatric war casualties. Pediatr Emerg Care. 2012;28(12):1361–5.
60. Zarka S, Lerner A. Complicated war trauma and care of the wounded: the Israeli experience in medical care and humanitarian support of Syrian refugees. New York: Springer; 2017.
61. Chao NS, Liu CS, Chung KL, Tang PM, Tai DK, Lee KY, et al. Retroperitoneal pelvic packing for haemodynamically unstable pelvic fractures in children and adolescents: a level-one trauma-centre experience. J Pediatr Surg. 2012;47(12):2244–50.
62. Vo NJ, Althoen M, Hippe DS, Prabhu SJ, Valji K, Padia SA. Pediatric abdominal and pelvic trauma: safety and efficacy of arterial embolization. J Vasc Interv Radiol. 2014;25(2):215–20.
63. Klein Y, Arieli I, Sagiv S, Peleg K, Ben-Galim P. Cervical spine injuries in civilian victims of explosions: should cervical collars be used? J Trauma Acute Care Surg. 2016;80(6):985–8.
64. Schoenfeld AJ, Laughlin MD, McCriskin BJ, Bader JO, Waterman BR, Belmont PJ Jr. Spinal injuries in United States military personnel deployed to Iraq and Afghanistan: an epidemiological investigation involving 7877 combat casualties from 2005 to 2009. Spine (Phila Pa 1976). 2013;38(20):1770–8.
65. Arishita GI, Vayer JS, Bellamy RF. Cervical spine immobilization of penetrating neck wounds in a hostile environment. J Trauma. 1989;29(3):332–7.
66. Keller MS, Mitchell ICS, Wakeman D, Trappey F, Jeziorczak P, Bass KD, et al. Cervical spine trauma. In: American Pediatric Surgical Association: Not A Textbook. 2017. https://www.pedsurglibrary.com/apsa/view/Pediatric-Surgery-NaT/829476/all/Cervical_Spine_Trauma.
67. USAISR, Burn care - joint trauma system clinical practice guideline. 2016.

Case Study: Boston Bombings, a Surgeon's View

37

David R. King

Introduction

The injuries resulting from the two improvised explosive devices detonated on Boylston Street during the running of the 117th Boston Marathon at 14:49 on April 15, 2013, changed our lives forever. As a surgeon, soldier, Bostonian, 50+ time chronic marathoner, and participant in the 117th Boston Marathon (3:12 marathon, roughly an hour before the blasts), I will forever remember the events of that day and how they altered our city, and our country, in perpetuity. I remember those who died (29-year-old Krystle Campbell, 23-year-old Lu Lingzi, 8-year-old Martin Richard, and 27-year-old Sean Collier) and celebrate those who lived: the survivors. This chapter is dedicated to the survivors of the Boston Marathon bombing.

The Bombing

Two ground-level improvised explosive devices were detonated on Boylston Street during the running of the 117th Boston Marathon, at 14:49:43 and 14:49:57 on April 15, 2013. A total of 243 injured patients presented with a myriad of injuries (Fig. 37.1). Of the total population of 243 injured casualties, 152 patients presented to the emergency department (ED) within 24 hours of the explosions. Among the 152 patients presented within 24 hours, there were 66 patients who suffered from at

D. R. King (✉)
Harvard Medical School, Division of Trauma, Emergency Surgery, and Surgical Critical Care, Boston, MA, USA

Knight Surgical Research Laboratory, Boston, MA, USA

Massachusetts General Hospital and Harvard Medical School, Boston, MA, USA
e-mail: dking3@mgh.harvard.edu

D. W. Callaway, J. L. Burstein (eds.), *Operational and Medical Management of Explosive and Blast Incidents*, https://doi.org/10.1007/978-3-030-40655-4_37

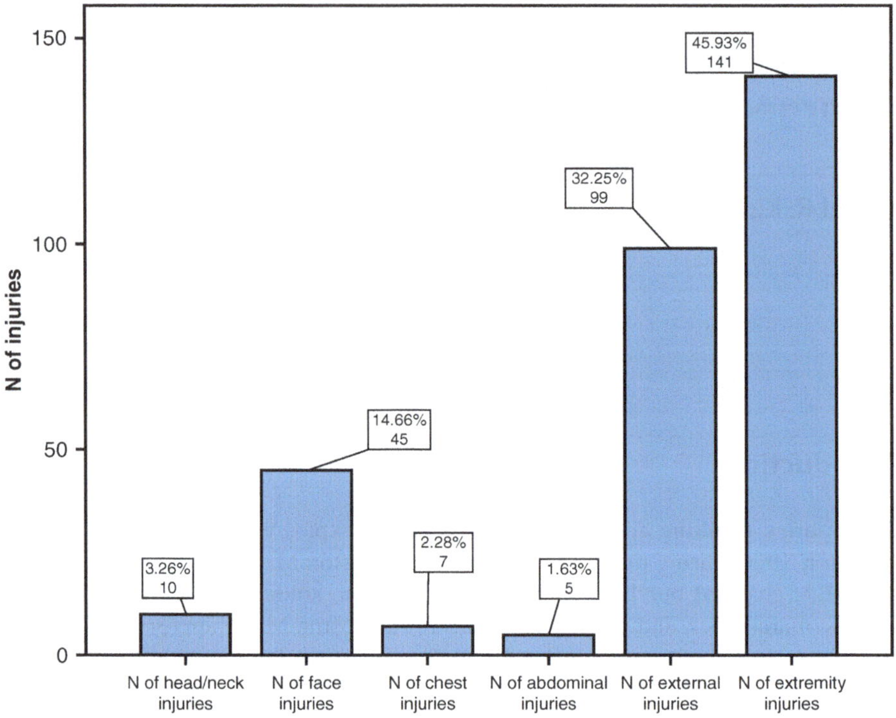

Fig. 37.1 Distribution of total injuries per body region among all 243 presenting patients

least one extremity injury. Figure 37.2 depicts the additional injury burden among all patients presenting with extremity injuries.

Of the 66 patients with extremity injury, 4 patients had upper extremities affected, 56 patients had only lower extremities affected, and 6 patients had combined upper and lower extremity injuries. There were 17 lower extremity traumatic amputations (LETA) in 15 patients, of whom 10 suffered below-knee traumatic amputation (BKA), 3 suffered above-knee traumatic amputation (AKA), 1 patient suffered bilateral BKA, and 1 suffered a BKA and an AKA.

There were additionally 10 patients with severe soft tissue injury (without traumatic amputation) having 12 lower extremities with 14 major vascular injuries (MVI). Seven of the latter were arterial (one femoral, two popliteal, and four other named arteries), and seven were venous (one femoral, three popliteal, and three other-named veins). Two lower extremities had combined arterial-venous injuries (one combined femoral arteriovenous and one combined popliteal arteriovenous injury). The burden of extremity injury is presented in Fig. 37.3.

Of all 66 patients with extremity injuries, 29 (44%) were recognized and documented as having life-threatening extremity exsanguination at the point of injury, including all 15 (100%) LETA patients, 7 of 10 (70%) MVI patients, and 7 of 41 (11%) non-LETA and non-MVI patients with other massive soft tissue and open long-bone fractures.

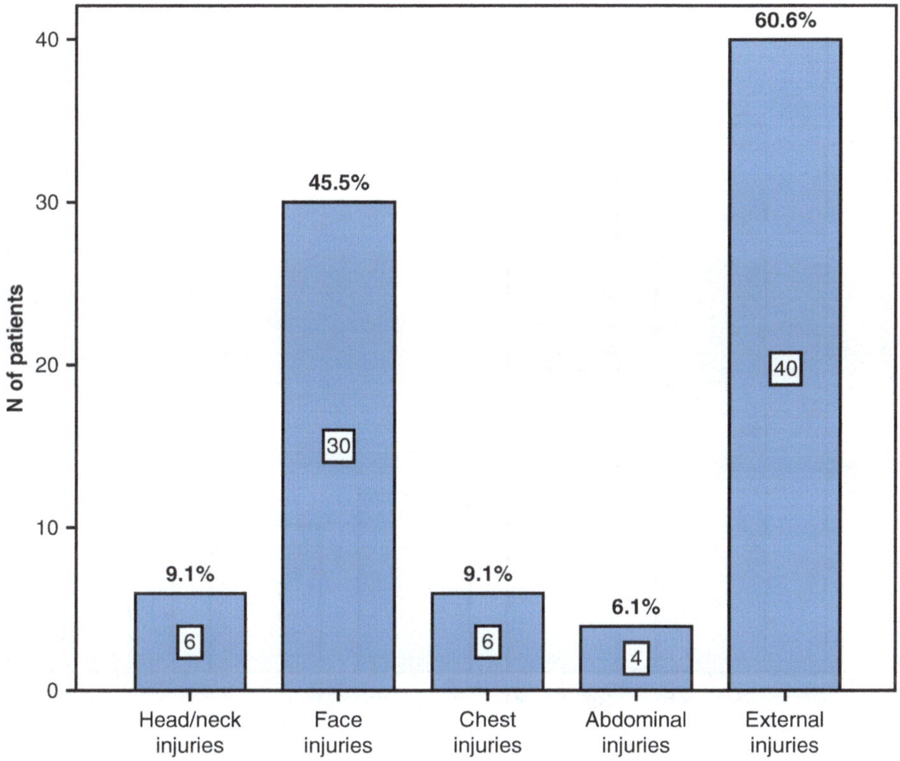

Fig. 37.2 Distribution of non-extremity injuries per body region among the 66 patients with extremity injuries

Among the 29 patients with recognized exsanguination, 27 tourniquets were applied at the point of injury: 94% of the LETA extremities, 42% of the lower extremities with major vascular injuries, and 6 of the 7 additional extremities with major soft tissue injury. No patient had more than one tourniquet per extremity, and no junctional injuries with significant hemorrhage were identified (although two patients who died on the scene had severe junctional injuries). Of the 16 LETA patients with tourniquets, 4 had improvised tourniquets applied by EMS, 7 had improvised tourniquets applied by non-EMS responders (some of whom had known medical training but were not acting as part of the official EMS response, including physicians, off-duty soldiers, etc.), and 5 had improvised tourniquets of unknown origin. Of the five lower extremities with MVI, two had improvised tourniquets applied by EMS, two had improvised tourniquets applied by non-EMS responders, and one had an improvised tourniquet of unknown origin. Of the six additional extremities with major soft tissue injury and exsanguination, four had improvised tourniquets applied by EMS, and two had improvised tourniquets of unknown origin. Figures 37.4 and 37.5 reflect the sources of the tourniquets recovered. In total, 37% of tourniquets were applied by EMS. Eight

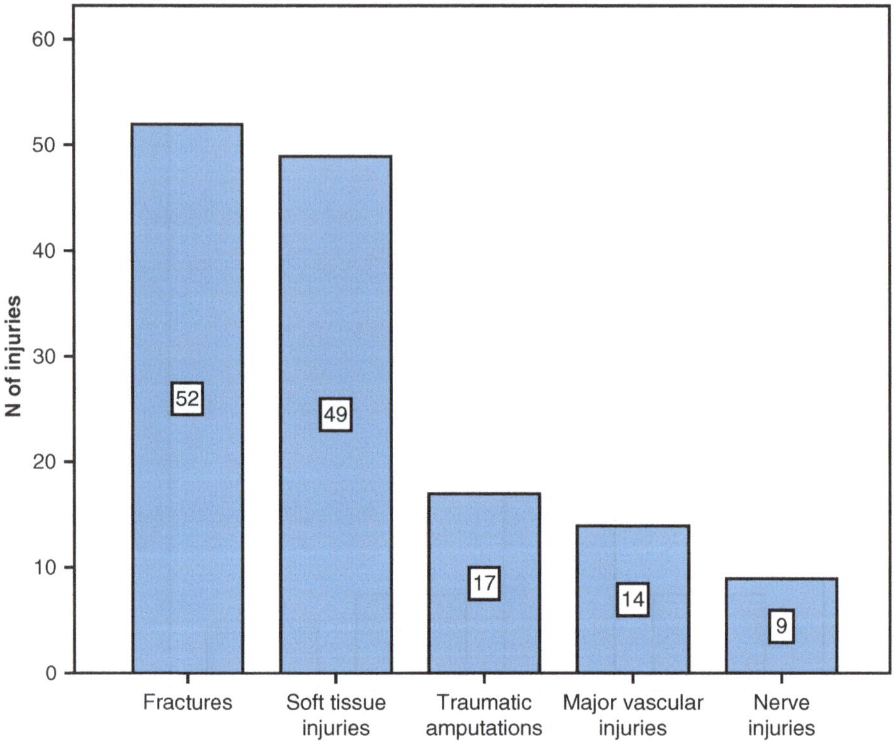

Fig. 37.3 Distribution of extremity injuries by type among the 66 patients with injured limbs

Fig. 37.4 Sources of the 27 tourniquets

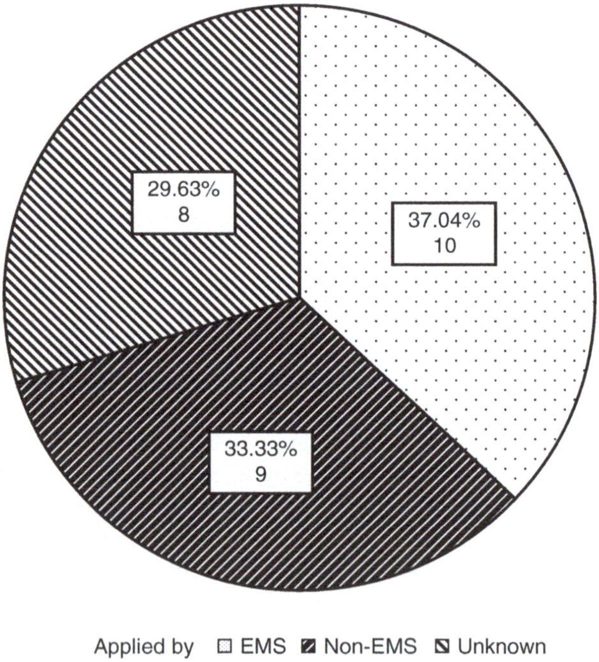

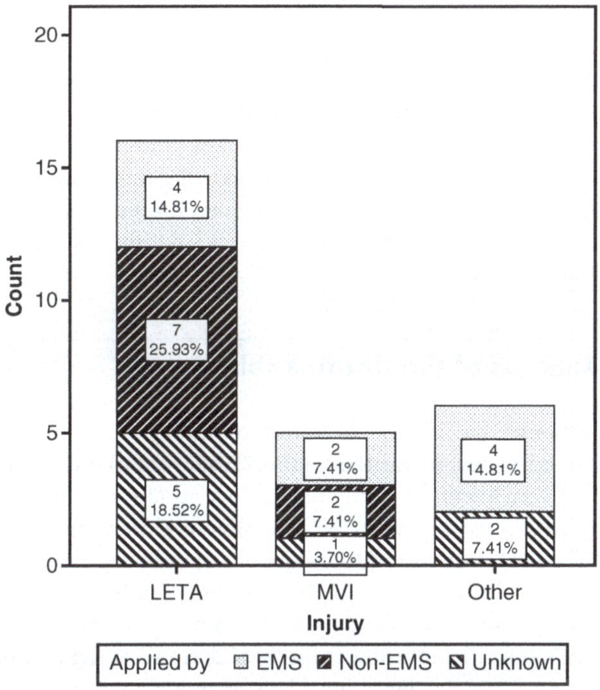

Fig. 37.5 Sources of the 27 tourniquets among 66 patients with extremity injury categorized by injury type

limbs presented to the ED with life-threatening exsanguination and had no pre-hospital tourniquet in place on arrival.

All tourniquets were improvised, including those applied by EMS, and no commercially available and purpose-designed tourniquets were identified. A review of photography and video from the scene response demonstrates a single extremity with soft tissue injury (but not a LETA) identified with a Combat Application Tourniquet (CAT) in place. We have no knowledge of this patient's trauma burden or outcome. At the Massachusetts General Hospital, all six improvised tourniquets encountered were venous tourniquets and required replacement with a commercial tourniquet to prevent ongoing extremity exsanguination. Similar reports exist from other Boston hospitals. Among the 66 patients with extremity injuries, mortality was 0%.

Triage and Index Surgery

Patients were repeatedly triaged, first at the point of injury, then at the EMS staging area near the bombing, then on the ambulance ramps of our hospital, and finally again in each of our trauma resuscitation rooms. Triage decisions are imperfect, by their very nature, and frequent re-evaluation allows for an opportunity to identify developing changes in conditions that will alter triage decisions. The decision to move a patient to the operating room is binary and generally irreversible, which commits those resources to that patient until the operation is done. Consequently, repeated preoperative triage is necessary to ensure that only the sickest patient (who have salvageable injuries) make it to the operating room. Importantly, patients with isolated limb injuries who have effective hemostasis with well-placed tourniquets do not need emergent surgery for their limb injuries. Caution is necessary, however, since these patients often have coexisting torso injuries that may be overlooked due to the visually stimulating (and distracting) extremity injuries. Attention should be directed to cavitary triage of the torso, not the striking limb injury with an effective tourniquet in place.

Analysis of the Unthinkable

Although the Boston Marathon bombing was not the first terrorist event in the United States, it was the first modern event to create mass casualties with a pattern of severe lower extremity blast injury commonly seen on the battlefield from improvised explosive devices [9]. The Boston experience demonstrated the nearly universal use of improvised tourniquets as a primary prehospital and presurgical attempt at hemostatic intervention for life-threatening extremity hemorrhage: an attempt at damage control that largely failed. A recent study conducted in Boston describes the city's informal tourniquet protocol and use of the commonly seen improvised tourniquet after the bombing. This manuscript, however, conspicuously omits data regarding effectiveness of the improvised tourniquet or why this device was specifically selected over others [12]. Recent data derived from military experience does not support the use of improvised tourniquets as best practice, as multiple studies [3–8] have consistently reported superior hemostatic results with the use of commercial, purpose-designed tourniquets. Our collective military experience has also established the hemostatic superiority of the commercially available devices by directly comparing them to improvised devices [13–15]. As a result, US combat personnel are now trained in self- and buddy application of these purpose-designed tourniquets [1, 3–8], and each US military service member carries at least one commercial tourniquet (often two). The translation of this military posture (general availability of tourniquets and widespread training on how to apply them correctly) to the homeland has not been maximally realized, unlike other battlefield lessons such as early use of antifibrinolytics, high-ratio transfusion, and abbreviated surgery, which have gained far more translational traction [16]. Had translation been more successful, one may have expected far more than a single commercial tourniquet identified after the bombing. Hemorrhage control is the first step of damage control, and damage control must start at the point of wounding.

Additional evidence from the civilian community [15, 17] demonstrates an obvious deficiency in the translation of the military's extremity hemorrhage control posture. A retrospective study on trauma registries at two large level 1 trauma centers in Canada [15] revealed that of 190 patients who suffered isolated extremity injuries with arterial injury, only 4 patients had a tourniquet present upon arrival. Those were all improvised tourniquets (neck tie, belt, or handkerchief) applied by police or bystanders. In the non-tourniquet group, six deaths were recorded as a direct result of exsanguination. While statistically significant differences were difficult to observe given the small number of patients who received a prehospital tourniquet, this study highlights the profound absence of systematic use of tourniquets in the prehospital environment. Following this, the 2012 Adult Traumatic Hemorrhage Control Protocol was introduced to all EMS providers in the province of Alberta, Canada – a protocol that advises the use of a commercial tourniquet for uncontrolled extremity bleeding and completes the translation of battlefield lessons to the homeland. Each state in the United States should consider adopting a similar protocol.

Although it is certainly possible to improvise an effective arterial tourniquet, the data suggests this is uncommonly done appropriately, especially under stress [4, 10–17]. An improvised tourniquet should (1) be wide enough to compress arterial and venous vasculature without creating pressure necrosis of the skin or neuropraxia (as may occur with narrow tourniquets, such as rubber tubing) and (2) have a device attached to create a mechanical advantage to generate adequate circumferential pressure (such as a windlass). The improvised tourniquets used in Boston met only the second of these two fundamental criteria. It is important to note that as materials science and tourniquet technology advances, it may be possible to create an effective arterial tourniquet device without a windlass [18, 19].

While full translation of the military posture regarding extremity hemorrhage control and tourniquet use may be ideal, one must accept that, in the setting of sudden disaster, tourniquets will continue to be improvised despite all efforts at translation by policy-makers. It is clear that improvised tourniquets, and the temporary hemorrhage control they offer, will always be used in mass casualty scenarios, and their role should not be entirely discounted. An improvised venous tourniquet can provide temporary hemorrhage control [3, 5, 6]; however, a comprehensive review of emergency tourniquet use recently highlighted the significance of unintentional venous tourniquets as potentially deadly [2], particularly in the minutes following initial bleeding control. The experience in Boston, with apparent, initial, hemostasis with improvised tourniquets at point of injury, supports this notion and appears to echo that of known paradoxical bleeding after venous tourniquet application. Venous tourniquets can create initial adequate hemorrhage control that soon worsens, as a time-dependent function, until hemorrhage control is lost and supplanted by paradoxical hemorrhage, the worsening of hemorrhage than if no tourniquet were used at all [3]. Perhaps an educational campaign to teach the correct way to apply a purpose-designed tourniquet, as well as how to improvise an effective arterial tourniquet, may be appropriate since it is nearly certain that limbs will have improvised tourniquets applied after the next, unfortunate, bombing in the homeland. Several studies suggest that adequate training can be minimal (less than a minute) and still result in trainees who can apply effective tourniquets [18, 19].

Despite some possible limitations with respect to prehospital extremity hemorrhage control, there were no inhospital deaths. The mean transport time from point of injury to ED was 24 min, substantially faster than the range of commonly reported evacuation times in the military and civilian literature, which could vary from well under 1 hour to over 2 hours after time of wounding, depending on the setting and circumstances [10, 13, 20–23]. The high number of Boston area metropolitan trauma centers all co-located in a very small geographic area in close proximity to the Boston Marathon finish line likely contributed to this rapid evacuation time, as well as the robust medical infrastructure already in place at the finish line for the expected event-related illnesses.

The Boston bombing experience suggests that (1) instances of multiple exsanguinating extremity injuries, similar to battlefield wounds, can occur in the homeland and (2) improvised tourniquets likely provided initial hemorrhage control, but the absence of purpose-designed devices in the bombing response probably created some cases of paradoxical bleeding. When contrasted to the wealth of evidence gathered from the last decade of military experience, these findings call for a reconsideration of our practices. We recommend that all EMS services translate a military posture with an extremity hemorrhage control protocol that emphasizes appropriate training with liberal availability of commercial, purpose-designed tourniquets. Proper tourniquet application techniques should be presented in the Advanced Trauma Life Support and Prehospital Trauma Life Support training manuals, among others. Several notable organizations, including the Hartford Consensus and the American College of Surgeons, are recommending translation and adoption of military posture toward prehospital extremity hemorrhage control [24, 25]. Physician leaders and policy-makers should insist on translation of a prehospital extremity hemorrhage control posture similar to the ubiquitous adoption and presence of automated external defibrillators in nearly every ambulance, federal building, cafeteria, and other public gathering area in the United States.

Lessons Learned

Although much attention has been given to the obvious absence of purpose-made tourniquets in the Boston bombing response, other lessons were also learned of significant importance. For the sake of completeness, the entire list of lessons learned is presented here.

- *Tourniquets work, are safe, require training, and need to be ubiquitous.* No purpose-designed tourniquets or advanced topical hemostatic agents were available. Although we must not discourage bystanders from responding to disaster to aid the injured, we must also be intellectually honest and recognize that (despite the lay press reporting) the improvised tourniquets applied on Boylston were likely not arterial tourniquets. Improvisation of an arterial tourniquet is a skill set that can be taught and should be widely incorporated into general first aid classes. If purpose-made tourniquets had been available, proper training to ensure correct application is necessary. The Committee for Tactical Emergency Casualty Care (C-TECC) and the Committee on Tactical Combat Casualty Care (CoTCCC) published guidelines regarding tourniquet use and formal training, and written protocols are widely available. These should be adopted as permanent part of the curriculum for every first responder.

- *There was too much "stay and play" in the medical tent at the finish line.* While the finish line medical tent instantly became the de facto triage area after the bombing, the transport time recorded for many severely injured patients was over an hour. Either by design or by a matter of mass confusion, some patients remained in the medical tent for an extended period. In a city with five level 1 trauma centers and hundreds of patients with surgical injuries, patients should be moved to hospitals in a swifter fashion.
- *Triage is dynamic.* Triage must be rapid and medical providers must accept that the triage process will be imperfect. Patients who are triaged as emergent may, in fact, not be dying. Other patients triaged as non-emergent may unexpectedly deteriorate. Frequent re-triage is required and may alter initial triage decisions. In the emergency department, patients should be re-triaged by a senior surgeon or senior emergency medicine physician. Utilization of the operating rooms is a finite resource, and only patients who truly need a life-saving operation should be triaged straight to the operating room. Care decisions should be made regarding axial imaging studies as many of these studies are initially unnecessary. A plain chest X-ray and a focused abdominal ultrasound exam are often the only imaging required to make informed inhospital triage decisions.
- *The most visually stimulating injury is often not the most life-threatening one.* The Boston bombing patients arrived with extremely devastating, and visually stimulating, limb injuries. These injuries, despite their appearance, were easily controlled with tourniquets. Some patients also had coexisting intracavitary hemorrhage. This can often be overlooked when the clinician inappropriately focused on the limb injury and neglects a complete trauma evaluation, particularly of the peritoneal and thoracic cavities. Once an effective tourniquet is in place, the limb injury becomes (temporarily) forgettable.
- *Damage control starts at the point of injury.* The damage control resuscitation (DCR) principles begin at point of injury, must be maintained during patient transportation, and should be aggressively implemented in the ED in order to prepare patients for best surgical survival. A low volume (or no volume) crystalloid fluid restrictive resuscitation strategy should be adopted. Patients waiting for less-than-emergent surgery should receive minimal crystalloid therapy. If resuscitation is required, volume expansion with a transfusion strategy that approximates fresh whole blood should be utilized. For many hospitals, this means adopting a strategy of high-ratio transfusion of packed red blood cells:plasma:platelets. All fluids and blood products should be warmed to normal body temperature. Antifibrinolytics should be liberally administered. For patients with limb injuries that have a tourniquet in place and are waiting for surgery, tourniquet conversion should be considered if time and manpower permit.
- *Damage control surgery is vital.* In the operating room, only hemorrhage control and contamination control are desired. Abbreviated surgery, vascular shunts, bowel stapled and left in discontinuity, and temporary abdominal closures should dominate the landscape. Ideally, only warmed blood and blood products should

be administered during damage control surgery. The operating room should be made as warm as possible; the surgeon should become exceedingly uncomfortable with the temperature in the room. When in doubt, all body cavities should be surgically interrogated. Bilateral tube thoracostomy, pericardial window, and laparotomy are the imaging methods of choice during damage control in disasters. Patients should be rapidly transferred to the intensive care unit and the operating room reset for the next patient. Once all index operations are complete, the entire team should reassemble to re-triage and regroup resources.

- *Sequential medical record numbers are dangerous.* Assigning patients sequential medical record numbers in simple escalating numerical fashion creates an unacceptable margin of error since there will be many simultaneous patients with medical record numbers differing by only a single digit (1,234,567, 1,234,568, 1,234,569…). This creates an unacceptable environment for a potential clerical error, single keystroke mistake, that would potentially result in a surgeon looking at the hemoglobin value of the wrong patient or (worse yet) ordering tests or procedures on the wrong patient. Medical record numbers during disasters should vary widely to prevent this error.
- *Don't go home just yet: the tertiary trauma survey is extremely important.* In disasters, it is a common urge to "take a break" once each patient's index operation is complete and all the bleeding and contamination are controlled. This, however, is a mistake. Once the initial surgery is done, the entire trauma team should reassemble to go over each patient again, in extreme detail. The purpose of this is twofold. First, the entire team needs to understand each patient's condition and status, so appropriate planning for operative take-backs, additional imaging, and other interventions can be planned and prioritized. Second, small injuries are commonly missed and will only be identified by a careful tertiary survey. Although most of our patients had non-life-threatening ruptured tympanic membranes, for example, these were largely not identified until posttrauma day 2 on a careful tertiary exam. This is, of course, an appropriate injury to miss on initial evaluation in a mass casualty situation; however, failure to recognize and treat this injury (and others like it) could result in long-term disability.
- *Human resource management is critical.* If the disaster is expected to become protracted, rest and sleep cycles should be mandated so that human resources do not become all simultaneously exhausted. Responders will not go home or rest voluntarily; this becomes a leadership imperative.

Conclusion

The Boston Marathon bombing solidified multiple lessons for our city. First, damage control starts at the point of injury. No one should die from a preventable cause of death such as limb exsanguination. The prehospital response to extremity exsanguination after the Boston Marathon bombing demonstrates that our current practice is an approach, lost in translation, from the battlefield to the homeland. Proper tourniquet application techniques should be presented in the Advanced Trauma Life Support and Prehospital Trauma Life Support training manuals, among others. Second, triage becomes the most important decision that is made on the scene of a disaster. That decision should be revisited often following initial triage of all casualties. Third, re-triage at the hospital is important to prevent inappropriate utilization of human and physical plant infrastructure on patients who are not truly dying. Finally, abbreviated surgery with attention to high-ratio transfusion, use of antifibrinolytics, vascular shunts, contamination control, and temporary abdominal (or chest) closure is necessary.

References

1. Welling DR, McKay PL, Rasmussen TE, Rich NM. A brief history of the tourniquet. J Vasc Surg. 2012;55(1):286–90.
2. Kragh JF Jr, Swan KG, Smith DC, Mabry RL, Blackbourne LH. Historical review of emergency tourniquet use to stop bleeding. Am J Surg. 2012;203(2):242–52.
3. Kragh JF Jr, O'Neill ML, Walters TJ, Dubick MA, Baer DG, Wade CE, et al. Minor morbidity with emergency tourniquet use to stop bleeding in severe limb trauma: research, history, and reconciling advocates and abolitionists. Mil Med. 2011;176(7):817–23.
4. King DR, van der Wilden G, Kragh JF Jr, Blackbourne LH. Forward assessment of 79 prehospital battlefield tourniquets used in the current war. J Spec Oper Med 2012;12(4):33–38.
5. Beekley AC, Sebesta JA, Blackbourne LH, Herbert GS, Kauvar DS, Baer DG, et al; 31st Combat Support Hospital Research Group. Prehospital tourniquet use in Operation Iraqi Freedom: effect on hemorrhage control and outcomes. J Trauma. 2008;64(2 Suppl):S28–37.
6. Kragh JF Jr, Walters TJ, Baer DG, Fox CJ, Wade CE, Salinas J, et al. Survival with emergency tourniquet use to stop bleeding in major limb trauma. Ann Surg. 2009;249(1):1–7.
7. Kragh JF Jr, Littrel ML, Jones JA, Walters TJ, Baer DG, Wade CE, et al. Battle casualty survival with emergency tourniquet use to stop limb bleeding. J Emerg Med. 2011;41(6):590–7.
8. Lakstein D, Blumenfeld A, Sokolov T, Lin G, Bssorai R, Lynn M, Ben-Abraham R. Tourniquets for hemorrhage control on the battlefield: a 4-year accumulated experience. J Trauma. 2003;54(5 Suppl):S221–5.
9. Kapur GB, Hutson HR, Davis MA, Rice PL. The United States twenty-year experience with bombing incidents: implications for terrorism preparedness and medical response. J Trauma. 2005;59(6):1436–44.
10. Gates JD, Arabian S, Biddinger P, Blansfield J, Burke P, Chung S, et al. The initial response to the Boston marathon bombing: lessons learned to prepare for the next disaster. Ann Surg. 2014;260(6):960–6.
11. King DR, Larentzakis A, Ramly EP, Boston Trauma Collaborative. Tourniquet use at the Boston Marathon bombing: lost in translation. J Trauma Acute Care Surg. 2015;78(3):594–9.
12. Kalish J, Burke P, Feldman J, Agarwal S, Glantz A, Moyer P, et al. The return of tourniquets. Original research evaluates the effectiveness of prehospital tourniquets for civilian penetrating extremity injuries. JEMS. 2008;33(8):44–6, 49–50, 52, 54.
13. D'Alleyrand JCG, Dutton RP, Pollak AN. Extrapolation of battlefield resuscitative care to the civilian setting. J Surg Orthop Adv. 2010;19(1):62–9.
14. Evaluation of self-applied tourniquets for combat applications, second phase. 2013. http://archive.rubicon-foundation.org/xmlui/handle/123456789/6870?show=full. Accessed 19 Sept 2013.
15. Passos E, Dingley B, Smith A, Engels PT, Ball CG, Faidi S, et al; Canadian Trauma Trials Collaborative. Tourniquet use for peripheral vascular injuries in the civilian setting. Injury. 2014;45(3):573–7.

16. Duchesne JC, Islam TM, Stuke L, Timmer JR, Barbeau JM, Marr AB, et al. Hemostatic resuscitation during surgery improves survival in patients with traumatic-induced coagulopathy. J Trauma. 2009;67, 33(1):–7; discussion 37–9.
17. Dorlac WC, DeBakey ME, Holcomb JB, Fagan SP, Kwong KL, Dorlac GR, et al. Mortality from isolated civilian penetrating extremity injury. J Trauma. 2005;59(1):217–22.
18. Wall PL, Duevel DC, Hassan MB, Welander JD, Sahr SM, Buising CM. Tourniquets and occlusion: the pressure of design. Mil Med. 2013;178(5):578–87.
19. Wall PL, Welander JD, Singh A, Sidwell RA, Buising CM. Stretch and wrap style tourniquet effectiveness with minimal training. Mil Med. 2012;177(11):1366–73.
20. Ingalls N, Zonies D, Bailey JA, Martin KD, Iddins BO, Carlton PK, et al. A review of the first 10 years of critical care aeromedical transport during Operation Iraqi Freedom and Operation Enduring Freedom: the importance of evacuation timing. JAMA Surg. 2014;149(8):807–13.
21. Ball CG, Williams BH, Tallah C, Salomone JP, Feliciano DV. The impact of shorter prehospital transport times on outcomes in patients with abdominal vascular injuries. J Trauma Manag Outcomes. 2013;7(1):11.
22. Crandall M, Sharp D, Unger E, Straus D, Brasel K, Hsia R, et al. Trauma deserts: distance from a trauma center, transport times, and mortality from gunshot wounds in Chicago. Am J Public Health. 2013;103(6):1103–9.
23. Bulger EM, Guffey D, Guyette FX, MacDonald RD, Brasel K, Kerby JD, et al; Resuscitation Outcomes Consortium Investigators. Impact of prehospital mode of transport after severe injury: a multicenter evaluation from the Resuscitation Outcomes Consortium. J Trauma Acute Care Surg. 2012;72(3):567–73; discussion 573–5.
24. Jacobs LM, McSwain NE Jr, Rotondo MF, Wade D, Fabbri W, Eastman AL, et al; Joint Committee to Create a National Policy to Enhance Survivability from Mass Casualty Shooting Events. Improving survival from active shooter events: the Hartford Consensus. J Trauma Acute Care Surg. 2013;74(6):1399–400.
25. Bulger EM, Snyder D, Schoelles K, Gotschall C, Dawson D, Lang E, et al. An evidence-based prehospital guideline for external hemorrhage control: American College of Surgeons Committee on Trauma. Prehosp Emerg Care. 2014;18(2):163–73.

Part V

ICU Management

ICU Management of Blast Victims: Scope of the Problem and Operational Considerations

38

Valerie G. Sams and Alexander D. Malloy

Introduction

Both terrorist activity and industrial incidents can result in complex blast injuries which have demonstrated a high rate of mangled extremities with the potential for multiple limb amputations, pelvic trauma, and genitourinary injuries [1]. These types of injuries are also a combination of penetrating, blast, burn, and blunt mechanisms which can lead to multisystem trauma and significant skin, soft tissue, muscle, and boney involvement [2]. Blast incidents have become increasingly common in recent years [3, 4]. These patients present with injury severity scores (ISS) of higher value on average than other trauma victims and have a higher transfusion requirement [5–9]. The decrease in mortality observed in military casualties who suffer these types of injuries is likely a combination of improved logistical support, equipment availability, experience and expertise of the critical care team, avoidance of coagulopathy and acute respiratory distress syndrome (ARDS), and proximity of advanced care to the point of injury [10, 11]. There are challenges to providing exceptional critical care in explosion-related mass casualty incidents (MCI) despite evolving and improving methods to provide balanced resuscitation [12]. Elements contributing to these challenges include limited ability for supply and resupply of equipment, resuscitation products, triage necessity and accuracy, ancillary support, and wound care.

V. G. Sams (✉) · A. D. Malloy
Division of Trauma, Department of Surgery, Brooke Army Medical Center, San Antonio, TX, USA
e-mail: Valerie.g.sams.mil@mail.mil

D. W. Callaway, J. L. Burstein (eds.), *Operational and Medical Management of Explosive and Blast Incidents*, https://doi.org/10.1007/978-3-030-40655-4_38

Challenges of Blast Incidents and MCI

When patients arrive to the intensive care unit, the roles of the critical care providers are to restore hemostasis in the patient and prevent loss of life, limb, or eyesight. Integrated teams of intensivists and critical care surgeons, executing evidence-based (or evidence-guided) and goal-directed therapies, improve mortality [13, 14].

Blast injuries often present as mass casualty incidents. Triage is a challenge in the explosion-related MCI setting, as resources are prone to depletion and the security situation remains fluid long after the initial patients arrive in the ICU. In addition, the extent of injury is often difficult to ascertain initially as mechanisms of injury can result from direct contact with the blast, concussive blast, and severe burns [15, 16]. Multisystem injury is almost always present and thus makes accurate triage challenging. Recognition of complex injury patters and specific organ system disruption must be accomplished quickly. In patients who undergo damage control surgery (DCS) and subsequent transfer to a critical care team for ongoing damage control resuscitation (DCR), the use and allocation of resuscitation products during the dynamic process of DCR may affect triage, especially if there are extended times for transfer to tertiary centers or if available resources are severely limited. In the battlefield setting, DCR may be prolonged due to distant evacuation routes or lack of immediate transportation, and the dynamic resuscitation that occurs could be significantly altered by such factors. Uncommon intensive management of manpower and resources, complex staffing arrangements, damage control techniques and practices to preserve supplies and resources, ongoing needs with multiple operations, and prolonged hospitalization all impact care of these types of patients. This coupled with the element of surprise that often exists with these types of incidents such that there is no warning of event and there must be rapid mobilization of personnel and resources both prehospital and in-hospital.

There are some differences between civilian and military evacuation thought processes in terms of resource limitations (i.e., personnel, supplies, and equipment), security of evacuation platforms (e.g., response risk tolerance), timing of patient movement, and injury evolution. The US military experience has developed ways to learn lessons from these challenges that can be useful to civilian systems. In general, the evolution of the injury patterns is not observed or known by prehospital providers, but is seen once the patient arrives at tertiary centers and intensive care units. The US military's Joint Trauma System developed a weekly teleconference to discuss combat casualty care through the continuum from point of injury to definitive care and even rehab [17–19]. This provides the opportunity to share insight and feedback from every level to include the intensive care management and thus the development of prehospital and in-hospital practices that improve patient care.

Patients are frequently transported to the ICU after damage control procedures with persistent hypovolemic shock resulting in acidosis and hypothermia. These conditions along with coagulopathy are associated with the lethal triad or "bloody vicious cycle" of trauma [20]. Intensive care teams must use aggressive warming techniques and goal-directed correction of coagulopathy and acidosis during prolonged resuscitations. Restoration of physiologic parameters is the primary outcome for any critical care team. Care should be taken when considering use of crystalloid infusions in the multisystem-injured patient as excess administration or over-resuscitation can be detrimental in patients with extensive burns, pulmonary contusion, or head injury. Crystalloids in sufficient amounts can result in dilutional coagulopathy, acute respiratory distress syndrome (ARDS), and abdominal compartment syndromes [3]. Damage control resuscitation principles to prevent the lethal triad require consideration in terms of equipment and supplies such as rapid fluid and blood infusers, point of care blood testing, warming blankets, blood bank products, and massive transfusion protocols. Activation of a walking whole blood bank may be necessary, and protocols implementing such are already in place within the US military system. Though major legal, logistical, and financial challenges exist, some civilian trauma centers are testing the walking blood bank concept [21–23].

Often, the acuity of blast victims requires a nursing to patient ratio of 1:1, limiting an intensive care unit's functional capacity for active care without bringing in additional nursing and technician staff. From an operational standpoint, the dynamic security situation, extent of MCI, or hospital lockdown procedures may impede the healthcare system's ability to rapidly surge staff from external sources. Intensive care teams should therefore consider internal options for cross-training staff, pushing advanced capabilities to wards outside of the ICU, and creating effective work-rest cycles.

Often, upon arrival to the ICU, the extent of blast injuries is difficult to ascertain. Injury patterns and evolution vary depending on a variety of factors (e.g., location and body position of the casualty relative to the blast, enclosed versus open air blast, comorbid conditions, etc.). Fragmentation of the materials (i.e., metal, wood, soil, human remains, etc.) may penetrate deep into the soft tissues, muscle, and bone. Routine serial debridement has become the mainstay of wound care in blast injuries to decrease bacterial load and to examine and debride nonviable tissue planes. Invasive bacterial and fungal infections have become very common in these injuries and are increasingly difficult to treat; additional soft tissue loss and amputation are often results of staving off sepsis from these infections. This reality requires sufficient surgical staff skilled in aggressive debridement techniques, amputations, and fasciotomies. Integrated surgical teams involving orthopedic, general, vascular, burn, and plastic surgeons should be routine at most trauma centers. But if they do not exist, a plan for ad hoc team creation should be in place. The operating theater must be staffed to accommodate repeat trips to the operating room for these patients over the span of several days. Wound care, dressing, and irrigation supplies will need to be managed and monitored closely. Penetrating injuries from fragments that are from the weapon itself or fragments that are a result of the explosion are the leading cause of death and injury in both military and civilian terrorist attacks with the exception of building collapse [15].

Many acutely injured blast victims will remain hospitalized and in the intensive care unit for several days following the event. The resulting high census and low patient throughput will likely impact the facility's ability to receive additional "routine" trauma or critical care patients. In order to mitigate impact on the regional trauma system, it is imperative that health systems, not just trauma centers, have operational plans in place to manage this type of acute surge in resource-intense, polytrauma patients. In the clinician's realm, prevention of abdominal compartment syndrome, acute kidney injury, acute respiratory distress syndrome, ventilator-associated pneumonia, and sepsis contribute to decreased rates of mortality and decreased length of stay in the injured patient. These outcomes can be accomplished by adhering to protocols and guidelines for ongoing resuscitation and critical care management in accordance with damage control resuscitation and clinical practice guidelines created by organizations such as the US military.

Facial trauma from a blast can quickly compromise an airway. These patients may require an invasive airway or a surgical airway. Additionally, blast injuries are notorious for pulmonary contusion, pulmonary edema, and "blast lung," resulting in additional barotrauma. These scenarios can quickly progress to acute respiratory distress syndrome (ARDS) particularly in the setting of blood and fluid resuscitation. Aggressive ventilator management with advanced modalities and settings is key for treating blast lung and ARDS [24]. This will require experienced and well-staffed respiratory therapy personnel, bronchoscopic capabilities, and possibly additional pulmonology colleagues to assist. In severe cases, extracorporeal membrane oxygenation (ECMO) therapy may be required [25, 26].

Cerebral injuries will require adequate cerebral perfusion pressure and possibly intracranial pressure monitoring to guide therapy and intervention. These types of injuries require neurosurgical specialists as well as staff familiar with monitoring equipment. Intracranial monitoring devices may be exhausted in a mass casualty incident and clinicians instead will rely on neurologic examination for clinical assessment of the severely head-injured patient. Hypertonic solutions, osmotic diuretics, and other medications used specifically for neurologic injury may be in limited supply or unavailable. While there is a paucity of evidence to suggest these therapies improve morbidity and mortality in blast TBI, they remain the mainstay of treatment of increased intracranial pressure [27]. Emergency decompressive procedures may be indicated without immediate available neurosurgical support. There are several instances in the literature where decompressive craniectomies and craniotomies have been performed by providers other than neurosurgeons; these instances are rare but must be in the skill set of an experienced critical care team [28, 29].

A frequently encountered injury in blasts is the ruptured tympanic membrane [30]. This occurs from the primary blast injury and can occur up to one-third of blast-injured patients [15, 31]. Of significance to the intensivist, the presence of tympanic membrane rupture should heighten the suspicion of other blast-related injuries. Every blast-injured patient should undergo otoscopic examination to evaluate for tympanic membrane injury, which has a strong correlation with associated multisystem injury, and should prompt a thorough tertiary survey [32, 33]. The concussive wave of a primary blast injury associated with ruptured tympanic membranes also has a stronger correlation with gas-filled anatomical structures, such as the lung or gastrointestinal tract, both of which may suffer barotrauma or perforation [32].

Similarly, ocular injury is common in blasts. Proximity to the explosion can result in primary globe rupture; secondary injury patterns can occur from fragmentation or debris deposited within the eye [15]. Most ocular injuries should be handled strictly by an ophthalmologist. The current practice guidelines for ocular blast injuries in a military setting are "shield and ship," i.e., placing a hard shield or securing existing protective eyewear if globe rupture or ocular injury is present. Immediate triage evaluation should include a slit lamp exam with fluorescein to evaluate for ruptured globe which would warrant an urgent ophthalmology consult. Urgent evaluation and surgical management are needed to prevent infection, vision loss, and possibly enucleation of the eye. Once triaged and in the ICU, these patients should be managed with the ophthalmologist to determine need for continued shielding of globe, types of intraocular medications, and frequency of medication administration and examinations. Despite improved eye protection, ocular blast injuries still comprise approximately 8–10% of all military blast injuries [34]. While maintaining vigilance and conducting serial examinations, clinicians can prevent vision loss which is the sequelae of undiagnosed increased intraocular pressure (IOP). A bedside ultrasound can be utilized to measure IOP and diagnose ocular compartment syndrome. If ocular compartment syndrome is suspected and imminent loss of the eye is a concern, an experienced physician may perform lateral canthotomy in an attempt to save the patient's vision. Otherwise, all injuries are typically evaluated by an experienced ophthalmologist.

Rhabdomyolysis is a more frequently seen condition in blast injuries due to traumatic amputations, massive soft tissue loss, and severe burns. Despite appropriate wound care and surgical management and balanced resuscitation to maintain adequate urine output in an effort to restore physiologic parameters, muscle breakdown can unfortunately lead to acute kidney injury and renal failure. Standard treatment for rhabdomyolysis includes intravascular volume resuscitation with crystalloid infusion and strict urine output monitoring with an endpoint resuscitation goal of 1–2 ml/kg of urine output per hour. Some institutions also attempt to alkalinize the urine with bicarbonate administration which is based on level 3 evidence as described in recent guidelines [35, 36]. Much like the standards of care with significant burns, the administration of large volumes of crystalloid for rhabdomyolysis can have paradoxical effects on the polytrauma patient, increasing the likelihood of abdominal compartment syndrome, pulmonary edema, and dilutional coagulopathy. Goal-directed resuscitation in these highly complex blast victims requires aggressive monitoring with conventional labs, thromboelastography, and physiologic parameters of resuscitation. Coupled with severe burns, patients with rhabdomyolysis may require continuous renal replacement therapy, continuous veno-venous hemofiltration, or hemodialysis, another labor-intensive intervention that requires close nursing support and resources that may or may not be available.

Significant total body surface area second- and third-degree burns have an association with blast injuries. These patients may require heroic resuscitative efforts, prolonged intubation, multiple surgical debridement, renal replacement therapy, prone positioning, and extensive skin grafting that may not be feasible in a combat intensive care unit due to limited resources and resupply.

Focus on Systems Approach

Blast-injured victims almost always arrive to the intensive care unit in extremis. These patients have multisystem trauma and can have occult hollow viscus injury from concussive blasts, severe burns, pulmonary contusions, ocular and otic injuries, and massive soft tissue injury or limb loss. They usually arrive intubated with the potential for an open abdomen, a mangled extremity, brain injury, or a combination of the above. The first step in preserving life in these patients is establishing clear communication with the pre-ICU teams (i.e., pre-hospital, emergency department, and surgical teams). Quantifying resuscitation, describing interventions, establishing venous access, and reevaluating ATLS measures are key lifesaving maneuvers. If a patient arrives with poor documentation or unclear communication based on resuscitative efforts, the patient's life could be at risk. Even in the absence of MCI, treatment of blast-injured patients can be chaotic due to the association of higher injury severity scores (ISS) and multifactorial hemodynamic instability. In the setting of MCI, this chaos can be logarithmically amplified; thus, clear communication, focus on assigned roles, appropriate triage, and adherence to care algorithms are paramount to maximize preservation of life.

System-based practices and goal-directed therapies developed over the last several years can aid in decreasing morbidity, mortality, over- and underresuscitation, and restoration of hemostasis. The largest limitation in goal-directed therapies and best practice measures can be lack of available resources.

What Is Currently Best Practice?

The US military Joint Trauma System has established clinical practice guidelines (CPG) that direct intensivists and surgeons in current best practice measures for treatment, resuscitation, and surgical management of the blast-injured patient [37]. These guidelines are updated periodically and provide a streamlined method for patient care that is widely agreed upon, but is not a substitute for best clinical practice in a given scenario. These guidelines have proven invaluable when treating blast-injured patients and mass casualties. Through the experience of multiple combat surgeons and physicians, coupled with comparative civilian data in blast injury and mass casualties, the advent of balanced resuscitation and administering whole blood products have proven to be effective in decreasing mortality and morbidity from over-resuscitation [12]. The best practice measures for blast-injured patients with multisystem trauma are widely accepted; intensive care system-based practices to restore homeostasis, minimize morbidity, and prevent mortality are the primary goals.

Many civilian institutions have developed their own MCI protocols. Frequently, these protocols are a direct result of lessons learned from domestic terroristic acts and bombings. Prior mass casualty protocols have been in existence for instances such as natural disasters and are maintained by Federal Emergency Management Agency (FEMA), state governments, and healthcare systems [38]. Recent hurricanes, forest fires, and mass shootings have all activated emergency responses invoking MCI plans. These protocols emphasize the need for a unified response from first responders, emergency room personnel, surgeons, intensivists, and ancillary staff to perform effective triage, resuscitative measures, and treatment plans to minimize mortality in scenarios that can quickly overwhelm available resources.

Conclusion

Catastrophic injuries and multiple amputations that would have made patients expectant in earlier times are now being managed with aggressive, multitiered intensive care. The development of evidence-based guidelines by healthcare providers, surgeons, intensivists, and ancillary staff promotes improved mortality rates, which have never been observed in prior military conflicts. The role of an intensive care unit is to maintain life and limb that has been compromised and to restore homeostasis. These objectives continue to be achieved, through the efforts of armed forces in creating walking blood banks, constant resupply chains that remain uninterrupted due to air superiority, and innovative measures performed by physicians in the absence of resources and supplies, which will be described in the following chapter.

Pitfalls

Special patient populations: There are special populations of patients or casualties that require certain considerations and are often the areas in which we see failures.

- Pediatric patients exposed to acts of terrorism "require more resources of intensive care units, have higher injury severity scores (scores for severity of injury in patients with multiple injuries), and have longer hospital stays than children who survived traumatic events unrelated to terrorism" [15].
- In pregnant patients, while the fetus is protected by amniotic fluid, the placental attachments can be disrupted from the blast wave and result in placental abruption. Women beyond the first trimester of pregnancy should be admitted for fetal monitoring [15].

Failure of communication, coordination, and triage

- Robust communication is important to allow for dynamic planning during ongoing operations.
- "Meticulous coordination of manpower and medical resources are among the greatest challenges" [3]. If areas do not have coordinated plans and processes that are reviewed and practiced, then it can be very chaotic and disorganized and morbidity increases. This is especially true in the high-resource ICU.
- Patients with injury to four or more body areas, facial and skull fractures, and peripheral vascular injury suggest severe trauma and the need for ICU admission [6]. Full-spectrum coordination of health systems is important to align critical resources with patient needs.

References

1. Wolf SJ, Bebarta VS, Bonnett CJ, Pons PT, Cantrill SV. Blast injuries. Lancet. 2009;374(9687):405–15.
2. Blast Injury SJH. Translating research into operational medicine. In: Lenhart MK, editor. Military quantitative physiology: problems and concepts in military operational medicine (textbooks of military medicine): US Army Medical Department and The Borden Institute; 2012. p. 267–302.
3. Kashuk JL, Halperin P, Caspi G, Colwell C, Moore EE. Bomb explosions in acts of terrorism: evil creativity challenges our trauma systems. J Am Coll Surg. 2009;209(1):134–40.
4. Mellor SG. Military surgery in the 21st century. J R Nav Med Serv. 2006;92(3):109–13.
5. Wightman JM, Gladish SL. Explosions and blast injuries. Ann Emerg Med. 2001;37(6):664–78.
6. Bala M, Willner D, Keidar A, Rivkind AI, Bdolah-Abram T, Almogy G. Indicators of the need for ICU admission following suicide bombing attacks. Scand J Trauma Resusc Emerg Med. 2012;20:19.
7. Spinella PC, Perkins JG, McLaughlin DF, Niles SE, Grathwohl KW, Beekley AC, et al. The effect of recombinant activated factor VII on mortality in combat-related casualties with severe trauma and massive transfusion. J Trauma. 2008;64(2):286–93.
8. Spinella PC, Cap AP. Whole blood: back to the future. Curr Opin Hematol. 2016;23(6):536–42.
9. Simpson E, Lin Y, Stanworth S, Birchall J, Doree C, Hyde C. Recombinant factor VIIa for the prevention and treatment of bleeding in patients without haemophilia. Cochrane Database Syst Rev. 2012;3:CD005011.
10. Mannucci PM, Levi M. Prevention and treatment of major blood loss. N Engl J Med. 2007;356(22):2301–11.
11. Perkins JG, Schreiber MA, Wade CE, Holcomb JB. Early versus late recombinant factor VIIa (rFVIIa) in combat trauma patients requiring massive transfusion. J Trauma. 2007;62:1095–101.
12. Holcomb JB, et al. PROMMTT Study Group. The prospective, observational, multicenter, major trauma transfusion (PROMMTT) study: comparative effectiveness of a time-varying treatment with competing risks. JAMA Surg. 2013;148(2):127–36.
13. Lettieri CJ, Shah AA, Greenburg DL. An intensivist-directed intensive care unit improves clinical outcomes in a combat zone. Crit Care Med. 2009;37(4):1256–60.

14. Grathwohl KW, Venticinque SG. Organizational characteristics of the austere intensive care unit: the evolution of military trauma and critical care medicine; applications for civilian medical care systems. Crit Care Med. 2008;36(7 Suppl):S275–83.
15. DePalma RG, Burris DG, Champion HR, Hodgson MJ. Blast injuries. N Engl J Med. 2005;352(13):1335–42.
16. Gans L, Kennedy T. Management of unique clinical entities in disaster medicine. Emerg Med Clin North Am. 1996;14:301–26.
17. Eastridge BJ, Jenkins D, Flaherty S, Schiller H, Holcomb JB. Trauma system development in a theater of war: experiences from Operation Iraqi Freedom and Operation Enduring Freedom. J Trauma. 2006;61(6):1366–72; discussion 1372–3.
18. Blackbourne LH, Baer DG, Eastridge BJ, Butler FK, Wenke JC, Hale RG, et al. Military medical revolution: military trauma system. J Trauma Acute Care Surg. 2012;73(6 Suppl 5):S388–94.
19. Palm K, Apodaca A, Spencer D, Costanzo G, Bailey J, Fortuna G, et al. Evaluation of military trauma system practices related to complications after injury. J Trauma Acute Care Surg. 2012;73(6 Suppl 5):S465–71.
20. Kashuk JL, Moore EE, Millikan JS, Moore JB. Major abdominal vascular trauma—a unified approach. J Trauma. 1982;22(8):672–9.
21. Fisher AD, Miles EA, Cap AP, Strandenes G, Kane SF. Tactical damage control resuscitation. Mil Med. 2015;180(8):869–75.
22. Yazer MH, Jackson B, Sperry JL, Alarcon L, Triulzi DJ, Murdock AD. Initial safety and feasibility of cold-stored uncrossmatched whole blood transfusion in civilian trauma patients. J Trauma Acute Care Surg. 2016;81(1):21–6.
23. Hauser CJ, Boffard K, Dutton R, Bernard GR, Croce MA, Holcomb JB, et al. Results of the CONTROL trial: efficacy and safety of recombinant activated factor VII in the management of refractory traumatic hemorrhage. J Trauma. 2010;69:489–500.
24. Mackenzie IM, Tunnicliffe B. Blast injuries to the lung: epidemiology and management 366. Phil Trans R Soc B Biol Sci. 2011;366(1562):295–9. https://doi.org/10.1098/rstb.2010.0252.
25. Ried M, Bein T, Philipp A, Müller T, Graf B, Schmid C, Zonies D, Diez C, Hofmann HS. Extracorporeal lung support in trauma patients with severe chest injury and acute lung failure: a 10-year institutional experience. Crit Care. 2013;17(3):R110. https://doi.org/10.1186/cc12782. PubMed PMID: 23786965; PubMed Central PMCID: PMC4056791.
26. Cordell-Smith JA, Roberts N, Peek GJ, Firmin RK. Traumatic lung injury treated by extracorporeal membrane oxygenation (ECMO). Injury. 2006;37(1):29–32. Epub 2005 Oct 21.
27. Berger-Pelleiter E, Emond M, Lauzier F, Shields JF, Turgeon AF. Hypertonic saline in severe traumatic brain injury: a systematic review and meta-analysis of randomized controlled trials. CMED. 2016;18(2):112–20. https://doi.org/10.1017/cem2016.12.
28. Wester K. Decompressive surgery for "pure" epidural hematomas: does neurosurgical expertise improve outcome? Neurosurgery. 1999;44(3):495–500.
29. US Department of Defense. Emergency war surgery, 4th United States Revision. Office of the Surgeon General, United States Army, vol. 20. Washington, DC: Borden Institute; 2014. p. 233.
30. Ballivet de Regloix S, Crambert A, Maurin O, LIsan Q, Marty S, Pons Y. Blast injury of the ear by massive explosion: a review of 41 cases. J R Army Med Corps. 2017;163(5):333–8.
31. Dougherty AL, MacGregor AJ, Han PP, Viirre E, Heltemes KJ, Galarneau MR. Blast-related ear injuries among U.S. military personnel. J Rehabil Res Dev. 2013;50(6):893–904.
32. Shah A, Ayala M, Capra G, Fox D, Hoffer M. Otologic assessment of blast and nonblast injury in returning Middle East-deployed service members. Laryngoscope. 2014;124(1):272–7.
33. Darley DS, Kellman RM. Otologic considerations of blast injury. Disaster Med Public Health Prep. 2010;4(2):145–52.
34. Mohammad NK, Al-Mahdi AH, Mohammed OM. Ophthalmic injuries related to maxillofacial trauma due to urban warfare. J Craniofac Surg. 2018;29(7):1804–8.

35. Rhabdomyolysis – Surgical Critical Care. Net www.surgicalcriticalcare.net/Guidelines/pdf_view.php?id=46. 24 July 2018.
36. Holt SG, Moore KP. Pathogenesis and treatment of renal dysfunction in rhabdomyolysis. Intensive Care Med. 2001;27:803–11.
37. Joint Trauma System. https://jts.amedd.army.mil.
38. Center for Domestic Preparedness. https://cdp.dhs.gov/about.

Ventilator Strategies

39

Douglas Frederic Powell

Introduction

Alveoli like air....

This simple statement heard on rounds in a trauma ICU is at the heart of all mechanisms of respiratory failure. When substances other than air enter the alveoli or when carbon dioxide is not expelled, gas exchange is impaired and hypoxic, hypercapnic, or mixed respiratory failure ensues. Substances that replace air in alveoli are, in increasing viscosity, fluid (pulmonary edema), blood (alveolar hemorrhage), pus (pneumonia), and protein (from alveolar hyaline membrane formation). The viscosity can predict the tenacity of the alveolar infiltrate and duration of respiratory support required to resolve the lung injury. Air entry can also be impaired by physical damage to (penetrating lung injury) or collapse of (atelectasis) alveoli.

Blast lung injury (BLI) shares much of the pathophysiology of acute respiratory distress syndrome (ARDS). However, explosions can also cause respiratory failure by every means by which alveoli cannot fill with air, often by multiple mechanisms. Before discussing ventilator strategies, it is important to understand that many causes of hypoxia and hypercapnia can occur in blast-injured patients, frequently simultaneously and often evolving over the course of a casualty's ICU care (as in the case with pulmonary contusion and ARDS). Blast patients frequently have other traumatic injuries that can impact the respiratory system, such as inhalation of particles or noxious substances, penetrating missiles, burns, or sequelae from massive blood transfusions. Other concomitant blast injuries may place constraints on ventilator management. Hemorrhagic shock may limit the

D. F. Powell (✉)
University of West Virginia, Heart and Vascular Institute, Morgantown, WV, USA

D. W. Callaway, J. L. Burstein (eds.), *Operational and Medical Management of Explosive and Blast Incidents*, https://doi.org/10.1007/978-3-030-40655-4_39

amount of intrathoracic pressure tolerated before global perfusion is impaired. Severe traumatic brain injury (TBI) may limit several ventilator stratigies used in severe lung injury. Peak end-expiratory pressure (PEEP) may need to be limited in severe TBI to reduce intrathoracic pressure and facilitate cerebral perfusion pressure. Permissive hypercapnea can cause cerebral vasodilation and increase intracranial pressure (ICP) and permissive hypoxia could result in increasing the ischemic penumbra around a focus of intracerebral injury.

Thus, while the primary problem in BLI is straightforward – not enough alveoli filling with air – the mechanisms and management are some of the most complex confronted in the intensive care unit. To optimally manage these casualties, ICU teams must understand which mechanisms of respiratory failure are at play in each casualty, tailor initial support to each casualty's pattern of respiratory system and other traumatic injuries, and be vigilant for the evolution or development of new respiratory injuries during the patient's ICU course.

Overview of Respiratory Injuries in Explosions

Much of the literature regarding lung injury in explosions is focused on primary BLI, defined as injury to the lungs by the primary pressure wave. It should be emphasized that it is rare to encounter BLI in the absence of other mechanisms and locations of blast-related traumatic injury. Explosions are a subset of polytrauma, and it is the rule, not the exception, that blast exposure causes multiple diverse injuries that sometimes affect or limit the choice of respiratory therapy. An understanding of blast lung injuries is important for the critical care physician because in patients who survive their initial blast exposure, primary blast injuries, primarily to the lung, contribute to a significant proportion of injuries that must be addressed in the ICU and as high as 86% of injuries that result in delayed fatalities [1].

The incidence of BLI is higher in confined-space explosions due to the greater proximity of victims to the center of the blast and the concentration, magnification, and prolongation of blast wave exposure due to containment by and reflection off of interior surfaces. Overall injury severity and mortality is higher in confined-space explosions due both to an increased incidence of primary lung injury and secondary and tertiary injuries due to structure collapse and concentration of thermal and inhalation injuries.

In open-space explosion, blast waves follow a predictable, exponential deterioration, ceasing to be a significant cause of primary blast injury beyond ~ 10–20 meters, while injuries due to propelled fragments can occur at up to 100 times that distance [2]. In open-space explosions, casualties close enough to the blast to receive BLI are usually killed by the force of the blast or propelled fragments.

In US military data from 2003 to 2006, only 3.6% of blast casualties had PBLI, likely reflecting the high incidence of open-space explosions due to a high prevalence of dismounted IEDs and indirect fire explosions [3]. In data from blast fatalities in Ireland from 1970 to 1984, 45% of victims had evidence of BLI and 17% had only lung damage on autopsy, likely due to a higher incidence of confined-space explosions in buildings and vehicles in this more urban conflict environment [4]. Israeli data published in 1996 found an 8% mortality in open-air blasts and a 49% mortality in closed-space bus bombings [5].

Primary blast injuries in the lung are caused by the action of the blast wave on the lung tissue. Lungs are comprised of high-density (capillaries) and low-density (alveoli) tissues. The blast wave has two components: a high-frequency, longitudinal stress wave and a low-frequency, transverse shear wave [6]. The initial stress wave causes damage when its force exceeds the tensile strength of lung tissues, typically the denser capillaries, resulting in alveolar hemorrhage. The subsequent shear wave affects lower-density tissues, causing tears in alveoli and the interstitium leading to enlarged air pockets that range in size from emphysema-like alveoli to pneumatoceles and pneumothoraces [7]. In an autopsy series of confined-space blast victims, the primary findings were alveolar distension ("blast emphysema") and diffuse alveolar, perivascular and subpleural hemorrhages [8].

Air embolism is a less common but potentially catastrophic complication of blast lung injury, likely caused by the translocation of air across permeable or ruptured alveolar membranes into associated vessels. Tsokos and colleagues report findings of venous air, fat and bone marrow embolism on their histologic examination of lungs of blast fatalities. In that series, fat embolism is a significant risk factor for the development of ARDS and was seen on 62% of the casualties, while air embolism was found on 50% of the cases [8]. The incidence of emboli in blast survivors will likely be lower than in these casualties who died immediately due to proximity to the blast; however the findings are instructive of the possible complications clinicians can encounter in the most seriously injured blast patients. In an Israeli case series of bus bombing victims, air emboli occurred in nearly 50% of the casualties with the most serious lung injuries and may have contributed to the high mortality rate (75%) in this cohort [9].

Other less common but serious complications of blast exposure are injuries to the large airways and pleura. Bronchopleural fistula and bronchial and tracheal disruption can be caused by primary, secondary or tertiary blast effects. Regardless of cause, their effect can be to prolong hypoxemia until recognized and managed. Both diagnosis and management of these complications may require specialized techniques.

Table 39.1 demonstrates the mechanisms of injuries to respiratory anatomy. It is organized by the mechanisms of blast injury defined and discussed elsewhere in this manuscript. A section on complications has been added, since it is most likely that if complications are manifest, it will be while patients are being cared for in the ICU.

Table 39.1 Mechanism and nature of blast lung injuries

Type	Mechanism	Injuries
Primary	Blast wave pressure	
Alveoli	Barotrauma, shear trauma	Pulmonary edema, alveolar hemorrhage, blast emphysema
Small airways		Pneumatocele
Vascular	Capillary rupture	Contusion, alveolar hemorrhage, air embolism
	Large-vessel disruption	Pulmonary hemorrhage, hemothorax
Large airways	Shear, burst injury	Tracheal, bronchial disruption, massive air leak
Pleura		Pneumothorax, pneumomediastinum, subcutaneous emphysema, bronchopleural fistula
Secondary	Projectiles, blunt or penetrating injury	
Alveoli		Pulmonary hemorrhage, hematoma
Large airways		Tracheal, bronchial disruption
Vascular		Pulmonary hemorrhage, hemothorax
Pleura		Pneumothorax
Tertiary	Victims thrown by blast, usually blunt impact/deceleration injury	
Alveoli		Contusion, pulmonary edema
Large airways		Tracheal, bronchial disruption
Vascular		Pulmonary hemorrhage, hemothorax
Pleura		Pneumothorax
Quartenary	Other mechanisms than direct blast forces[a]	
Burns		Thoracic eschar, thermal airway injury, inhalation
Chemicals		Pneumonitis, secretions, chemical burns
Spinal cord		Respiratory muscle paralysis/ventilatory failure
Exacerbations of underlying diseases		COPD, asthma exacerbations due to inhaled particles or inflammatory effects of lung trauma
Traumatic injuries affecting respiratory therapy		
Hemorrhagic shock		Lower tolerance for PEEP/intrathoracic pressure
TBI		Lower tolerance for PEEP/intrathoracic pressure due to cerebral perfusion pressure requirements, lower tolerance for permissive hypercapnea
Complications		

Air emboli, fat emboli, ARDS, pneumonia, pulmonary emboli, aspiration pneumonitis/pneumonis, abscess/pneumonia from contaminated fragments

[a]A "quinary" category of injuries due to weaponized chemical, biologic, and radiation agents is used by the US Department of Defense

Assessment and Monitoring of Respiratory Status in Blast Casualties

In patients who can provide a subjective exam, symptoms of blast lung injury include severe chest pain and dyspnea. Cough may or may not be present. Although rare, BLI can occur in the absence of other traumatic and thoracic injuries, and these symptoms in a patient exposed to a blast, especially in a confined space, should be taken as signs of occult PBLI and prompt further workup with imaging, arterial

Table 39.2 Monitoring recommendations for pulmonary blast injuries

Minimum: SpO_2, $EtCO_2$, clinical exam, pulmonary US
Better: Minimum + ABG, CXR
Best: Minimum + better + chest CT

blood gas (ABG) measurement, and close observation as these patients have a significant risk of deterioration to respiratory failure.

Hemoptysis in the blast patient should prompt concern for alveolar hemorrhage. Other signs of BLI that can be present are tachypnea, cyanosis, and confusion and agitation, due either to hypoxia or cerebral effects of the blast such as concussion or cerebral air embolism.

As mentioned previously, blast casualties commonly suffer from a multitude of traumatic injuries. Many of these will have been addressed prior to admission to the ICU; however, hypovolemic shock may require ongoing monitoring, resuscitation, and close observation for uncontrolled bleeding amenable to further procedural or surgical intervention. Severe TBI may require clinical monitoring for deterioration of mental status, pupillary exam, or intracranial pressure if admitted to the ICU with a pressure-monitoring device.

For respiratory monitoring, Table 39.2 presents minimum, better, and best recommendations, recognizing that many blast victims may be cared for in resource-limited environments for a variety of reasons such armed conflict, acts of terror, and natural disasters.

Critical care ultrasound (CCUS) has long been used to diagnose pneumothorax, pleural effusion, and hemothorax. Recently, CCUS has been shown to have good accuracy when compared to chest CT for diagnosing pulmonary contusion in blunt trauma to the chest. The presence of the alveolar-interstitial syndrome (B-lines), peripheral parenchymal lesion (C-lines), confluent consolidations/hepatization, or parenchymal disruption with localized pleural effusion [10, 11] are sonographic indications of acute lung injury.

Initial measurement and monitoring of the partial pressure of oxygen to fraction of inspired oxygen (PaO_2:FiO_2) ratio is used to assess the initial severity of blast lung injury, prognosis, and need for more aggressive ventilator support. Initial PaO_2:FiO_2less than 60 has been correlated with severe PBLI and worse prognosis [9]. PaO_2:FiO_2 less than 60 for more than 4 hours of conventional ventilator support has responded to earlier initiation of high-frequency oscillatory ventilation (HFOV) in some centers [7]. It is also important to track to assess for the development of ARDS (Table 39.3).

In absence of other injuries, some reports warn that patients in close proximity to blast are at high risk of occult pulmonary injuries [7, 12]. Casualties exposed to blast in enclosed spaces are at especially high risk of primary or occult pulmonary injuries due to (1) magnification of blast forces in enclosed space; (2) reflection of blast forces off of walls, prolonging exposure to damaging shock waves; and (3) greater likelihood of inhalation injury due to heat, particles, or noxious gases. Pulmonary contusion and inhalation injuries can develop insidiously in a patient who initially has mild or even no respiratory signs or symptoms. Close monitoring is therefore required for survivors of enclosed-space explosions or those in close proximity to open-air blasts who somehow escape other injuries because of the possibility of developing latent pulmonary injury and respiratory decompensation.

Table 39.3 ARDS criteria

ARDS severity	PaO_2:FiO_2 criteria[a]
Mild	200–300
Moderate	100–200
Severe	<100
Additional criteria:	
Acute onset: within 7 days of a defined clinical event	
Chest imaging: bilateral opacities not fully explained by effusions, collapse, nodules	
Origin of edema: respiratory failure not fully explained by cardiac failure or fluid overload	

[a]With PEEP >/= 5 cmH_2O

Ventilator Strategies

There is no prospective literature comparing ventilator modes or settings in blast patients. What literature exists are institutional or organizational (e.g., military) reports of ventilator management in particular series of casualties. All ventilator strategies in the blast population are extrapolated from studies of other conditions, principally ARDS and thoracic trauma.

Respiratory failure in blast lung injuries is almost always hypoxic. There are some special cases where hypercapnic or mixed respiratory failure may occur that will be discussed in the section "Other ICU Management Considerations." The basic strategy of ventilator management is lung-protective ventilation. This makes sense, because in blast patients the lungs are likely to be more seriously injured and have a wider variety of injuries than any other lung-injured or lung-diseased population. Because lung injury in blast casualties can be so extensive, a balance must be made when selecting ventilator strategies and settings between oxygenating, ventilating and minimizing risk of further damage.

Another consideration in blast-injured patients is the high incidence of alveolar hemorrhage, which may preclude use of extracorporeal membrane oxygenation (ECMO) for refractory hypoxemia due to its anticoagulation requirement. Salvage should be attempted with conventional ventilator therapy with maximum PEEP as tolerated and salvage or experimental techniques such as neuromuscular blockade, inhaled nitric oxide (INOX), inhaled prostacyclines, prone positioning and inhaled activated recombinant factor VII (rFVIIa), or advanced ventilator therapy, with high-frequency oscillatory ventilation (HFOV) being the most reported.

Lung-Protective Ventilation

The initial ventilator mode and settings for lung injuries in blast patients follow the recommendations of the landmark 2000 ARDSNet study [13], which found a mortality benefit from volume assist control ventilation using lower tidal volumes, PEEP titrated to FiO_2, and tidal volume and PEEP titrated to maintain plateau pressures less than 30 cm of water. It is worth reviewing the methods of this study before applying

Table 39.4 ARDSNet PEEP/FiO_2

FiO_2	0.3	0.4	0.5	0.6	0.7	0.8	0.9	1.0
PEEP (mmHg)	5	5 or 8	8 or 10	10	10, 12, 14	14	14, 16, 18	18, 20, 22, 24

its recommendations to blast lung injury because the settings, especially of tidal volume and PEEP, are more nuanced and individualized than is commonly understood.

Specifically, tidal volumes in low tidal volume cohort started at volume of 6 cc/kg/ideal body weight (IBW) but were titrated down to a minimum of 4 cc/kg/IBW as needed to maintain plateau pressure less than 30 cm of water. For patients with severe dyspnea (e.g., due to metabolic acidosis), tidal volumes could be titrated up to 7–8 cc/kg/IBW as long as plateau pressures remained at 30 cm of water or less [13]. Thus, tidal volume for lung-protective ventilation in ARDS patients can range from 4 to 8 cm of water depending on patient variables of plateau pressure and dyspnea.

PEEP in the ARDSNet study is titrated to FiO_2 as shown in Table 39.4. PEEP in the low tidal volume cohort in the ARDSNet study was generally higher than conventionally used at the time. It is thought that one of the mechanisms of reduced lung injury in the low tidal volume group was a reduction in the opening and closing stresses on the alveoli due to less of a pressure differential between plateau (open) and end-expiratory (closing) pressures, a benefit that could be especially useful in the setting of even more severe alveolar injury in PBLI than in ARDS.

Although the ARDSNet study is also associated with the concept of permissive hypercapnea (and, by extension, respiratory acidosis), the investigators attempted to strictly control pH by increasing minute ventilation or giving sodium bicarbonate. They discuss that less controlled pH may have contributed to the lack of benefit shown from low tidal volume strategies in previous studies.

Basic Ventilator Principles in Managing Blast Lung Injury

Tidal Volume

The tidal volume is based upon precise ideal body weight. Estimations generally overestimate weight and thus start at higher-than-ideal tidal volumes. Initial tidal volume has been shown to correlate with the risk of acute lung injury [14], so selecting a carefully calculated initial tidal volume is vital in this population with an already high risk of developing ARDS. Begin at the 6 cc/kg/IBW target. Measure plateau pressure initially, and then monitor every 4 hours. Titrate down in 1 cc/kg/IBW increments for plateau pressure greater than 30 cm of water to a minimum of 4 cm of water.

FiO_2

There is some evidence in animal studies that maintaining a high concentration for the first 24 hours of resuscitation can reduce air emboli [15], which are a high risk in moderate and severe blast lung injury [8, 9]. If initial radiography shows extensive bilateral pulmonary infiltrates and a PaO_2:FiO_2ratio consistent with severe ARDS (<100), consider maintaining FiO_2 at 80% for the first 8–24 hours. Titrate down at the early end of this range for rapidly improving PaO_2:FiO_2, and maintain to the latter end of this range for poorly improving PaO_2:FiO_2. Do not maintain high FiO_2 if oxygenation goals are met beyond this period due to the risk of hyperoxic lung injury.

PEEP

The risk of damaging friable alveoli in blast lung injury from higher mean airway pressures seen with increased PEEP is likely offset by the risk of damage from greater stress of opening and closing seen with larger differences between opening and closing pressures with low PEEP. Current practice in military hospitals familiar with blast casualties is to set PEEP according to FiO_2 (see Table 39.4) to meet plateau pressure and modest oxygenation (PaO_2 > 60 mmHg) goals [7].

Permissive Hypercapnea and Acidosis

Although some expert recommendations include toleration of pH in a range of 7.15 to 7.25, this acidosis increases the risk of coagulopathy that can prolong or worsen both pulmonary bleeding and bleeding from other traumatic injuries. For the global optimization of the polytrauma patient, it is preferred to keep pH at 7.3 or greater using either increased minute ventilation or sodium bicarbonate.

Strategies for Refractory Hypoxemia in Blast Lung Injury

Extensively damaged lungs in blast casualties often require advanced ventilator strategies (Table 39.5). In a cohort of survivors of two bus bombings in Israel, all four of the patients with the most severe blast lung injury required salvage ventilator modes (one dual lung, one ECMO, two HFOV) [9]. The British Military Hospital experience reports improved outcomes with early PaO_2:FiO_2 </ = 60 mmHg for more than 4 hours [7].

Several strategies have been shown to improve oxygenation using conventional ventilator equipment in ARDS patient. Neuromuscular blockade with cisatracurium for

Table 39.5 Stepwise approach to refractory hypoxemia in blast lung injury

1.	Maximize PEEP as tolerated by plateau pressure
2.	Consider prone positioning, neuromuscular blockade
3.	Change to advanced ventilator mode: HFOV is the best supported in blast literature
4.	Consider inhaled prostacyclines or nitric oxide if available
5.	Consider ECMO if no evidence of bleeding

48 hours improved outcomes in a cohort of patients with moderate-to-severe ARDS, possibly by reducing oxygen demand from respiratory muscles, improving recruitment and reducing barotrauma due to improved patient-ventilator synchrony [16].

Another strategy for improving oxygenation is prone positioning, which is easily accomplished even in resource-limited facilities. In a study where patients with severe ARDS were placed in the prone position for 16 hours or more per day and ventilator settings were applied according to the ARDSNet protocol, mortality and ventilator days were decreased with no increase in complications [17]. The physiologic rationale is that prone positioning improves alveolar recruitment by removing the weight of the heart from the left lower lobe and placing more parenchymal area in West zone 1 of the lung, where it is less prone to atelectasis and alveolar collapse (note: in West zone 1, the pressure in the alveoli is greater than the arteries and veins, meaning there is the lowest atelectatic force).

HFOV is the most-reported advanced ventilator mode with some centers using cuff deflation to improve clearance of CO_2 without recourse to higher amplitudes and frequencies that could increase risk of ventilator-induced lung injury (VILI) [12].

There are few reports of airway pressure release ventilation (APRV) in the treatment of refractory hypoxemia in blast lung. This may be due to a perceived increased risk of VILI due to high mean airway pressures and the opening and closing stress of spontaneous breathing which is required in APRV to adequately clear CO_2. However, if oxygenation is poor after other maneuvers such as neuromuscular blockade and prone positioning and a facility does not have HFOV capability, APRV can be attempted, starting on the lower end of P-high, e.g., 20 cm of water. As with all blast lung-injured patients, monitoring should be performed for signs of VILI such as subcutaneous emphysema or worsening air leak.

Evidence for inhaled prostacyclines and nitric oxide exists only as case reports with mixed success in improving oxygenation in severely hypoxic patients with blast lung injury.

ECMO must be used cautiously in blast lung injury due to a high incidence of small and large pulmonary vessel injury manifest as alveolar and pulmonary hemorrhage when compared with other causes of hypoxic respiratory failure such as ARDS or severe pneumonia. The requirement for anticoagulation of the ECMO circuit can trigger or worsen existing pulmonary bleeding. ECMO may be considered for refractory hypoxemia if there is no evidence of pulmonary or other traumatic bleeding.

Other ICU Management Considerations

Pneumothoraces are common in blast casualties and can occur by a variety of mechanisms. Large pneumoratheces and pneumothoraces with tension physiology should be relieved with tube thoracostomy or emergent needle decompression followed by tube thoracostomy. Recent evidence has shown that non-tension pneumothoraces <35 mm (measured perpendicularly on axial CT scans) in trauma patients can be managed noninvasively [18]. Hemothoraces require tube drainage and can cause significant hemorrhage that requires blood product resuscitation.

Air embolism is a significant risk (in some reports greater than 50%) [9] in patients with severe blast lung injury and a risk in patients with moderate injury. Symptoms are acute neurologic deterioration, focal neurologic deficits, or cardiovascular collapse. Treatment is immediate left-lateral decubitus, head down positioning, followed by hyperbaric oxygen therapy. Animal studies have suggested that an initial (8–24 hours) period of high FiO_2 can attenuate the risk of air embolism [15].

Inhalation and upper airway thermal injuries are common. Early placement of definitive airway is important for casualties with burns to the face or mouth, stridor, or hoarse voice. Diagnosis is by bronchoscopy. If significant body surface area is involved with full- or partial-thickness burns, transfer to a specialized burn center should be considered.

Although rare, several complications of blast injury to the lung can require single or independent lung ventilation:

Tracheal, bronchial disruption and bronchopleural fistula can be caused by barotrauma or shear trauma. Signs, symptoms, evaluation, and management of all three conditions are similar. Large airway leak should be suspected if a collapsed lung is slow or resistant to reinflation after tube thoracostomy or if a significant, persistent air leak is present. The presence of subcutaneous emphysema or pneumomediastinum can also suggest disruption of the large airways, but this can also occur on a more microscopic level due either to initial injury in the blast or exacerbation of small airway leaks under positive pressure ventilation. If sub-Q emphysema does not improve, evaluate for a large airway leak. Diagnosis is by bronchoscopy. Management is complex and may require surgical or interventional bronchoscopy repair and one-lung or independent lung ventilation [19].

Severe single lung injury in which providing the same ventilator volumes or pressures to both lungs can result in overdistention and further damage to the injured lung and underventilation of the uninjured or less-injured lung. Dual-lung ventilation is a strategy where a dual-lumen endotracheal tube is connected to two ventilators, one providing minimal support to the injured lung, the other full support, adjusted to the reduced volume of a single lung, to the healthier lung. This strategy was used in a case of severe unilateral penetrating chest trauma with survival and successful ventilator liberation after 30 days of a complicated ICU course that included neuromuscular blockade, inhaled prostacyclines, proning and APRV [20].

In *severe TBI* with the presence or risk of increased intracranial pressure (ICP), permissive hypercapnea is not recommended due to cerebral vasodilation that can exacerbate ICP. "Permissive hypoxia" (60 mmHg) is also contraindicated due to recommendations that brain-injured patients receive normal levels of oxygenation. If increased ICP develops, blood pressure may need to be optimized to provide adequate cerebral perfusion pressure. This could contraindicate higher levels of PEEP due to the negative effect of increased intrathoracic pressure on systemic blood pressure.

Alveolar hemorrhage is a frequent finding in blast lung injury. Case studies have reported management of severe, persistent alveolar hemorrhage with activated recombinant factor VII (rFVIIa). A novel therapy for alveolar hemorrhage is intrapulmonary administration of rFVIIa in a dose of 50 mcg/kg by nebulizer which in one case of diffuse alveolar hemorrhage resolved bleeding after intravenous rFVIIa had failed [21].

Hypercapnic respiratory failure. As discussed, this is relatively rare in blast casualties. Situations in which this can develop are:

- Third-degree burns that cause thoracic eschar, restricting tidal volume. Treatment is escharotomy.
- Spinal injury causing respiratory muscle paralysis. Treatment is mechanical ventilation to ensure adequate ventilation that may be required in the absence or after resolution of lung injury causing hypoxic respiratory failure.
- Exacerbation of underlying pulmonary diseases such asthma or chronic obstructive pulmonary disease (COPD) due to inflammatory insult of blast lung injury or inhaled gases or particles. Treatment is with inhaled bronchodilators and IV corticosteroids if not contraindicated by wound healing considerations and respiratory support.

Conclusion

Lung injuries in blast result from a variety of mechanisms and usually present a heterogenous pattern of injuries that range from small airways and vessels to large airway and vessel disruption. BLI due to the pressure and shearing effects of the primary blast wave is the most reported pulmonary condition resulting from explosions. BLI is characterized primarily by rupture of capillaries leading to pulmonary contusion and hemoptysis and tearing of alveoli leading to pulmonary edema due to inflammation and airspace abnormalities that range from smaller, emphysema-like blebs to larger disruptions such as pneumatoceles and pneumothoraces [7, 9]. Serious complications of BLI include venous air embolism, which can be rapidly fatal if not recognized and emergently managed, fat embolism which increases risk for ARDS later in the ICU course, and large airway disruptions such as bronchopleural fistula and tracheal disruption.

Evaluation of lung injuries in blast should include chest radiography, ideally computerized chest tomography, and arterial blood gas measurements to enable calculation of the PaO_2:FiO_2 ratio. Much like ARDS, BLI is characterized from mild to severe based on a composite of more extensive lung injury on imaging and worsening PaO_2:FiO_2 ratio. BLI is severe when PaO_2:FiO_2 is less than 60 mmHg and bilateral infiltrates or other injury is extensive on radiography. BLI is moderate when the P:F ratio is between 60 and 200 and bilateral or unilateral injury is moderate on imaging and mild when the P:F is greater than 200 and infiltrates are mild [9]. Casualties with moderate or severe BLI will almost always experience hypoxic respiratory failure, requiring intubation and mechanical ventilation.

Ventilator strategy for managing hypoxic respiratory failure in BLI must walk a fine line between optimizing oxygenation, ensuring adequate ventilation, and not causing further damage to what are already extremely damaged and fragile lungs.

The hallmark of ventilator management of BLI is low tidal volume ventilation as outlined in the ARDSNet protocol [13] with strict adherence to tidal volume selection based on a calculated ideal body weight (IBW) and adjustment of settings to maintain plateau pressures below 30 mm of mercury. Salvage strategies for refractory hypoxia (PaO_2 less than 60 mmHg after optimization of ARDSNet settings) include neuromuscular blockade [16], prone positioning [17], inhaled prostacyclines or nitric oxide and high-frequency oscillatory ventilation (HFOV). ECMO is often not an option due to the high incidence of hemoptysis and pulmonary hemorrhage in BLI which would be exacerbated by the requirement for anticoagulation.

Care must be taken when managing ventilator settings to be mindful of other traumatic injuries that are likely in blast polytrauma victims. Hemorrhagic shock may limit the tolerance of PEEP. Severe TBI may also limit tolerance of PEEP and proscribe permissive hypercapnea and permissive hypoxia.

In conclusion, the management of blast casualties with moderate or severe lung injury presents one of the most complex respiratory conditions that can be encountered in an ICU. The pattern of injury is diverse, the underlying structure of the blast-injured lung is fragile and easily prone to further iatrogenic injury, numerous pulmonary complications can be present initially or develop over the ICU course, and other traumatic injuries may limit the ventilator strategies available to the clinician.

Pitfalls

- Overestimating tidal volume based on a subjective estimation instead of an objective calculation of ideal body weight (IBW) with which to set an accurate tidal volume of 6 cc/kg/IBW and make IBW-based adjustments from there.
- Not following plateau pressures at regular enough intervals. These should be checked at a minimum of every 4 hours during the initial resuscitation of moderate-to-severe BLI.
- Be vigilant for acute symptoms of venous air embolism. A sudden decline in global neurologic status, development of acute focal neurologic deficits, or the acute onset of cardiovascular collapse should prompt a diagnosis of venous air embolism. Immediate left-lateral decubitus, head down positioning is the emergency response. Hyperbaric oxygen therapy should be administered after stabilization.

References

1. Mayorga MA. The pathology of primary blast overpressure injury. Toxicology. 1997;121:17–28.
2. Champion HR, Holcomb JB, Young LA. Injuries from explosions: physics, biophysics, pathology and required research focus. J Trauma. 2009;66:1468–77.
3. Ritenour AE, Blackbourne LH, Kelly JF, McLaughlin DF, Pearse LA, Holcomb JB, et al. Incidence of primary blast injury in US military overseas contingency operations: a retrospective study. Ann Surg. 2010;251:1140–4.

4. Mellor SG, Cooper GJ. Analysis of 828 servicemen killed or injured by explosion in Northern Ireland 1970–1984: the hostile action casualty system. Br J Surg. 1989;76:1006–10.
5. Leibovici D, Gofrit ON, Stein M, Shapira SC, Noga Y, Heruti RJ, et al. Blast injuries: bus versus open-air bombings. A comparative study of injuries in survivors of open-air versus confined-space explosions. J Trauma. 1996;41:1030–5.
6. Weightman JM, Gladish SL. Explosions and blast injuries. Ann Emerg Med. 2001;37:664–78.
7. Mackenzie I, Tunnicliffe CJ, Mahoney P, Kirkman E. What the intensive care doctor needs to know about blast-related lung injury. JICS. 2013;14(4):303–12.
8. Tsokos M, Paulsen F, Petri S, Burkhard M, Puschel K, Turk E. Histologic, immunohistochemical, and ultrastructural findings in human blast lung injury. Am J Respir Crit Care Med. 2003;168:549–55.
9. Pizov R, Oppenheim-Eden A, Matot I, Weiss YG, Eidelman LA, Rivkind AI, et al. Blast lung injury from and explosion on a civilian bus. Chest. 1999;115:165–72.
10. Soldati G, Testa A, Silva FR, Carbone L, Portale G, Silveri NG. Chest ultrasonography in lung contusion. Chest. 2006;130(2):533–8.
11. Helmy S, Beshay B, Abdel Hady M, Mansour A. Role of chest ultrasonography in the diagnosis of lung contusion. Egypt J Chest Dis Tuberculosis. 2015;64:469–75.
12. Mackenzie IM, Tunnicliffe B. Blast injuries to the lung: epidemiology and management. Phil Trans R Soc B. 2011;366:295–9.
13. The Acute Respiratory Distress Syndrome Network. Ventilation with lower tidal volumes as compared with traditional tidal volumes for acute lung injury and the acute respiratory distress syndrome. N Engl J Med. 2000;342:301–8.
14. Edens JW, Chung KK, Pamplin JC, Allan PF, Jones JA, King BT, et al. Predictors of early acute lung injury at a combat support hospital: a prospective observational study. J Trauma. 2010;69 Suppl 1:S81–6.
15. Kirkman E, Watts S, Cooper G. Blast injury research models. Philos Trans R Soc Lond Ser B Biol Sci. 2011;366:144–59.
16. Papazian L, Forel J-M, Gacouin A, Penot-Ragon C, Perrin G, Loundou A, et al. Neuromuscular blockers in early acute respiratory distress syndrome. N Engl J Med. 2010;363:1107–16.
17. Guerin C, Reignier J, Richard JC, Beuret P, Gacouin A, Boulain T, et al. Prone positioning in severe acute respiratory distress syndrome. N Engl J Med. 2013;368:2159–68.
18. Bou Zein Eddine S, Boyle KA, Dodgion CM, Davis CS, Webb TP, Juern JS, et al. Observing pneumothoraces: the 35-millimeter rule is safe for both blunt and penetrating chest trauma. J Trauma Acute Care Surg. 2019;86(4):557–64.
19. Mikita JA, Powell DF. Ventilation for tracheal disruption and bronchopleural fistula. In: Bukenmaier III C, Mahoney PF, editors. Combat anesthesia: the first 24 hours, vol. c2015. San Antonio: Borden Institute. p. 315–9.
20. Rudder N, Marcos B. Independent lung ventilation in severe traumatic unilateral lung injury with refractory hypoxemia. Crit Care Med. 2018;46(1 suppl):S779.
21. Heslet I, Nelsen JD, Levi M, Sengeloev H, Johansson P. Successful pulmonary administration of activated recombinant factor VII in Diffuse Alveolar Hemorrhage (DAH). Crit Care. 2006;10:R177.

ICU Management: Extended Resuscitation Considerations

40

Craig R. Ainsworth

Introduction

Blast-related injuries can be easily missed in the chaos of triage that can follow mass casualty explosive events [1]. Resuscitative efforts should be initiated as soon as possible and can occur during primary and secondary trauma surveys and other diagnostic procedures. As information is obtained about the nature of injuries, the resuscitation should be adjusted in real time using previously established targets of resuscitation such as systolic blood pressure, mean arterial blood pressure, urine output, lactate level, and venous oxygen saturation.

The hallmark weapon used by terrorists and insurgents in the wars in Afghanistan and Iraq has been the improvised explosive device (IED). These devices are responsible for over 60% of military deaths in the conflict in Iraq [2]. Improvised explosive devices have also been extensively used against civilians in recent years in Israel, London, Madrid, Africa, and Mumbai [3]. This discussion is mainly geared to treatment of those suffering from such injuries, but other blast injuries are similar.

Extended Resuscitation

While much of the literature on managing blast injuries focuses on initial care, those who care for patients with blast injury should be familiar with managing those issues that arise after the initial injury. For example, a patient with shock early in the clinical course post injury should be extensively assessed for hemorrhage, and life-saving measures should be taken to replace hemorrhaged blood through balanced

C. R. Ainsworth (✉)
Burn Center, Clinical Division, US Army Institute of Surgical Research, JBSA Fort Sam Houston, San Antonio, TX, USA
e-mail: craig.r.ainsworth.mil@mail.mil

D. W. Callaway, J. L. Burstein (eds.), *Operational and Medical Management of Explosive and Blast Incidents*, https://doi.org/10.1007/978-3-030-40655-4_40

resuscitation in addition to finding the source of bleeding and stopping it. A patient who *remains* in shock despite hemorrhage control and an adequate resuscitation or who develops shock later in their clinical course should be reevaluated to verify that the resuscitation has been adequate and to rule out injuries such as pneumothorax, mediastinal trauma causing cardiac tamponade, pulmonary embolism, compartment syndrome, and/or infectious complications [4].

Apart from the damage that blasts can do to specific organ systems, they induce a systemic inflammatory response that causes capillary leak and uncompensated shock-like physiology [1]. An appropriate resuscitation using a balanced transfusion strategy is of the utmost importance so as to reverse the physiological derangements caused by hemorrhagic shock. A review of preoperative and postoperative acidosis, coagulopathy, and hypothermia, in 51 combat troops operated on for severe blast injury, demonstrated this fact [5]. In the series, patients were transfused an average of 27 units of packed red blood cells, 27 units of fresh frozen plasma, 2 units of cryoprecipitate, and 4 pheresis units of platelets. The pH, prothrombin time, and temperature average increased in all patients from 7.19 to 7.45 from 18 s to 14 s and from 36.1 °C to 37.4 °C, correspondingly. This relatively modern intraoperative resuscitation strategy corrected the physiological derangements caused by hemorrhagic shock [5].

The initial neurologic exam is of the utmost importance. If a patient does not have evidence of penetrating brain trauma, but presents with altered mentation, blunt brain and cerebrovascular trauma should be considered. Additionally, if the patient was the victim of a blast injury in an enclosed space, or was in that space after a fire broke out, and presents with altered mental status, carbon monoxide poisoning should be ruled out. This can be done by obtaining a carboxyhemoglobin level, and consideration should be made as to whether to empirically administer the antidote for cyanide toxicity. Cyanide toxicity occurs when patients inhale the by-products of burning plastics and other materials used in modern construction. If the patient initially presents with appropriate mentation and goes on to become agitated, lethargic, or confused, providers should screen the casualty for delirium. In one study of 50 combat trauma patients admitted to the ICU, 68% of whom were exposed to blast injury and screened for delirium, 36% were found to be delirious at the first assessment (average time to assessment was 7 hours from admission and 26 hours from point of injury) [6]. Many of these patients received fentanyl and ketamine for pain control and propofol for sedation. There was no relationship between the mechanism of injury or the use of ketamine and the development of delirium [6]. However, ventilator days and total length of stay increased delirium risk.

After experiencing a blast, concussive syndromes with accompanying memory impairment and cognitive disturbances are common and can be associated with the development of post-traumatic stress disorder [7, 8]. If significant traumatic brain injury (TBI) occurs after a blast, measures to prevent cerebral edema and optimize patient outcome should be taken. These can include maintenance of normal serum levels of sodium and glucose, avoidance of hyperthermia, the use of seizure and vasospasm prevention drugs, and measures to decrease intracranial pressure (osmotherapy, hyperventilation, elevating the head).

Blasts can cause direct barotrauma, hemorrhage, contusion, and arterial air embolism in the lung [1]. The incidence of blast injury to the lung increases three-fold when the blast occurs in an enclosed space. This highlights the importance of knowing the circumstances of a patient's blast injury as blast lung injury may manifest later in the patients ICU course [9]. Patients with a normal chest x-ray should be observed if they report pulmonary symptoms after a blast as the lung injury may not be apparent on chest X-ray, and clinicians should consider obtaining a computed tomography scan of the chest [1].

The implosion forces caused by a blast will traumatize the alveolar structure and cause blood and fluid to leak from the capillaries and into the alveolar space [1]. Resuscitation should be adequate to restore hemodynamic stability, but judicious enough to avoid worsening pulmonary edema. These injuries result in shortness of breath, hypoxia, cough, and hemoptysis. Injuries to the bronchial vasculature can result in air emboli, especially in patients who require positive pressure ventilation. These emboli can cause obstruction of blood flow to the heart, brain, intestines, or any soft tissue that the artery may supply, with devastating consequences for the patient. Experts suggest the placement of "prophylactic chest tubes" in patients with severe blast injury who require positive pressure ventilation [1]. Patients with blast lung injury can develop severe acute respiratory distress syndrome (ARDS), and this usually occurs after the initial resuscitation. Interventions that have been shown to benefit patients with ARDS include low tidal volume mechanical ventilation strategies that employ high levels of positive end expiratory pressure, use of neuromuscular blocking agents, and prone positioning. Prone positioning is beneficial in that lung inflation is more homogeneous from dorsal to ventral than in the supine position. This allows for more evenly distributed pressure and volume from a breath delivered by mechanical ventilation. In the last 20 years, large clinical trials have been conducted to compare the prone and supine positions in ARDS to see if there is an impact on mortality. The data from these trials demonstrate a survival benefit in patients with PaO_2/FiO_2 ratio less than 100 [10]. If the abovementioned measures fail, extracorporeal membrane oxygenation (ECMO) can be utilized to oxygenate and ventilate the patient until they recover from their blast injury-related severe ARDS. ECMO has been safely delivered in austere military environments and has been safely used on patients with traumatic injuries and thermal burns [11–13].

During resuscitation, the patient should undergo serial abdominal exams as abdominal organs are frequently injured during a blast, particularly in enclosed spaces. Implosion forces can cause rupture or separation of the layers of the bowel wall [1]. As with the lungs, arterial air emboli can occur and cause mesenteric ischemia. Hemorrhage from injured bowel can lead to shock. Resuscitative efforts should be balanced with the knowledge of other organ systems injured. In patients with injury isolated to the intestines, resuscitation to a target systolic blood pressure of 80–90 mm Hg has been suggested to improve outcome until hemorrhage control can be achieved [14]. A "balanced" or "controlled" resuscitation target may also be beneficial in concomitant intestinal and lung blast injury so as to prevent or minimize pulmonary edema. Patients with TBI will need a higher mean arterial pressure to maintain an adequate cerebral perfusion pressure.

Blast trauma to the extremities represented over 50% of combat injuries in recent conflicts [2]. In addition to an elevated injury severity score and massive transfusion requirements, the presence of an unstable pelvic fracture is known to independently raise mortality in patients with blast injury [15]. A key extended resuscitation consideration in these patients is compartment syndrome. Compartment syndrome and rhabdomyolysis can occur as a direct consequence of the blast injury or can be delayed and develop as a consequence of over-resuscitation, particularly in patients with concomitant burn injury [16]. For this reason, providers should follow a formula similar to existing burn fluid protocols such as the ISR rule of 10s, the modified Brooke, or the Parkland formula when resuscitating a patient with extremity trauma and burn injury from a blast so as to avoid fluid creep [17]. Palpation of a tense extremity compartment and loss of pulses are late physical exam findings in compartment syndrome. Practitioners can check pulses hourly, check compartment pressures with commercially available devices, and trend serum creatinine kinase levels to be vigilant for compartment syndromes. Early fasciotomy is recommended in high-risk patients as none of the diagnostic measures listed above are sensitive enough to prevent misdiagnosis [1].

Traumatic injuries, and particularly TBI, put the patient in a hypercoagulable state. The increased risk of forming deep vein thrombosis and suffering pulmonary emboli should be mitigated by the use of venous thromboembolism prophylaxis. Clinicians should balance the patient's risk of venous thromboembolism with the risk of major bleeding and decide whether to use mechanical or pharmacologic prophylaxis. Once hemostasis has been achieved, chemoprophylaxis should be initiated according to published guidelines [18]. Pharmacologic prophylaxis is not always associated with increased rates of bleeding or hemorrhage in the injured tissue. In a review of 67 patients with penetrating brain injury, 32 patients received their first dose of venous thromboembolism chemoprophylaxis within 24 hours. They were compared to 35 patients who did not receive early chemoprophylaxis. The incidence of worsened intracranial hemorrhage was 16% after early chemoprophylaxis compared to a rate of 17% when it was not given early. The incidence of DVT or PE was 12% after early chemoprophylaxis and 17% when it was not given early. Though this difference was not statistically significant, it demonstrates that there was a trend toward increased risk of thrombosis without a concomitant increased risk of bleeding with the use of chemoprophylaxis [19].

Providers should be mindful of the types of infections that can complicate blast injuries and give rise to distributive shock and cause an extended resuscitation. Often times, soil bacteria and fungus can be blasted into the soft tissues causing an initial and prolonged systemic inflammatory response and infection. Blast injuries during dismounted operations in Afghanistan that caused limb amputations and perineal injuries and required large blood volume resuscitation were associated with invasive fungal infections. This knowledge informed practitioners' aggressive use of antifungal therapies [20]. A Danish military review of 20 patients who had sustained serious blast injuries as a result of explosion revealed that infections after combat injuries were a major problem because of the different microbiological profiles in the region the soldiers were operating in. Knowledge of the microbiological flora of the geographical location of the conflict is essential to properly manage these patients after their initial resuscitation [21].

Conclusion

For those involved in the ICU management of patients with blast injury, knowledge of the circumstances of the blast injury and where the injury occurred will inform the immediate and extended care of the patient with respect to risk for different types of injury and/or infection. As the patients evolve clinically, so do the diagnoses that can account for persistent or recurrent shock. A balanced resuscitation is recommended for those with uncontrolled hemorrhage. Resuscitation pre-, post-, and intraoperatively with blood products should use ratios known to improve patient outcomes. Commonly injured organ systems such as the brain, lung, and intestines can be supported through evidence-based resuscitative efforts.

Pitfalls

- Assess the adequacy of resuscitation and whether or not hemostasis has been achieved in blast-injured patients who remain in shock.
- Resuscitation should be balanced so as to avoid fluid creep and pulmonary edema.
- Extremity compartment syndrome can be difficult to diagnose; liberal use of early fasciotomy in high-risk patients is appropriate.

References

1. Wolf SJ, Bebarta VS, Bonnett CJ, Pons PT, Cantrill SV. Blast injuries. Lancet. 2009;374:405–15.
2. Owens BD, Kragh JF Jr, Wenke JC, Macaitis J, Wade CE, Holcomb JB. Combat wounds in operation Iraqi Freedom and operation Enduring Freedom. J Trauma. 2008;64:295–9.
3. Krishnamurthy R, Daundkar BB, Malve ML. Successive explosions in Mumbai the economic center of India. J Clin Forensic Med. 2006;13:311–5.
4. Shamim F, Rizwan M, Aziz A. Bomb blast and its consequences: successful intensive care management of massive pulmonary embolism. J Coll Physicians Surg Pak. 2016;26(6 Suppl):S7–9.
5. Morrison JJ, Ross JD, Poon H, Midwinter MJ, Jansen JO. Intra-operative correction of acidosis, coagulopathy and hypothermia in combat casualties with severe haemorrhagic shock. Anaesthesia. 2013;68(8):846–50. https://doi.org/10.1111/anae.12316. Epub 2013 Jun 1.
6. Ingalls NK, Armstrong B, Hester M, Hatzfeld JJ, Robinson BR, Fortuna GR. The Fog of War: delirium prevalence in a combat intensive care unit. Mil Med. 2015;180(3 Suppl):33–6.
7. Cernak I, Wang Z, Jiang J, Bian X, Savic J. Ultrastructural and functional characteristics of blast injury-induced neurotrauma. J Trauma. 2001;50:695–706.
8. Hoge CW, McGurk D, Thomas JL, Cox AL, Engel CC, Castro CA. Mild traumatic brain injury in U.S. Soldiers returning from Iraq. N Engl J Med. 2008;358:453–63.

9. Arnold JL, Tsai MC, Halpern P, Smithline H, Stok E, Ersoy G. Mass-casualty, terrorist bombings: epidemiological outcomes, resource utilization and time course of emergency needs (Part 1). Prehosp Disaster Med. 2003;18:220–34.
10. Guérin C, Reignier J, Richard JC, Beuret P, Gacouin A, Boulain T, et al. Prone positioning in severe acute respiratory distress syndrome. N Engl J Med. 2013;368(23):2159–68.
11. Biscotti M, Gannon WD, Abrams D, Agerstrand C, Claassen J, Brodie D, Bacchetta M. Extracorporeal membrane oxygenation use in patients with traumatic brain injury. Perfusion. 2015;30(5):407–9.
12. Ainsworth CR, Dellavolpe J, Chung KK, Cancio LC, Mason P. Revisiting extracorporeal membrane oxygenation for ARDS in burns: a case series and review of the literature. Burns. 2018;44(6):1433–8. https://doi.org/10.1016/j.burns.2018.05.008.
13. Mohamed MAT, Maraqa T, Bacchetta MD, McShane M, Wilson KL. The feasibility of veno-venous ECMO at Role-2 facilities in austere military environments. Mil Med. 2018;183(9–10):e644–8. https://doi.org/10.1093/milmed/usx132.
14. Burris D, Rhee P, Kaufmann C. Controlled resuscitation for uncontrolled hemorrhagic shock. J Trauma. 1999;46:216–23.
15. Oh JS, Tubb CC, Poepping TP, Ryan P, Clasper JC, Katschke AR, Tuman C, et al. Dismounted blast injuries in patients treated at a role 3 military hospital in Afghanistan: patterns of injury and mortality. Mil Med. 2016;181(9):1069–74.
16. May J, Sadri A, Wood F. Stryker intracompartmental pressure monitor in the triage of circumferential limb burns. Ann R Coll Surg Engl. 2015;97(2):160–1.
17. Lundy JB, Chung KK, Pamplin JC, Ainsworth CR, Jeng JC, Friedman BC. Update on severe burn management for the intensivist. J Intensive Care Med. 2016;31(8):499–510.
18. Gould MK, Garcia DA, Wren SM, Karanicolas PJ, Arcelus JI, Heit JA. Prevention of VTE in nonorthopedic surgical patients: Antithrombotic Therapy and Prevention of Thrombosis, 9th ed: American College of Chest Physicians Evidence-Based Clinical Practice Guidelines. Chest. 2012;141(2 Suppl):e227S–77S.
19. Meyer RM, Larkin MB, Szuflita NS, Neal CJ, Tomlin JM, Armonda RA, Bailey JA, Bell RS. Early venous thromboembolism chemoprophylaxis in combat-related penetrating brain injury. J Neurosurg. 2017;126(4):1047–55.
20. Murray CK, Gross K, Russell RJ, Haslett RA. Dismounted complex blast injuries including invasive fungal infections. US Army Med Dep J. 2016;(2–16):24–8.
21. Wetterslev M, Rose-Larsen K, Hansen-Schwartz J, Steen-Andersen J, Møller K, Møller-Sørensen H. Mechanism of injury and microbiological flora of the geographical location are essential for the prognosis in soldiers with serious warfare injuries. Dan Med J. 2013;60(9):A4704.

Case Study from Afghanistan: Dismounted Complex Blast Injury

41

Jennifer M. Gurney

Scenario: Operational

In 2010 and 2011 in Afghanistan, foot patrols became more common as soldiers and Marines searched villages in northern Afghanistan, especially in places like the Korengal Valley. This area of Afghanistan has steep mountains, poorly maintained roads, and multiple villages nested in valleys. Soldiers and Marines would perform patrols through villages searching for insurgents and providing aid to the locals in the villages. Insurgents would bury improvised explosive devices (IEDs) on the roads and throughout villages. These IEDs injured scores of military personnel and Afghani civilians.

When IED/blast injuries occur while a service member (SM) is in a vehicle, it is referred to as a "mounted IED" injury. If the SM is on patrol, and is injured by an IED, it is referred to as a "dismounted IED" injury. Dismounted IED injuries became increasingly common after 2010. Because these injuries are so severe, with devastating soft tissue destruction and, frequently, high bilateral lower extremity amputations, they are referred to collectively as dismounted complex blast injury (DCBI) [1, 2]. Without immediate treatment including bilateral lower extremity tourniquets, these injuries are rapidly lethal secondary to rapid exsanguination.

In the scenario being presented, soldiers were on a foot patrol and an IED was detonated. After the IED blast, the troops encountered small arms fire. There were a total of seven casualties; five had minor fragment injuries to upper and lower extremities, one had a mangled left lower extremity, and the soldier closest to the blast had bilateral lower extremity amputations and a large arm laceration/fragmentation injury.

J. M. Gurney (✉)
Department of Surgery, Joint Trauma System, US Army Institute of Surgical Research/San Antonio Military Medical Center, San Antonio, TX, USA
e-mail: jennifer.m.gurney.mil@mail.mil

D. W. Callaway, J. L. Burstein (eds.), *Operational and Medical Management of Explosive and Blast Incidents*, https://doi.org/10.1007/978-3-030-40655-4_41

Scenario: Medical

Location: Role 3 (Combat Support Hospital) in Afghanistan

In the military continuum of care (Fig. 41.1), casualties are brought to the closest military treatment facility (MTF). The Role 2 MTF (forward surgical team) is the first place on the battlefield that has surgical capability [3, 4]. Ideally, casualties are within 1 hour of surgical care from point of injury [5, 6]. The Role 3 is the highest level of medical capability on the battlefield. There is a 10+ ICU bed capability, usually three to six operating rooms, surgical and medical subspecialty care, as well as a patient holding capacity. Additionally, there is a robust blood bank and

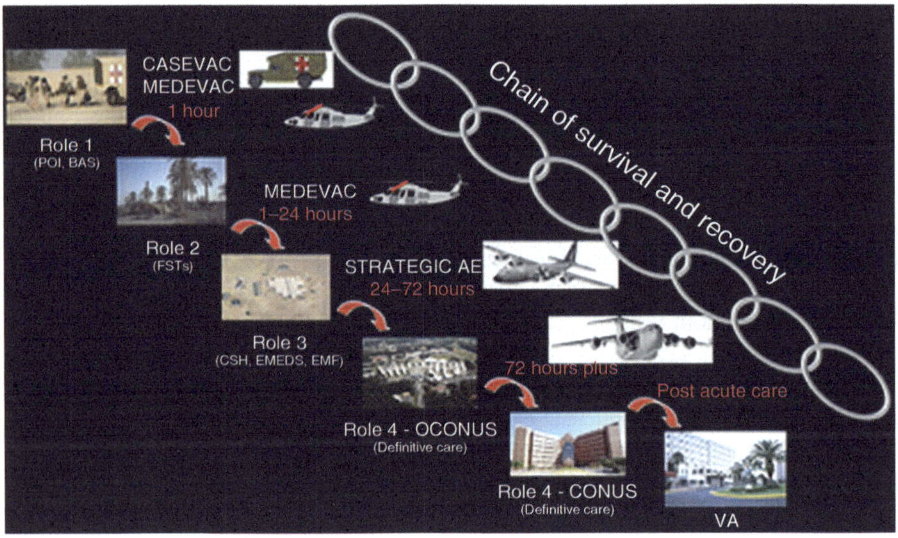

Fig. 41.1 The military trauma system's continuum of care. The roles of care on the battlefield start at point of injury (POI). Casualties move through increasing levels of care on the battlefield and then back to CONUS (Continental United States) facilities. At each level of care, the capabilities are increased. The DoD's Trauma System is embodied by the system of care referred to as the Joint Trauma System (JTS). The JTS has clinical practice guidelines for each level of care. Role 1 care (POI and BAS, Battalion Aid Station) is directed by the Tactical Combat Casualty Care (TCCC) guidelines. Role 2 care is the first level of surgical care on the battlefield. FST (forward surgical teams) are an example of a Role 2; they can range between 8 and 20 people and are placed strategically in the battlespace to provide damage control surgery in order to get the casualty to the next level of care. Examples of Role 3 military treatment facilities are the CSH (combat support hospital), the EMEDS (expeditionary medical support system), and the EMF (expeditionary medical facility). The Role 3 is the highest level of care on the battlefield and has surgical specialty capabilities. These are usually comprised of 60 to 300 personnel. There is currently one Role 4 OCONUS (Outside the Continental United States) in the military that is located in Germany, close to a large air base in order to facilitate evacuation. Casualties move along this continuum of care through multiple modes of transportation. What would be an elevator ride at a level 1 trauma center in the United States can be greater than a 10,000-mile journey in the current battlefield system of care

the capability to obtain warm fresh whole blood from a "walking blood bank," i.e., other troops as donors. Casualties usually arrive at Role 3 MTF by helicopters; however, ground transport can occur as well by means of military vehicles and vehicles of opportunity.

Role 3 MTFs, during times of high operational tempo, can see over 100 trauma patients/week and perform upward of 200 surgical procedures weekly [5]. Casualties frequently present to the Role 3 MTF as part of a multiple casualty incident.

Prehospital Care

The casualties from this incident were moved to a safe area. The patient with the isolated left lower extremity injury had a tourniquet placed and was triaged as delayed. The casualty with the bilateral lower extremity amputations had "high and tight" tourniquets placed on both thighs as well as the right arm [7, 8]. There was noted to be a large amount of blood at the scene prior to him being moved out of the firefight. His GCS was 8 (E2M4V2), and he noted to be "barely breathing"; he responded to deep sternal rub. A cricothyroidotomy was performed to protect the casualty's airway and to provide assisted ventilation if necessary. Point-of-injury vitals were HR 135, weak radial pulse, and respiratory rate 27. A MEDEVAC (Fig. 41.2) was called; there was a 20-minute ETA secondary to the troops remaining in a heavy firefight. A peripheral IV was attempted and not successful, sternal IO was then expeditiously placed, and the casualty received 500 of crystalloid. (Of note, this casualty was injured in 2011. Today, the casualty would have received prehospital low-titer Group O whole blood; this was not available in 2011 [8–10]).

A MEDEVAC arrived 30 minutes after injury. The patient was loaded onto the MEDEVAC. The flight to the Role 3 was 9 minutes. En route to the Role 3, the

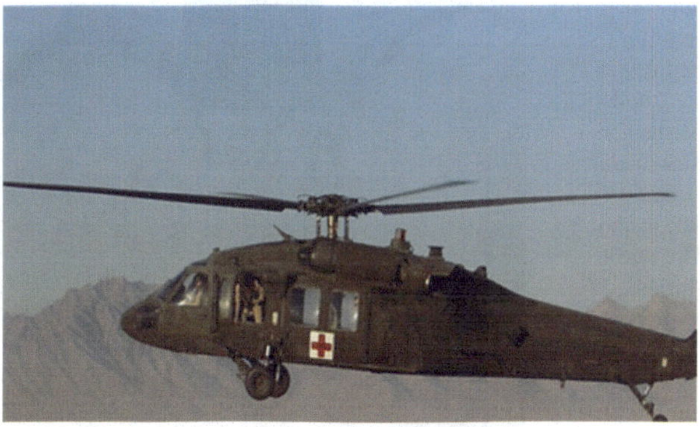

Fig. 41.2 MEDEVAC helicopter in Afghanistan. Casualty transport is most commonly by the Black Hawk helicopter. These helicopters can carry two litter patients and four non-litter patients depending on how they are configured. Certain configurations allow for four litter patients. The Black Hawk is the most common means for combat casualty transport from point of injury to the first role of care in the current battlefield system of care

patient became completely unresponsive and pulses were unable to be palpated. CPR was initiated in the MEDEVAC (Black Hawk helicopter).

Role 3

The patient arrived at the Role 3 (combat support hospital) with CPR in progress, beginning 5 minutes prior to arrival. The patient had a GCS of 3; HR was 50 bpm on the monitor and no pulse was palpated. CPR was continued and blood transfusion was started through the sternal IO catheter. A resuscitation line was then placed into the right subclavian vein and the massive transfusion protocol was initiated. Simultaneously, a resuscitative thoracotomy was performed and the descending thoracic aorta was cross-clamped. After approximately 60 seconds of cardiac massage, a perfusing cardiac rhythm was appreciated. The patient received 5 units of RBC and 5 units of FFP; he also required multiple doses of epinephrine. A walking blood bank was initiated to obtain warm fresh whole blood (WFWB). Of note, WFWB is used at all roles of care in the combat zone. It is used either as a platelet source, if there are not enough components, or if the patient's physiology is critical enough that WFWB is deemed necessary [11–14].

The patient proceeded to the operating room (Fig. 41.3). His aorta remained cross-clamped until there was evidence of cardiac filling and evidence of a MAP greater than 50 mmHg. An additional Cordis introducer catheter was placed in the right groin. He received TXA and antibiotics. In the operating room, the patient continued to demonstrate hemodynamically lability. Removal of the aortic cross-clamp

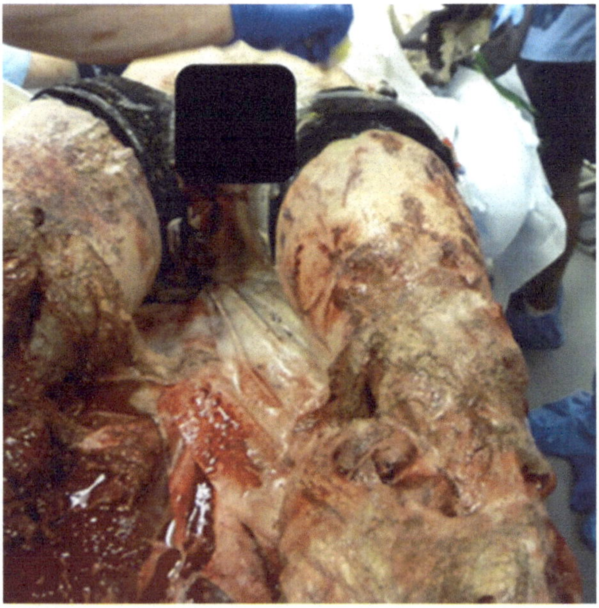

Fig. 41.3 Example of dismounted complex blast injury (DCBI) on day of injury. This casualty is already in the operating room with pneumatic tourniquets in place, and surgical prep is being performed. The significant amount of lower extremity soft tissue destruction can be appreciated. The blast effect of these injuries travels ominously more proximal than what is appreciated during the initial debridement

resulted in intraoperative cardiac arrest, and the patient required additional doses of epinephrine and cardiac massage. The patient developed coagulopathy of trauma and had large amounts of bleeding from the lower extremity wounds, making obtaining hemostasis of the large soft tissue wounds challenging. Hemostasis was obtained with packing, vascular control of visible vessels, and the liberal use of hemostatic agents.

The patient received 4 units of WFWB in the operating room and began to stabilize. He left the operating room with bilateral above-the-knee amputations, temporary closure of the left thoracotomy incision, and packing to the left arm wound. He continued to require vasopressors on initial arrival to the ICU. Over the next 6–8 hours, the patient began to stabilize and tolerated slow weaning from vasopressor support. He received a total of 9 units WBWB, 9 units of RBC, and 8 units of FFP within the first 10 hours after injury.

Early the next morning, approximately 14 hours after injury, the patient returned to the operating room. He had an additional 4 units of whole blood in reserve obtained from the walking blood bank the evening prior. In the operating room, he underwent washout and definitive closure of his left thoracotomy wound and simultaneous irrigation and debridement of his left arm wound and bilateral lower extremity amputation sites. The left arm wound required a moderate debridement secondary to contamination remaining in the muscle tissue. After debridement and washout, a negative pressure open pore sponge dressing was placed for temporary wound closure.

Both of the lower extremities had evidence of continued myonecrosis. The surgical team debrided dead muscle and salvaged as much viable skin and subcutaneous tissue as possible. The lower extremity wounds were irrigated with 0.25% Dakin's solution in addition to 9 L of warm normal saline. These wounds were placed in negative pressure open pore sponge vacuum dressing in order to prepare the patient for the critical care air transport (CCAT) flight to Germany. The patient required a small amount of epinephrine as a pressor in the operating room to tolerate anesthetic. He received 3 units of whole blood intraoperatively. Of note, if the patient were going to remain at the Role 3 for an additional 24 hours, then the wounds would have been packed with Dakin's solution and he would have returned to the operating room in 12–24 hours for repeat irrigation and debridement of the wounds prior to evacuation out of the combat zone [1, 15].

Role 4: Landstuhl, Germany

A critical care air transport team (CCAT) flew the patient to Landstuhl Regional Medical Center (LRMC) in Germany. LRMC is the first site out of the combat zone for casualties from Iraq and Afghanistan. In addition to getting US service members, LRMC gets international and NATO members; they are further stabilized prior to returning to their home country. The patient was at LRMC for just over 48 hours.

During the time at LRMC, the casualty underwent two additional lower extremity amputation site wound washouts and debridement. The team noted during each operative intervention that the lower extremity myonecrosis continued to progress and muscle debridement was required. The patient was on IV antibiotics and antifungals for his wounds, and there was a concern for aspiration pneumonia as well. He was getting continuous tube feeds for nutritional support.

During this time of very high operative tempo at LRMC, all intubated casualties would receive a post-pyloric nasoenteric feeding tube, usually placed within hours after arrival by the gastroenterology service. This practice was adopted early in the conflicts when it was observed that because of the frequent trips to the operating room and air transfer, casualties were not getting adequate nutrition. Because of the risk of aspiration in flight, casualties traveling by CCAT needed to have the enteric tube post-pyloric to continue enteral nutrition. Also, at LRMC, each casualty undergoes a screening ultrasound of upper and lower extremity venous systems to assess for DVT. Typically, patients that arrived at LRMC would get admitted to the ICU, have a screening DVT ultrasound, and return to the operating room for wound assessment within a few hours after arrival.

CONUS (Continental United States)

The patient left LRMC by CCAT just prior to post injury day 4. He arrived to the SICU at Walter Reed Army Medical Center. He returned to the operating room shortly after arrival for assessment of the lower extremity amputation sites. Over the course of the following weeks, the patient underwent multiple surgeries, to include a left hip disarticulation secondary to a failed left AKA due to infection. Fig. 41.4 demonstrates the wound at 16 days post injury and 7 months after injury; note the heterotopic ossification. Heterotopic ossification is relatively common in the combat casualty population. This casualty suffered from significant pain from

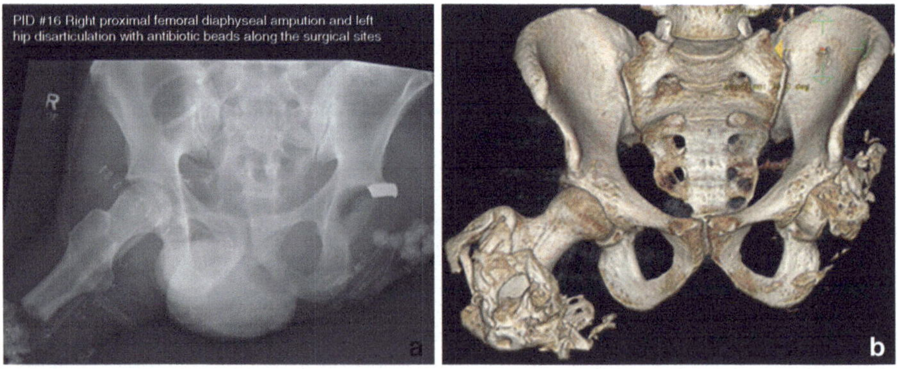

Fig. 41.4 (**a**, **b**) Progression of wounds. Depending on the intensity of the blast injury, wound progression resulting in much higher amputation levels occurs. Serially operative debridement of all areas of myonecrosis is needed to prevent overwhelming infection, including fungal infections, which can be lethal

the heterotopic ossification. His left arm healed without consequence, and he was able to move around in a wheelchair. He underwent years of rehabilitation. Most remarkably, on recovery, he was neurologically and cognitively intact. The casualty went back to school and pursued a graduate educational degree.

Lessons Learned

- Modern care for the explosive-injured casualty is exceptionally complex and resource-intensive.
- The battlefield standards for care are guided by the Joint Trauma System Clinical Practice Guidelines.
- DCBI is devastating and requires multiple surgeries. The final amputation site usually ends up being at a higher level secondary to the zone of injury from the blast and evolving myonecrosis.
- In the operating room, multiple surgical teams are required for the first few operative interventions to appropriately manage the large wound burdens in these casualties.
- Whole blood is the preferred resuscitation therapy for hemorrhage. Over 10,100 units of WFWB have been transfused in the current conflicts in the Middle East. LTOWB was introduced into the military trauma system in November 2016 and is the standard for resuscitation in hemorrhagic shock.
- The military's trauma system is global. Casualties will move from point of injury through multiple roles of care. Each role of care has increasing capabilities. During the recent conflicts, most seriously injured casualties were evacuated from the area of operations within 48 hours.

References

1. Gordon W, Talbot M, Fleming M, Shero J, Potter B, Stockinger ZT. High bilateral amputations and Dismounted Complex Blast Injury (DCBI). Mil Med. 2018;183(suppl_2):118–22.
2. Cannon JW, Hofmann LJ, Glasgow SC, Potter BK, Rodriguez CJ, Cancio LC, et al. Dismounted complex blast injuries: a comprehensive review of the modern combat experience. J Am Coll Surg. 2016;223(4):652–64.e8.
3. Hahn C, Staudt AM, Brockmeyer J, Mann-Salinas EA, Gurney JM. Characteristics of Iraqi patients treated during operation inherent resolve by a forward surgical team. Mil Med. 2019;184(Suppl 1):301–5.
4. Kotwal RS, Staudt AM, Mazuchowski EL, Gurney JM, Shackelford SA, Butler FK, et al. A US military role 2 forward surgical team database study of combat mortality in Afghanistan. J Trauma Acute Care Surg. 2018;85(3):603–12.
5. Kotwal RS, Howard JT, Orman JA, Tarpey BW, Bailey JA, Champion HR, et al. The effect of a Golden Hour Policy on the morbidity and mortality of combat casualties. JAMA Surg. 2016;151(1):15–24.
6. Turner CA, Stockinger ZT, Gurney JM. Combat surgical workload in Operation Iraqi Freedom and Operation Enduring Freedom: the definitive analysis. J Trauma Acute Care Surg. 2017;83(1):77–83.

7. Butler FKTCCC. Updates: two decades of saving lives on the battlefield: tactical combat casualty care turns 20. J Spec Oper Med. 2017;17(2):166–72.
8. Montgomery HR, Butler FK, Kerr W, Conklin CC, Morissette DM, Remley MA, et al. TCCC guidelines comprehensive review and update: TCCC guidelines change 16-03. J Spec Oper Med. 2017;17(2):21–38.
9. Bennett BL, Littlejohn LF, Kheirabadi BS, Butler FK, Kotwal RS, Dubick MA, et al. Management of external hemorrhage in tactical combat casualty care: chitosan-based hemostatic gauze dressings – TCCC guidelines-change 13-05. J Spec Oper Med. 2014;14(3):40–57.
10. Butler FK, Holcomb JB, Schreiber MA, Kotwal RS, Jenkins DA, Champion HR, et al. Fluid resuscitation for hemorrhagic shock in tactical combat casualty care: TCCC guidelines change 14-01 – 2 June 2014. J Spec Oper Med. 2014;14(3):13–38.
11. Vanderspurt CK, Spinella PC, Cap AP, Hill R, Matthews SA, Corley JB, et al. The use of whole blood in US military operations in Iraq, Syria, and Afghanistan since the introduction of low-titer Type O whole blood: feasibility, acceptability, challenges. Transfusion. 2019;59(3):965–70.
12. Bassett AK, Auten JD, Zieber TJ, Lunceford NL. Early, prehospital activation of the walking blood bank based on mechanism of injury improves time to fresh whole blood transfusion. J Spec Oper Med. 2016;16(2):5–8.
13. Spinella PC, Perkins JG, Grathwohl KW, Beekley AC, Holcomb JB. Warm fresh whole blood is independently associated with improved survival for patients with combat-related traumatic injuries. J Trauma. 2009;66(4 Suppl):S69–76.
14. Cap AP, Beckett A, Benov A, Borgman M, Chen J, Corley JB, et al. Whole blood transfusion. Mil Med. 2018;183(suppl_2):44–51.
15. Murray CK, Gross K, Russell RJ, Haslett RA. Dismounted complex blast injuries including invasive fungal infections. US Army Med Dep J. 2016(2–16):24–8.

Part VI

Special Considerations

Chemical, Biological, Radiological, or Nuclear Event (CBRNE): Prehospital and Hospital Management

42

Douglas A. Romney

Introduction

The prehospital and hospital management of blast events involving hazardous materials requires attention as it deviates from standard practice. Hazardous materials (HAZMAT) are generally considered to include chemical, biological, radiological agents and nuclear waste (CBRN). A CBRN incident is one involving the threat of exposure to a chemical or biological agent or to a source of nuclear contamination or radiation. Release of the agent may be intentional or unintentional, requiring different response patterns, and the threat to the public from these agents will, in many cases, exceed the danger from the initial blast incident.

HAZMAT materials pose a potential threat to human life and health but are otherwise unrelated. Each category of agents has its own characteristics, within each category are numerous subcategories often containing many individual agents. A comprehensive review of all hazardous materials is fortunately not required for the medical provider to render lifesaving aid. However, knowledge of the existence and nature of these threats as they pertain to a blast incident response is necessary to protect the responder and the public from potential harm or death.

Although CBRN incidents all carry inherent hazard to human life, the characteristics of these agents and the mechanism of their toxic effects vary widely. It is important to understand some basic features of each. Chemical agents are the most varied and may be classified based on their effects on the human body. Onset of symptoms is rapid, generally within seconds to hours. These agents will persist on survivors and must be removed to prevent contamination of other areas. They can

D. A. Romney (✉)
Harvard Medical School, Boston, MA, USA

Department of Emergency Medicine, Beth Israel Deaconess Medical Center, Boston, MA, USA
e-mail: dromney@bidmc.harvard.edu

D. W. Callaway, J. L. Burstein (eds.), *Operational and Medical Management of Explosive and Blast Incidents*, https://doi.org/10.1007/978-3-030-40655-4_42

have effects on any organ system of the body and often multiple systems simultaneously. Each family of agents will have a characteristic clinical course and identifying features. Some agent families have specific antidotes or treatment strategies.

Biological warfare agents are unique in that they can introduce a disease outbreak into the larger population, leading to an epidemic and causing damage far beyond the initial attack. These agents require special training to handle and are often sensitive to environmental factors. The delivery of such an agent without compromising its survival poses logistical challenges, particularly in the setting of a blast incident. When possible, access to dangerous pathogens is highly controlled, although some exist in the human population globally or are periodically introduced into the human population through contact with an animal or insect carrying the pathogen. Onset of symptoms after exposure to a biological agent will be delayed for hours to weeks after an exposure. Often, there are no signs that an agent is present at the scene of a blast. Terrorists have been reported to employ suicide bombers infected with HIV or other infectious diseases [1, 2].

Nuclear radiation and contamination are often poorly understood by providers and may present little imminent threat to life. Detection of radiation emission should prompt extreme caution and specialized resources. Source and waste control, including decontamination of patients, are the key to the initial management of nuclear events. Effects of radiation poisoning may be immediate in severe cases, but even lethal doses may be minimally symptomatic at onset [3].

All HAZMAT agents are potentially fatal to humans and may also result in prolonged and incomplete recovery after exposure. Initial actions must be taken to secure the best outcome for the greatest number of survivors while ensuring responder safety. Efforts should also focus on minimizing property and financial loss as well as damage to the environment. Each class of agents requires altering standard procedures to account for the hazard.

Biological Agents

Biological warfare agents are pathogens or their toxins that may be used intentionally as weapons. Weaponized agents, including bacteria, viruses, fungi, parasites, and the toxins they produce, share certain characteristics that make them effective for wartime use (see Table 42.1) [4]. The Centers for Disease Control and Prevention categorizes potential biological weapons into categories based on transmissibility, virulence, and lethality, special actions required for preparedness, as well as the potential for public panic and social disruption [5]. Category A contains the highest priority weapons, including anthrax, botulism, plague, smallpox, tularemia, and the viral hemorrhagic fevers. Category B, of moderate concern, includes brucellosis, glanders, melioidosis, psittacosis, Q fever, typhus fever, viral encephalitis, ricin toxin, staphylococcal enterotoxin B, *Clostridium perfringens* epsilon toxin, and food safety and water safety threats. Category C agents include emerging infectious diseases such as Nipah virus and hantavirus [5]. This and other classification systems, as well as information on specific agents, can be found on official websites and treated at length in other texts.

Table 42.1 Characteristics of effective biological warfare agents [2]

Characteristics of biological warfare agent	Weaponized qualities
Infectivity	Effective bioagents can establish infection with only a few organisms
Virulence	The ideal bioagent causes very severe or prolonged disease in its host
Toxicity	Specific to toxins, a highly toxic agent produces very severe effects in its victims
Incubation	A longer incubation period allows time for a biological agent to spread in a population and conceals the origin of the outbreak
Transmissibility	An ideal bioagent is spread easily from person to person
Lethality	Bioagents are typically chosen because they cause death in many of their victims
Stability	Stable bioagents can be produced, stored, and released in a target population while remaining infectious; sensitivity to environmental factors at any stage may impact the effectiveness of the attack

Pathogens are unique in that they carry the risk of causing disease outbreak or pandemic in the larger population. Their incubation period complicates the recognition and control of these agents after an attack. Fortunately, most agents are heat sensitive and degrade in the environment, making their application in the setting of blast incidents more difficult. However, the threat of biological contamination remains real and discovery of a biological attack may be catastrophically delayed by the absence of evidence from the scene of the incident unless specifically disclosed by the perpetrators. The first responder and emergency medical provider must maintain situational awareness and be vigilant for these agents, alerting authorities to any suspicious substances encountered. Compliance with personal protective equipment, including the use of CBRN respirators, and decontamination protocol is the most important measure the medical provider can take to reduce the likelihood of infection and the spread of disease. In many cases, it may be impossible to detect a biological attack on scene or in the immediate aftermath. Clinicians must report suspicious cases to public health authorities so that unusual disease patterns can be identified in the population and a common exposure among victims can be identified.

The response to a biological attack must begin as soon as the threat has been identified. Vaccination programs can augment the population's acquired immunity and are available for many agents including anthrax, botulinum toxin, tularemia, plague, Q fever, and smallpox. However, vaccines require several weeks before they are effective, and mass vaccination campaigns must be carefully implemented to avoid increased human interaction and exposure to the disease. In some cases, quarantine and isolation protocols must be implemented to prevent further transmission. Treatment of many but not all these diseases is possible using modern antibiotic, antiviral, or antifungal medications. For some viral agents and toxins or in the case of antibiotic resistance, only supportive care may be available. In the United States, antivirals, antibiotics, and other essential medications are stockpiled by the federal government in preparation for such an event. Public health authorities would authorize the release of such caches and disseminate treatment protocols after an incident.

Chemical Agents

The effects of hazardous chemical exposure are typically first identified on scene or, in some cases, in the hours after an incident occurs. Agents may be classified according to the adverse effects they have on the human body (see Table 42.2). Toxic syndromes (toxidromes) overlap, and, in many cases, identification of the agent will not be immediately possible. Many treatment algorithms have been developed to assist providers in using the clinical signs and symptoms of each agent class to aid in rapid identification and treatment of patients [6]. While most chemical incidents are caused by inappropriate handling and storage of product or transportation mishaps, not all incidents involving toxic industrial chemicals (TICS) or toxic industrial materials (TIMs) are accidental. TICs and TIMs are commonly used in terror attacks due to their prevalence and accessibility, including agents such as ammonia, chlorine, fluorine, phosgene, nitric acid, and hydrogen cyanide, among others [7]. Terrorists can obtain these materials and incorporate them into an explosive device or identify and target large storage or transport vessels. Certain features of a release should raise suspicion of an attack, including an incident occurring in a symbolic or strategic location, at a time of high population density, involving multiple sites, or

Table 42.2 Classification of chemical weapon agents [4]

Agent class	Toxidrome	Immediate treatment
Nerve agents	Confusion, diaphoresis, increased secretions and incontinence, miosis, fasciculation, paralysis, respiratory distress, seizure, coma	Atropine, pralidoxime, supportive care
Metabolic toxins (asphyxiants)	Shortness of breath, seizure, coma	Cyanide antidote, supportive care
Opioids	Confusion, miosis, sedation, respiratory depression, coma	Naloxone, supportive care
Anesthetic agents	Confusion, respiratory depression, sedation, coma	Naloxone trial if unclear, supportive care
Anticholinergic/ antimuscarinic agents	Confusion, hallucination, mydriasis, fever, dry skin, coma	Consider physostigmine, supportive care
Blistering agents (vesicants)	Mucus and skin irritation, coughing, blistering, seizure, coma	Supportive care, eye irrigation
Caustic agents	Mucus and skin irritation, eye irritation, coughing	Supportive care, eye irrigation
Riot control agents	Mucus irritation, coughing, shortness of breath, vomiting	Supportive care, eye irrigation
Trichothecene mycotoxins (T2 mycotoxins)	Mucus irritation, rash, delayed vomiting, bleeding	Supportive care, eye irrigation
Centrally active pulmonary agents	Mucus irritation, coughing, shortness of breath, collapse, lung injury	Supportive care, eye irrigation
Peripherally acting pulmonary agents	Delayed shortness of breath and lung injury	Supportive care
Botulinum	Double vision, difficulty swallowing, delayed paralysis, and respiratory depression	Supportive care

causing more destruction than would typically be expected. More efficient and portable weaponized agents designed to kill human beings exist but are scarce and heavily regulated. These chemical weapons are designed to be highly lethal and difficult to detect and have specific properties related to volatility, solubility, and onset of symptoms so they can be employed to maximal effect.

The effects of exposure to any hazardous material may be immediate or delayed but, except for certain carcinogens and related agents ill-suited for intentional release, will always be identifiable within hours after the attack. Patients in the aftermath of a blast incident should always be evaluated for unusual symptoms that do not match typical patterns of injury and illness after a blast. For example, patients with significant respiratory symptoms after an outdoor explosion, those with altered mental status or neurologic effects unrelated to head injury or blast effects, and patients with significant unexplained gastrointestinal symptoms or other unusual behavior should prompt the responder to consider the presence of a chemical agent.

While chemical agents cannot cause disease outbreak, contamination of the environment can cause injury or death to humans or animals and destruction of natural resources. Efforts must always be made to contain and/or remove hazardous product in the aftermath of an event.

Caution should also be taken when moving patients into the enclosed space of an ambulance, particularly when vaporization and off-gassing of residual product are a concern. All patients exposed to chemical product must be decontaminated on scene or prior to entering the hospital to avoid secondary contamination of treatment spaces. Providers receiving patients at the hospital should be aware that many patients will self-present for care after a mass casualty incident and will not have been evaluated or decontaminated on scene.

Nuclear and Radiation Incidents

Terminology regarding radiation and nuclear incidents can be confusing, particularly for the nonspecialist. Nuclear radiation refers to the emission of nuclear particles and energy caused by nuclear fission or nuclear decay. Ionizing radiation is the emission of particles or energy that can change or damage the atomic structure of its target. In human cells, this damage may result in the immediate death of the cell or may cause significant damage to DNA or other structures, resulting in the development of cancer or reduced function of the organ. Types of ionizing radiation may include alpha and beta particles, positrons, neutrons, and gamma radiation, each of which has certain properties (see Table 42.3) [7].

In the case of nuclear radiation exposure, the patient's tissue has been exposed to ionizing radiation and is subject to damage, but like thermal injury from infrared radiation exposure, the patient carries no risk to the medical provider. Routine care and hygiene protocols are adequate to ensure patient and provider safety, and decontamination of irradiated patients is not required. Contamination, on the other hand, involves the introduction of radioactive material into or onto the patient. Such material could be inhaled, ingested, absorbed, or embedded and may contaminate the

Table 42.3 Types of ionizing nuclear radiation and properties [8]

Radiation type	Description	Shielding	Potential for ionization
Alpha	Two large positively charged particles (protons), two large neutral particles (neutrons)	May be blocked by paper	High
Neutron	One large neutral particle	Meters of concrete or water	Low
Beta	One small negatively charged particle (electron)	3 mm aluminum	Medium
Positron	One small positively charged particle	Similar to beta radiation, released together	Medium
Gamma and X-ray	Electromagnetic energy wave (high energy)	Meters of concrete or lead	Low

external surface of the patient's body. This material continues to undergo nuclear decay, emitting radiation and causing ongoing injury to the patient. Any individual contaminated by contact with the agent will be similarly affected. Thus, decontamination of the patient is essential to prevent further injury as well as secondary contamination of care providers and the environment.

Injury from nuclear incidents always occurs because of exposure to nuclear radiation and accumulates in a dose-dependent fashion (see Table 42.4). Some tissues, particularly the reproductive organs, blood and bone marrow, lymphatic tissues, and intestines, are highly sensitive to radiation exposure and will rapidly accumulate lasting damage [9]. Patients suffering from altered mental status, seizure, or significant gastrointestinal effects on scene due to radiation exposure have likely received a lethal dose of radiation. If the exposure is ongoing, all individuals in the area are in immediate danger and must evacuate. Access to the area must be denied until the source is contained.

There is a substantial risk of a dirty bomb, conventional explosives packed with radioactive material, being detonated in a civilian population. The sale and transportation of nuclear material is heavily regulated, but international compliance is uneven and the material cannot be detected without specialized equipment. Radiation sources are used heavily in science, healthcare, technology, and industry; material could be stockpiled without alerting authorities. Dirty bombs expose victims to radiation during the blast and contaminate the skin, lungs, and mucous membranes' nuclear material, leading to ongoing radiation exposure until removed by decontamination. The primary challenge with response to a "dirty bomb" is that regardless of the actual danger from the contaminants, the triggering of radiological response protocols will create a significant operational burden and may incite general panic.

Because humans have no natural means of detecting nuclear radiation, first responders and emergency medical providers should always maintain awareness of the potential for radiation injury. Part of establishing scene safety in the aftermath of the blast incident, particularly an intentional incident or an incident occurring at

Table 42.4 Dose-dependent effects of nuclear radiation [8]

		Whole-body absorbed dose (1 Gray = 100 rad)				
Phase		1–2 Gy	2–6 Gy	5–10 Gy	10–30 Gy	>30 Gy
Prodromal	Symptoms	Vomiting, headache	Vomiting, diarrhea, mild headache, mild fever, transient cognitive effects	Copious vomiting, heavy diarrhea, headache, fever, prolonged cognitive impairment	Copious vomiting, heavy diarrhea, headache, fever, incapacitating cognitive impairment	Copious vomiting, heavy diarrhea, severe headache, severe fever, seizures, neurologic dysfunction
	Time to onset	2–6 hours	1–2 hours	<1 hour	<10 minutes	Immediate
	Duration	<1 day	1–2 days	<2 days	<2 days	N/A
Latent period		1 month	1 week to 1 month	Less than 1 week	None	None
Manifest	Symptoms	Mild leukopenia, fatigue, mild damage to bone marrow	Moderate leukopenia, bleeding, infection, alopecia	Pancytopenia, fever, vomiting and diarrhea, electrolyte disturbance, hypotension	Pancytopenia, fever, vomiting and diarrhea, CNS effects, electrolyte disturbance, shock	N/A
	Sequelae	Mild damage to marrow	Moderate to severe damage to marrow, mild gastrointestinal damage	Severe damage to marrow, moderate gastrointestinal damage	Severe damage to marrow and gastrointestinal, cardiovascular, pulmonary, nervous systems	N/A
Time to death		6–8 weeks	4–6 weeks	2–4 weeks	Days to weeks	Immediate to 2 days
Likelihood of death		Low	High without care, moderate with care	Nearly universal without care, high despite care	Nearly universal despite care	Rapid and universal regardless of care

a site where nuclear material is present, includes using a radiation detector to check for potential hazards. If there is no radiation detected, this does not indicate that patients will not develop radiation injury or that a nuclear event has not occurred; only ongoing emission is detected. The purpose of radiation detection is to help establish that the scene is safe for responders to enter and that patients do not require decontamination from radioactive substances. First responders should also note that personal protective equipment does not shield the provider from radiation. Special equipment is required to safely evacuate survivors from the radioactive site. If equipment on scene indicates ongoing nuclear emission, patients and responders evacuated from the scene should be checked again to evaluate for any potential contamination.

Providers receiving patients at the hospital should be aware that many patients will self-present for care after a mass casualty incident and will not have been evaluated or decontaminated on scene. It is also not safe to assume that all incidents will have been appropriately screened for radiation by first responders as not all emergency response vehicles carry this equipment. Finally, not all hospitals routinely screen patients and visitors for radiation, particularly at sites where radiation therapy is delivered or nuclear diagnostic procedures are performed, as the false-positive rate using standard equipment is unacceptable. On the other hand, many providers also fail to understand the difference between radiation exposure and contamination, leading to unnecessary decontamination and delay in care for critically injured irradiated patients.

Unlike a dirty bomb, a true nuclear detonation, one in which nuclear fission or fusion is the source of the blast, will also release a large pulse wave of electromagnetic energy that will result in failure of the electrical grid and cellular networks as well as destroying electronic devices including modern vehicles. Able-bodied survivors will have to escape on foot, limiting the ability of the population to evacuate from the area. First responders and healthcare facilities in the area will likely be incapacitated at least by equipment failure, and additional supplies will have to be mobilized for the response. Healthcare facilities spared from the worst of the damage will be overwhelmed by the volume of patients with burn injuries and radiation toxicity. Radiation toxicity and burns require large treatment teams with ample supplies to provide specialized intensive care. Unreliable communication and transportation will hamper relief efforts, and the response to such an event will necessarily be coordinated at the national or international level. The site of any nuclear attack would remain contaminated for a prolonged period, adding to the symbolism and psychological impact of the event.

Prehospital Considerations

One of the greatest challenges in managing a CBRN incident is recognizing that a scene carries the potential for exposure to these agents. First responders should assume that all blast incidents, whether intentional or unintentional, carried the potential for exposure to hazardous materials. Whether intentional or unintentional, whether primary or secondary effect of the blast, all potentially hazardous materials must be contained, and all exposed survivors must be assessed and treated for toxic effects.

First responders should be vigilant for unusual or atypical features of any blast incident scene, such as patients with unusual complaints or illness patterns that do not fit typical patterns for blast-injured patients. Examples might include coughing or suffocating patients outdoors, individuals with vomiting and diarrhea, altered mental status, seizures outside the blast zone, or skin blistering without burn injuries. Unusual liquids, vapors, medical supplies, laboratory samples, containers, or other suspicious materials should also be identified as potential hazards. Any unusual odors or sounds should also be noted. The area should also be checked for nuclear radiation with a radiation detector.

If there are concerns for provider health and safety, including a potential CBRN event, access to the scene should be prevented and efforts made to secure the area. Commanding officers and other responding agencies should also be made aware of the threat, so a coordinated response can be arranged. Patients and responders should gather at a safe distance and uphill, upwind, and upstream from any potential source of release. It is important to remember that, in the case of intentional events, a secondary attack may be planned targeting first responders or the perpetrator may be planning a separate incident once local resources are committed.

Once the access to the scene is controlled, trained HAZMAT responders wearing appropriate protective equipment can access the scene. In most cases, access to the HAZMAT scene requires Level A personal protective equipment with a fully enclosed self-contained breathing apparatus (SCBA). For medical responders, on-scene priorities include discovery of survivors, performing lifesaving interventions as required and when circumstances permit, decontamination and extrication of affected survivors, and triage and evacuation of patients. It is crucial to thoroughly decontaminate patients prior to transfer when highly toxic agents are involved. The environment of the ambulance is enclosed and warm, ideal conditions for evaporation and off-gassing of hazardous product that is contaminating a patient's body or vaporized from the lungs. Responders must shield survivors from adverse environmental conditions such as extreme temperature and precipitation, as well as accommodating special needs populations and animals and preserving the privacy and dignity of patients to the extent possible.

Hospital Considerations

Medical management in the aftermath of a blast incident involving hazardous materials is complex and dangerous. Challenges include the surge in patient presentations, safety and security of the facility and those on-site, and management of severe and unusual illness and injury patterns. Immediately available staff, medication, and supplies used for critical care, surgical, and respiratory interventions will be rapidly depleted by the increased demand. Experienced staff members and additional resources must be requested as soon as possible to avoid interruption or delay in care. Additional space can be created by utilizing alternate care sites, canceling elective procedures, facilitating rapid discharge of existing patients, and moving patients from areas of high demand to other suitable locations. Enhanced security must be coordinated with law enforcement. The distribution of patients among hospitals should be coordinated regionally using existing relationships to avoid overwhelming the resources of a single institution. Considering these challenges in advance facilitates appropriate planning and minimizes disruption of care.

The primary goal at any hospital site must be the safety and security of staff, patients, and visitors and protection of clinical resources. It is in the interest of all patients to maintain continuity of operations, which requires decontamination and isolation as appropriate to ensure safety. Hospital-based providers, particularly in the emergency department, should remain aware of protocols for their local response agencies and maintain clear channels of communication so that critical decisions can be informed by information on scene. Accessing news and social media reports may provide corroborating information.

While some victims may die due to exposure or the delay in care, decontamination protocols must be considered an essential part of patient care. Decontamination to remove radioactive material, biological agents, or other hazardous material should occur prior to entering patient care areas to avoid contamination of the clinical space. Like the ambulance, the hospital environment is warm and enclosed, so thorough decontamination to prevent direct contamination and off-gassing of hazardous material is required and should be regularly drilled in advance. Patients requiring isolation to prevent the spread of infectious disease should also enter the clinical space with appropriate measures in place. In cases where the threat of bioagent exposure is undefined or significant concern exists for potential exposure, it may not be possible to isolate each patient due to the constraints of physical space. In these cases, isolating the cohort of potentially exposed individuals may be an effective measure to protect staff and other patients. Transportation to radiology and inpatient settings, as well as handling of laboratory samples, should be given special consideration when planning isolation protocols at the facility.

Care for blast incidents with HAZMAT contamination is in many ways similar to typical care. Patients with neurologic injury or derangement of vital signs will receive supportive care. Life- and limb-threatening injuries will receive operative intervention. Burns, inhalational injury, and traumatic injury will be managed according to protocol. Additionally, patients may require specific antidotes or treatments for chemical exposure and may require prolonged sedation with respiratory and nutritional support. Patients exposed to biological agents will be managed with appropriate antibiotic prophylaxis, isolation, and monitoring and treatment for illness as it arises. Patient suffering from radiation poisoning may require specific treatment depending on the type of radiation, designed to bind or remove the radioactive agent, prevent damage to vulnerable tissues, or stimulate recovery of marrow and other tissues. Survivors of radiation poisoning will also require prolonged supportive care, requiring isolation precautions for neutropenia as well as transfusions and nutritional support [10].

When receiving patients from the emergency department, it is always prudent to ensure that appropriate decontamination and isolation precautions have been implemented prior to receiving a patient on the unit to avoid contamination of inpatient spaces and hallways. For patients with extensive injury or after exposure to a biological agent, nuclear radiation, or other hazardous material, prolonged treatment courses and high resource utilization should be expected. Normal stocks of medication and supplies will be rapidly exhausted and must be replaced. As alluded to previously in this section, disease outbreak in the aftermath of a biological attack would far exceed capacity in the system. Measures taken to prevent and control the spread of disease early will be critical in protecting the population. Certain antibiotics, pain and sedation medications, antidotes, resuscitation fluids, blood products, wound dressings, antiarrhythmics and vasoactive medications, respiratory medications, and ventilators may be in high demand and adequate backup supplies secured in advance.

In the long term, like all blast victims, survivors' functional limitations due to injury or illness will need to be met with the use of medical assist devices, prosthesis, medication, or surgical revision. Sight and hearing may be affected; respiratory, digestive, nervous function, and orthopedic disabilities are possible. Psychological trauma is certain to occur among survivors, responders, and in the community at large. Measures should be taken early to identify those at risk of disability or lasting trauma so that steps can be taken to mitigate the damage.

General Considerations

Certain assumptions are often made when planning for CBRN events to provide actionable guidance to clinical providers. While strategic assumptions are unavoidable, the prudent responder is aware of these assumptions and checks their application to each incident. For example, biological agents are heat sensitive and are often presumed to be incompatible with a blast attack by an individual or nonstate actor. While this is not technically accurate, delivery of an active biological agent in the context of a blast incident is technically challenging, nearly impossible to detect, and highly unlikely to occur.

Another basic assumption is that the effects of a chemical agent will occur rapidly enough to be identified on scene by the observant provider. Since decontamination after every blast incident would result in the death of many critically ill patients, it is a reasonable screening strategy in most cases but might fail in cold or other extreme conditions. It is also reasonable to assume that any nuclear/radiation event in most developed countries is likely intentional because the oversight of nuclear material storage and transportation is very stringent. Despite this oversight, unintentional releases have occurred even in highly developed and regulated countries even in recent years. Some biological weapons, such as smallpox, should not ever be present in a population in the absence of an intentional release. For other bioagents such as anthrax, hantavirus, Ebola, and others, periodic outbreaks of disease are the norm in some populations.

It is also helpful to consider intentional and unintentional CBRN blast events separately. Both intentional and unintentional attacks carry the risk of contamination. However, an unintentional release is more likely to involve an agent that is less hazardous to human life and the environment, is less likely to occur in a densely populated area, may occur off-hours, and is often related to equipment failure, mishaps in handling or transportation, or as secondary effect of damage after a blast. Particularly in industrial or transportation settings, mitigation strategies and countermeasures can be pre-staged in preparation for an accidental release. Similarly, identification of the agent in industrial settings is often provided visually on safety placards or documents and should be known to personnel on scene and site managers.

By contrast, intentional events are more likely to occur in a densely populated or sensitive area during peak hours and will involve an extremely hazardous material spread in a manner designed to cause maximum injury. While these classic patterns are helpful when planning for events, the effects of a secondary release may be so dramatic as to obscure their intentional origin, or an intentional attack may have entirely unexpected secondary effects. The quantity of material will vary widely from incident to incident and is not necessarily reflective of whether an incident was intentional. If any doubt exists, it is always better to assume an incident is intentional until proven otherwise. This helps the responder maintain awareness for the possibility of a secondary attack or a second incident.

Conclusion and Pitfalls

Lessons can be learned from recent experience with chemical attacks on civilian populations in Syria and other war zones. While it is always dangerous to generalize lessons from a specific conflict, healthcare workers serving these populations have identified many common experiences in the aftermath of chemical attack blast incidents that can provide valuable insight to aid in preparation. The tactics used by terrorists in the Middle East and other conflict zones represent the current state of the art and are likely to be exported or emulated.

One surprising finding is that terrorists seem to be specifically targeting vulnerable populations such as children and the elderly and that these populations are particularly vulnerable to the effects of hazardous agents. Schools, daycares, and other sites where these populations gather are common targets for attack and often lack hardened security measures [11]. After a blast, heavy gases and airborne materials will not immediately dissipate, increasing the exposure of shorter individuals such as children and those knocked to the ground. Explosives detonating at ground level which would cause lower extremity injuries to adults may be fatal to children. Burn and blast injuries are more severe at extremes of age, while metabolic differences make these populations particularly susceptible to the effects of hazardous materials.

After a blast incident involving hazardous materials, the chaos and social upheaval in the affected community have predictable impacts on the healthcare system. Access to healthcare facilities is often limited by infrastructure damage or the risk of attack. Often patients are not able to reach hospitals to receive care, while healthcare institutions are rapidly depleted of supplies and available staff. Personal protective equipment, antidotes, intravenous fluids, antibiotics, surgical supplies, and dressing materials are rapidly consumed, and their absence prevents the delivery of effective care [12].

In recent years, access to hospitals in conflict regions has been further complicated as terrorists across the globe are specifically targeting healthcare facilities in primary or secondary attacks, hoping to disrupt essential medical services and deny access to care for the injured. This reinforces the fear of patients and providers, causing the population to view hospitals not as places of safety and healing but rather strategic assets and potential targets of attack. It is no surprise that, living and working under these conditions, providers across the region consistently identify deterioration of mental health and stressful, dangerous living and working conditions to be a significant barrier in their systems [13].

The presence of hazardous materials at the scene of a blast event threatens the lives of survivors and responders alike. Knowledge of these agents and familiarity with their effects provide the responder with the ability to act efficiently and confidently, minimizing the loss of life and improving outcomes for survivors. Recognizing the features of a CBRN incident and acting appropriately save lives on scene and in the hospital. Whether the release is intentional or unintentional and regardless of which agent is released, strategies do exist to mitigate the damage.

References

1. Eshkol Z, Katz K. Injuries from biologic material of suicide bombers. Injury. 2005;36(2):271–4.
2. Braverman I, Wexler D, Oren M. A novel mode of infection with hepatitis B: penetrating bone fragments due to the explosion of a suicide bomber. Isr Med Assoc J. 2002;4(7):528–9.
3. CDC Radiation Emergencies. Acute radiation syndrome: a fact sheet for physicians [Internet]. Emergency preparedness and response. 2017 [cited 16 October 2018]. Available from: https://emergency.cdc.gov/radiation/arsphysicianfactsheet.asp.
4. NATO handbook on the medical aspects of NBC defensive operations AMedP-6(B). [Washington, D.C.]: Depts. of the Army, the Navy, and the Air Force; 1996.
5. CDC Bioterrorism Agents/Diseases (by category). Emergency preparedness & response [Internet]. 2017 [cited 16 October 2018]. Available from: https://emergency.cdc.gov/agent/agentlist-category.asp.
6. Ciottone G. Toxidrome recognition in chemical-weapons attacks. N Engl J Med. 2018;378(17):1611–20.
7. U.S. Department of Justice. Guide for the selection of chemical agent and toxic industrial material detection equipment for emergency first responders, vol. 1. Washington, DC: Government printing Office; 2000. www.ncjrs.org/pdffiles1/nij/184449.pdf.
8. CDC Bioterrorism Agents/Diseases (by category). Emergency preparedness & response. 2018. Retrieved April 30, 2019, from https://emergency.cdc.gov/agent/agentlist-category.asp.

9. Radiation Theory: Nature of Radiation [Internet]. Introduction to radiation safety. 2018 [cited 16 October 2018]. Available from: https://www.nde-ed.org/EducationResources/CommunityCollege/RadiationSafety/theory/nature.htm.
10. Bushberg J. Radiation exposure and contamination. In: Porter R, Kaplan J, Lynn R, Reddy M, editors. Merck manual professional edition [Internet]. Kenilworth, NJ: Merck Sharp & Dohme, Corporation; 2018. [cited 16 October 2018]. Available from: https://www.merckmanuals.com/professional/injuries-poisoning/radiation-exposure-and-contamination/radiation-exposure-and-contamination.
11. Gee P. Chemical weapons are intentionally deployed against the most vulnerable groups of people. BMJ. 2018;361:k1672. https://doi.org/10.1136/bmj.k1672.
12. Footer KHA, Clouse E, Rayes D, Sahloul Z, Rubenstein LS. Qualitative accounts from Syrian health professionals regarding violations of the right to health, including the use of chemical weapons, in opposition-held Syria. BMJ Open. 2018;8(8):e021096. https://doi.org/10.1136/bmjopen-2017-021096. PubMed PMID: 30082351; PubMed Central PMCID: PMC6078235.
13. World Health Organization. Mental health: evidence and research team. Mental health of populations exposed to biological and chemical weapons: World Health Organization; 2005. https://www.who.int/mental_health/media/bcw_and_mental_heath_who_2005.pdf.

Burn Management

43

Bradley Michael Golden and John G. McManus

Introduction

Explosions or blasts may precipitate disasters and usually arise from either industrial accidents or terrorist origins. Most explosive events, whether intentional violence or non-intentional and accidental, can cause burn injuries. It is notable that, terrorism aside, deaths from fires and burns are the third leading cause of fatal home injury. The mortality rate from burn injury ranks eighth among the 25 developed countries [1]. According to the American Burn Association National Burn Repository 2012 statistics, over 450,000 victims received medical treatment for burns in the United States in the last decade [1]. The majority of burns result from fire and/or flame injuries and contact with hot objects. Chemical burns account for approximately 3% of burns and 7% of burn admissions annually. Approximately 3400 deaths occurred (most from smoke inhalation), including 2550 deaths from residential fires (most from cooking), 300 from vehicle crash fires, and 550 from other sources (approximately 150 deaths from flame burns or smoke inhalation in nonresidential fires, 400 from contact with electricity, scalding liquids, or hot objects). Although the number of fatalities and injuries from residential fires has declined gradually, many residential fire-related deaths remain preventable and pose a significant public health problem. Almost 60% of acute burn hospitalizations in the United States were admitted to 127 burn centers [1]. Burn centers average over 200 annual admissions for burn injury and skin disorders requiring similar treatment. The other 4500 US acute care hospitals average fewer than three burn admissions each per year [1–4]. Fire and burn injuries represent 1% of the incidence of

B. M. Golden (✉)
Department of Emergency Medicine, Medical College of Georgia at Augusta University, Augusta, GA, USA
e-mail: bgolden@augusta.edu

J. G. McManus
Augusta University, Evans, GA, USA

D. W. Callaway, J. L. Burstein (eds.), *Operational and Medical Management of Explosive and Blast Incidents*, https://doi.org/10.1007/978-3-030-40655-4_43

injuries and 2% of the total costs of injuries, or $7.5 billion each year [5]. Risk factors for burn injuries in the United States include extremes of age (<4 years and >65 years), poverty, African and Native American descent, and rural area dwellers.

With regard to explosive events, burn injuries from terrorist bombings will continue to be a problem into the foreseeable future [6]. Terrorist bombs, typically improvised explosive devices (IEDs), are usually custom-made, may use any number of designs or explosives, and are of two types: (1) conventional, which are filled with chemical explosives, and (2) dispersive, which are filled with chemicals and/or other projectiles such as nails, steel pellets, screws, and nuts designed to disperse [6]. Temperatures from direct contact and the explosive gases can reach 3000 degrees Centigrade (5432 degrees Fahrenheit) and result in burns in victims close to the detonation [6].

Pathophysiology

Most adults have sustained burns during their lives. The skin is the largest organ in the body and serves as a barrier to outside insults and injuries. The skin protects against water loss, entrance of microorganisms, toxins, mechanical shock and forces, extreme environmental temperatures, and ultraviolet light damage to keratin and melanin. Furthermore, the skin is involved in sensory perception, temperature regulation, and biochemical activities (e.g., vitamin D synthesis).

The skin is made up of three basic layers. The outer layer, the epidermis, is the thin outer layer of the skin which consists of the stratum corneum containing fully mature keratinocytes which produce fibrous proteins (keratins) that are continuously shed (prevents the entry of most foreign substances as well as the loss of fluid from the body), the keratinocyte layer containing living keratinocytes (squamous cells), and the basal layer, the deepest layer of the epidermis, containing basal cells (continually dividing and forming new keratinocytes). The middle layer of the skin, the dermis, contains blood vessels, lymph vessels, hair follicles, sweat glands, fibroblasts, and nerves. The dermis is held together by collagen, made by fibroblasts, and gives skin flexibility and strength. The dermis also contains pain and touch receptors. The subcutis is the deepest layer of skin and consists of a network of collagen and fat cells that aid in conserving the body's heat and protect the body from injury by acting as a "shock absorber."

Severity of Burn

Accurate assessment of the burn patient and appropriate institution of early care are critical to optimal outcomes. Although burn size and depth are obvious factors in determining burn severity, the location of the burn, age of the patient, preexisting disease, and presence of trauma, including inhalation injury, may complicate treatment. Specific anatomical locations of burns often result in significant morbidity and mortality disproportionate to burn size (i.e., head, neck, hands, feet, perineum, and genitalia).

Furthermore, patients <2 years or >50 years of age are at higher risk of complications and death [1]. Infants' thin skin, limited reserve, and high surface area-to-mass ratio contribute to this risk, whereas thinning skin and coexisting medical problems commonly associated with aging are major factors in older individuals. Young children are also at risk for burns caused by abuse. There are several ways to classify burns, involving depth, severity, and surface area.

Depth

Burn depth is a product of temperature, duration of exposure, and skin thickness, with depth being described in its relationship to total skin thickness. Most burns have areas that are of mixed depth, with deeper burns often occurring in areas of thinner skin. The older classification of describing "degrees" of burn is not often used any more. Rather, the American Burn Association now uses the total body surface area and the severity (partial verses full thickness) of injury as a modern descriptor (Table 43.1). The old descriptive terms are paired with the newer classification system in order to understand the changes.

First-degree burns also known as superficial burn injuries involve only the epidermis of the skin and are recognized by their erythematous appearance and lack of blisters or skin separation. The classic first-degree injury is the sunburn or superficial scald burn from spills. These burns usually have morbidity restricted only to pain and are therefore not classified by burn size.

Second-degree burns, now called superficial or deep partial thickness burn injuries, involve the epidermis and part way through the dermis. Epithelial elements remain in the undestroyed dermal appendages and spontaneous healing usually occurs in 7–28 days. Second-degree burns are very painful and are usually blistered.

Third-degree burns, also known as full-thickness burn injuries, are those that extend through the dermis, destroying all epidermal and dermal elements. They may initially have blisters containing hemorrhagic fluid and/or dead tissue (eschar). The presence or absence of pain is an unreliable indicator of depth and severity.

Table 43.1 Burn description

Burn thickness	Deepest skin structure involved	Appearance	Pain	Prognosis (without surgical intervention)
Superficial (first-degree)	Epidermis	Dry, blanching erythema	Painful	Heals without scarring, 5–10 days
Superficial partial thickness (second-degree)	Upper dermis	Blisters; wet, blanching erythema	Painful	Heals without scarring, <3 weeks
Deep partial-thickness (second-degree)	Lower dermis	Yellow or white, dry, nonblanching	Decreased sensation	Heals in 3–8 weeks; likely to scar if healing >3 weeks
Full-thickness (third-degree)	Subcutaneous structures	White or black/brown, nonblanching	Decreased sensation	Heals by contracture >8 weeks; will scar

Burn Size

Accurate initial assessment of burn size is essential for optimal patient care. Burn size is expressed as total body surface area (TBSA) or body surface area (BSA), where approximately 1% of a patient's surface area is equal to the palmar surface of the patient's hand with the fingers closed. This measurement is most useful for small (<5% TBSA) or spotty burns. For larger areas, the rule of nines (Fig. 43.1) for adults provides a simple and rapid estimation of burn size in the adult.

When calculating burn size using any method, first-degree burns are not counted, and only the proportion of area with at least a partial-thickness burn is calculated. Thus, for an upper extremity to be considered 9% TBSA, the entire extremity from the shoulder to the finger tips must be burned at least to the blistering level. If only the posterior half of the upper extremity is burned, then burn size is considered to be 4.5% TBSA.

Calculating pediatric burns is often challenging and can be inaccurate if the provider is not appropriately trained. The rule of nines (see Fig. 43.1) has also been used for pediatric patients. However, the Lund and Browder classification can also be used to more precisely calculate the percentage of BSA burned by mapping the injured areas of the body on charts detailing age-appropriate measurements. This method identifies the different body proportions according to the age of the patient (with children having larger heads and smaller lower extremities than adults) and through dividing the body into smaller units, such as dividing the upper extremity

Child body Part	% of total BSA
Arm	9%
Head and neck	18%
Leg	14%
Anterior trunk	18%
Posterior trunk	18%

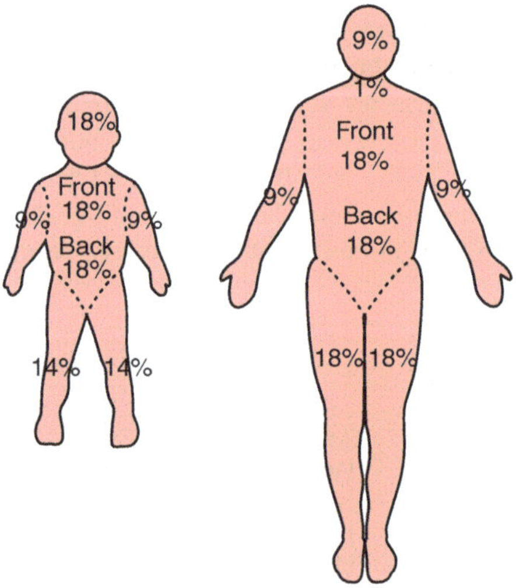

Adult body Part	% of total BSA
Arm	9%
Head	9%
Neck	1%
Leg	18%
Anterior trunk	18%
Posterior trunk	18%

Fig. 43.1 Burn percentage

into the upper arm, lower arm, and hand. Computer programs are now being used to estimate surface area calculations.

Inhalation Injury

Inhalation injury is a complex set of pathophysiological reactions that occur from exposure to smoke and/or chemical products. Systemic and respiratory damage can result in significant morbidity and mortality as well as permanent dysfunction [7, 8]. When combined with thermal injury, inhalation injury increases pulmonary compliance and fluid requirements and doubles mortality. Technically, injury is a misnomer, and inhalation injury is really the result of fluid shifts caused by external burns. These conditions do not necessarily imply pulmonary injury, because they also occur with scald and chemical burns. Edema formation in the posterior pharynx, glottic, and subglottic areas associated with deep burns of the upper chest, neck, and lower face has the potential to occlude the upper airway. Tachypnea and stridor are often late signs and when absent are unreliable in ruling out airway injury.

Airway injury is diagnosed by fiber-optic bronchoscopy [9]. Early grading of inhalation injury severity is often inaccurate. The injury is basically a chemical burn from which resulting edema of the small airways creates distal microatelectasis and a clinical picture identical to acute respiratory distress syndrome. Lower airway or "smoke inhalation" injury is caused by the patient inhaling the products of combustion, often as a result of being in a confined space. Specific injuries resulting from specific toxins, cyanide and carbon monoxide, are discussed elsewhere in this text.

Chemical Burn

A caustic or corrosive agent is a chemical capable of causing tissue and mucous membrane injury upon contact. These agents are generally made up of extreme pH values (<3 or >11). The American Burn Association National Burn Repository reported in 2012 that over a 10-year period, chemicals represented 3.3% of all burns in the United States [1]. The majority of these burns resulted from accidental exposure at work. Chemical burns have higher complication rates in the very young and old populations with the most common complications being cellulitis, pneumonia, and respiratory failure. Common household and industrial products that result in burns include hydrochloric acid, potassium hydroxide, sodium hydroxide, sulfuric and phosphoric acids, and many others. Hydrofluoric acid (HF) is a weak acid that requires special consideration and treatment with specific antidotes. Although the most commonly affected body areas are the face, eyes, and extremities, almost all fatalities are as a result of ingestion [10].

Specific Training Requirements

The central concepts for prehospital providers and EMS physicians caring for burn patients include the following:

- Thorough training on a consistent, organized patient assessment algorithm that can be applied to all burn patients, regardless of injury severity, is foundational. It should provide hierarchical management that focuses on life threats, yet incorporates full, sequenced evaluation and integrated management options for actual and potential injuries. Frequent reassessments and ability to integrate information and recognize trends that require urgent intervention are essential.
- Efficient and appropriate use of local resources (air evacuation, hazardous materials teams, specialized rescue units), knowledge of hospital capabilities, and specific destination policies (e.g., specialty burn care center) can improve patient outcomes in patients with significant injuries where time is of the essence. EMS systems should have policies and procedures to identify such patients and promote primary transport to the appropriate facility when available. This concept, pioneered by trauma systems, is now being extended effectively to non-trauma disease processes.
- Proper use of spinal motion restriction, splinting, fluid resuscitation, and pain management to limit additional morbidity. Knowing how and when to properly use infrequent invasive procedures such as cricothyrotomy, needle thoracostomy, and escharotomy is essential for patient safety and care.
- Recognition of a chemical exposure and proper use of protective equipment is essential in limiting exposure to bystander and healthcare personnel.

Burn-Specific Patient Assessment and Care

The mechanism of injury, while not entirely predictive of actual injury sustained, often alerts the astute clinician to potential injuries that may be encountered during the assessment and management of burn patients. The importance of integration of local EMS and hospital resources with tailoring guidelines to optimize patient care within these parameters cannot be overemphasized. Newer telemedicine applications that allow concurrent assessment by EMS and receiving emergency physicians may facilitate triage, continuity of care, and expedited care at the receiving facility for a number of time-sensitive medical complaints, certainly including burn injuries.

Burn management differs significantly from routine trauma care. Traumatic injuries occur in 5–15% of admitted burn patients [1]. Evaluation and treatment of traumatic injuries take precedence over treatment of the burn, with the caveat that maintenance of body temperature, airway protection, and appropriate burn fluid resuscitation must be achieved.

Distance to the destination burn or trauma center should influence the plan for airway management. If transport time is short (e.g., <10 minutes) and if able to achieve adequate oxygenation and ventilation with basic measures such as a face mask or bag-valve-mask ventilation, time should generally not be taken at the scene for endotracheal intubation (ETI), including pharmacologically assisted intubation. However, in patients with suspected inhalation injury or impending obstruction, prehospital personnel should consider immediate ETI. ETI can be particularly challenging in the burn victim due to altered mental status and/or combativeness, airway secretions or debris, and potential swelling and distortion of anatomy.

The EMS provider must decide if the delay in transport due to placing an advanced airway in a specific patient and situation is clinically beneficial, specifically, if the delay outweighs the potential risk to the patient from either deterioration due to the injuries or due to secondary complications that could occur if the airway cannot be secured in a timely manner [11]. While orotracheal intubation is the preferred route, edema and debris in a burn patient's airway may require a cricothyrotomy to be performed as a last resort. Training EMS personnel in alternative airway techniques may be extremely useful for complicated airway management [12].

Secure the tube with cotton umbilical ribbon. Do not use adhesive tape on the endotracheal tube or any other important device or tube in the burn patient. The patient will become very edematous, the burned skin will slough off, and the endotracheal tube will fall out if secured only with tape. If this happens, it is very difficult to reestablish the airway due to extensive airway edema. If the patient is not intubated, closely observe for early indicators of impending airway obstruction such as swelling of the face or tongue and hoarseness. Be prepared to intubate the patient if these signs appear.

Careful monitoring of respiratory parameters including pulse oximetry, end-tidal carbon dioxide, ventilatory compliance, and circulation will provide trending that can alert the provider to developing complications in a critical patient [11]. High-flow oxygen should be used in all patients who show signs of respiratory distress and/or hypoxia. Beta-agonists have been used in cases of inhalation injury resulting in increased oxygen delivery and decreased bronchospasm [8]. Outcome prediction metrics based on currently available high-level noninvasive monitoring may help refine destination choices and in-hospital trauma management. Burn eschar on the chest may interfere with ventilation, and if this is the case, chest escharotomy should be performed during this assessment.

Those with burn injuries have higher fluid requirements than other trauma patients [8, 9, 13]. However, prehospital personnel must avoid excessive fluid resuscitation that could paradoxically lead to worsening hemorrhage and/or pulmonary function. Fluid resuscitation is the cornerstone of early burn care. The microvascular structures beneath a burn wound develop increased permeability immediately after injury, resulting in capillary leakage. Capillary leak is roughly proportional to burn size and becomes hemodynamically significant in burns larger than 20% TBSA (10% TBSA in young children or elderly patients). The objective of resuscitation is to replace lost intravascular fluid with the minimal amount of fluid required to maintain normal bodily function [13].

Guidelines in the current literature instruct providers to calculate predicted 24-hour fluid requirements and initiate fluid resuscitation based on these formulas

[13]. Half of the fluid should be given in the first 8 hours and the other half over the next 16 hours. Although there are multiple formulas for predicting the first 24 hours of fluid required in burn patients, two of the most advocated formulas are as follows:

Modified Brooke: Initial 24 hours: no colloids. Ringer's lactated (RL) solution 2 mL/kg/% burn in adults and 3 mL/kg/% burn in children.

Parkland Formula: Initial 24 hours: RL solution 4 mL/kg/% burn for adults and 3 mL/kg/% burn for children. RL solution is added for maintenance for children:

- 4 mL/kg/hour for children weighing 0–10 kg
- 40 mL/hour +2 mL/hour for children weighing 10–20 kg
- 60 mL/hour +1 mL/kg/hour for children weighing 20 kg or higher

A randomized study of adult military burn patients comparing these two formulas demonstrated that the modified Brooke formula was successful in lowering fluid requirements without increased mortality [13]. Another burn formula to simplify fluid delivery was also advocated in prehospital patients, labeled "the rule of 10" [14].

- Estimate burn size (using the rule of nines) to the nearest 10% TBSA.
- Multiply that by 10 to calculate the initial fluid rate for patients weighing 40–80 kg.
- Increase fluid rate weight above 80 kg by 100 cc/hour for every 10 kg of body.

Under-resuscitation may result in renal failure, hypotension, and multiple organ dysfunction, whereas over-resuscitation results in pulmonary and cardiac overload and excessive edema formation [8, 10]. The extremes of age are especially sensitive to poor estimation of fluid needs. Resuscitation requires an accurate estimation of the time of burn, burn size, and measurement of patient weight. Factors that increase fluid requirements include inhalation injury, late initiation of resuscitation, deep burns, acute intoxication, and preexisting malnutrition [1].

Burn fluid formulas are merely starting points in resuscitation. Individual changes to fluid administration rates must be made hourly (or half-hourly in infants and small children) based on urine output, vital signs, and other markers of perfusion. Most utilize the formula recommended by the burn center to which the patient is being transferred [14].

Regardless of the type and volume of fluid used in resuscitation of burn patients, awareness and prevention of hypothermia are essential in maintaining circulation. Hypothermia increases burn mortality. Administration of significant volumes of IV fluids at or below room temperature can exacerbate the problem. Preventing heat loss and providing warm fluids to a patient in need of volume resuscitation or rewarming can diminish this potential effect [15–17]. Several commercially available fluid warmers have been studied [18].

All wounds should be exposed for evaluation. In patients with extensive burns, overlying clothes and jewelry should be removed. These items may have melted onto the skin. If this is the case, the burn team may need to excise these items along with the burned skin. Jewelry may have to be cut off with wire cutters or similar devices. Decontamination from toxins and chemicals should also begin during this phase of assessment. Saturated clothing should be removed, powdered chemicals should be brushed off the skin, and the contaminated area(s) irrigated with copious amounts of water until the patient experiences a decrease in pain in the wound. The use of neutralizing solutions in treatment of chemical burns is not routinely recommended except for burns involving hydrogen fluoride. Chemical injuries to the eye are treated by forcing the eyelid open and flushing the eye with water or saline.

Special Considerations

Compartment Syndrome

Formation of edema beneath full-thickness (usually circumferential) burn eschar has the potential to occlude arterial inflow to the extremity or restrict chest motion and hence ventilation, resulting in respiratory failure [19]. If available, Doppler signals should be followed; if not, check pulses, skin temperature, and capillary refill at regular intervals. Diminution of the signal or a change in its character may suggest compartment syndrome. Patients receiving massive amounts of fluid may also develop compartment syndrome. This results from an increase in the tissue pressure in a restricted compartment of the body. If compartment syndrome is suspected, decompression of the involved compartments with appropriate escharotomy and fasciotomy is indicated as soon as possible [19]. Treatment with escharotomy may be performed in the prehospital setting with either local anesthesia or conscious sedation. Incisions are placed on the medial and lateral portions of affected extremities or on the midaxillary lines of the trunk connected by an inverted "V" (chevron) incision along the costal margins (Fig. 43.2). Escharotomies of the fingers are seldom, if ever, required.

Pain Management

The prehospital environment provides unique challenges in treatment of acute pain such as the lack of supplies and equipment, delayed or prolonged evacuation times and distances, devastating injuries, provider inexperience, and dangerous tactical situations [20, 21]. Studies have shown an increase in the incidence of chronic pain and posttraumatic stress disorder (PTSD) with failure to recognize and treat acute pain appropriately. In addition, studies have seen a reduction in PTSD incidence when pain is adequately managed, particularly with early use of ketamine [22, 23].

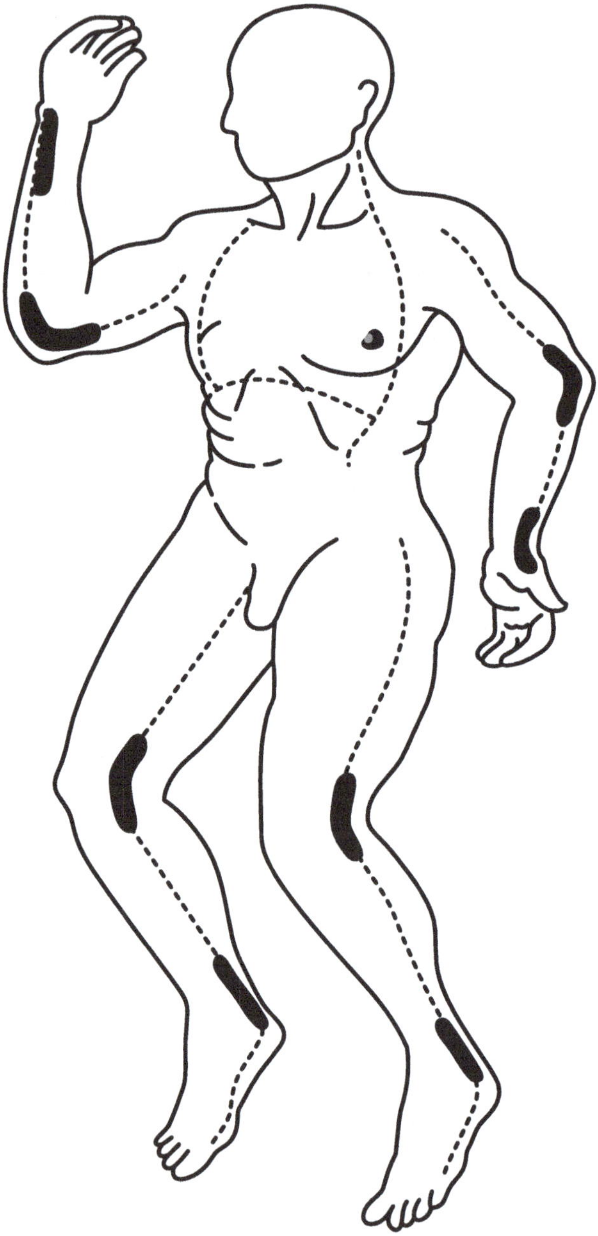

Fig. 43.2 Location of escharotomy incisions. (Source: US Army Institute of Surgical Research)

Hydrofluoric Acid

Hydrofluoric acid (HF) is an aqueous solution of the inorganic acid of elemental fluorine and will dissolve anything that has glass or silica content. HF and related products may cause dermal, ocular, pulmonary, gastrointestinal, and systemic injury [1]. When in contact with skin, HF dissociates into hydrogen ions and free fluoride ions. There may be a latent period before a clinically evident burn is apparent, dependent on the concentration of the acid and the length of time it is in contact with the skin. Fluoride ions penetrate tissues deeply, causing tissue damage and the potential for systemic toxicity depending on the HF concentration. In general, exposure to HF solutions of greater than 50% concentration results in immediate pain and tissue destruction. The skin appears blanched, and within 1–2 hours the dermal lines are obliterated by edema. Dermal contact with concentrations of 20–50% HF usually results in burns that develop within a few hours [9, 24].

Concentrations greater than 20% HF have a potential for serious toxicity regardless of the degree of surface area involved [24]. Contact with solutions of less than 20% HF concentration results in dermal injury that usually develops within about 24 hours [25]. The clinical presentation of exposure to strong HF solutions of greater than 20% begins with pain at the site that is characteristically intense [25] and often described by patients as "burning," "deep," "throbbing," or "exquisite." Local erythema and edema may or may not be present initially, but later a pale, blanched appearance of the skin is apparent in more severe burns from concentrated HF (e.g., >50%) [9, 24, 25]. Extensive bullae and maceration of tissue may be seen. Gray areas may develop and progress to frank necrosis and deep ulceration within 6–24 hours. HF exposure results in hypocalcemia, hypomagnesia, and hyperkalemia. These electrolyte disturbances can be profound and lead to death. The mainstay of treatment is calcium, both systemically and locally as a paste or solution.

Guidelines for Prehospital Management

Guidelines for management of the burn patient should be focused on providing necessary interventions, together with rapid transport to the closest appropriate facility. Triage guidelines should also address burn/trauma patients who need different types of specialty care by identifying regional facilities with special capabilities such as pediatric trauma, burn care, hyperbaric therapy, and extremity replantation. Scene time should not be delayed while the provider waits for direct medical oversight. Patient outcomes are significantly better at burn centers than non-burn centers [26]. Burn centers have teams of professionals dedicated to optimal burn care. The American Burn Association has established criteria for transfer of a patient to one of these centers.

Requirements for Transfer

Patients with major burns (>20% TBSA) require IV access, preferably two large-bore peripheral lines. Catheters may be placed through the burned tissue. Central venous access should be avoided because of its high complication rate in the early postburn period when vasospasm, low flow, and a hypercoagulable state contribute to complications. A urinary catheter and a nasogastric tube are recommended for long or delayed transport. Use of ice on a burn wound is absolutely contraindicated because of the risk of a cold injury superimposed on the burn. Continual efforts must be made to keep the patient warm. No burn debridement is required before transfer, and the burns should be wrapped in dry sterile, clean sheets, or burn-specific water-based gel dressings and further covered with warm blankets.

Prevention

The prehospital environment offers a unique "teachable moment" for clinicians to educate patients and their families about preventing burns in the future. Prevention programs and safety legislation have made substantial contributions to decreasing the incidence and severity of burn injury, especially for parents and school-age children.

In addition, several initiatives are targeting vulnerable segments of the population for prevention efforts. Mothers with less than high school education who are younger than 20 years old and have more than two children are at a much higher risk for fatal fire events [1]. Although prevention initiatives are reaching increasing numbers of people, there is still the need for further education of the public and in particular those subsegments of the population at high risk for burn injury.

Pitfalls

- Not taking control of the airway early. A focused physical exam needs to be completed to look for any signs suggestive of inhalation injury, such as neck burns, singed nasal hairs, carbonaceous sputum, voice changes, or soot in the upper airways. If the patient has any signs of airway compromise, it clearly necessitates intubation, even ones who appear well initially can rapidly deteriorate.
- Missing systemic poisoning. Not only do patients suffer direct pulmonary injury, they are also at risk for hypoxemia from CO and cyanide, especially if the fire occurred in an enclosed space. It should be presumed the patient is suffering from systemic poisoning unless it can be ruled out with carboxyhemoglobin testing. Cyanide levels are rarely available in the acute setting; however, a lactate level greater than 10 mmol/L is highly predictive of poisoning.
- Not managing the traumatic issues first. While the burn injuries can appear grotesque and can be the patients' focus due to the pain, traumatic injuries must be managed first. Missed traumatic injuries are more likely to cause increased mortality and, therefore, ATLS protocols should be followed prior to burn-specific management.

References

1. American Burn Association. 2012 National burn repository report of data from 2002–2011. Available at: www.ameriburn.org/2012NBRAnnualReport.pdf.
2. Ahrens M. Home structure fires. National Fire Protection Association: Quincy, MA; 2011.
3. Karter MJ. Fire loss in the United States during 2010. Quincy, MA: National Fire Protection Association, Fire Analysis and Research Division; 2011.
4. Centers for Disease Control. Fire deaths and injuries fact sheet. Available at: www.cdc.gov/homeandrecreationalsafety/fire-prevention/fires-factsheet.html.
5. Corso P, Finkelstein E, Miller T, Fiebelkorn I, Zaloshnja E. Incidence and lifetime costs of injuries in the United States. Inj Prev. 2006;12(4):212–8.
6. Atiyeh BS, Gunn SW, Hayek SN. Military and civilian burn injuries during armed conflicts. Ann Burns Fire Disasters. 2007;20(4):203–15.
7. Palmieri TL. Inhalation injury: research progress and needs. J Burn Care Res. 2007;28:549–54.
8. Colohan SM. Predicting prognosis in thermal burns with associated inhalational injury: a systematic review of prognostic factors in adult burn victims. J Burn Care Res. 2010;31:529–39.
9. Shirani KZ, Pruitt BA Jr, Mason AD Jr. The influence of inhalation injury and pneumonia on burn mortality. Ann Surg. 1987;205:82–7.
10. Stuke LE, Arnoldo BD, Hunt JL, Purdue GF. Hydrofluoric acid burns: a 15-year experience. J Burn Care Res. 2008;29:893–6.
11. Wang HE, Kupas DF, Hostler D, Cooney R, Yealy DM, Lave JR. Procedural experience with out-of-hospital endotracheal intubation. Crit Care Med. 2005;33:1718–21.
12. Kurola JO, Turunen MJ, Laakso J, Gorski JT, Paakkonen HJ, Silfvast TO. A comparison of the laryngeal tube and bag-valve mask ventilation by emergency medical technicians: a feasibility study in anesthetized patients. Anesth Analg. 2005;101:1477–81.
13. Chung KK, Wolf SE, Cancio LC, Alvarado R, Jones JA, McCorcle J, et al. Resuscitation of severely burned military casualties: fluid begets more fluid. J Trauma. 2009;67:231–7.
14. Chung KK, Salinas J, Renz EM, Alvarado RA, King BT, Barillo DJ, et al. Simple derivation of the initial fluid rate for the resuscitation of severely burned adult combat casualties: in silico validation of the rule of 10. J Trauma. 2010;69:S49–54.
15. Hildebrand F, Giannoudis PV, van Griensven M, Chawda M, Pape HC. Pathophysiologic changes and effects of hypothermia on outcome in elective surgery and trauma patients. Am J Surg. 2004;187:363–71.
16. Mizushima Y, Wang P, Cioffi WG, Bland KI, Chaudry IH. Should normothermia be restored and maintained during resuscitation after trauma and hemorrhage? J Trauma. 2000;48:58–65.
17. Segers MJ, Diephuis JC, van Kesteren RG, van der Werken C. Hypothermia in trauma patients. Unfallchirurg. 1998;101(10):742–9.
18. Dubick MA, Brooks DE, Macaitis JM, Bice TG, Moreau AR, Holcomb JB. Evaluation of commercially available fluid-warming devices for use in forward surgical and combat areas. Mil Med. 2005;170:76–82.
19. Kupas DF, Miller DD. Out-of-hospital chest escharotomy: a case series and procedure review. Prehosp Emerg Care. 2010;14:349–54.
20. Black I, McManus JG. Pain management in current combat operations. Prehosp Emerg Care. 2009;13:223–7.
21. Wedmore IS, Johnson T, Czarnik J, Hendrix S. Pain management in the wilderness and operational setting. Emerg Med Clin N Am. 2005;23:585–601.
22. Otis JD, Keane TM, Kerns RD. An examination of the relationship between chronic pain and post-traumatic stress disorder. J Rehabil Res Dev. 2003;40:397–405.
23. McGhee LL, Maani CV, Garza TH, Gaylord KM, Black IH. The correlation between ketamine and posttraumatic stress disorder in burned service members. J Trauma. 2008;64:S195–8.

24. Seyb ST, Noordhoek L, Botens S, Mani MM. A study to determine the efficacy of treatments for hydrofluoric acid burns. J Burn Care Rehabil. 1995;16:253–7.
25. Centers for Disease Control and Prevention. Hydrogen fluoride systemic agent. Available at: www.cdc.gov/niosh/ershdb/Emergency ResponseCard_29750030.html.
26. Holmes JH 4th, Carter JE, Neff LP, Cairns BA, d'Agostino RB Jr, Griffin LP, et al. The effectiveness of regionalized burn care: an analysis of 6,873 burn admissions in North Carolina from 2000 to 2007. J Am Coll Surg. 2011;212:487–93.

Wound Management

44

Alexander Hart

Introduction

The subacute and chronic management of wounds suffered through blast injuries is critical to decreasing morbidity and mortality. While basic wound care principles form the basis of management, blast injuries require caregivers to manage wounds differently than they might for other types of injuries.

History of Wound Management

Ancient Wound Care

Humanity has been attempting to manage wounds since prehistory. The Mesopotamians produced clay tablets ~2500 BCE detailing methods of wound care from the time [1, 2]. These describe the washing of wounds, making of plasters, and bandaging of wounds. Early wound care methods heavily featured the use of plants as astringents, honey, and alcohol for antimicrobial effects and for other properties. Interestingly, the effects of substances such as honey were likely discovered separately by various cultures, suggesting empirical, observatory learning.

The Greeks were advanced in their stress on cleanliness, washing wounds with boiled water, followed by acetic acid (vinegar), and alcohol (wine). The Romans were noted for describing the importance of rubor, tumor, calor, and dolor (redness, swelling, heat, and pain) as cardinal signs of inflammation [1]. In ancient times, suturing was an uncommon occurrence, with most cultures leaving wounds open

A. Hart (✉)
Department of Emergency Medicine, Beth Israel Deaconess Medical Center, Boston, MA, USA
e-mail: ahart1@bidmc.harvard.edu

D. W. Callaway, J. L. Burstein (eds.), *Operational and Medical Management of Explosive and Blast Incidents*, https://doi.org/10.1007/978-3-030-40655-4_44

during their treatment. Hippocrates (460–377 BCE) is noted for describing the debridement of necrotic material in wound healing. He recommended using wool which had been boiled in water or wine as a useful dressing. He also documents the knowledge of the Greeks that a bandage used too tightly could cause gangrene.

In the Middle Ages, the most advanced wound care was that which had been set down by Galen and Celsus and was mostly practiced in the Middle East. Celsus recommended the use of dry pledgets to stop hemorrhage, with progression to a moist sponge if that did not suffice. Cobwebs were a remedy of choice for small, oozing wounds. The use of ligature on a vessel was described, with cautery used as a last resort. Galen also wrote about the use of finger pressure on a blood vessel to stop arterial bleeding. He also used ligatures for arterial bleeding and styptic substances on venous bleeding. The knowledge of the Arabic-speaking world was written down by Albucasis (also known as Abu al-Qasim al-Zahrawi [936–1013 CE]), which is the method in which it passed to the European medical community. The Arabic world is where distillation, crystallization, and the science of pharmacy were first performed, all important advances in the production of wound care materials.

Theodoric, a disciple of the Bologna school of medical thought, argued in his writings against the idea of probing, packing, and dressing wounds. Although Maitre Henri de Mondeville (1260–1320 CE) attempted to question these teachings and believed that contagion caused wound infection, his teachings were not adopted widely throughout the Middle Ages. Guy de Chauliac (1300–1368 CE) proposed five principles of wound treatment which are recognizable to today's clinicians: the removal of foreign bodies, re-approximation of separated parts, maintenance of apposition, conservation of substance, and treatment of complications. As gunpowder was introduced to the West, cautery took on a larger role, being used even for smaller, non-bleeding wounds [2].

Civil War Wound Care

Sterile technique was not recognized as important even through the Civil War, leading to high rates of wound infections. Antiseptic technique was a major breakthrough of the late 1800s, improving surgical outcomes, which through the end of the American Civil War, were dismal [1]. This is because the germ theory of disease would not be established until 1870 [3]. The Civil War was when the first early-modern surgical techniques were developed for arterial ligation. During this conflict, Union Army surgeons performed ~30,000 amputations on ~175,000 extremity wounds. Those who underwent amputation had a greater than 25% mortality rate. Surgeons of the time noted that the amputations done under 24 hours from the time of injury had a significantly lower mortality than those performed over 48 hours later, an early indication of the later focus on early surgical management of severe traumatic injuries [3]. This time period saw the progression from cautery and tourniquets as a primary approach to hemorrhage control to the increased use of ligature. However, fatality rates from abdominal (87%) and chest (62%) wounds remained high given the high infection rates and lack of antibiotics.

Throughout this time period, postoperative infections killed many soldiers, given the lack of antibiotics. Surgeons also saw a type of necrotizing fasciitis called hospital gangrene, with a 45% mortality in postoperative wounds. Management of the time was to dissect away the dead tissue and inject wound margins with bromine, followed by packing with bromine-soaked dressings and isolation from other patients. The nurses caring for these patients dressed their wounds last and washed their hands in chlorinated soda in an effort to reduce the transmission of infection to those who were not yet suffering from it. Although the techniques have changed, these same principles of management pertain to today's blast injury care [3].

Korean War and Vietnam Conflict Wound Care

By the late 1900s, while the United States was embroiled in conflicts in Korea and Vietnam, combat medics were applying pressure dressings for hemorrhage control, with tourniquets as a backup option. The usefulness of early antibiotics had been elaborated, and field antibiotics were used in cases where transport was delayed.

Specialty surgery by vascular and orthopedic surgeons became more common during the Vietnam conflict, with highly sophisticated vascular repairs. Fractures were reduced and put either in traction or casts. Additionally, the prevalent use of antibiotics decreased mortality from abdominal wounds to 4.5%, down from 21% during World War II [4].

Wound Care in Today's Conflicts

The prevalence of improvised explosive devices (IEDs) and suicide bombers in Afghanistan and Iraq have transformed the approach to blast injuries in combat, which has been translated to the civilian arena. High-velocity weapons and IEDs account for more than 75% of all wounds in these conflicts. Limbs with massive tissue damage from these mechanisms frequently require amputation. Advanced hemostatic agents such as hemostatic dressings are used in conjunction with tourniquets, which have taken on a significantly more prevalent role in blast care. Vascular care has also advanced significantly, and autologous veins can be used for early temporizing repair of vascular injuries to prevent devitalization of injured tissue. External fixation is used more frequently in cases that will require multiple debridements, decreasing the need for amputations.

Biologic Basis of Wound Care

Histology

Wound healing occurs in four overlapping phases: hemostasis, inflammation, proliferation, and maturation/remodeling. Hemostasis begins within seconds of a wound occurring. Platelets are exposed by the injury, causing them to start the process of clot formation and to begin releasing multiple cytokines, chemokines, and hormones, which induce the other phases of healing. Fibrin polymerizes to form the mature clot and as a scaffold for cells which will start the next steps in healing. Catecholamines act on the endothelium to induce vasoconstriction, limiting the hemorrhage. Small vessels vasodilate to allow in leukocytes, red blood cells, and plasma proteins.

Inflammation is caused as neutrophils, macrophages, and lymphocytes flood the injured area. Neutrophils arrive within 24 hours, and the by-products of their apoptosis attract phagocytes, including lymphocytes and macrophages. These clear out the debris and bacteria in the wound. Inhibition of inflammation, using anti-inflammatory medications, can result in improper healing. However, a prolonged inflammatory phase can also impair healing, leading to chronic wounds and severe scarring. High bacterial load, repeated trauma, and foreign bodies have been shown to impair this phase.

Proliferation begins with reepithelialization, capillary budding, and the production of an extracellular matrix to fill the defect in the tissue. Keratinocytes proliferate and produce a new basement membrane near the edge of the wound as the healing advances. The next row of keratinocytes then attaches, digesting the extracellular matrix which previously filled that space. An uninfected exudate will cover the wound during this phase to prevent loss of moisture and hold growth factors. One key factor in wound care is the maintenance of this layer, as its destruction can delay healing. Any wound that is healing by secondary intention will at this point fill in with granulation tissue. Angiogenesis continues throughout this phase.

Angiogenesis and maturation occur as vessels sprout to repopulate the new dermis. The cells from previous phases undergo apoptosis as this remodeling phase begins. Type I collagen is produced, which causes the tensile strength of the wound to improve significantly. This phase requires a significant nutrient load, and any issues with nutrition can negatively affect the process [5].

Wound healing from any event requires the coordination of a cascade of biochemical processes involving multiple cell types to manage the degradation and regeneration of tissue. Growth factors are a type of cytokine, a class of proteins which allow cells to communicate with one another. Within this class, growth factors stimulate the migration (chemotaxis) and proliferation of cells, as well as signaling them to create new tissue. Growth factors also induce epithelial cells to grow, blood vessels to form, and the formation of a cell matrix. They can act by endocrine transmission through the blood to a remote site, through direct paracrine action on adjacent cells, and by autocrine self-regulatory roles on the excreting cell. Growth factors only affect cells which have their particular receptor, which then activates intracellular processes to cause individual effects. These receptors can have direct catalytic activity or may act through G-protein coupling. The exact methods of growth factor-receptor binding and cell stimulation are still areas of intense study [6]. Several of the best elucidated growth factors that play major roles in wound healing are discussed in Table 44.1.

Table 44.1 Major growth factors in wound healing

Growth factor	Function	Locations	Method of action
Epidermal growth factor (EGF)	Granulation tissue development, maturation of epidermal cells	Most body fluids	Paracrine
Transforming growth factor-α (TGF-α)	Granulation tissue development, epidermal regrowth	Most body fluids	Paracrine
Platelet-derived growth factor (PDGF)	Chemotaxis of fibroblasts/monocytes, mitogenesis of fibroblasts/vascular smooth muscle	Released from platelets, macrophages, endothelium, vascular smooth muscle, fibroblasts	Paracrine, autocrine
Transforming growth factor-β (TGF-β)	Mitogenesis and regulation of cell matrix production, angiogenesis	Platelets, macrophages, bone, monocytes, lymphocytes	Paracrine
Fibroblast growth factors (FGFs)	Chemotaxis of endothelium/leukocytes, mitogenesis of endothelium	Endothelium, macrophages, fibroblasts	Endocrine, paracrine, autocrine
Tumor necrosis factor-α (TNF-α)	Cell survival and cell death signaling	Macrophages	Autocrine, paracrine

Types of Repair

Wounds can close via several mechanisms. Closure by primary intention refers to a wound in which the provider closes the wound during initial intervention. This can be done with sutures, clips, skin closure strips, glue, or staples. The wound is typically closed within 48–72 hours without infection or other complicating factors. Primary intention is less common with blast wounds than many other types of injuries owing to the frequency of debris and infection with these wounds. Delayed primary closure refers to the closure of wounds by the provider after this timeframe. In blast injuries, the most common reason for this delay is the need for further debridement prior to closure.

Wounds can also heal by secondary intention. This method is typically chosen when the amount of damaged tissue precludes realignment of the wound edges or when infection/debris makes the likelihood of infection too high for a primary closure. Thus, this is a very common method in blast injuries. The wound will heal from the base, as it fills in with granulation tissue, and epithelialization progresses from the edges.

Careful debridement is important due to the presence of devitalized tissue, debris, and bacteria. This can be done through several methods. Autolytic debridement is a slow method that requires keeping the injury moist and allows the body to clear the devitalized tissue through its own biochemical processes. Mechanical debridement is quicker and occurs through a physical process such as irrigation with pressure or debridement with pads or with bandages that can debride the wound during removal. Biosurgical debridement refers to the application of larvae to the wound to quickly debride an injury. Conservative sharp debridement is the use of scalpel or scissors to remove dead tissue outside the operating room. Surgical debridement occurs in the operating room and is a quicker method of debridement, which will frequently be required of blast injuries.

Dressings

There are a number of types of dressings in use for varying wounds, each with their own benefits and drawbacks. Nonadherent fabrics (absorptive) include gauze, foams, and alginates. Hydrophobic fabrics have some occlusive properties, but do not allow for fluid drainage. These include Vaseline gauze (the Kendall Co., Mansfield, MA), Xeroform (the Kendall Co.), and Telfa (the Kendall Co.). Hydrophilic dressings (e.g., Adaptic [Johnson & Johnson Medical, Arlington, TX]) allow for excellent drainage of fluids and exudates into any dressings above them. Gauze is a very commonly used bandage and is frequently used to cover other non-occlusive, nonadhering dressings, with its main benefit being its absorption of discharge. However, gauze directly in contact to the wound frequently adheres to the surface, causing pain and unintentional debridement of the healing wound. For this reason, it is more typically used in wounds closed by primary intention or as a secondary dressing.

Occlusive or moisture-retentive dressings include the traditional non-biologics such as foams, films, hydrocolloids, hydrogels, and alginates, as well as the newer non-biologics, including hydrofiber, collagen, and hyaluronic acid dressings. This group also includes the biologic dressings, also known as grafts, and the biosynthetic skin substitutes, such as cultured epidermal grafts, dermal replacements, and composite skin substitutes. Finally, antimicrobial dressings fall into this category. These are bactericidal and maintain the moisture of the wound. Many bactericidal dressings use silver impregnation to create bactericidal properties and are useful for 3–7 days. There are not yet enough data to determine if silver-impregnated dressings actually prevent or treat infection.

Non-biologic occlusive dressings vary widely in their uses. Foams are absorbent and easy to form to the wound, but they require a secondary covering dressing. Due to their absorbency, they should not be used on dry wounds. If they dry to the wound, saline should be used to dampen it prior to removal to prevent damage to the underlying epithelium. They are excellent for partial-thickness, moderately exudative wounds, especially when pressure relief is desired. Films create an excellent bacterial barrier and are adhesive without a secondary dressing, but can cause a collection of fluid and may adhere to the wound itself. They are excellent for donor sites, superficial burns, or partial-thickness wounds without significant exudates. They are not frequently used in the care of blasts due to the tendency for bacteria to become trapped under them if the wound is not sterile. Hydrocolloids give some autolytic debridement, enhance angiogenesis, and create a physical barrier for bacteria. They can be used on partial- or full-thickness wounds, especially those with a mild-moderate amount of exudate such as pressure ulcers, venous ulcers, or acute surgical wounds. However, in the contaminated wounds created by blasts, they have less of a place. They can make it harder to determine the presence of infection, as they cause the formation of a yellow gel with an unpleasant aroma, which can be confused with an infected wound. Hydrogels are soothing and hydrating and do not adhere to wounds. They require a secondary dressing and frequent dressing changes, but are useful in painful, partial-thickness wounds. In the arena of blast injuries, they would likely be used mostly for donor sites and other dry wounds [7]. They typically are not used for wounds undergoing primary closure [8]. Alginates are highly absorbent and hemostatic, do not adhere, and require comparatively few dressing changes. They should not be used in dry wounds, as they can overly dry the area. They do require a secondary dressing and also often come with an unpleasant aroma. They can be used in highly exudative wounds of partial or full thickness and after surgery.

Newer non-biologic occlusive dressings include hydrofibers, collagens, and hyaluronic acid dressings. Hydrofibers are useful for moderate-heavily exudative wounds and those prone to further bleeding. They can be used for packing cavities and are useful on a wide range of wounds. They require an overlying secondary dressing and, when being removed, often require saline to prevent stripping of granulation tissue. Collagens are useful in exudative wounds on slowly healing ulcers. They can cause some irritation and may initially increase the drainage from the wound. Hyaluronic acid dressings are absorbent and biodegradable. They accelerate granulation tissue and reepithelialization.

Grafts are frequently used in blast wounds. Autografts are taken from the patient; allografts come from a human donor, usually a cadaver; and xenografts come from another species, usually pigs. Xenografts are temporary dressings that will be rejected. Partial- or split-thickness grafts consist of epidermis and a portion of the dermis. Full-thickness skin grafts contain the entirety of the epidermis and dermis and often contain some subcutaneous tissue as well [7]. Grafts may be used extensively in blast injuries, as the surrounding tissue is often so macerated as to be difficult to close or cover an injury appropriately. However, this benefit must be balanced with the fact that autografts cause new injuries to the patient and they can often not be taken from the ideal areas to the diffuse injuries suffered by many blast patients.

Continuum of Care Considerations

Systemic changes to the physiology of the patient due to the severity of their wounds and the frequently associated multisystem trauma from blasts require changes in the methods of management [9]. The often unstable nature of these patients and the severity of their injuries commonly require patients to have multiple operations in the acute and subacute phases of their recovery, usually every 24–72 hours [10]. These may include fasciotomies due to the difficulty of the vascular exam and the dissection up fascial planes caused by blasts, which sends contamination deeper than the initial visible wound [9]. These associated injuries and surgical wounds from which a patient suffers will dictate the timing for serial visits to the operating room. The physiologic changes to the patient may also affect the immune system and wound healing, so nutrition and infection risk must be carefully monitored.

Restoration of the soft tissue overlying fractures has been shown to improve bone healing as well as decrease complications [11]. However, the timing and type of coverage remains controversial among surgeons [9, 12]. There is often marginally viable soft tissue, which requires staged operations and frequent examinations to determine overall viability [9, 13]. Clinicians managing wounds from blast injuries should also be cognizant of the irritation from the serial, thorough debridements that are frequently required to achieve a clean wound capable of healing. The need for serial debridements has led to controversy over optimal timing of coverage for blast wounds. While wounds would ideally be closed early, the need for multiple surgical procedures means that most of this tissue will require delayed reconstruction. Optimizing the exact timing of closure versus further debridements remains a topic for further study [9].

Broad-spectrum antibiotics are a mainstay in the treatment of blast injuries [10]. Studies have shown again and again that the earlier the administration of antibiotics, the lower the complication rate of the wound. Current recommendations suggest introduction of intravenous antibiotics within 1 hour, as studies have shown that those who received them under 66 minutes from the time of injury have improved wound healing and overall outcomes [14]. All patients with blast injuries should receive tetanus prophylaxis, as the impregnation of blast wounds with soil causes them to be high risk for this complication.

The damaged tissue from a blast has also been shown to have a higher than otherwise expected incidence of fungal infections. These invasive fungal infections are thought to be caused due to the aerosolized debris from the explosion, which impregnates in the devitalized tissue and causes fungal infections [15]. The clinician's index of suspicion for fungal infections must always be high in these cases, due to the high mortality associated with fungal infection of wounds. These infections are typically diagnosed late in the course of the patient's care. Patients are at higher risk for invasive fungal infection from a blast if they are not walking; if they have extensive injuries to the perineum, genitourinary system, or rectum; if they require >25 units of either whole blood or packed red blood cells; if they have an above-knee amputation in the field; or if they undergo progressive, more proximal amputations. One sign that clinicians should be sensitive to is any progressive tissue necrosis noted over consecutive debridements, as it can be a sign of fungal infection [16, 17]. Patients with suspected or confirmed fungal infections should be started immediately on broad-spectrum antifungal coverage, with liposomal amphotericin B and triazoles (e.g., Voriconazole) being commonly recommended. However, the mainstay of treatment in invasive fungal infection is thorough debridement and topical antifungal application of Dakin's solution. These should be supplemented with an infectious disease specialist consultation in any patient with suspected invasive fungal infection. Surgical debridement may also include the application of antibacterial and antifungal beads intraoperatively.

Clinical Treatment of Casualties

Surgical wounds and those from traumatic injuries can often benefit from being treated with negative pressure wound therapy. Early on, negative pressure gives temporary coverage over wounds that for any reason may not be appropriate for full closure. While applied, it has been shown to diminish edema as well as promote granulation and angiogenesis, and it decreases the wound surface area. This can improve the chances of having a delayed primary closure. It can also decrease the amount of tissue needed for flaps or other surgical closures [18].

Controversies remain within the realm of negative pressure wound therapy. Some studies have shown that use in blast injuries can cause sepsis if the granulation tissue overgrows an infected area and walls off dead space, causing an abscess. The use of deep drains under a negative pressure wound dressing has been advocated as a method for allowing closure of deep cavities without this causing abscess formation, but this still requires further study [19]. While silver-impregnated dressings are being used in many settings today, the use of silver impregnation in conjunction with negative pressure therapy remains a new field with significant controversy [20, 21].

While the literature on embedded foreign bodies is minimal, current recommendations from the CDC state that small foreign bodies embedded only in soft tissue and associated with small, uninfected wounds do not likely require surgical removal [10]. More proximal, large foreign bodies that can be removed without disturbing large underlying structures should be removed, especially in dirty wounds, where they can be a nidus for infection.

HEENT Injuries

Blast Injuries to the Head and Neck (HEENT) require special subacute management. Since such a small portion of these injuries that survive to hospital arrival are life-threatening, they can be easily overlooked and mismanaged by a clinician without experience. External ear or pinna injuries should have any exposed cartilage covered. This is most commonly done with primary closure, which prevents the exposed cartilage from becoming devitalized. Depending on the severity of the injury and the survival of vitalized tissue in the area, this may require a flap or other more advanced surgical procedure. If the pinna is devitalized from an avulsion injury, debridement and secondary reconstruction at a later date are likely necessary [13, 22].

Eye injuries are very common (28% of survivors) in blast injuries and typically will require ophthalmology evaluation of the globe. In the subacute setting, providers should remember that even if the eye is the only injury a patient suffers from a blast, the patient should still receive tetanus prophylaxis. Additionally, any injury to the eye requires broad-spectrum intravenous antibiotics in the acute phase; ceftazidime and vancomycin, with or without clindamycin, are recommended by the CDC [23].

Injuries to the face can also include the facial nerve, which is typically non-salvageable. Thus, facial nerve injuries are not repaired primarily. Vascular injuries to the face most commonly require no specific management, as the extensive collateralization of the facial vasculature means the majority of tissues are difficult to devitalize. However, any necrotic tissues require significant debridement. Areas of questionable viability are managed conservatively and given 24–72 hours to declare themselves as viable or in need of debridement, as salvaging even small parts of the face can make significant differences in long-term cosmetic outcomes. Like many blast injuries, facial injuries require early antibiotics to prevent significant facial infections [13].

Long-Term Rehabilitation

Over the past 20 years, due to US military involvement in Afghanistan and Iraq, significant information has come out of the US military medical establishment regarding the importance of long-term rehabilitation. Blast injuries to the lower extremities frequently cause alterations in movement and mechanical loading patterns. This has been associated with long-term issues with low back pain, osteoarthritis, and cardiovascular issues [24]. Management of these risks with prostheses and rehabilitation is critical to the long-term outcomes of blast patients.

Nutrition

Rapid and appropriate wound healing and the prevention of chronic wounds require appropriate patient nutrition. Wound healing requires a heavy energy burden, which can quickly exhaust the energy and protein stores of a severely wounded or undernourished patient. Malnutrition and other nutritional deficiencies are among the many factors that can negatively affect wound healing, raising the likelihood of a chronic (>6 weeks) wound [25].

In addition to total energy requirements, protein stores are of massive importance given the requirement to form and deposit large amounts of protein in rebuilding the extracellular matrix and cells of a wound. Severe trauma and sepsis have been found to lead to loss of body protein up to 150–250 g (which correlates to 0.6–1.0 kg of muscle tissue) daily. A deficit in either of these intake needs can lead to delayed vascularization, decreased collagen deposition, prolonged inflammatory phase, and decreased tensile strength of the newly created skin. Some amino acids such as arginine and methionine are thought to be especially important for wound healing due to their high presence in many proteins involved in the process [25, 26]. Additionally, protein malnutrition can decrease the levels of complement and antibodies, leading to increased rates of wound infection. Some studies have shown up to 42% of patients being malnourished, even in high-resource regions, suggesting that patients may require nutritional supplementation despite lacking an appearance of malnutrition clinically [26].

In addition to energy and protein, wound healing requires a steady supply of fatty acids, used to create cell membranes and for eicosanoid synthesis. Vitamin C (ascorbic acid) is used by the body to hydroxylate proline and lysine during collagen production and cross-linking, making it vital to patients undergoing wound healing [25, 26]. Vitamin A is also vital to wound healing, as it stimulates epithelialization and collagen deposition. It is especially important in those with decreased wound healing due to long-term steroid use [26]. Zinc is a cofactor for a number of biosynthetic enzymatic reactions and thus is necessary for proliferating cells. Lack of iron, which is a cofactor for proline and lysine hydroxylation enzymes in collagen synthesis, as well as it's roll in oxygen transport, can also decrease the quality of wound healing [25, 26].

Scar Management

Scarring outcomes are vital to patient evaluations of their wound care and can be determinants of functional outcomes as well. Hypertrophic scarring is a common finding in large wounds, especially in burn injuries, where rates can reach 80% [27]. Common interventions to improve scarring outcomes include topical antibiotic ointments such as bacitracin, which provides moisture as well as antimicrobial effects. Petroleum jelly also provides moisture to decrease scarring. Scar massage can be initiated after 2–3 weeks of healing, once the wound has developed enough tensile strength. This degrades excess, nonpliable collagen, leading to softer, more supple scars. Pressure dressings use compressive forces to disrupt collagen bundles, which can flatten the scar and decrease hypertrophy in select patients. Dermabrasion has also been used to resurface and decrease the size of scars, though careful selection is required, as it can cause prolonged bleeding if used in some patients [28].

Topical scar management creams using silicone gel have been shown to decrease pathologic scarring, as well as paresthesias, erythema, and keloids, when compared to controls. High-tension wounds can benefit from mechanomodulatory therapy using the Embrace device on trunk and extremity incisions. Despite short-term side effects, there is some preliminary data to suggest that nonablative fractional laser therapy improves texture, pigmentation, and pliability of incisions and grafts in some selected patients. Sunscreen and sun avoidance also has shown improvement in scarring outcomes [29]. However, there are some data that burns do not respond as well to many of these therapies as non-burn wounds [27].

Newer therapies are currently being studied that show promise in the healing of burns. One such intervention is the injection of localized interferon (IFN), which has been shown to decrease the T_{H2} immune response, increasing the T_{H1} response and thus decreasing the likelihood of creating hypertrophic scars [27].

Conclusion

Blast events can cause significant, multisystem injury. Failure to consider the physiologic changes to a patient due to these injuries can negatively affect their ability to recover. Once the acute phase of care has occurred, many of these patients will require multiple returns to the operating room and will have multiple wounds of a surgical nature as well as from the initial blast injury. Understanding the potential for infection of these wounds, as well as how to prevent complications and to manage their dressings and debridement, is critical to the long-term outcomes of every patient involved in a blast injury.

Pitfalls

- Failure to return to basic wound care principles for all contaminated wounds
- Failure to initiate antibiotics and debride appropriately in frequently infected wounds
- Failure to continuously repeat evaluations for complications of wounds

References

1. Shah JB. The history of wound care. J Am Col Certif Wound Spec. 2011;3:65–6. Available from: https://www.ncbi.nlm.nih.gov/pmc/articles/PMC3601883/pdf/main.pdf.
2. Forrest RD. Early history of wound treatment. Vol. 75, J Royal Soc Med. 1982. Available from: https://www.ncbi.nlm.nih.gov/pmc/articles/PMC1437561/pdf/jrsocmed00251-0064.pdf.
3. Reilly RF. Medical and surgical care during the American Civil War, 1861–1865. Proc (Bayl Univ Med Cent). 2016;29(2):138. Available from: https://www.ncbi.nlm.nih.gov/pmc/articles/PMC4790547/.
4. Manring MM, Hawk A, Calhoun JH, Andersen RC. Treatment of war wounds: a historical review. Clin Orthop Relat Res. 2009;467(8):2168. Available from: https://www.ncbi.nlm.nih.gov/pmc/articles/PMC2706344/.
5. Gantwerker EA, Hom DB. Skin: histology and physiology of wound healing. Scarring Scars Facial Wounds Heal Ski Histol Clin Plast Surg. 2012;39:85–97.
6. Ganapathy N, Venkataraman SS, Daniel R, Aravind RJ, Kumarakrishnan VB. Molecular biology of wound healing. J Pharm Bioallied Sci. 2012;4(Suppl 2):S334. Available from: https://www.ncbi.nlm.nih.gov/pmc/articles/PMC3467878/.
7. Siegel DM, Robinson JK, Hanke CW, Fratila A. Surgery of the skin: procedural dermatology. 856 p.
8. Davies P. Wound care. Oxford Handbook of Surgical Nursing Vol. 1. Oxford University Press; 2016. https://doi.org/10.1093/med/9780199642663.001.0001.
9. Sheean AJ, Tintle SM, Rhee PC. Soft tissue and wound management of blast injuries. Curr Rev Musculoskelet Med. 2015;8(3):265–271. https://doi.org/10.1007/s12178-015-9275-x.
10. Blast Extremity Injuries. Available from: https://www.emergency.cdc.gov/BlastInjuries.
11. Byrd HS, Cierny G, Tebbetts JB. The management of open tibial fractures with associated soft-tissue loss: external pin fixation with early flap coverage. Plast Reconstr Surg [Internet]. 1981 [cited 2018 Oct 3];68(1):73–82. Available from: https://journals.lww.com/plasreconsurg/Citation/1981/07000/The_Management_of_Open_Tibial_Fractures_with.15.aspx.
12. Tintle SM, Gwinn DE, Andersen RC, Kumar AR. Soft tissue coverage of combat wounds. J Surg Orthop Adv. 2010;19(1):29–34. Available from: http://www.ncbi.nlm.nih.gov/pubmed/20371004.
13. Kumar V, Singh AK, Kumar P, Shenoy YR, Verma AK, Borole AJ, et al. Blast injury face: an exemplified review of management. Natl J Maxillofac Surg [Internet]. 2013. [cited 2018 Sep 30];4(1):33–39. Available from: https://www.ncbi.nlm.nih.gov/pmc/articles/PMC3800382/.
14. Lack WD, Karunakar MA, Angerame MR, Seymour RB, Sims S, Kellam JF, et al. Type III open tibia fractures: Immediate Antibiotic Prophylaxis Minimizes Infection. J Orthop Trauma

[Internet]. 2015 Jan [cited 2018 Oct 3];29(1): p 1-6. Available from: https://journals.lww.com/jorthotrauma/Abstract/2015/01000/Type_III_Open_Tibia_Fractures__Immediate.1.aspx.
15. Fanfair RN, Benedict K, Bos J, Bennett SD, Lo Y-C, Adebanjo T, et al. Necrotizing cutaneous mucormycosis after a Tornado in Joplin, Missouri, in 2011. N Engl J Med. 2012;367(23):2214–2239. Available from: https://www-nejm-org.ezp-prod1.hul.harvard.edu/doi/pdf/10.1056/NEJMoa1204781.
16. Warkentien T, Rodriguez C, Lloyd B, et al. Invasive mold infections following combat-related injuries. Clin Infect Dis. 2012;55(11):1441–1449. https://doi.org/10.1093/cid/cis749.
17. Rodriguez CJ, Tribble DR, Malone DL, Murray CK, Jessie EM, Khan M, et al. Treatment of suspected invasive fungal infection in war wounds. Mil Med. 2018 Sep 1;183(suppl_2):142–6. Available from: https://academic.oup.com/milmed/article/183/suppl_2/142/5091143.
18. Streubel PN, Stinner DJ, Obremskey WT. Use of negative-pressure wound therapy in orthopaedic trauma. J Am Acad Orthop Surg [Internet]. 2012 [cited 2018 Oct 3];20(9):564–74. Available from: https://journals.lww.com/jaaos/Abstract/2012/09000/Use_of_Negative_pressure_Wound_Therapy_in.3.aspx.
19. Rispoli DM, Horne BR, Kryzak TJ, Richardson MW. Description of a technique for vacuum-assisted deep drains in the management of cavitary defects and deep infections in devastating military and civilian trauma. J Trauma [Internet]. 2010 [cited 2018 Oct 3];68:1247–52. Available from: https://journals.lww.com/jtrauma/Abstract/2010/05000/Description_of_a_Technique_for_Vacuum_Assisted.33.aspx.
20. Elliott C. The use of silver-impregnated dressings in blast injuries. Br J Nurs [Internet]. [cited 2018 Sep 30];19(13):835–9. Available from: http://www.ncbi.nlm.nih.gov/pubmed/20606613.
21. Stinner DJ, Waterman SM, Masini BD, Wenke JC. Silver dressings augment the ability of negative pressure wound therapy to reduce bacteria in a contaminated open fracture model. J Trauma [Internet]. 2011 [cited 2018 Oct 3];71:S147–50. Available from: https://journals.lww.com/jtrauma/Abstract/2011/07001/Silver_Dressings_Augment_the_Ability_of_Negative.25.aspx.
22. Ear Blast Injuries [Internet]. [cited 2018 Sep 30]. Available from: http://www.emergency.cdc.gov/BlastInjuries.
23. Blast injuries: fact sheets for professionals [Internet]. [cited 2018 Oct 3]. Available from: http://emergency.cdc.gov/BlastInjuries.
24. Butowicz CM, Dearth CL, Hendershot BD. Impact of Traumatic Lower Extremity Injuries Beyond Acute Care: Movement-Based Considerations for Resultant Longer Term Secondary Health Conditions. Adv Wound Care (New Rochelle). 2017;6(8):269–278. https://doi.org/10.1089/wound.2016.0714.
25. Wild T, Rahbarnia A, Kellner M, Sobotka L, Eberlein T. Basics in nutrition and wound healing. Nutrition [Internet]. 2010; 26(9):862-866. [cited 2019 May 9]. Available from: https://www.sciencedirect.com/science/article/abs/pii/S0899900710001668?via%3Dihub.
26. Arnold M, Barbul A. Nutrition and wound healing. Plast Reconstr Surg [Internet]. 2006 [cited 2019 May 9];117(7S Supplement):42S–58S. Available from: https://insights.ovid.com/pubmed?pmid=16799374.
27. Tredget EE, Levi B, Donelan MB. Biology and principles of scar management and burn reconstruction. Surg Clin North Am. 2014;94(4):793–815. https://doi.org/10.1016/j.suc.2014.05.005.
28. Commander SJ, Chamata E, Cox J, Dickey RM, Lee EI. Update on Postsurgical Scar Management. Semin Plast Surg. 2016;30(3):122–128. https://doi.org/10.1055/s-0036-1584824.
29. Perez JL, Rohrich RJ. Optimizing postsurgical scars: a systematic review on best practices in preventative scar management. Plast Reconstr Surg. 2017;140(782e):1017–25. Available from: https://insights.ovid.com/pubmed?pmid=28806293.

Psychological Consequences: Responders and Community

45

Ann Payne and John G. McManus

Introduction

Mental health disorders exist prior to disasters and are a major public health issue. Broadly speaking the adult population has a prevalence of 10–15% of depression and anxiety, 1% psychosis, and a variable prevalence of alcohol and drug misuse, while up to 10% of children experience mental health disorders at any one time [1]. Shortages of personnel in psychiatry in an area prior to a disaster can place an exceptional burden in the aftermath, especially in developing countries [1].

Explosions or blasts may precipitate disasters and usually arise from either industrial accidents or terrorist origins. There is evidence to suggest that explosive events, whether it is intentional violence or non-intentional and accidental, can influence the burden of adverse mental health outcomes in the community [2, 3]. Explosive incidents are violent encounters, which threaten harm or death to individuals, families, and communities with additional disruption to invaluable resources, services, and social networks [3–5]. Research in mental health incidence, recognition, mitigation, and treatment from explosive events has been evolving with much of the current science having military origin [6]. For an individual, the risk of posttraumatic psychopathology is elevated depending on the duration and degree of exposure to the trauma scene (i.e., dose-related). The response to any disaster must include not only the initial assessment of individual needs but also the psychological, social, cultural, economic, and structural needs of the affected communities as a whole [3, 7].

A. Payne (✉)
Department of Psychiatry/University College Cork (UCC), St. Stephen's Hospital, Glanmire, Cork, Ireland

J. G. McManus
Augusta University, Evans, GA, USA

D. W. Callaway, J. L. Burstein (eds.), *Operational and Medical Management of Explosive and Blast Incidents*, https://doi.org/10.1007/978-3-030-40655-4_45

Mental Health in Disaster Planning

It is essential that disaster planners are aware of the possible psychological impact on responders, citizens, and the community from explosive events. Responders of all types and members of the community require psychological support across a broad range of areas in the aftermath. The scale of an event such as a large explosion can have an immediate psychological impact and erode procedures and common protocols. This usually results in the review of actions and consequences such as the very obvious adequacy of personal protective equipment (PPE) and practice protocols and how best they can be improved [7]. However, mental health needs may be somewhat ignored or neglected. While not all individuals are adversely affected by a particular disaster, the evidence shows we can expect a range of mental and physical health consequences both in the acute and longer-term aftermath. The World Health Organization (WHO) states clearly that "there is no health without mental health" and mental health is determined by a range of socioeconomic, biological, and environmental factors [8]. One can see from this premise that in order to manage individuals and communities experiencing a disaster, it is necessary to address not only the more obvious physical aspects but also the mental health needs. Psychiatrists should now take a leadership role in preplanning and coordination of a multidisciplinary response to the crisis, to anticipate the immediate-, medium-, and long-term psychological needs [3].

Disasters due to terrorist events, impact directly on the individual responders, indirectly on their families and their community as a result of the loss of loved ones. The risk of the loss of responder colleagues is very real. Both the individual grief and the grief experienced by the community may be quite complicated; as a result the recovery period is somewhat less predictable as people need to process complex perceptions regarding the attackers, such as politics, culture, and religion. Lemieux et al. report that disaster responders report satisfaction in being able to do something to help [9]. It is felt that responders tend to follow the emotional states and pathways that the victims and survivors experience close to the event. Individuals in the affected community tend to be more vulnerable to mental health disorders if they have prior mental health issues, chronic medical illness substance abuse or poor coping mechanisms. Responders equally may be overwhelmed with compassion fatigue and vicarious trauma [10].

Table 45.1 displays the practical timeline for potential psychological intervention during specific phases. These phases of the event and recovery are variable especially with regard to their duration. Within each phase, there is significant individual variation in the reactions of workers and survivors. Math et al. have described the phases as the heroic, honeymoon, disillusionment, and restabilization phases [10]. Most of the acute and intermediate phase (heroic and honeymoon) reactions and disorders are usually self-limiting. The long-term phase (disillusionment and restabilzation) disorders may benefit the most from mental health professional intervention. Although prophylactic use of psychotropic medication is very limited in actually preventing mental health morbidity, in established injury or illness medication most certainly plays an important role in recovery. The use of cognitive behavior therapy (CBT) in mitigating mental health morbidity appears to be promising.

As the phases progress, posttraumatic stress disorder (PTSD) and compassion fatigue can develop when the so-called honeymoon period ends. Facing the reality

Table 45.1 Practical timeline for disaster phases

Heroic phase	0–1 weeks	*Acute and immediate response work:* characterized by individuals and the community directing inordinate levels of energy into the activities of rescuing, helping, sheltering, emergency repair, and cleaning up
Honeymoon phase	2–8 weeks	*Intermediate response work:* characterized generally by community and survivor optimism because of the massive influx of help
Disillusionment phase	2–36 months	*Long-term response work:* characterized by fatigue, irritating experiences, and the knowledge of diminishing resources
Restabilization phase	Variable > 6–36 months	*Continued recovery work:* characterized by individual variance that occurs within this phase. Some individuals are able to regain equilibrium within 6 months. For some individuals, the first-year anniversary of the disaster precipitates or exacerbates posttraumatic stress symptoms

of rebuilding and recovery in the community requires endurance and an ability to deal with disparities with the lack of available appropriate resources in the disillusionment period. Secondary traumatic stress can develop at any time for a responder if they are vulnerable to the graphic material they are exposed to by victims and survivors. Alternatively, responders may experience compassion satisfaction as they effect change and produce positive outcomes in the face of adversity alongside the community [11].

Disaster planning is the blueprint for a multiagency response, and mental health needs may be addressed by a psychiatrist's participation in the overall framework for the emergency response, as stated by Ng [12]. Risk reduction and timely supportive measures in the context of mental health of both the affected community and emergency responders may be considered as part of the overall preparedness by planning a logistical approach in the above phases: pre-event, acute response, and post-event.

Pre- event During this phase preparation includes education around structures, agencies, and hierarchies in the community that may be anticipated to be required for emergency interventions. From a mental health point of view, first responders, fire department, emergency medical services (EMS), and police need coordinated information to link appropriately with the key hospitals in the area. Psychiatrists and allied professionals can tap into a network of agencies in the community to volunteer in times of a disaster. Along with doctors, this would also include nursing staff and allied professionals, e.g., social workers occupational therapists, pharmacists, and psychologists, in order to respond to the immediate needs following the event.

Acute phase It is important to recognize that there may be a range of emotional, cognitive, behavioral, and spiritual reactions in response to a blast or disaster. Individuals and even first responders may experience physical trauma personally and losses of significant family members, friends, and colleagues. People are usually displaced and may need evacuation. The vulnerable, like the elderly, children, or those with enduring mental health disorders in the area may be separated from their supports. Mental health triage is important in the post-disaster setting and can be led and provided by psychiatrists [12].

Interestingly, in the analysis of crowd behavior at the time of an incident or disaster, the common assumption was that "panic" would ensue. However, evidence lately has shown that rather than mass panic, there can be a sense of cohesion and often altruistic behavior as a result of the shared experience. In the face of a common threat there may be unity among survivors. This is an important reference point for rescue services [11]. More recently, crowd behavior analysis technology has been developed, and many countries use computational methodologies which may prove useful in both disaster planning and assisting in the immediate aftermath in crowd management and facilitate flow of people and resources [13, 14].

Post-event Here the challenge is to meet the needs of those affected individuals in the disaster zone for their assessment, diagnosis, treatment, and their appropriate multidisciplinary management, using the bio-psycho-social approach, while ensuring confidentiality and removing barriers to care.

Psychological First Aid

Survivors of disasters face barriers to care. Most do not appear to access the services available, and those who do, 50% will default and drop out of the service [15]. The need to respond to distressed survivors and first responders following a critical incident is quite powerful. The aim is not to re-traumatize the affected individual, family members, or first responder by requesting that they debrief and ventilate cathartic emotions, as contrary to initial reports, research has shown that in a small number of individuals this is potentially harmful [16–19].

Psychological first aid (PFA) has become a blueprint for the delivery of psychosocial interventions in the aftermath of a critical event. PFA tools aim to be practical, empathic, and respectful of various cultures, settings, and needs [20]. PFA was first described over 60 years ago [21], and the principles have recently been updated by Young et al. [22]. In early intervention screen and treat programs, the aim is primarily to screen and identify all trauma-exposed individuals with properly validated measures to determine who develops persistent symptoms of psychopathology and then provide evidence-based treatment.

There are a number of PFA tools available, and despite widespread acceptance of their effectiveness, research in this area has proven difficult for obvious strategic and ethical reasons. Over the years, since the middle of the last century, there have been attempts to delineate the best response in major incidents [23]. However, it is fair to say that literature review processes have led to a peer consensus of "evidence informed but without proof of effectiveness" for the use of PFA [24]. It is clear that there is enough to suggest PFA's overall usefulness in times of crisis, but the PFA is not a "one size fits all" and as such must be backed up with substantial mental health expertise close to the field [24]. The components of the available PFA packages

Table 45.2 Components of PFA

A sense of safety
Calm
A sense of self-efficacy and collective efficacy
Connectedness
Hope

Table 45.3 PFA plan to address needs

Providing practical care (which does not intrude) including basic needs like food, shelter, and information
Assess any other needs and concerns
Listen to people, provide comfort and calm
Protect from further harm
And help people to connect with the appropriate services, social and health supports

were reviewed by Hobfoll et al. and are described to have five essential elements, or core components, seen in Table 45.2 [25].

According to Sphere and IASC, the PFA is a human support for those suffering and includes needs described in Table 45.3 [26].

Additionally, PFA plans must be accessible and allow for swift training of humanitarian volunteers prior to their deployment to the explosive incident. The PFA is not only for trained professionals and is not a "psychological debriefing" to put time and events in chronological order. For example, the WHO publication, War Trauma Foundation and World Vision International Psychological First Aid (2011), uses the above principles in a very simple and easy-to-read format. This publication describes the when, where, and how to deliver psychological support even by providers with limited training [27].

In this, it is explicit that one should "help responsibly" involving four main principals:

- Respect safety, dignity, and rights
- Adapt to take account of people's culture
- Be aware of other emergency response measures
- Look after oneself

Preparing in advance of deployment and using these principles can help triage and decrease chaotic situations due to explosive and disaster events.

Evidence Supporting PFA

In London, July 2005, four bombers attacked the London transport system, resulting in 56 deaths and 775 casualties out of 4000 passengers [28]. Experience had shown the need to provide immediate support and counseling, which would then be followed by a formal outreach program to identify trauma-exposed individuals believed to be at high risk for mental health disorders like PTSD and major depression. However, many individuals at risk may be unlikely to self-refer [29].

A screen-and-treat approach after the London bombings was also endorsed and reported by Brewin et al. [28]. After PFA was initiated, screening or intervention teams targeted all trauma-exposed individuals to identify psychopathologies and then offer appropriate evidence-based treatment. The Trauma Screening Questionnaire (TSQ) was utilized and is an excellent 10-item, yes-or-no screening tool. Those individuals found to be positive with the TSQ tool went on for a more detailed assessment that included a structured clinical interview, the CAGE alcohol abuse screening instrument, the SF-12 Health Survey, and, where appropriate, the Short McGill Pain Questionnaire and the Inventory of Complicated Grief-Revised. Use of advanced screening and intervention resulted in significant reduction in long-term PTSD symptoms [30–33].

After the World Trade Center (WTC) attack, the general population around lower Manhattan had a 12% prevalence of PTSD up to 3 years following the event [34]. Project Liberty provided crisis counseling to almost 690,000 individuals. Stuber et al. found after 6 months that in relation to PTSD and depression, there was a surprisingly significant unmet need for individuals with no past history of mental health issues prior to the WTC event [35]. Donahue et al. also reported that the use of screening instruments and cognitive behavioral interventions resulted in reduction of grief and depression overall, but not PTSD [36].

Emergency Responders and Mental Health

The definition of an emergency responder in any disaster but also after a blast or explosion can be considered to be part of an expanded response team. A large-scale man-made or industrial blast incident can precipitate the influx of personnel from firefighters, emergency medical services (EMS), police, construction and utility workers, and even local volunteers along with individuals from government agencies. The process of putting one's own life at risk for the sake of others is at the very heart of first-responder actions.

First responders do not appear to have a higher prevalence of mental health disorder compared to other occupations, but they are more often exposed to multiple traumatic events. Exposure to trauma increases the risk of experiencing a new-onset mental health disorder, particularly in the early stages of their careers. Teaching curricula which include targeted coping skills could potentially assist in timely interventions in early career first responders and may help reduce future psychiatric morbidity [37].

In 2001, at the World Trade Center terrorist attacks, 450 emergency responders died, which was one-sixth of the total number of victims at the scene [38]. Hundreds more suffered serious physical injuries. However, even more suffered longitudinal mental health difficulties.

Wild et al. found in fact that early screening during training of EMS personnel can help identify those individuals at high risk for mental health disorders like

PTSD or depression and allow for targeted interventions and strategies around these risk factors to improve resilience to traumatic experiences [39].

To examine the consequences of trauma-like explosions, we can use the *Diagnostic and Statistical Manual of Mental Disorders*, 5th ed. or DSM-5 [40]. The range of criteria specialists use to formalize a diagnosis is quite intricate, but if we take the criteria for PTSD as a reference point, we can perhaps consider the other presentations as part of a spectrum of injury and illness. Put simply, acute stress disorder (ASD) is an earlier version of the PTSD, occurring shortly after the trauma and lasting at least 3 days to 1 month. Individuals with ASD present with intrusive symptoms, such as memories, nightmares, and flashbacks, and experience physiological or psychological responses to certain triggers. They also may use avoidance techniques to block thoughts and emotions and/or people. Arousal issues are common, like irritability and aggression, difficulties concentrating and sleeping, and also hypervigilance with increased startle response. Along with this, the person may report very negative cognitions and mood manifesting as guilt, blame (self or others), anger, loss of interests and connection with people, and overall an inability to experience positive emotions. Dissociative symptoms such as amnesia or altered sense of reality of self or surroundings can also occur.

The above criteria assume that there are no other confounding causes for the previously described behavior like traumatic brain injury (TBI), substance misuse, or other organic illness.

Although quite complex, these DSM-5 criteria for ASD may assist in prediction of individuals who will subsequently develop PTSD. It follows then that in acute trauma settings, triage and identifying at-risk individuals could promote early intervention or allow for suitable subsequent monitoring [41]. ASD may progress to PTSD after 1 month, but it may also be a transient condition that resolves within 1 month of exposure to traumatic event(s) and does not lead to PTSD. In about 50% of people who eventually develop PTSD, the initial presenting condition was ASD [40]. Symptoms of ASD may worsen over the initial month, often as a consequence of ongoing stressors or additional traumatic events. The PTSD criteria are described in Table 45.4.

In the responder community of 9/11, firefighters experienced an elevated risk of PTSD over the general public up to 11% in one study by Berninger et al. [38]. Nearly 12.9% of police responders to 9/11 also were shown to have PTSD, with up to 50% of these individuals experiencing comorbid depression and anxiety [42]. Furthermore, Stellman et al., in a 5-year follow-up study using self-screening questionnaire of over 10,000 WTC workers, found the prevalence of probable PTSD to be 11.1% (which is similar to the prevalence in soldiers returning from Afghanistan) [43]. Overall, 8.8% had depression, 5% panic disorder, while 45% fulfilled criteria for prolonged stress reaction [43]. Most of these workers reported psychological/behavioral changes in their children at the time of working at the disaster site as well. This risk of mental health difficulties can be found to be associated with an exposure-response gradient, i.e., those who arrived earlier and were at the scene

Table 45.4 PTSD criteria

PTSD	Description	Specific examples
Criterion A	Exposure to trauma	Direct exposure Repeated exposure, e.g., *responders retrieving dead bodies*
Criterion B	Intrusion symptoms	Recurrent memories Nightmares Flashbacks Distress response to cues
Criterion C	Avoidance of	Trauma-related *(internal)* thoughts or feelings Trauma-related reminders *(external) – people, places, or activities*
Criterion D	Negative cognition and mood	Dissociative amnesia Negative beliefs ∗Negative emotions: *fear, horror, guilt, shame, and anger* Inability to experience joy ∗Loss of interest Blame of self or others for cause of trauma Detachment or withdrawal from others
Criterion E	Arousal	Irritability or aggression Reckless/self-destructive behavior Hypervigilance Increased startle Concentration and Sleep disturbance
Criterion F	Duration	Must experience criteria B, C, D, and E for >1 month
Criterion G	Impaired function	Social, occupational, or other
Criterion H	Exclusion	Not due to medication, substance use, or other illness
Dissociative subtype: used when depersonalization and derealization occur in tandem with other symptoms described above. *Delayed subtype:* occur post trauma after a period in which symptoms were not present or were present at a subthreshold level		

Adapted from American Psychiatric Association [40]

longer experienced more difficulties, which suggests that screening may assist appropriate targeted responses in at-risk populations [37–43].

Special Populations

Previous studies have shown that the psychological reactions of many women and children in disasters zones highlight certain gaps in awareness and preparedness. The most significant finding in studies from Bangladesh shows that children and women were more distressed psychologically than adult men either due to the practical limitations of their situation or due to a lack of awareness of disaster mental health [44]. Efforts to recognize particular mental health needs of women and children should be considered during all phases of disasters: mitigation, preparedness planning, response, and recovery.

Military Responders

Active Duty Service Members (ADSM) in the military are exposed to traumatic events in the course of deployments or combat. There are a number of programs within the armed forces that aim to prepare the individual for mental health consequences secondary to trauma [45]. Combat and Operational Stress First Aid (COSFA) was adapted from PFA principals for use in theaters of operation, but with some significant differences. There is a different mind-set, though, compared to civilian PFA in a number of ways. Combat exposure contributes to ongoing predictable and cumulative stressors. Unlike civilians, the military prepare in advance and train for potentially overwhelming stressors. Combatants seldom experience the stress of combat and other operations passively; combatants are usually not considered victims. Dealing with psychological consequences due to trauma must be an inherent part of the leadership and military structures. Leaders at all levels must be engaged in COSFA at every level in an operation. Often military leadership and unit cohesion potentially provide more powerful healing and recovery resources than the clinical skills of counselors or therapists.

The stress continuum model (Fig. 45.1) is a very useful visual guide for individuals and leaders to help identify mental health issues and perhaps signpost appropriate interventions. This has also been adapted for use in civilian organizations such as firefighters, paramedics, and other first-responder units [46, 47].

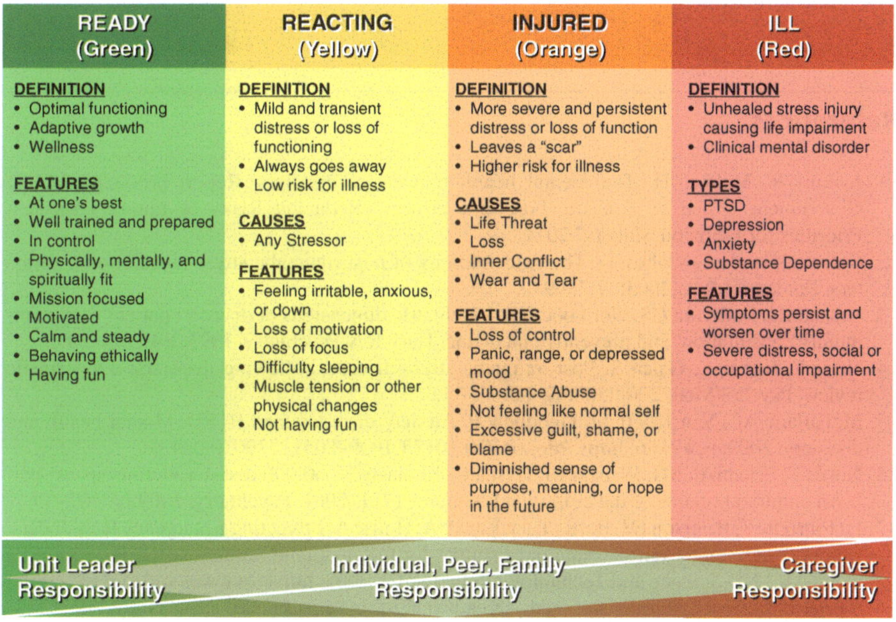

Fig. 45.1 Stress continuum model (COSFA)

Conclusion

Disasters cannot be avoided completely, but we need to learn how to prepare, respond, recover, rehabilitate, and reintegrate. There is a need to understand the effects of disaster on health so that precautionary measures can be adopted to mitigate the suffering. Research in mental health incidence, recognition, mitigation, and treatment from explosive events has been evolving, with much of the current science having military origin. Further investigations are required to document the effectiveness of the most common methods and to develop mental health as well as household disaster preparedness. Community mental health disaster preparedness may play a vital and supportive role and enable a suitable response when facing disasters. Disaster management is a continuous and integrated cyclical process of planning, organizing, coordinating, and implementing measures to prevent and to manage disaster effectively. Thus, now it is time to integrate disaster mental health into public health principles.

Pitfalls

- Lack of mental health specialists involvement in preparedness in the pre-event systems and teams, in preventive medicine and disaster planning
- Barriers to appropriate, timely mental health care- difficulties with self recognition, screening, referral to specialist services and identification of those at risk for long term disorders.
- Lack of preparation for special at risk populations such as elderly, women, and children

References

1. Jenkins R, Meltzer H. The mental health impacts of disasters. Report produced for the Government Office of Science, Foresight Project "Reducing Risks of Future Disasters: Priorities for Decision Makers" 2012.
2. Galea S, Nandi A, Vlahov D. The epidemiology of post-traumatic stress disorder after disasters. Epidemiol Rev. 2005;27:78–91.
3. Ursano RJ, Fullerton CS, Norwood AE. Psychiatric dimensions of disaster: patient care, community consultation, and preventive medicine. Harv Rev Psychiatry. 1995;3(4):196–209.
4. Neria Y, Nandi A, Galea S. Post-traumatic stress disorder following disasters: a systematic review. Psychol Med. 2008;38:467–80.
5. McFarlane AC, Van Hooff M, Goodhew F. Anxiety disorders and PTSD. Mental health and disasters; 2009. p. 47–66. https://doi.org/10.1017/CBO9780511730030.004.
6. Norris F, Friedman MJ, Watson PJ, Byrne C, Kaniasty K. 60,000 disaster victims speak: part I. An empirical review of the empirical literature: 1981–2001. Psychiatry. 2002;65:207–39.
7. LaTourrette T, Peterson DJ, Bartis T, Jackson BA, House A. Protecting Emergency Responders. Centre for Disease Control. National Institute for Occupational Safety and Health (NIOSH) and the RAND Science and Technology Policy Vol 2, 2003. https://www.google.ie/url?sa=t&rct=j&q=&esrc=s&source=web&cd=4&cad=rja&uact=8&ved=2ahUKEwiTmpjM7Z_eAhUKVsAKHQVpB8sQFjADegQIBhAC&url=https%3A%2F%2Fwww.cdc.gov%2Fniosh%2Fdocket%2Farchive%2Fpdfs%2FNIOSH-010%2F0010-010103-Book.pdf&usg=AOvVaw3d0PeEK9qvnyovhDj4KPMg. Accessed November 2018.

8. Saxena S, Funk M, Chisholm D. World health assembly adopts comprehensive mental health action plan 2013-2020. Lancet. 2013;381(9882):1970–1.
9. Lemieux CM, Plummer CA, Richardson R, Simon CE, Ai AL. Mental health, substance use, and adaptive coping among social work students in the aftermath of Hurricanes Katrina and Rita. J Social Work Educ. 2010;46(3):391–410.
10. Math SB, Nirmala MC, Moirangthem S, Kumar NC. Disaster management: mental health perspective. Indian J Psychol Med. 2015;37(3):261–71.
11. Naturale A. Chapter 6. In: Quitangon G, Evces MR, editors. Vicarious trauma and disaster mental health: understanding the risk and promoting resilience. New York: Rutledge; 2015. p. 73–9.
12. Ng AT. Disaster psychiatry: what psychiatrists need to know. Psychiatr Times. 2010; 27(11).
13. Cocking C, Drury J, Reicher S. The psychology of crowd behaviour in emergency evacuations: results from two interview studies and implications for the Fire and Rescue Services. Irish J Psychol. 2012;30(1–2):59–73.
14. Joshi KY, Vohra SA. Crowd behavior analysis. Intl J Sci Res. 2014;3(12):835–7.
15. Rodriguez JJ, Kohn R. Use of mental health services among disaster survivors. Curr Opin Psychiatry. 2008;21(4):370–8.
16. Schultz JM, Forbes D. Psychological first aid. Rapid proliferation and the search for evidence. Disaster Health. 2014;2(1):3–12. https://doi.org/10.4161/dish.26006.
17. Raphael B, Meldrum L, McFarlane AC. Does debriefing after psychological trauma work? BMJ. 1995;310(6993):1479–80.
18. Rose S, Bisson J, Churchill R, Wessely S. Psychological debriefing for preventing post traumatic stress disorder (PTSD). Cochrane Database Syst Rev. 2002;2:CD000560.
19. Van Emmerik AAP, Kamphuis JH, Hulsbosch AM, Emmelkamp P. Single session debriefing after psychological trauma: a meta-analysis. Lancet. 2002;360:766–71.
20. Uhernik JA, Husson MA. Psychological first aid: an evidence informed approach for acute disaster behavioral health response. In: Walz GR, Bleuer JC, Yep RK, editors. Compelling counselling interventions. Alexandria: American Counselling Association; 2009. p. 271–80.
21. Drayer CS, Cameron DC, Woodward WD, Glass AJ. Psychological first aid in community disasters—prepared by the American Psychiatric Association Committee on Civil Defense. JAMA. 1954;156:36–41.
22. Young BH. The immediate response to disaster: guidelines to adult psychological first aid. In: Ritchie EC, Friedman MJ, Watson PJ, editors. Mass violence and early intervention. New York: Guilford Press; 2006. p. 134–54.
23. Lindemann E. Symptomatology and management of acute grief. Am J Psychiatry. 1994;151(6 Suppl):155–60.
24. Fox JH, Burkle FM Jr, Bass J, Pia FA, Epstein JL, Markenson D. The effectiveness of psychological first aid as a disaster intervention tool: research analysis of peer-reviewed literature from 1990-2010. Disaster Med Public Health Prep. 2012;6(3):247–52.
25. Hobfoll SE, Watson PJ, Bell CC, Bryant RA, Brymer MJ, Friedman MJ, et al. Five essential elements of immediate and mid-term mass trauma intervention: empirical evidence. Psychiatry. 2007;70(4):283–315; discussion.
26. The Sphere Project. Humanitarian Charter and Minimum Standards in Disaster Response. Geneva: The Sphere Project; 2011. Found at: http://www.sphereproject.org. Accessed Nov 2018.
27. Van Ommeren M, Snider L, Schafer A. (World Health Organization, War Trauma Foundation and World Vision International). Psychological First Aid: Guide for Field Workers. World Health Organization. Geneva. 2011. Available at: http://whqlibdoc.who.int/publications/2011/9789241548205_eng.pdf. Accessed Nov 2018.
28. Brewin CR, Scragg P, Robertson M, Thompson M, d'Ardenne P, Ehlers A. Psychosocial Steering Group, London Bombings Trauma Response Programme. Promoting Mental Health following the London bombings: a screen and treat approach. J Traum Stress. 2008;21(1):3–8.
29. Turner SW, Thompson JA, Rosser RM. The King's cross fire: planning a "phase two" psychosocial response. Disaster Manag. 1989;2:31–7.

30. Mayfield D, McLeod G, Hall P. The CAGE questionnaire: validation of a new alcoholism instrument. Am J Psychiatry. 1974;131:1121–3.
31. Ware J Jr, Kosinski M, Keller SD. A 12-item short-form health survey: construction of scales and preliminary tests of reliability and validity. Med Care. 1996;34:220–33.
32. Melzack R. The short-form McGill pain questionnaire. Pain. 1987;30:191–7.
33. Prigerson HG, Jacobs SC. Traumatic grief as a distinct disorder: a rationale, consensus criteria, and a preliminary empirical test. In: Stroebe MS, Hansson RO, Stroebe W, Schut H, editors. Handbook of bereavement research: consequences, coping, and care. Washington, DC: American Psychological Association; 2001. p. 588–613.
34. DiGrande L, Perrin MA, Thorpe LE, Thalji L, Murphy J, Wu D, et al. Posttraumatic stress symptoms, PTSD, and risk factors among lower Manhattan residents 2–3 years after the September 11, 2001 terrorist attacks. J Traum Stress. 2008;21:264–73. https://doi.org/10.1002/jts.20345.
35. Stuber J, Galea S, Boscarino JA, Schlesinger M. Was there unmet mental health need after the September 11, 2001 terrorist attacks? Soc Psychiatry Psychiatr Epidemiol. 2006;41(3):230–40.
36. Donahue SA, Lanzara CB, Felton CJ, Essock SM, Carpinello S. Project liberty: New York's crisis counseling program created in the aftermath of September 11, 2001. Psychiatr Serv. 2006;57(9):1253–8.
37. Kaufmann C, Rutkow L, Spira P, Mojtabai R. Mental health of protective services workers: results from the national epidemiologic survey on alcohol and related conditions. Disaster Med Public Health Prep. 2013;7(1):36–45.
38. Berninger A, Webber MP, Cohen HW, Gustave J, Lee R, Niles JK, Prezant DJ. Trends of elevated PTSD risk in firefighters exposed to the World Trade Center disaster: 2001–2005. Public Health Rep. 2010;125(4):556–66.
39. Wild J, Smith KV, Thompson E, Béar F, MJ L, Ehlers A. A prospective study of pre-trauma risk factors for post-traumatic stress disorder and depression. Psychol Med. 2016;46(12):2571–82.
40. American Psychiatric Association. Diagnostic and statistical manual of mental disorders. 5th. ed. Washington, DC: American Psychiatric Association; 2013.
41. Bryant RA, Creamer M, O'Donnell M, Silove D, McFarlane AC, Forbes D. Comparison of the capacity of DSM-IV and DSM-5 acute stress disorder definitions to predict posttraumatic stress disorder and related disorders. J Clin Psychiatry. 2015;76(4):391–7.
42. Bowler RM, Kornblith ES, Li J, Adams SW, Gocheva VV, Schwarzer R, Cone JE. Police officers who responded to 9/11: comorbidity of PTSD, depression, and anxiety 10-11 years later. Am J Ind Med. 2016;59(6):425–36.
43. Stellman JM, Smith RP, Katz CL, Sharma V, Charney DS, Herbert R, et al. Enduring mental health morbidity and social function impairment in world trade center rescue, recovery, and cleanup workers: the psychological dimension of an environmental health disaster. Environ Health Perspect. 2008;116(9):1248–53.
44. Choudhury WA, Quraishi FA, Haque Z. Mental health and psychosocial aspects of disaster preparedness in Bangladesh. Int Rev Psychiatry. 2006;18(6):529–35.
45. Nash WP, Westphal RJ, Watson P, Litz BT. Bureau of Medicine and Surgery, Department of the Navy, in cooperation with the Combat and Operational Stress Control, Manpower & Reserve Affairs, Headquarters Marine Corps, the Navy Operational Stress Control, Chief of Naval Personnel, TotalForce N, and the National Center for PTSD, Department of Veterans Affairs. Combat and Operational Stress First Aid (COSFA) Field Operations Manual. Washington, DC: U.S. Government. 2010. Available at: http://www.alsbom-gm.org/files/COSFA%20NAVY%20TM.pdf. Accessed Jan 2019.
46. Gist R, Watson P, Taylor V, Elvander E. Curbside manner: stress first aid for the street (student manual). National Fallen Firefighters Association, 2013. Available at: http://www.fireherolearningnetwork.com/Training_Programs/Curbside_Manner__Stress_First_Aid_for_the_Street.aspx. Accessed Jan 2019.
47. Watson P, Taylor V, Gist R, Elvander E, Leto F, Martin B, et al. Stress first aid for firefighters and emergency medical services personnel student manual. National Fallen Firefighters Association, National Center for PTSD, Department of Veterans Affairs, 2013.

Index

D. W. Callaway, J. L. Burstein (eds.), *Operational and Medical Management of Explosive and Blast Incidents*, https://doi.org/10.1007/978-3-030-40655-4

W

The manufacturer's authorised representative in the EU is Springer Nature Customer Service Centre GmbH, Europaplatz 3, 69115 Heidelberg, Germany. If you have any concerns regarding our products, please contact ProductSafety@springernature.com

Printed and bound by CPI Group (UK) Ltd, Croydon, CR0 4YY
05/10/2026
02228126-0018